Fast Facts for the Final FFICM and EDIC

This comprehensive revision guide breaks down complex critical care concepts into over 200 essential topics, strategically designed in accessible bullet points and tables. It delivers only the most exam-relevant information, focusing specifically on past questions to maximize the chances of success, and the concise format allows for quick assimilation during crucial revision periods, making every study minute count.

Knowledge retention is enhanced through the guide's systematic approach to each topic, presenting aetiology, pathophysiology, diagnosis, and treatment in a logical sequence that reinforces understanding. This structured method ensures that facts don't exist in isolation but connect meaningfully, building the robust foundation of high-yield information that is invaluable during those critical final weeks before examinations.

Confidence is the ultimate key to exam success, and this guide is the pathway to achieving it. By enabling efficient revision of the entire curriculum, it ensures candidates for the FFICM and EDIC enter their exams not just prepared but empowered. With comprehensive coverage of the essential basic sciences required by anaesthetists, this guide transforms anxiety into assurance and preparation into performance. Due to the emphasis of this book on learning the basics, it will be helpful to other medical staff members working in intensive care, like nurses, ACCPs, and foundation year doctors as well.

Dr Amit Sharma is currently working at Royal Stoke University Hospital, Stoke-on-Trent, UK. He postgraduated in anaesthesia from the prestigious Maulana Azad Medical College, New Delhi, one of the top 3 medical colleges in India. After that, he cleared European Diploma in Anaesthesiology and Intensive Care (EDAIC) and registered with GMC to work as a Junior Specialist Doctor in the NHS. During this time, he completed his FRCA examination with distinction in both primary and final Fellowship of the Royal college of anaesthetists (FRCA) and joined training in the UK. He cleared his Fellowship of the Faculty of Intensive Care Medicine (FFICM) and European Diploma in Intensive Care (EDIC) examinations during his dual intensive care medicine and anaesthesia training and has been appointed as honorary lecturer at the University of Plymouth for the Advanced Critical Care Practitioners (ACCP) programme. He has an active interest in use of point-of-care ultrasound and staff well-being initiatives.

Fast Facts

Fast Facts for the Primary FRCA and EDAIC: Basic Science for Anaesthetists
Amit Sharma

Fast Facts for the Final FFICM and EDIC: Core Concepts in Critical Care Medicine
Amit Sharma

Fast Facts for the Final FFICM and EDIC

Core Concepts in Critical Care Medicine

Amit Sharma

CRC Press
Taylor & Francis Group
Boca Raton London New York

CRC Press is an imprint of the
Taylor & Francis Group, an **informa** business

Designed cover image: Shutterstock

First edition published 2026
by CRC Press
2385 NW Executive Center Drive, Suite 320, Boca Raton, FL 33431

and by CRC Press
4 Park Square, Milton Park, Abingdon, Oxon, OX14 4RN

CRC Press is an imprint of Taylor & Francis Group, LLC

© 2026 Amit Sharma

ISBN: 978-1-032-75922-7 (hbk)
ISBN: 978-1-032-75927-2 (pbk)
ISBN: 978-1-003-47621-4 (ebk)

DOI: 10.1201/9781003476214

Typeset in Minion
by Apex CoVantage, LLC

Contents

Supportive Care in ITU
The Most Important Chapter

ITU is a game of inches. The success or failure of a treatment depends upon attention to detail and the cumulative impact of small steps. I wanted to write many facts of this chapter in the preface of the book, but then I wasn't sure if people still read the preface, hence a separate section to emphasize the importance of supportive care in ITU.

We don't have any magical pill in the ITU, and most of the management revolves around supporting organ systems till the time the original pathology is resolved. High-quality supportive care consists of doing basic things right, and recovery from critical illness is a race between recovery from the precipitants of critical illness and accumulating ICU complications. In all the chapters of this book, I have avoided repeating the same supportive care everywhere, unless something specific had to be mentioned. Hence, you can add the following tenets in every answer during viva sessions.

Supportive Care in ITU

✓ **Fever in ICU**
- Avoid checking an endotracheal aspirate in intubated patients, unless there is clinical suspicion of pneumonia.
- Avoid urinalysis and culture from an indwelling Foley catheter, unless there is a urinary obstruction or recent urinary tract manipulation, as cystitis is rarely the cause of new-onset fever.
- Avoid treating fever with acetaminophen with the sole intention of treating fever as it can conceal the true fever curve.
- Avoid empirical antibiotics in an episode of fever, unless there is a high index of suspicion for a specific focus of infection or fever associated with hypotension, signifying septic shock.

✓ **Fluid overload**
- Critically sick patients typically retain fluid and tend to develop fluid overload.
- Maintenance fluids should be avoided, unless specifically indicated, such as in diabetic ketoacidosis or rhabdomyolysis.
- For patients who are >5 L positive, use of diuresis can be helpful, and to furosemide add a thiazide as well, to avoid hypernatraemia.

✓ **Gastrointestinal (GI) prophylaxis**
- Use GI prophylaxis only for intubated patients and when used, the agent is a proton pump inhibitor, like omeprazole or pantoprazole PO or IV.
- Enteral nutrition should be given whenever possible, and established enteral feeding provides a protective effect against stress ulcers.

✓ **Nutritional support**
- Adequate nutrition through enteral or parenteral nutrition helps boost immunity and promotes healing.
- Enteral nutrition, unless contraindicated, should be started as early as possible within the first 48 h of ICU stay.

✓ **DVT prophylaxis**
- All ICU patients should receive pharmacological DVT prophylaxis, unless contraindicated, like for platelets <50,000/mm^3 or INR >1.5.
- Low-molecular-weight heparin, like enoxaparin, is preferred.

✓ **Glycaemic control**
- Avoid hypoglycaemia as it is more dangerous.
- Use variable-rate insulin infusion for blood sugar >10 mmol/L.

✓ **Anaemia**
  - Give blood transfusion if haemoglobin is <70 g/L, unless patient is having active cardiac ischaemia.
  - Acute fall in haemoglobin is mostly due to either bleeding or haemolysis, and check for bruising, haematomas, or melaena.
  - Investigations needed may include complete blood count with LDH and haptoglobin to exclude haemolysis, clotting studies to exclude bleeding, and imaging like CT angiography to look for potential source of bleeding.

✓ **Hypokalaemia**
  - Target >4 mmol/L to prevent atrial fibrillation.
  - Use oral supplementation wherever possible, and be careful in renal failure.
  - Correct concomitant hypomagnesaemia as they both usually co-exist.

✓ **Hypomagnesaemia**
  - Treat with intravenous magnesium, as oral magnesium can cause diarrhoea.

✓ **Hypernatraemia**
  - It can make the patient delirious and thirsty if they are awake; treat it with free water in the form of oral water via enteral tube or as 5% dextrose solution.

✓ **Hyponatraemia**
  - Mild hyponatraemia (Na^+ between 125 and 135 mEq/L) is common in critical care setup and doesn't require aggressive treatment.

✓ **Hypocalcaemia**
  - Hypocalcaemia is also very common in ICU, and unless ionized calcium is <0.7 mmol/L or patient is having symptoms of hypocalcaemia, don't treat it.

✓ **Troponins**
  - Troponins are elevated in most critically ill patients and levels should be done only in patients with suspicion of myocardial ischaemia based on ECG changes or history.

✓ **Skin integrity**
  - Prevent pressure ulcers through regular repositioning, specialized mattresses, and meticulous skin care.

✓ **Mobility and physical therapy**
  - Early mobilization prevents muscle weakness and improves circulation.

✓ **Infection control**
  - Prevents infection, and measures like hand hygiene are effective.

✓ **Pain management**
  - Assess pain and manage it to avoid prolonged mechanical ventilation, increased ICU length of stay, pulmonary complications, and the development of post-traumatic stress disorder.
  - Paracetamol and oral morphine are good painkillers and commonly used in ICU.

✓ **Delirium management**
  - Delirium is common in patients on prolonged sedation and increases ICU length of stay.
  - Minimize sedation, promote sleep, and encourage orientation to time and place.

✓ **Medications to avoid in ICU**
  - **ACE inhibitors/angiotensin receptor blockers:** AKI and hypotension.
  - **NSAIDs:** kidney dysfunction and gastrointestinal bleeding.
  - **Benzodiazepines:** cause delirium.

Ward Round in ITU

✓ **FAST HUGS BID (quick patient review)**
  - F → Feeding
  - A → Analgesia
  - S → Sedation
  - T → Thromboprophylaxis
  - H → Head-up position
  - U → Ulcer prophylaxis
  - G → Glycaemic control
  - S → Spontaneous breathing trial
  - B → Bowel care
  - I → Indwelling catheter removal
  - D → De-escalation of antibiotics

✓ **A–Z assessment (comprehensive review of patient)**
  - A → Airway
  - B → Breathing
  - C → Circulation
  - D → Drugs/disability (GCS assessment)
  - E → Electrolytes (Na^+, K^+, Mg^{2+}, Ca^{2+}, PO_4^{3-})
  - F → Feeding/fluids/fluid balance
  - G → Gut (stools)
  - H → Haematology (anticoagulants)
  - I → Infusions/infection/inflammatory markers
  - J → Jaundice (LFTs)
  - K → Kidneys (renal function)
  - L → Lines
  - M → Microbiology (antibiotics)/mobilize (sit out)
  - N → Next of kin (update family)

- O → Other specialities/outreach team
- P → Pain/pharmacy/physio/pressure sores
- Q → Questions (from MDT)
- R → Radiology/rehab
- S → Sedation/SALT
- T → Temperature/transfer to specialist centre
- U → Understanding (Do we know why the patient is in ITU?)
- V → Ventilator bundle
- W → Weaning (tracheostomy)/withdrawal of care
- X → X-rays
- Y → Yeast (any risk factor for fungal infection)
- Z → Zzzzz (sleep)[1]

✓ **Aetiology of pathology.** Always look for the cause of the signs and symptoms in a patient newly admitted to critical care. **Nothing happens randomly.**

Pneumonic for Viva Purposes: VINDICATE

- V → Vascular
- I → Infection
- N → Neoplasm
- D → Degenerative
- I → Idiopathic/inflammatory/intoxication
- C → Congenital
- A → Autoimmune
- T → Trauma
- E → Endocrine

NOTE

1 Big thanks to Dr Jagtar Pooni, Consultant Anaesthesia and Intensive Care at Royal Wolverhampton Trust, for introducing me to this method of assessment and helping me improve my practice. You hardly miss anything in your ward rounds after using this method.

Preface

The Fellowship of the Faculty of Intensive Care Medicine (FFICM) exam comprises of passing the MCQs first, followed by OSCE and SOE viva. The European Diploma of Intensive Care (EDIC) exam involves MCQs initially and then an OSCE-format exam that utilizes both clinical case scenario (CCS) and computer-based scenario (CBS) stations. Both the exams are highly standardized and require both theoretical and practical knowledge to ace them. Covering all the questions asked in the past are the pillars of success for these exams, and the "fast facts" content presents all of them in a concise manner to both help build confidence for the exams and ace them without stress.

This book covers all the high-yield facts in an antegrade fashion that helps you retain the information more and for longer periods of time. The concepts of critical care have been woven around all the MCQs asked in the past to make sure that you benefit from this book both practically and academically. The point-based format of the book will help to memorise study material for the OSCE and viva part and ease the art of communication. All the latest guidelines have been included, and it's a perfect companion to practise evidence-based medicine. The emphasis of this book on just the relevant facts ensures that you cut the clutter in those valuable last few days before the exam and sit in it after covering the entire breadth of the course.

Critical care is a team game and involves not just the doctors but the advanced critical care practitioners (ACCPs), critical care outreach team (CCOT), and nurses as well. The basic nature of this book will make sure that not just the exam-going trainees but all the key people working in the intensive care department will benefit from it and improve their understanding of the tenets of critical care.

Acknowledgements

There is a saying that "family comes first," and I couldn't agree more. Every inch of this book has been written with the immense help and support of my wife, Dr Kritika Vats; my daughter, Aaryana Meera Sharma; and my parents, Mr Viney Bhushan Sharma and Mrs Sandhya Sharma, who have always shown great pride in my work.

Working in an intensive care unit in the UK has helped me build my confidence in critical care, and I would like to thank Dr Ranjna Basra for supervising me through it right from my start, when I arrived in Birmingham in the middle of the two Covid waves. She helped me understand both the clinical and the non-clinical parts of working here, and a lot of my comprehension of the chapters written in this book comes from her.

No clinical field is complete without being backed by research, and thanks to Professor Tonny Veenith for instilling the question in my head, before starting any treatment, is it evidence based? I have used that approach to provide clinical trials for all the important treatment protocols in the book.

A big thanks to my current educational supervisor, Dr Salman Islam, for helping me through the last few months of writing this book and believing in me. His skills in motivating people to get the best out of them can be utilized by any manager in top-tier sports.

As anaesthetists who are practising intensive care medicine, we sometimes tend to manage the patients in an ABCDE manner and ignore an important aspect of "what is causing all this". I absolutely value the constant questioning by Dr Shameer Gopal and Dr Saibal Ganguly on the ward rounds and over the phone, shifting my focus from just "ABCDE assessment" to "a complete patient assessment". Thanks a lot for correcting my radar.

The Department of Critical Care at Queen Elizabeth Hospital, Birmingham, has played a huge role in building my basics as an intensivist, and I would like to thank Prof. Nicholas Murphy, Prof. Tony Whitehouse, Dr David Riddington, Dr Deborah Turfrey, Dr Kaye England, Dr Mav Manji, Dr Bill Tunnicliffe, Dr Zahid Khan, Dr Brian Pouchet, Dr Alejandro Barrios, Dr Catherine Snelson, Dr Nilesh Parekh, Dr Tessa Oelofse, Dr Steffen Kroll, Dr Sandeep Walia, Dr David Balthazor, Dr Ravi Hebballi, Dr Nandan Gautam, Dr Harjot Singh, Dr Neil Abeysinghe, Dr Tomasz Torlinski, Dr Randeep Mullhi, Dr Jeremy Willson, Dr Mario Cibelli, Dr Mansoor Bangash, Dr Jaimin Patel, Dr Dhruv Parekh, Dr Laura Tasker, Dr Ravi Chauhan, Dr Andy Johnston, Dr Abby Ford, Dr Richard Browne, Dr John Kelly, Dr Asif Arshad, Dr Phillip El-Dalil, Dr Carla Richardson, Dr Gregory Packer, Dr Fayaz Roked, Dr Nicholas Talbot, Dr Shraddha Goyal, Dr Phillip Howells, Dr Claire Keene, Dr Andrew Owen, Dr Mario Ferrante, Dr Mitali Chakravarty, and Dr Muzzammil Ali for their constant guidance.

I have worked with many hospitals across the UK and give the highest amount of gratitude towards Dr Jagtar Pooni, Dr Mamta Patel, Dr Anand Damodaran, Dr Ron Daniels, Dr Andrew Macduff, Dr Ramesha Giri, Dr Alexander Ng, Dr Pratap Makam, Dr Cyril Chacko, Dr Antonella Meraglia, Dr Asha Ramkumar, Dr Chakravarthy Tutika, Dr Kesavan Dhamodaran, Dr Matthew Ilchyshyn, Dr Nick Coleman, Dr Stephen Kreuper, Dr Moses Chikungwa, Dr Christopher Thompson, Dr Fernando Rodriguez-Albarran, Dr Ramprasad Matsa, Dr Nehal Patel, Dr Andrew Disney, Dr Mohamed Shoaeir, Dr George Mathew, Dr Prabhjoyt Kler, Dr Shashank Danndhiganaahalli, Dr Stephen Lord, Dr Paul Vincent, Dr Jonathan Messing, Dr Ranjit

Bains, Dr Prashant Nasa, and Dr Sukhpreet Sihota for always being supportive and kind to me.

Thanks to Dr Pooja Chopra Wadwa, Dr Munish Chauhan, Dr Samir Malik, Dr Priteema Chanana, and Dr Madhur Arora for preparing me at Fortis Memorial Research Institute, India, for practising critical care in the UK.

I would take this opportunity to thank my critical care colleagues for helping me through my shifts and in preparing for the exams, making sure I am always well backed up. Big thanks to Dr Stelios Chatzimichail, Dr Carl Groves, Dr Philip Harrington, Dr Jeremy Hing, Dr Katie Archer, Dr Rosie Worrall (always leading with a solution), Dr Anandh Balu, Dr Lloyd Edwards, Dr Prakash Vadukul, Dr Steve Mclaren (always the saviour), Dr Gemma Talling, Dr James Gorham, Dr Umar Kaleem, Dr Michael Burns, Dr Rachel Olive, Dr Tarek Hassan, Dr Vasant Patil, Dr Palnisamy Matheswaran, Dr Robert Crichton, Dr Wasim Mir, Dr Kerrie Aldridge, Dr Nikiesha Lee Dunbar, Dr Ahmed Abdelmohsen, Dr Hannah Leadbetter, Dr Andrew Pearson, Dr Ahmed Elsayed, Dr David Fotheringham, Dr Ranveer Cheema, Dr Jonathan Durbin, and Dr Surpreet Grewal.

There is a saying amongst surgeons that whenever in doubt, ask the anaesthetist at the head end, and in ITU we can easily say that if a registrar is in doubt, they can ask the friendly neighbourhood ACCP. Hence, I would like to thank Alan Clethro (The Big Al), James Sherwin, Nigel Manning, Poonam Rani, Amanda Bingham, Heather Jones, Rebecca Boot, Alison Fowler, Mark Horner, Lottie Poulton, David Nice, Stevie Park, Kathleen Ford, Laura Foster, Nicki Paver, Katie Humphries, James Lacey, Dileep Mullakudiyil, Samuel Harris, Rhea Elizabeth, Amy Watts, Susie McManus, Bill Allen, Katie Betts, Alex Villaplaza, Madison Larden, Shaveta Devesar, Kathleen Holden, Nicola Howarth, Ian Lewis, Daniel Mahaffey, Ashley Louise, Scott Hawkins, Andrew Simmons, Kate McCormick, Emily Brownsill, Charlene Parton, Charlotte Cox, Lydia Sterland, Stephanie Walker, Nicola Bradshaw, Maria Stanyer, Michael Kington-Moore, Amii Knight, Rebecca Burkard, and David Cartlidge for making lives easier for us.

Thanks to my friends like family, Dr Saurabh Taneja, Dr Rahul Sapra (brother from another mother), Dr Sadhana Sapra Saini, Dr Suneesh Thilak, Dr Melanie Sahni, Dr Krishna Navaneetham, Dr Pranav Osuri, Dr Carl Van Miegham, Dr Rohan Sikka, and Dr Manan Bajaj, for always listening to me and being there.

Last but not the least, I can't thank enough my father-in-law, Mr Puneet Kumar Vats; my mother-in-law, Mrs Udita Vats; my brother, Dr Ankit Sharma; my sisters-in-laws, Kanika Vats and Dr Noor Dharmarha; my brother-in-law, Udbhav Vats; and baby Saanvi, for the constant encouragement.

And finally, I would really like to express my absolute appreciation for my amazing editors, Miranda Bromage and Paige Loughlin, and editorial assistant, Hudson Greig, for their wonderful guidance and amazing patience. You guys are absolute heroes in helping to get these books out in great shape and on a timely schedule.

Dedication

I would like to dedicate this book to all NHS staff members, for treating every patient with dignity and compassion and providing state-of-the-art care, regardless of their circumstances.

Surgical Problems

ABDOMINAL COMPARTMENT SYNDROME

Epidemiology

✓ **Intra-Abdominal Hypertension (IAH)**
- As per the Abdominal Compartment Society, *intra-abdominal hypertension* is intra-abdominal pressure (IAP) >12 mmHg on more than one occasion.
- Prevalence of IAH in ICU patients is almost 30–50%.

✓ **Abdominal Compartment Syndrome (ACS) (Exam favorite in all differential diagnosis)**
- IAP >20 mmHg with new organ dysfunction or failure[Q].
- Prevalence of abdominal compartment syndrome in ICU patients is around 6%.
- **Risk factors:** High BMI, **acute pancreatitis**[Q] (60% of severe acute pancreatitis will develop abdominal compartment syndrome), **ruptured aortic aneurysms**, burns, fluid resuscitation, abdominal surgery, ascites, vasoactive therapy, ARDS, and hypothermia.

Clinical Features and Diagnosis

✓ **Normal Intra-Abdominal Pressure (IAP)**
- 5–7 mmHg.

✓ **World Society of the Abdominal Compartment Syndrome (WSACS) Classification:**

Intra-abdominal hypertension[Q]	• Grade I: IAP 12–15 mmHg
	• Grade II: IAP 16–20 mmHg
	• Grade III: IAP 21–25 mmHg
	• Grade IV: IAP >25 mmHg

Abdominal compartment syndrome[Q]	IAP >20 mmHg with new organ dysfunction or failure
	• **Primary:** Intra-abdominal process
	• **Secondary:** Illness not directly related to abdomen and pelvis

✓ **Monitoring**
- Intravesical measurement is gold standard currently.
- Good correlation, but may be inaccurate in the presence of adhesions, bladder haematoma, and pelvic fractures. Intragastric techniques can be used in contraindications.
- With patient supine, transducer zeroed at the point midaxillary line meets **iliac crest**.
- 25 mL of 0.9% NaCl is used. Wait for 30–60s for temperature to be in equilibrium. Three readings should be taken.
- **IAP measurement every 4 h, or more frequently in unstable patients, is recommended.**
- Challenging in awake patient and obese patient.
- **Poor sensitivity (40%) of raised intra-abdominal pressure, with clinical abdominal girth measurement.**

✓ **Organ Failure**[Q]
- More likely at pressure >25 mmHg.
- **Neurological failure:** Raised JVP and, hence, intracranial pressure.
- **Respiratory failure:** Diaphragm is elevated and causes atelectasis. Plateau and peak pressures increase.
- **Cardiovascular failure**
  - ❖ Decreased preload, contractility, and increased afterload.

❖ Elevation of diaphragm constricts vena caval opening, and IVC size can't be used for assessing volume responsiveness.

❖ Pulse pressure variability and stroke volume variation also lose responsiveness.

- **Renal failure:** Decreased renal flow leads to acute kidney injury.

✓ **Abdominal Compartment Syndrome Triad**
- A tense distended abdomen, respiratory distress, and oliguria.

Prevention and Treatment[Q]

✓ **Step 1: Avoid Fluid Overload and Prone Position**
- **Adequate sedation and analgesia.**
- NG tube decompression, rectal tube, and prokinetics[Q].
- USG abdomen.

✓ **Step 2: Fluid Removal Using Diuresis**
- Albumin infusion can be given in severe burn injury to prevent gut swelling.
- Reverse Trendelenburg positioning.
- **Reduced enteral nutrition should be considered in case of IAH grade I or II.**
- **CT abdomen and percutaneous drainage** of intra-abdominal or retroperitoneal fluid collections in carefully selected patients.

✓ **Step 3: Dialysis to Remove Fluid**
- Temporary **neuromuscular blockers**.
- Stop enteral feeding and **colonoscopy, with bowel decompression** or neostigmine in cases of Ogilvie syndrome.
- Pressure >20 mmHg with multiorgan failure may require surgery. No specific cutoff pressure required for surgery, and complete clinical picture required for the decision to go for surgery.
- Primary closure isn't always attempted post-surgery.

✓ **Open Abdomen**
- Abdomen is left open for high intra abdominal pressures after laparotomy for ischaemic colitis and abdominal aortic aneurysm.
- *Indications for an open-abdomen post-trauma are transfusion of >10 units of RBCs or >15 L of crystalloids.*
- However, it is no longer recommended in patients with acute pancreatitis.

- **Delayed closure should be considered if surgeon is struggling to close a laparotomy wound.**
- Goal should be to close within 8 d, as delay can lead to entero-atmospheric fistula. Closure can be done by direct fascial closure or using biological/synthetic mesh bridge repair.
- **Bogota bag** used in the past to suture to borders of skin. It didn't allow drainage of fluid from abdomen.
- **Vacuum-assisted closure devices**
  ❖ Are newer devices and have improved outcomes in patients with open abdomen.
  ❖ Prevent intra-abdominal viscera from adhering to the abdominal wall.
  ❖ Negative pressure allows active drainage of fluid and exudate.
  ❖ Dressing changes performed every 3 to 4 d and, hence, simplifying wound management.
- **Complications** include recurrence of abdominal compartment syndrome, abdominal abscesses, entero-cutaneous fistulae, and ventral hernias.

Prognosis

✓ Untreated ACS can lead to mortality between 40 and 100%.

EMERGENCY LAPAROTOMY

Basic Concepts of GIT

✓ **Daily Fluid Turnover**
- **Total input in GI Tract:** Water intake of 2,000 mL + endogenous secretions of 7,000 mL = 9,000 mL.
  ❖ **Endogenous secretions (mL):** Salivary gland 1,500 mL, stomach 2,500 mL, bile 500 mL, pancreas 1,500 mL, small intestine 1,000 mL.
- **Total reabsorbed by GI tract:** 8,800 mL.
  ❖ Jejunum 5,500 mL, ileum 2,000 mL, colon 1,300 mL.
- **Passed in stools:** 200 mL.

✓ **Gut Arterial Supply[Q]**
- **Celiac trunk:** T12. Left gastric, common hepatic, splenic artery.
- **Superior mesenteric artery (SMA):** L1. Distal duodenum till proximal transverse colon.

- **Inferior mesenteric artery (IMA):** L3. Left colic, sigmoid, and rectal arteries.

✓ **Gut Venous Drainage**
- **Portal vein**[Q]: Superior mesenteric vein + splenic vein.
- **Superior mesenteric vein:** Right gastro-omental vein, jejunal vein, ileal vein, right colic vein, and middle colic vein.
- **Splenic vein:** Left gastro-omental vein, pancreatic vein, and inferior mesenteric vein (left colic vein, sigmoidal vein, and superior rectal vein).
- Left gastric, right gastric, cystic, and para-umbilical veins drain directly into portal vein.
- Oesophageal, rectal, paraumbilical, and retroperitoneal veins are key collateral veins between portal veins and systemic veins.

Investigations

✓ **Ultrasound**
- First-line investigation. Can detect free fluid in abdomen, solid and hollow organ structure, and perfusion.

✓ **Abdominal X-ray**
- **Normal anatomy**
  - ❖ Gastric bubble is normal.
  - ❖ The larger solid organs of the abdomen are usually outlined by fat, which, being of lower density, allows us to see the organ edge.
  - ❖ Ascending and descending colons are fixed. Transverse colon is free and can be seen across the X-ray.
  - ❖ **Small bowel** can be recognised by **valvulae conniventes** (across the bowel). **Large bowel** will show haustral pattern.
  - ❖ Gas in small and large bowel is also common if bowel is of a normal calibre. Bowel dilatation is diameter >3 cm, >6 cm, >9 cm for small bowel, large bowel, and caecum, respectively. The risk of perforation increases exponentially if caecal diameter exceeds 12 cm.
- **Pathology**
  - ❖ An erect chest radiograph will demonstrate free air under the diaphragm[Q] if a perforation is present.
  - ❖ Gas with fluid levels suggests ileus, but not necessarily obstruction.

- ❖ Gas in small bowel and rectum and absent in large bowel is diagnostic of mechanical large bowel obstruction.
- ❖ **Rigler's sign:** Within the peritoneal cavity following a perforated viscus, the supine abdomen film may demonstrate gas on both sides of the bowel wall.
- ❖ **Pneumobilia:** Gas can also be seen around the biliary tree.
- ❖ **Thumbprinting**[Q]: Thickened haustral folds (oedema) seen in large colon due to colitis.
- ❖ **Pneumatosis:** Presence of gas bubbles in a linear pattern in the bowel wall. It can be benign but in an unwell patient can signify bowel infarction.
- ❖ **Sentinel loop**[Q]: A short segment of adynamic ileus which is in proximity of an intra-abdominal inflammatory process, e.g. pancreatitis, appendicitis.

✓ **CT Scan**
- Can detect free air or fluid, increased thickness of bowel wall, increased bowel diameter, intestinal pneumatosis, and disrupted mesenteric blood flow.
- Variations in contrast
  - ❖ **Intravenous contrast:** Highlights the blood vessels of liver, kidney, and spleen.
  - ❖ **Oral contrast:** Improves visualization of oesophagus, stomach, and intestines.
  - ❖ **Rectal contrast:** Improves visualization of large intestines and pelvic organs.
- **Variations in timing of IV contrast**
  - ❖ **Non-enhanced contrast:** No contrast used. Used for detecting calcifications, like kidney stones.
  - ❖ **Early arterial phase:** 15–20 s post-injection. Contrast is still in the arteries and has not enhanced the organs and other tissues.
  - ❖ **Late arterial phase:** 35–40 s post-injection. Called **arterial phase** or early portal phase as well. Enhances organs with blood supplies from arteries.
  - ❖ **Hepatic or late portal phase:** 70–80 s post-injection. Enhancement of liver[Q] parenchyma through blood supply by portal vein.
  - ❖ **Nephrogenic phase:** 100 s post-injection. Enhances renal parenchyma, including medulla.
  - ❖ **Delayed phase:** 6–10 min post-injection. Wash out of contrast from

all abdominal structures except fibrotic tissues, which become relatively dense compared to the normal tissue.

Causes of Acute Abdomen

✓ **Ileus**
- *Ileus* is failure of peristalsis without mechanical obstruction.
- In **ileus**, large bowel and small bowel are involved. Causes are as follows:
  - ❖ **Gastrointestinal:** Acute peritonitis, diverticulitis, post-operation, pancreatitis.
  - ❖ **Systemic:** Sepsis, trauma, hypovolaemia.
  - ❖ **Metabolic imbalance:** Uraemia, hyponatraemia, hypokalaemia, hyperglycaemia.
  - ❖ **Medications:** Opioids, calcium channel blockers, anticholinergics like TCAs, loperamide.
- **Abdominal X-ray:** Air fluid levels and distended bowel.
- Presents with abdominal pain/distension, vomiting, intolerance of enteral feeding, and absence of defecation.
- **Treatment**
  - ❖ Rule out bowel obstruction, and involve surgical team.
  - ❖ Avoid lying flat, and use NG decompression.
  - ❖ Reduce dose of opioids, and stop other offending drugs.
  - ❖ *Reduce feeding rate by 50% for next 6–8 h and then try progressively increasing it over 1–2 d.*
  - ❖ **Consider trophic feeding** if tolerated, and consider **parenteral nutrition** if prolonged.
  - ❖ GI motility drugs like metoclopramide/ erythromycin.
  - ❖ Correct electrolytes like potassium and magnesium.

✓ **Small Bowel Obstruction**
- **Bowel obstruction** is generally referred to mechanical obstruction.
- **Commonest cause is adhesions[Q].** Hernia and tumours are other causes.
- **Bowel obstruction:** 90% of cases have obstruction only (small bowel 75%, and large bowel 15%).

- **Bowel strangulation (obstruction + ischaemia)**
  - ❖ About 10% of obstruction cases will have strangulation (small bowel 7%, and large bowel 3%).
  - ❖ Bowel is strangulated if the blood supply of its contents becomes compromised, leading to risk of bowel ischaemia.
  - ❖ It's a surgical emergency[Q] and seen in adhesions and volvulus.
- Presents with abdominal pain/distension, vomiting[Q], intolerance of enteral feeding, inability to pass gas or have bowel movements, and possibly diarrhoea.
- **Investigations**
  - ❖ On abdominal X-ray, the more visible the small bowel, the more likely it's pathological
  - ❖ *CT scan is investigation of choice.* Dilated loops: >3 cm for small bowel and >6 cm for large bowel.
- **Treatment**
  - ❖ **Treatment is mostly conservative** initially, with nasogastric drainage initially for 72 h in the absence of bowel ischaemia.
  - ❖ Inflammatory conditions like Crohn's disease may benefit from medical therapy before surgery.
  - ❖ *Surgery: Signs of ischaemia, like pneumatosis, volvulus, and incarcerated hernia, and risk of perforation like bowel dilatation should be looked for and surgery should be done for these indications urgently.*

✓ **Large Bowel Obstruction**
- This is a surgical emergency.
- **Causes:** Malignancy, diverticular disease, and volvulus.
- **Symptoms:** Absolute constipation, bloating, and lower abdominal pain.
- *CT with oral and IV contrast to demonstrate complete from partial obstruction.*
- Chronic colitis shows thumbprinting sign with thickened mucosa.
- **Treatment**
  - ❖ **Treatment is surgical.** Pseudo-obstruction can be managed conservatively with low threshold for suspicion of perforation or ischaemia.

❖ Treatment also includes NG tube on free drainage, fluid and electrolytes and antibiotics.

✓ **Acute Colonic Pseudo-Obstruction/Ogilvie's Syndrome[Q]**

- Ileus of the large intestine. Clinical and radiological evidence of large bowel obstruction in the absence of mechanical obstruction.
- History of recent surgery maybe there.
- Abdominal pain and distension, failure to pass stools are clinical signs.
- Abdominal X-rays will show dilated colon:
  ❖ The bigger the diameter of the dilated bowel, the higher the risk of perforation.
  ❖ Ischaemia and perforation will be seen in 15% of patients if caecal diameter >12 cm and duration >6 d.
- **CT scan is the investigation of choice.** No transition point on CT scan or gradual transition seen near splenic flexure.
- Intra-abdominal pressures should be checked regularly.
- **Treatment**
  ❖ IV neostigmine is used: 0.4–0.8 mg/h up to a maximum of 2.5 mg.
  ❖ Gastrografin given rectally can be therapeutic as well as diagnostic.
  ❖ Endoscopic decompression, radiologically guided percutaneous cecostomy, and surgery are invasive procedures that can be done.

✓ **Acute Mesenteric Ischaemia (AMI)**

- The dreaded complication when lactates are rising but the morale of the team is not.
- **Aetiology**
  ❖ **SMA embolism (25%)[Q]:** Caused by AF, endocarditis.
  ❖ **SMA thrombosis (40%)[Q]:** Due to atherosclerosis, and these patients have history of chronic mesenteric ischaemia like postprandial pain, weight loss or food fear.
  ❖ **Non-occlusive mesenteric ischaemia (25%):** Due to hypoperfusion because of hypovolaemia, vasoconstrictive agents.
  ❖ **Mesenteric venous thrombosis (10%)[Q]:** Hypercoagulability due to sepsis, pancreatitis, inflammatory bowel disease.

- *Typically, the splenic flexure is the commonest site for bowel ischaemia, as this a "watershed" territory.*
- **Risk factors:** Age >70 yr, atrial fibrillation, ischaemic heart disease, stroke, smoking, high-dose vasopressors.
- **Presentation:** Severe abdominal pain, nausea, vomiting, diarrhoea (bloody stool).
  ❖ Raised WBCs. *Severe lactic acidosis resistant to fluid therapy[Q].*
  ❖ Signs of peritonitis mean irreversible intestinal ischaemia with bowel necrosis.
- CT scan (contrast enhancement in arterial and venous phases) is investigation of choice. Shows wall thickening, bowel dilation, mesenteric stranding, portal venous gas. **Pneumatosis intestinalis is the most specific sign.**
- **Treatment**
  ❖ Fluid resuscitation and broad-spectrum antibiotics.
  ❖ Nasogastric decompression.
  ❖ **Prompt laparotomy (damage control surgery)** in cases of overt peritonitis[Q].
  ❖ **Revascularization:** Embolic disease is treated with angioplasty or embolectomy. Atherosclerotic disease is treated with open or endovascular stenting or surgical SMA bypass.
- In patients receiving vasopressors, enteral nutrition should be started at low dose and increased slowly, monitoring lactates and IAP.
- A 50–80% mortality rate.

✓ **Peritonitis**

- The *peritoneum* is the largest and most complex serous membrane in the body.
- Parietal peritoneum lines the abdominal wall, and visceral peritoneum lines the abdominal organs, with a potential space between them known as the peritoneal cavity.
  ❖ The peritoneal cavity is divided incompletely into compartments by mesenteric attachments and secondary retro-peritonealization of certain visceral organs.
  ❖ The greater omentum functions as a fat storage organ and a mobile immune organ.

- **Types of peritonitis**
  - ❖ **Primary peritonitis:** Contamination of peritoneal cavity due to translocation of bacteria across the gut wall or haematogenous spread – e.g. spontaneous bacterial peritonitis.
  - ❖ **Secondary peritonitis:** Due to perforation of an organ – e.g. appendix, duodenal ulcer.
  - ❖ **Tertiary peritonitis:** Peritonitis persisting after 48 h of surgical treatment.
- **Signs and symptoms**
  - ❖ Abdominal pain, distended abdomen, dehydration, paralytic ileus, fever, tachycardia.
  - ❖ High WBCs, high CRP, and rising lactates.
- **Diagnosis:** Abdominal X-ray, CT scan and peritoneal fluid analysis.
- **Treatment:** Early source control, including damage control surgery, antibiotics, fluids, nutritional support, and managing complications of organ dysfunction.

✓ **Abdominal Abscess**
- Localized abscesses are amenable to ultrasound- or CT-guided drainage.

Emergency Laparotomy

✓ **Epidemiology**
- Approximately 30,000 emergency laparotomies are performed in the UK every year.
- The timing of emergency surgery is a cornerstone for improved outcome.

✓ **Indications**
- Intestinal perforation
- Intestinal obstruction
- Peritonitis
- Ischaemia
- Abdominal abscess
- Colitis
- Abdominal compartment syndrome
- Intestinal fistula
- Haemorrhage

✓ **Timing of Emergency Surgery**
- The timing of emergency surgery is a cornerstone for improved outcome:
  - ❖ **Immediate:** Intra-abdominal haemorrhage.
  - ❖ **Within an hour of diagnosis:** Acute mesenteric ischaemia, strangulated hernia, bowel perforation leading to peritonitis.

- ❖ **Within 6 h of diagnosis:** Localized peritonitis, abscess.
- ❖ **Within 24 h of diagnosis:** Acute appendicitis.

✓ **Risk Stratification Specific for Emergency Laparotomy**
- **National Emergency Laparotomy Audit (NELA) score:** Mortality risk score of >10% should be admitted to ITU.
- **National Surgical Quality Improvement Program (NSQIP):** Database of the USA.
- **P-POSSUM score:** Mortality risk of 5% or frailty indicates high-risk surgery.

✓ **Other Risk Stratification Scores Used in Surgery**
- **American Society of Anesthesiologists (ASA) physical status classification.**
- **Lee's Revised Cardiac Risk Index:** Risk of cardiac complications after non-cardiac surgery.
- **Duke Activity Status Index:** Estimates functional capacity of patients.
- **Surgical Outcome Risk Tool (SORT):** Risk of death within 30 d of inpatient surgery.

✓ **Preoperative Problems**
- Hypovolaemia, sepsis, acute kidney injury, pulmonary atelectasis.

✓ **Intraoperative Surgical Considerations**
- Avoid primary anastomosis if on significant vasopressor support.
- Consider open abdomen if intrabdominal hypertension likely.
- Avoid prolonged surgery in elderly.
- Large-bore NG tube for gastrointestinal obstruction prior to closure of abdomen, which is checked by surgeon.

✓ **Post-Operative Issues**
- **Analgesia**
  - ❖ Poorly controlled pain can lead to atelectasis, pneumonia, myocardial ischaemia.
  - ❖ Central neuraxial blockade, like epidural and spinal analgesia, can be used but is mostly contraindicated due to coagulation and systemic sepsis.
  - ❖ Transversus abdominus plane (TAP) block or posterior rectus sheath blocks either as single shot or catheter placed by surgeon or anaesthetist can be used.
  - ❖ Intraoperative use of lidocaine (1–2 mg/kg, followed by an infusion of

0.5–3 mg/kg/h), ketamine, or magnesium can reduce the need of opioids post-operatively.

- ❖ Fentanyl or morphine patient-controlled analgesia (PCA) can be used post-operatively.
- **Post-abdominal surgery sepsis causes**
  - ❖ 0–2 d: Tissue necrosis, UTI, pulmonary embolus.
  - ❖ 3–5 d: Wound infection, intra-abdominal abscess.
  - ❖ 5 d: Anastomotic leak.
- **Paralytic ileus**
  - ❖ Common till 4 d post-surgery.
  - ❖ After 4 d, it can be because of peritonitis, abscess, leak.
- **Relook laparotomy**
  - ❖ Mortality risk of a negative laparotomy in the critically ill patient is about 15%, whereas unrecognized intra-abdominal sepsis can have a mortality rate above 50%.
  - ❖ Relaparotomy should be based on careful consideration of possible benefits and harms in the individual patient.

✓ **Enhanced Recovery After Surgery (ERAS)**
- Multimodal perioperative care pathway for early recovery of patients undergoing major surgery.
  - **Some methods involved**
    - ❖ Optimal fluid management
    - ❖ Early start of enteral nutrition
    - ❖ Removal of indwelling catheters
    - ❖ Early mobilization
    - ❖ Physiotherapy

✓ **National Emergency Laparotomy Audit (NELA)**
- NELA is a joint national audit of the Royal College of Anaesthetists, Royal College of Surgeons, and Health Quality Improvement Project (HQIP).
- Purpose is to improve the quality of care for patients undergoing emergency laparotomy through the provision of high quality of data. Children, trauma, and vascular laparotomies are excluded.
- **NELA score:** Risk assessment tool to predict 30 d mortality in patients undergoing emergency laparotomy. A score of 5% or more is considered high-risk.
- **Key quality standards** from the ninth NELA report 2024:

- ❖ Proportion of patients who had a **CT scan that was reported by senior radiologist** and communicated with the team in the correct time scale before surgery.
- ❖ Proportion of patients with suspected infection or sepsis that have **antibiotic** administration within the correct time frame.
- ❖ Proportion of patients arriving in **theatre within a time scale appropriate to urgency.**
- ❖ Proportion of patients in whom **a risk assessment was documented preoperatively AND post-operatively.**
- ❖ **Proportion of high-risk patients (risk of death ≥5%) with consultant surgeon and consultant anaesthetist present in theatre.**
- ❖ Proportion of patients **admitted directly to critical care post-operatively when risk of death is >10%.**
- ❖ Proportion of patients **aged 65 or older and frail or aged 80 and older** who receive **post-operative assessment and management by a member of a perioperative team with expertise in comprehensive geriatric assessment (CGA).**
- ❖ **Proportion of patients aged 65 or older where a formal assessment of frailty was made.**
- **Key outcome measures**
  - ❖ **Mortality:** Goal to reduce national 30 d mortality to below 8.7%
  - ❖ **Outcome:** Goal to reduce national mean length of stay to below 15 d

POST-SURGICAL COMPLICATIONS

Surgical Site Infection (SSI)
- Infection that occurs within 30 d of surgery or 12 months of implants.
- **Classification (CDC) of SSI**
  - ❖ **Superficial incisional infections:** Skin and superficial part of subcutaneous tissue involved.
  - ❖ **Deep incisional infections:** Soft tissues deeper than subcutaneous tissue, like muscle and fascial planes.
  - ❖ **Organ/space infections:** Involving organ or anatomical space beyond the incision site.

- Stitch abscess, episiotomy, and infected burn wound are not considered as SSIs[Q].
- **Surgical procedures can be classified as**
  - ❖ **Clean:** Wounds that are uninfected, are without inflammation, and do not involve respiratory, gastrointestinal, or genitourinary tracts.
  - ❖ **Clean-contaminated:** Controlled entry into the respiratory, gastrointestinal, or genitourinary tracts, but without gross contamination.
  - ❖ **Contaminated:** Wounds with a break in sterile technique, gross spillage from gastrointestinal tract, or traumatic wounds older than 12 h.
  - ❖ **Dirty:** Wounds with an existing infection at the time of surgery, such as perforated viscera or wounds with pus; traumatic wounds older than 24 h.
- ✓ **Clinical Features**
  - **Risk factors for SSI: Prolonged hypotension**[Q], advanced age, haematoma, malnutrition, dirty surgery, diabetes mellitus, **blood transfusion**[Q], **razors**[Q], C-arm, surgery >5 h.
  - Colonization with MSSA[Q] increases the risk of post-operative wound infection.
  - *Enterobacter cloacae* develops mutation fast and is a known case of SSI.
  - **Elevation of temperature above 38.5°C on post-operative day 3 suggests infection**[Q].
  - Diagnosis is predominantly clinical, with imaging like ultrasound and CT scan used for assistance.
- ✓ **Prevention and Treatment**
  - **Preoperative phase (NICE guidelines):**
    - ❖ **Nasal decolonization:** Nasal mupirocin and CHG body wash before procedures in which *Staphylococcus aureus* is a likely cause of surgical site infection.
    - ❖ **Hair removal:** Not recommended routinely, and if have to be removed, electric clippers to be used with a single-use head on the day of surgery.
  - **Preoperative antibiotic prophylaxis**
    - ❖ Antibiotics prophylaxis only for patients before clean surgery involving an implant, clean-contaminated surgery, and contaminated surgery.

- ❖ Give antibiotics 30–60 min before surgery, except vancomycin and quinolones, which can be given 120 min before incision.
- ❖ Extra dose for surgical prophylaxis is essential for prolonged surgery (operation longer than half-life of the antibiotic given)[Q].
- ❖ *Prophylactic antibiotics should be discontinued within 24 h.*
- ❖ For cardiac surgeries, antibiotics should be given for 48 h post-operatively.
- **Skin preparation**
  - ❖ Use of 2% chlorhexidine gluconate (CHG) or 10% povidone-iodine reduces the burden of SSI.
  - ❖ Povidone-iodine solutions are not as effective as 2% CHG, as chlorhexidine has a broader spectrum of antimicrobial activity and longer-lasting effects.
- **Regional anaesthesia**
  - ❖ Beneficial for post-operative pain and modifies inflammatory response.
  - ❖ Morphine, fentanyl, and remifentanil have immunosuppressive properties.
  - ❖ *Oxycodone and buprenorphine both do not have immunosuppressive effects*[Q].
- Keep post-operative blood glucose level less than 10 mmol/L in cardiac patients[Q].
- **Definitive treatment**[Q]: Broad-spectrum antibiotics and source control by wound debridement.

Short Bowel Syndrome (SBS)

- Small bowel less than 180–200 cm of length leading to nutritional supplementation.
- ✓ **Physiology**
  - Normal bowel length is 275–850 cm. Water and sodium absorption occurs throughout the bowel.
    - ❖ **Jejunum:** Absorbs most nutrients in first 100 cm.
    - ❖ **Ileum:** Vitamin B12 and bile salts in last 100 cm.
    - ❖ **Terminal ileum and proximal colon:** Magnesium absorption.
- ✓ **Causes**
  - **Adults:** Crohn disease, mesenteric ischaemia, radiation enteritis, post-surgical adhesions.
  - **Children:** Volvulus, necrotizing colitis, intestinal malformations.

✓ **Anatomical Classification**
- **End-jejunostomy:** Jejunum, ileum, and colon resected, with stoma arising from jejunum.
- **Jejunocolic anastomosis:** Jejunum in continuity with left colon.
- **Jejunoileal anastomosis:** Some part of jejunum is resected, and rest is anastomosed with ileum.

✓ **Clinical Features**
- **Three phases of SBS**
  - ❖ **Acute phase (3–4 wk):** Metabolic derangements (water and salt loss) and gastric hypersecretion.
  - ❖ **Adaptive phase (1–2 yr):** Slow motility and hyperphagia.
  - ❖ **Maintenance phase:** Special diet and pharmacological supplementation.
- Malabsorption (vitamin B12, other fat-soluble vitamins), weight loss, diarrhoea, steatorrhoea, gall stones, renal stones.

✓ **Complications**
- **Intestinal failure**
  - ❖ Reduced gut absorption requiring supplementation of macronutrients and water.
  - ❖ **Classification**
    - **Mild:** Oral nutritional supplementation
    - **Moderate:** Enteral nutrition
    - **Severe:** Parenteral nutrition
  - ❖ Those with less than 60 cm of small bowel and parenteral nutrition-related complications are candidates for **intestinal transplant.** Five-year survival post-intestinal transplant is 50%.
- **Liver cholestasis:** Treatment involves switching from soy-based lipid emulsions to fish oil-based emulsions.
- **D-lactic acidosis**
  - ❖ Due to fermentation of unabsorbed carbohydrates by colonic bacteria. Can lead to D-lactate encephalopathy, presenting as slurred speech, ataxia, altered mental status.
  - ❖ Treatment includes reducing enteral feeds with carbohydrates and antibiotics, like metronidazole.

✓ **Treatment**
- Good nutritional status.
- Prevent complications, like intestinal failure.
- Prevent complications of parenteral nutrition, like metabolic bone disease, by giving magnesium, vitamin D, and bisphosphonates.

✓ **Prognosis**
- Those with >180 cm bowel do not require parenteral nutrition.
- Those with <60 cm will likely require lifetime parenteral nutrition.

SPLENECTOMY

✓ **Asplenism**
- Loss of spleen. Post-traumatic or therapeutic surgical removal of the spleen is most common cause[Q] of asplenism.
- Spleen may **not be functionally working**[Q] due to recurrent thrombotic events in haemoglobinopathies, like sickle cell disease and thalassemia.
- Asplenism produces a state of immunodeficiency[Q] by the following ways:
  - ❖ Impaired production of immunoglobins.
  - ❖ Insufficient opsonizing filter function of the spleen.
  - ❖ Reduced phagocytosis due to lack of splenic macrophages.
  - ❖ Removal of RBCs infected with malaria and *Babesia*.

✓ **Causes of splenectomy/asplenia**
- **Congenital haemolytic anaemias:** Hereditary spherocytosis, sickle cell disease (functional asplenism), thalassemia.
- **Acquired immunological disorders:** Immune thrombocytopaenic purpura (ITP), autoimmune haemolytic anaemia.
- **Malignancies:** Leukaemias, lymphoma, myelofibrosis.
- **Hypersplenism:** Cirrhosis, malaria, Felty syndrome, metabolic storage disorders like Gaucher or Niemann–Pick disease.
- **Trauma:** Blunt abdominal trauma, road traffic accident, penetrating trauma, spontaneous rupture (infectious mononucleosis)[Q].
- **Anatomical necessity:** En bloc with stomach in radical gastrectomy, en bloc with distal pancreas for pancreatic cancer involving head and tail.

✓ **Splenectomy Post-Operative Changes**
- **Increased risk of infections by encapsulated organisms**[Q]: *Streptococcus pneumoniae, Neisseria meningitidis, Haemophilus influenzae* type b, influenza virus, *Salmonella*, malaria, *Babesia*[Q].
- **Full blood count and blood film changes**: Leucocytosis, thrombocytosis, pitted RBCs, Howell–Jolly bodies (nuclear fragments within RBCs), Heinz bodies, target cells, basophilia.
- **Thrombosis risk**: Risk post-splenectomy is high, and portal splenic mesenteric thrombosis and pulmonary embolism are seen.

✓ **Immediate Vaccination**
- **Initial vaccines**
  - ❖ Pneumococcal polysaccharide vaccine (PPV23)
  - ❖ Meningococcal group A, C, W135, Y (ACWY) conjugate vaccine
  - ❖ Meningococcal group B vaccine
  - ❖ Influenza vaccine
- **One month after initial vaccine**
  - ❖ Meningococcal group B vaccine booster dose
- **Elective splenectomy**
  - ❖ Immunize with first four vaccines at least 2 wk (ideally 4–6 wk) before surgery.
  - ❖ Fifth vaccine (meningococcal group B booster dose) should be given after a month or at least 2 wk post-operatively.
- **Emergency splenectomy**: Immunize with first four vaccines at least 2 wk after surgery or when patient is feeling sufficiently well.

✓ **Follow-Up Vaccination**
- Seasonal influenza vaccine every year. Pneumococcal (PPV 23) every 5 yr

✓ **Prophylactic Antibiotics**
- Penicillin V 250 mg PO BD for at least the first 2 y post-splenectomy, possibly for life.
- Erythromycin (penicillin allergy) 500 mg PO BD for at least the first 2 y post-splenectomy, possibly for life.

✓ **Fever Management**
- **Overwhelming post-splenectomy infection (OPSI)** should be considered in any febrile patient with splenectomy.
- Infection by encapsulated organisms[Q] which are normally protected against by spleen.

- Risk of sepsis is highest in first 2 yr after splenectomy.
- If untreated, fulminant septic shock happens and death over 2 to 5 d.
- Empirical antibiotics (third-generation cephalosporins) as soon as possible, with management of patient according to surviving sepsis guidelines.

✓ **Thrombocytosis**
- If $>1000 \times 10^9$, start on aspirin 200 mg PO once a day.

CORONARY ARTERY BYPASS GRAFT

✓ **Coronary Artery Bypass Graft (CABG) Surgery**
- Most performed adult cardiac surgical procedure.
- On-pump CABG and off-pump CABG (OPCAB) are two ways of performing it.
- OPCAB comprises around 15% of all CABG procedures in UK.

✓ **Left Internal Mammary Artery (LIMA)[Q] to Left Anterior Descending (LAD) Artery Anastomosis**
- Superior as compared to stenting of LAD; hence, left internal mammary arterial grafts are preferred in proximal left coronary artery lesions.
- Saphenous vein grafts are commonly used to bypass other vessels.
- Stenting is non-inferior to venous bypass grafts for non-LAD territories.

✓ **Tenets of Good Post-Operative Care in Patients Undergoing Cardiac Surgical Procedures**
- Post-operative course is influenced by intraoperative events, adequate haemostasis, and haemodynamic optimization (transoesophageal echocardiography used). Chest drains are inserted in mediastinal and pleural cavities, and temporary epicardial pacing wires used.
- Good cardiovascular function is of prime importance for recovery of other organs.
- Warm extremities with strong pulses and good urine output are reassuring.
- Restore lung volumes by minimizing lung water.
- Control post-operative pain to prevent infections and chronic pain.
- Preservation of renal function is important for minimizing post-operative morbidity.

Intraoperative Event	Sequelae
Aortic cannulation	• Atheroembolic stroke, mesenteric ischaemia • Aortic dissection leading to organ ischaemia
Femoral artery cannulation	• Distal leg ischaemia, vascular trauma
Femoral vein cannulation	• Deep vein thrombosis
Right atrial cannulation	• Bleeding, atrial fibrillation
High-dose heparin	• Coagulopathy, heparin-induced thrombocytopaenia
Crystalloids for priming of CPB circuit	• Dilutional coagulopathy, anaemia, and volume overload
Cardioplegia	• Myocardial injury and conduction defects
Extracorporeal circulation	• Systemic inflammatory response leading to vasoplegia^Q and coagulopathy • Microemboli leading to stroke, renal and mesenteric impairment
Hypothermia	• Splanchnic vasoconstriction leading to mesenteric and renal ischaemia • Coagulopathy

Preoperative Phase

✓ **Aspirin Cessation**

- Unless there is an indication for non-cessation of aspirin (recent drug eluting stents, left main stem disease, critical proximal stenosis, symptoms at rest), all elective patients should have aspirin discontinued 5 d prior to surgery.
- For patients receiving dual antiplatelet therapy (DAPT), aspirin should be continued around the time of surgery and clopidogrel/prasugrel stopped 5 d before surgery.
- Warfarin should be discontinued 5 d before surgery. Patients with mechanical heart valves and those at high risk of thromboembolism should have bridging therapy with heparin.

- Direct oral anticoagulants should be stopped at least 48 h preoperatively.

✓ **ACE Inhibitors, Angiotensin Receptors/Blockers, Diuretics, and Digoxin**

- Should be omitted on the day of surgery.
- Anti-anginal drugs like beta-blockers, calcium channel blockers, nitrates, and ivabradine should be given on day of surgery.

Post-Operative Phase

✓ **Cardiovascular Complications**

- **Low cardiac output**
  - ❖ Low CO is defined as cardiac index < 2.2 L/min/m².
  - ❖ **Risk factors:** Impaired LV dysfunction, emergency surgery, incomplete revascularization.
  - ❖ **High-risk cases** like severe LV dysfunction with EF <30%, RV dysfunction, pulmonary hypertension, or severe renal insufficiency may warrant the use of pulmonary artery catheter.
  - ❖ Haemodynamic liability is the rule in the early post-operative period, and not overreacting to disquieting yet self-limited haemodynamic swings is the key.
  - ❖ Appropriate fluid resuscitation should be the first-line therapy for early haemodynamic instability^Q. Crystalloids are preferred. Aim for CVP 4–12 mmHg and Hb 80 g/L in low-risk and 90 g/L in high-risk cases.
  - ❖ Optimize preload and afterload, and if still no improvement, inotropic support might be needed. Dobutamine in combination with noradrenaline is used to compensate for vasodilatory effects of dobutamine. Phosphodiesterase III inhibitors like milrinone can be used for RV dysfunction or low CO state with vasoconstriction. An inodilator and calcium channel sensitizer, levosimendan, is used at some centres as well.
  - ❖ Inhaled NO can be used for RV dysfunction and pulmonary hypertension as it selectively produces pulmonary vasodilation and decreases RV afterload. However, no mortality benefit has been determined.

- ❖ Intra-aortic balloon pump (IABP), VA-ECMO, or ventricular assist device (VAD) may be needed in refractory shock.
- **Cardiac arrhythmias**
  - ❖ Peak between second and fifth post-operative day.
  - ❖ Supraventricular tachyarrhythmias (SVTs) occur in 20–50% of patients, and AF is the commonest SVT seen.
  - ❖ **Ventricular arrhythmias may signify ongoing myocardial ischaemia**.
  - ❖ Patients with severe LV dysfunction and repeated ventricular arrhythmias may benefit from implantable cardioverter defibrillator (ICD).
- **Myocardial ischaemia:** ST-T changes seen in two or more contiguous leads indicate an acute graft failure.
- **Cardiac tamponade**
  - ❖ It should be suspected when low cardiac output is accompanied by sudden cessation of chest tube drainage^Q. Transoesophageal echo may be needed to rule it out.
  - ❖ *Beck's triad*^{Q} (hypotension, distended neck veins, and muffled heart sounds) has poor sensitivity.
  - ❖ Rate and not volume of fluid accumulation is important as **a volume of 100 mL acutely can cause tamponade whereas volumes of up to 1,500 mL may accumulate during chronic causes.**
  - ❖ Tachycardia, high CVP with reduced "*y*" descent, hypotension, low-voltage QRS, beat-to-beat QRS variation, known as **electrical alternans (pathognomonic)**^{Q}.
  - ❖ A drop in SBP >10 mmHg during inspiration is a sign of **pulsus paradoxus**.
  - ❖ CXR shows enlarged cardiac silhouette with clear lung fields.
  - ❖ **Echocardiography**^{Q} is the best investigation in an awake patient showing diastolic collapse of heart chambers.
  - ❖ Diastolic right ventricular collapse (highly specific). Systolic right atrial collapse (earliest sign). LV/LA collapse is a very late sign.
  - ❖ **Pericardiocentesis: For large effusions**^{Q} (>20 mm) without haemodynamic compromise or smaller effusions (<10 mm) with haemodynamic compromise on echocardiography. Performed with **subxiphoid approach**^{Q} under fluoroscopy, except in emergency situations. Continuous ECG monitoring is done to prevent cardiac damage.
  - ❖ **Surgery** is done for clots or loculated effusions.
- ✓ **Post-Operative Bleeding**
  - • Either medical (coagulation defects) or surgical (anastomotic leaks) bleeding.
  - • Thromboelastography (TEG) or other point-of-care (POC) viscoelastic tests may be used to diagnose medical bleeding.
- ✓ **Pulmonary Complications**
  - • Medial sternotomy decreases functional residual capacity and vital capacity.
  - • Atelectasis and pleural effusions are seen in 90% of patients.
  - • Cardiac surgery is a risk factor for ARDS and can be minimized by use of lung protective ventilation.
- ✓ **Renal Dysfunction**
  - • Acute kidney injury (AKI) ranged from 1 to 5% of cardiac surgical patients.
  - • AKI requiring renal replacement therapy increases the length of ICU and hospital stay along with risk of mortality by 27 times compared to patients without AKI.
- ✓ **Gastrointestinal Complications**
  - • Paralytic ileus, upper GI bleeding, mesenteric ischaemia might be seen post-operatively.
  - • CT angiography is diagnostic study of choice in acute mesenteric ischaemia and antibiotics should be started early if suspected.
- ✓ **Sepsis**
  - • Sternal wound infections, pneumonia, UTIs, and CVC infections can happen. Hyperglycaemia and blood transfusions are risk factors.
  - • NICE-SUGAR study found better survival with blood glucose targets of less than 10 mmol/L.
- ✓ **Neurological Dysfunction**
  - • From mild cognitive dysfunction to cerebrovascular accident (2–4%). Delirium occurs in 50% of patients above 60 yr of age.

✓ **Weaning and De-Escalation**
- Weaning from ventilator can be done in 4–6 h in most uncomplicated CABG procedures.
- Inotropic weaning, removal of PAC, removal of chest drains and Foley catheter can be done post-operative day 1.
- Excessive chest tube drainage is commonly defined as bleeding >200 mL/h to 1,500 mL/8 h, and chest drains can be taken out if drain output drops to <100 mL/8 h or <30 mL/h for two consecutive hours after chest physiotherapy.
- **Post-operatively, all patients should be administered aspirin (rectal 300 mg) within first 6 h, when chest drain output is satisfactory (<100 mL/h).** Aspirin 150 mg should be started within the first 24 h and continued lifelong. Clopidogrel 75 mg daily should be given to patients who are aspirin intolerant.
  - ❖ **DAPT** should be restarted in patients within one year of ACS/PCI whenever it is safe.
  - ❖ Statin and beta-blockers should be started early in post-operative period.
- Central venous catheters can be removed when patient hasn't received inotropic support >12 h and urine output >0.5 mL/kg/h.
- Patients can gain up to 6 L of volume from intraoperative period to post-operative day 1 and low-dose IV diuretics (e.g. furosemide 20 mg BD can be started in patients).
- Maintenance fluids should be avoided and after checking patient's swallowing reflex, oral intake of fluids can be started on day 1.
- Patients are mobilized and ambulated on post-operative day 1.
- Epicardial pacing can usually be removed on post-operative day 1 or 2.
- All this explained in so much detail keeping in mind your posting to cardiac ICU, where I don't want both the patient and the treating physician simultaneously to have a tachycardia.

Additional Questions

✓ **Aetiology of Pericardial Effusion**
- Post-cardiac surgery
- Post-traumatic
- Aortic dissection
- Iatrogenic (TAVI, PCI)
- Renal failure
- Neoplasm
- Infections (TB, HIV)

PNEUMONECTOMY

Epidemiology

✓ **Pneumonectomy**
- Surgical removal of an entire lung performed via thoracotomy.

✓ **Indication for Pneumonectomy**
- Bronchial carcinoma is the most common indication.
- Other indications are uncontrolled haemorrhage, chronic infective lung disorder, and fungal infections.

Physiology

✓ **One-Lung Ventilation (OLV)**
- Depends upon lateral decubitus position, open chest, and collapse of non-dependent lung, all of which cause increased shunt.
- During two-lung ventilation in the lateral position, blood flow to the non-dependent lung is 40% compared to 60% to dependent lung.
  - ❖ Patient in lateral decubitus position with dependent lung receiving greater blood flow due to effect of gravity. The non-dependent lung will receive more ventilation due to improved compliance.
- A 5% physiological shunt in lateral position in each lung makes it effective, with 35% blood flow in non-dependent lung compared to 55% in dependent lung.
- Hypoxia causes hypoxic pulmonary vasoconstriction[Q] (HPV) and diverts blood from area of low ventilation.
  - ❖ Fall in alveolar PO_2 leads to less nitric oxide (NO) being synthesized and, hence, vasoconstriction.
- OLV involves ventilating the dependent lung. HPV creates at least 50% shunt[Q] and hence blood flow to non-dependent lung becomes halved, 35/2 = 17.5%. As this blood goes to dependent lung, it has now 55 + 17.5 = 72.5% blood flow.
- So dependent lung gets 72.5% of blood flow but compliance is decreased because of

elevated diaphragm, pressure from abdominal and mediastinal structures. This causes V/Q mismatch.

✓ **NICE Recommendations**
- NICE recommends that post-pneumonectomy FEV_1 and DLCO should be >30%. Those with <30% values should have formal exercise testing using CPET.
- VO_2 peak[Q] >15 mL O_2/kg/min is defined as good physiological function, whereas values less than 10 mL O_2/kg/min[Q] is defined as a contraindication.
- Anaerobic threshold[Q] <11 mL/kg/min is associated with poorer outcome.

Intraoperative Management

✓ **Double-Lumen Tube or Bronchial Blocker**
- Used for one-lung ventilation.

✓ **Indications for One-Lung Ventilation (OLV)[Q]**
- **Absolute indications for OLV**
  ❖ Lung protection from blood, pus.
  ❖ Control of ventilation (e.g. bronchopleural fistula, traumatic damage to a major bronchial airway, bullae that may rupture with IPPV).
- **Relative indications for OLV**
  ❖ Thoracic aortic aneurysm, oesophagectomy, pneumonectomy.

✓ **Intraoperative Hypoxaemia**
- Fractional inspired oxygen can be increased to 100%.
- Check double-lumen tube (DLT) for cuff hernia/block/kink.
- Check anaesthetic circuit and connections.
- Ensure adequate cardiac output.
- Insufflate O_2 to non-ventilated lung.
- Apply CPAP to non-ventilated lung: 5–10 cm H_2O.
- Apply PEEP to ventilated lung.
- Intermittent insufflation of non-ventilated lung.
- Clamping appropriate pulmonary artery to reduce shunt.
- Two-lung ventilation may need to be restarted.

Early Post-Operative Complications

✓ **RV Failure[Q]**
- May be seen due to increased pulmonary vascular resistance.

- Judicious fluid use. Diuretic/RRT if significant tricuspid regurgitation.
- Milrinone for supporting right ventricle contractility combined with vasopressin/noradrenaline for systemic vasoconstriction.
- Nitric oxide (NO) and prostacyclin (endothelin receptor antagonist) to decrease right-sided afterload.

✓ **Cardiac Arrhythmias**
- Seen in 5–40% cases. Atrial fibrillation is common.

✓ **Post-Pneumonectomy Pulmonary Oedema**
- Remaining lung gets double the usual pulmonary flow. Seen 12–96 h post-operatively.

✓ **Bronchopleural Fistula**
- More than 90% of air leaks stop within several weeks after operation.

✓ **Cardiac Herniation**
- Seen on right-sided pneumonectomy and that too, if the pericardium is debrided on the right side.
- Raised JVP/CVP and presence of heart sounds on the right side.

Late Complications

✓ **Post-Pneumonectomy Syndrome[Q]**
- Post-pneumonectomy space (PPS) will initially be filled with air.
- Within 24 h, the hemidiaphragm on the pneumonectomy side will elevate slightly, the mediastinum will shift towards the PPS, and fluid will begin to accumulate within the PPS.
- The lung on the opposite side will start hyperinflating.
- Initially, there will be a gas-fluid level in the PPS, and this level will gradually increase as more fluid accumulates.
- **Post-pneumonectomy syndrome:** Delayed complication with severe mediastinal shift, airway compression, and rotation of the heart.

Post-Pneumonectomy Care

✓ **Early Extubation and Avoiding Reintubation**
- Avoid positive pressure ventilation and chest drains OFF suction.

✓ **High Fowler's Position**
- Sitting upright with a 60–90° flexion at hips.
- No rolling over onto the side of the intact lung.

✓ **NG Tube**
- If right pneumonectomy, place an NG tube on free drainage as they may develop gastric distension that can put pressure on the remaining lung.

✓ **Analgesia**
- Multimodal with paravertebral block inserted by surgeon favoured over thoracic epidural.

✓ **Fluid Balance**
- Negative or neutral as predisposition to pulmonary oedema.

TRANSPLANT PATIENTS

✓ **Problems with Transplant Patients**
- Extensive past medical history with multiple comorbidities
- Polypharmacy
- Transplant-specific issues

✓ **Absolute Contraindications**[Q]
- CJD
- HIV active
- Infection, uncontrolled
- Cancer, metastatic, uncurable

Heart Transplant Patients

✓ **Description**
- Immunogenic organs with high exposure of immunosuppressive medication

✓ **Indications**
- Acute or chronic heart failure
  - ❖ **Routine:** Outpatients on oral medications for heart failure
  - ❖ **Urgent:** Patient requiring inotropic or intra-aortic balloon pump
  - ❖ **Super urgent:** Patient requiring temporary mechanical support either as ECMO or VAD

✓ **Specific Contraindications**
- Severe pulmonary hypertension with pulmonary artery systolic pressure >60 mmHg, transpulmonary pressure gradient >15 mmHg, and pulmonary vascular resistance (PVR) of >5 wood units
- Advanced kidney disease (GFR <30 mL/min/1.73 m^2)
- Chronic liver disease (cirrhosis)
- Severe pulmonary disease with FEV_1 <50% or recent pulmonary emboli

- Significant cerebrovascular or peripheral vascular disease
- Active infection, like hepatitis B, C, and HIV
- Active malignancy
- Active substance abuse
- Severe psychiatric illness or adverse psychosocial factors
- Morbid obesity with BMI >35 kg/m^2

✓ **Operative Management**
- CMV-free and leuco-depleted blood and blood products are arranged.
- Pulmonary artery catheter is used to calculate PVR and pharmacological measures to reduce PVR if high.
- Orthotropic heart transplant with bicaval anastomosis is preferred.
- Inotropic support with milrinone and noradrenaline is started to give time to heart to recover.

✓ **Early Complications**
- Right ventricular dysfunction[Q] is the most common problem with a newly transplanted heart.
- Anastomosis leakage or tamponade.
- Ischaemia of electrical guiding system (all of them get temporary pacemakers).
- Rejection represented by increasing cardiac markers or stiffening of the heart.
- Acute kidney injury.

✓ **Late Complications**
- **Cardiac allograft vasculopathy**[Q]: Narrowing of coronary arteries.
- Malignancy: New-onset solid organ malignancies seen in around 10% of patients within 1–5 yr of transplant.

✓ **Post–Heart Transplant Management**
- Early extubation is preferred with regular diuretics to offload right ventricle.
- **Physiological changes**
  - ❖ Resting heart rate of 90–100 bpm is maintained. No autonomic innervation.
  - ❖ No effect of Valsalva manoeuvre[Q] and carotid sinus massage[Q] and drugs like atropine[Q], glycopyrrolate, and digoxin, as vagal innervation is cut.
  - ❖ Ephedrine has a decreased response as there is no catecholamine store in the myocardial neurons.
  - ❖ *Adrenaline and noradrenaline have augmented inotropic response.*

- ❖ Dobutamine and isoprenaline maintain a normal response.
- ❖ Inhaled nitric oxide is given to decrease pulmonary hypertension.
- **Primary graft dysfunction**
  - ❖ Failure of graft function within the first 24 h after transplant in absence of hyperacute rejection, pulmonary hypertension, or known surgical complications.
  - ❖ Characterized by severe bi-/one-ventricular failure along with poor cardiac output and severe hypoperfusion state.
- **Rejection of transplant**
  - ❖ Cell-mediated vs antibody-mediated.
  - ❖ Intraoperatively, basiliximab is given along with methylprednisolone, with calcineurin inhibitors started in a couple of days, when renal function stabilizes.
  - ❖ A difficult-to-convert AF may be a sign of acute rejection.
  - ❖ Most patients are on three immunosuppressive agents during the first year and two immunosuppressive agents lifelong.
- **Antimicrobials**
  - ❖ **Valganciclovir** to cover CMV for 3–6 months.
  - ❖ **Cotrimoxazole** to cover *Pneumocystis jirovecii* till the time of intense immunosuppression.

Lung Transplant Patients

✓ **Description**
- Immunogenic organs with high exposure of immunosuppressive medication.

✓ **Indications**
- COPD, interstitial lung disease, bronchiectasis associated with cystic fibrosis, and pulmonary hypertension.

✓ **Specific Contraindications**
- They are almost the same if you see:
  - ❖ Active malignancy or recent history of malignancy.
  - ❖ Poorly controlled significant dysfunction of another major organ system like heart, liver, kidney, or brain.
  - ❖ Poorly controlled infection with a virulent or resistant microbe.
  - ❖ Chest wall or spinal deformity expected to cause severe deformity after transplantation.
  - ❖ Active substance abuse.
  - ❖ Severe psychiatric illness or adverse psychosocial factors.
  - ❖ Morbid obesity with BMI >35 kg/m².
  - ❖ Life expectancy <5 yr.

✓ **Operative Management**
- Thoracic epidural analgesiaᵠ as incisions can be bilateral thoracotomy, clamshell incision, or median sternotomy.
- One-lung ventilation may be used during single lung transplant.
- Surgical technique involves anastomosis of bronchi, right and left pulmonary arteries, and all pulmonary veins.
- Cardiopulmonary bypass may be used electively in patients with severe pulmonary hypertension and emergent in patients with cardiorespiratory compromise.

✓ **Early Complications**
- Post-surgical complications: Bronchial ischaemia, lung torsion, vascular anastomotic leak
- Bleeding, especially with patient on ECMO
- Anxiety, breathlessness, and cough while on ECMO
- High rate of fungal infections (prophylaxis given)
- Acute kidney injury

✓ **Late Complications**
- Bronchiolitis obliterans
- Post-transplant lymphoproliferative disease

✓ **Post–Lung Transplant Management**
- Early extubation is preferred once analgesia is adequate.
- Lung protective ventilation and fluid restriction to prevent oedema of graft.
- **Primary graft dysfunction**
  - ❖ Seen in up to 30% of patients. Acute hypoxaemia associated with bilateral radiological infiltrates.
  - ❖ Largest cause of early mortality, and pulmonary hypertension is a risk factor.
  - ❖ Surfactant therapy is used as a rescue therapy.
- **Rejection of transplant**
  - ❖ Cell-mediated vs antibody-mediated.
  - ❖ A pretransplant oral dose of cyclosporin is given, followed by IV mycophenolate and methylprednisolone on anaesthetic induction.

❖ Most patients are on three immunosuppressive agents, like in heart transplant.

Liver Transplant Patients

✓ **Description**
- Immunotolerant organ with lower exposure of immunosuppressive medication. Delayed introduction of calcineurin inhibitors is tolerated.

✓ **Indications**
- Acute liver failure and chronic cirrhotic liver disease

✓ **Specific Contraindications**Q
- Active substance abuse (alcohol or illicit drugs)
- Severe psychiatric illness or adverse psychosocial factors
- Severe cardiopulmonary disease
- Advanced age
- Extrahepatic cancer

✓ **Operative Management**
- Severe hyponatraemia is a poor prognostic indicator and should be corrected preoperatively by fluid restriction, spironolactone, and RRT.
- Liver transplant is a laparotomy with risk of major haemorrhage.
- Rapid infusion and cell salvage systems must be available with point of care testing to guide blood product administration.
- **Surgical phases:**
  - ❖ **Preanhepatic:** Initial incision to the isolation of native liver from circulation.
  - ❖ **Anhepatic:** From isolation of native liver to implantation of new liver.
  - ❖ **Neohepatic:** New graft reperfusion.

✓ **Early Complications**
- Portal vein or hepatic artery thrombosisQ (Doppler ultrasound on day 1 to ensure flow).
- Biliary complications (bile leak, anastomotic stenosis).
- Infections by enterococci and Gram-negative bacilli.
- Acute rejection (seen in first 6 months as fever, increased transaminases, bilirubin, thrombocytopaenia). Easily reversed.
- Acute kidney injury.

✓ **Late Complications**
- **Post-transplantation lymphoproliferative disorder (PTLD):** EBV, pyrexia of unknown origin, mononucleosis-like syndrome, infiltrative disease of the allograft.

✓ **Post–Liver Transplant Management**
- **Hepatic artery thrombosis (HAT)**
  - ❖ Can be early (<21 d) or late.
  - ❖ **Early HAT** presents with cardiovascular instability, coagulopathy, and elevated transaminases. Hyperlactataemia may be the first sign. Treatment is revascularization by transarterial thrombectomy, thrombolysis, or surgical exploration.
  - ❖ **Late HAT** presents with biliary complications like biliary strictures, leaks, and cholangitis.
- **Primary non-function of the graft:** Within first 24 h, failure of graft to start normal hepatic enzymatic processes. Seen in patients with acute liver failure. Retransplant is the treatment.
- **Rejection**
  - ❖ **Hyperacute:** Uncommon after ABO compatible liver transplant. Seen within first few days of transplant. Signs are thrombocytopaenia, rising bilirubin, and other signs of acute liver failure. Retransplant is needed.
  - ❖ **Acute:** T cell–mediated rejection, seen within first 3 months. Signs are tachycardia, fever, hepatomegaly, and ascites, with increased transaminases, bilirubin, and alkaline phosphatases. Increased immunosuppression is needed.
  - ❖ **Chronic:** Cell-mediated. Leads to hepatic fibrosis, leading to jaundice, portal hypertension, and loss of synthetic function. Increased immunosuppression is needed.
- **Immunosuppression**
  - ❖ Calcineurin inhibitors like cyclosporine/tacrolimus along with corticosteroids.
  - ❖ Mycophenolate may be used in acute rejection.

Immunosuppression for Solid Organ Transplants

✓ **Primary Graft Failure/Dysfunction**
- Severe dysfunction of the transplanted organ in the immediate post-operative period. Used in context of mostly dysfunctional heart or lung transplant.

- Causes are an inappropriate-sized organ, poor organ preservation, prolonged ischaemia, or reperfusion injury.

✓ **Immunosuppression in Solid Organ Transplant**
- Rejection is mainly by *cell-mediated immunity*. Antigen-presenting cell bind to antigens and present them to T cells, which releases IL-2 for further proliferation of lymphocytes.
- **Induction**
  - ❖ Polyclonal antibodies (thymoglobulin, ATGAM), monoclonal antibodies (basiliximab, alemtuzumab).
  - ❖ The purpose of induction is to prevent rejection and delay the introduction of calcineurin inhibitors, as they add to nephrotoxicity.
- **Maintenance:** Calcineurin inhibitors as monotherapy or in combination with steroids, or an antimetabolite is used.
- **Anti-rejection**
  - ❖ Drugs used to treat acute episode of ongoing rejection.
  - ❖ **T cell–mediated rejection:** Thymoglobulin and steroids.
  - ❖ **Antibody-mediated rejection:** Plasmapheresis and IVIG.

✓ **Pharmacological Agents**
- **Corticosteroids**
  - ❖ Inhibit T cell proliferation, antibody formation, and expression of cytokines.
  - ❖ **Side effects:** Glucose intolerance, hypertension, osteoporosis, hyperlipidaemia.
- **Cyclosporine (CSA)** (calcineurin inhibitor)
  - ❖ Blocks production of IL-2.
  - ❖ Has been used in kidney and liver transplant.
  - ❖ **Side effects:** *Nephrotoxicity*[Q], hypertension, neurological toxicity, like posterior reversible encephalopathy syndrome (PRES), hypertrichosis, hyperlipidaemia, and gingival hyperplasia.
- **Tacrolimus (TAC)** (calcineurin inhibitor)
  - ❖ Blocks production of IL-2.
  - ❖ Presence of bile in digestive tract doesn't affect absorption, unlike CSA. A 25% oral bioavailability.
  - ❖ *Better graft survival rates in kidney and liver transplant than CSA.* Used

in kidney, liver, heart, lung, and bowel transplant. *TAC has helped in using steroid-free regimen*[Q].
  - ❖ **Side effects:** *Nephrotoxicity*, hypertension, *neurotoxicity* (worse with TAC), diabetes mellitus. *Better lipid profile than CSA.*
  - ❖ Drug monitoring is routine (levels: 5–20 ng/mL).
- **Azathioprine (AZA)** (antimetabolite)
  - ❖ Prodrug of 6-mercaptopurine, which blocks purine synthesis.
  - ❖ **Side effects:** Well-tolerated mostly, and a common side effect is dose-dependent decrease in white blood cell count. *Liver necrosis* and *pancreatitis* also seen.
- **Mycophenolic acid (MMF)** (antimetabolite)
  - ❖ Blocks purine synthesis.
  - ❖ Used in kidney, liver, heart, lung, and pancreas transplants.
  - ❖ Side effects: *GI toxicity more than AZA.* Enteric-coated MMF has been used to mitigate GI toxicity. Neutropaenia and thrombocytopaenia also seen.
  - ❖ Drug monitoring is not routine.
- **Sirolimus (SRL)** (mTOR inhibitor)
  - ❖ *Reduces sensitivity of T cells and B cells to IL-2.*
  - ❖ Used in kidney transplant. Treatment of lymphangioleiomyomatosis as well.
  - ❖ **Side effects:** Less diabetogenic and nephrotoxic. Hyperlipidaemia, anaemia, leucopaenia, and thrombocytopaenia.
  - ❖ Drug monitoring is routine.

✓ **Biological Agents**
- **Polyclonal antibodies**
  - ❖ **ATGAM:** Prevents and treats acute rejection episodes. Prepared by immunizing **horses** with human thymocytes.
  - ❖ **Thymoglobulin (ATG):** Prevents and treats acute rejection episodes. Prepared by immunizing **rabbits** with human thymocytes.
- **Monoclonal antibodies**
  - ❖ **Basiliximab** (anti-IL-2): Prevents acute rejection.
  - ❖ **Rituximab** (anti-CD20): Used as a treatment of post-transplant lymphoproliferative disease (PTLD).

✓ **Infectious Complications**
  • **Description:** Anti-CMV prophylaxis (ganciclovir or valganciclovir) is standard practice.
    ❖ **0–1 month:** Recipient-derived or *hospital/ventilator-acquired infections*, like drug-resistant Gram-negative organisms, S. aureus, VRE, *Candida* (non-albicans), aspiration and secondary infections, *catheter infections*, *Clostridium difficile colitis.*
    ❖ **1–12 months:** *Opportunistic infection* and *reactivation of latent disease*, such as polyomavirus, PCP, *Nocardia*, tuberculosis, *Listeria*, CMV, *Varicella*, toxoplasmosis, EBV-related post-transplant lymphoproliferative disorder.
    ❖ **>12 months:** Severe form of *community-acquired pneumonia* (respiratory syncytial virus, influenza, and *Legionella*), *urinary tract infections*, or *opportunistic infections* (PML, PTLD, late-onset CMV, *Nocardia*).
✓ **Prevention of Neutropenia:** Antimicrobial prophylaxis for solid organ transplant patients.
  • PCP prophylaxis: All patients. TMP-SMX. Usually for a year.
  • CMV prophylaxis: Indication is CMV-positive donor or recipient. Ganciclovir. For first 3–6 months.
  • HSV/VZV prophylaxis: Indication is HSV/VZV seropositive patients. Acyclovir.
  • Hepatitis B: Indication is HBsAg seropositive patients. Lamivudine.

WHIPPLE PROCEDURE

✓ **Whipple Procedure**
  • Pancreaticoduodenectomy
  • Indication: Pancreatic cancer
✓ **Intraoperative Management**
  • Removal of the head of pancreas, duodenum, gall bladder, and bile duct, and then the bile duct, stomach stump, and pancreatic duct anastomosed to jejunum (three anastomosis).
  • Effective analgesia is important for post-operative respiratory function and preventions of complications. Mid thoracic (T5–T8) epidurals are used.
✓ **Post-Operative Management**
  • **Early ambulation:** Out of the bed on day 1.

  • **Pulmonary secretion clearance.**
  • **Pain control:** Thoracic epidural until third post-operative day. Regular paracetamol and naproxen for 5 d.
  • Gastric decompression by NG tube.
  • **Slow advancement of diet**
    ❖ Encourage clear fluids immediately and diet to commence from day 1 post-operatively as NJ feed at 15 mL/h.
    ❖ Remove NJ/NG tubes on post-operative day 2 if drain fluid amylase <2,000 IU/L and NG output <500 mL/24 h.
✓ **Complications**
  • **Cardiopulmonary complications:** Post-operative pneumonia, ARDS, and atrial fibrillation.
  • **Pancreatic fistulae/pancreatic leak:** Failure of healing of the pancreatic-enteric anastomosis and drain fluid amylase levels more than three times the serum amylase on the third post-operative days.
    ❖ **Grade A fistulas:** Short-lived, and management involves delayed removal of intraperitoneal drains.
    ❖ **Grade B fistulas:** Require use of TPN and antibiotics.
    ❖ **Grade C fistulas:** Clinically unwell patients who may be septic. Reoperation is required.
  • **Pseudoaneurysms**
    ❖ Gastroduodenal artery aneurysm haemorrhage may be seen. They present with abdominal pain, massive GI haemorrhage, and haemodynamic instability.
    ❖ CT angiogram can identify the bleeding, and IR-guided embolization can control the bleeding.
  • **Delayed gastric emptying**
    ❖ Inability to return to a standard diet by end of the first post-operative week and includes prolonged nasogastric use.
    ❖ Motility agents like metoclopramide and erythromycin are first-line agents.
    ❖ Enteral nutrition via naso-jejunostomy tube or gastrostomy tube, or **parenteral nutrition** should be considered.
  • **Exocrine and endocrine insufficiency**
    ❖ Post-operative exocrine insufficiency may present as weight loss or steatorrhoea and can be treated with oral enzyme supplementation.

❖ New-onset diabetes may be seen in 11–54% of patients.

✓ **Prognosis**
- **Complication rate** is 30%, and **mortality** post-PPPD is 1–4%.

COLORECTAL SURGERY

✓ **Colorectal Cancer**
- Second largest cause of cancer-related mortality in the UK.
- Colorectal surgeries, both elective and urgent, can require critical care support due to the risk of complications, like anastomotic leaks and sepsis.
- Factors like old age, male gender, social deprivation, heart failure, and type 2 DM are associated with a higher need for intensive care support.

✓ **Colorectal Resection**
- Done for colorectal cancers.
- **Right hemicolectomy:** Right side of the colon is removed, and end-to-end anastomosis.
- **Left hemicolectomy:** Left side of the colon is removed, and end-to-end anastomosis.
- **Sigmoid colectomy:** Sigmoid colon is removed, and end-to-end anastomosis.
- **Low anterior resection of rectum:** Lower portions of sigmoid colon and rectum are excised, and ends anastomosed. A temporary loop ileostomy is formed to protect the anastomosis and is reversed later.
- **High anterior resection of rectum:** A bigger portion of sigmoid and recto-sigmoid junction is excised, and anastomosis formed. Covering loop ileostomy or colostomy may be needed.
- **Abdominoperineal resection:** *Sigmoid colon, rectum, and anus* are removed in an abdominal and perineal wound, and formation of an end colostomy. **Done for rectal cancer.**
- **Hartmann's procedure:** The whole of sigmoid colon and the upper rectum are removed, and a descending colon end colostomy formed. **Anus is not dissected.** Performed mostly as an **emergency procedure** for sigmoid malignancy or perforation.
- **Total colectomy:** Colon is removed and only the rectum and anus left with an end ileostomy formed. Done more quickly in an emergency situation.

- **Pan-proctocolectomy:** Colon, rectum, and anus are removed. Commonly done for ulcerative colitis, Crohn's disease, and familial polyposis.

✓ **Intraoperative Management**
- Goal is to minimize stress response and prevent post-operative gut dysfunction.
- Laparoscopic techniques are preferred for faster recovery.
- Analgesia using thoracic epidural to prevent post-operative complications.
- Abdominal wall blocks with PCA pumps are getting increasingly popular for pain relief.

✓ **Post-Operative Care for Colon Surgeries**
- **Early ambulation:** Prevents loss of skeletal muscle, development of insulin resistance, lung atelectasis, and thromboembolic disease.
- **Liberal enteral feeding:** Early feeding <24 h prevents development of ileus.
- **Restricted intravenous fluids:** To avoid bowel congestion and anastomotic leakage.
- **Multimodal pain therapy:** Thoracic epidural analgesia (TEA) at the level of T6 to T12 for open surgeries, plus regular paracetamol and ketorolac. TEA is used in patients at high risk of pulmonary complications undergoing laparoscopic resection.

✓ **Specific Complications**
- **Anastomotic leak**
  - ❖ Leak seen in up to 20% of patients within first 7 d of surgery.
  - ❖ Fever, tachycardia, abdominal pain, signs of peritonitis.
  - ❖ Diagnosis confirmed by erect chest X-ray showing air.
  - ❖ Stable patients without peritonitis managed conservatively by bowel rest, antibiotics, and percutaneous drainage.
  - ❖ Unstable patients or those with peritonitis are managed with re-exploration.
- **Genitourinary dysfunction**
  - ❖ Injury to sacral splanchnic and hypogastric nerves during rectal mobilization can lead to urinary and sexual dysfunction.

OESOPHAGECTOMY

Oesophagectomy

✓ **Oesophagectomy**
- Done for oesophageal cancer.

- **Surgical approach:** Excision of the oesophagus and relocating the stomach in the mediastinum.
  - ❖ **Ivor Lewis oesophagectomy:** Laparotomy followed by right thoracotomy.
  - ❖ **McKeown oesophagectomy:** Tri-incisional technique which uses a cervical incision for upper anastomosis apart from laparotomy and thoracotomy incision.
  - ❖ **Trans-hiatal oesophagectomy:** Laparotomy and dissection of the lower oesophagus through an enlarged diaphragmatic hiatus, followed by removal of the oesophagus and re-anastomosis via left cervical incision, thereby avoiding thoracotomy totally.

✓ **Intraoperative Management**
  - *One-lung ventilation is required.*
  - Minimizing fluid overload, as it can lead to pulmonary complications.
  - Adequate analgesia for preventing postoperative respiratory failure. You might escape with a non-functional epidural in a Whipple procedure, but a good working epidural is a must for oesophagectomy.

✓ **Post-Operative Care**
  - **Early extubation**
    - ❖ Very high risk of aspiration in immediate post-operative period may justify transfer to the ICU with delayed extubation in patients post-gastrectomy and post-oesophagectomy.
    - ❖ *Avoid CPAP/HFNO immediately postoperatively to protect anastomosis[Q].*
  - **Early ambulation.**
  - **NG tube on free drainage:** To protect the anastomosis, identify GI bleeding, and monitor gastric secretion volume.
  - **Judicious fluid administration:** Anastomosis is away from the site of origin of its blood supply. Hence, excessive tissue oedema and vasoconstriction should be avoided.
  - **Chest physiotherapy:** To prevent secretions and atelectasis.
  - **Pain control optimization:** Thoracic epidural to be taken out on POD 4/5. Regular paracetamol and tramadol.
  - **Early diet initiation:** Start feeding jejunostomy with 30 mL/h water on POD1 and standard enteral feed at 30 mL/h on POD2.

✓ **Complications**
  - **Pulmonary complications:** Pneumonia is common and a potentially serious complication. Development of ARDS should prompt consideration for sepsis or unrecognized anastomotic leak.
  - **Cardiovascular complications:** Supraventricular arrhythmias like AF are common.
  - **Oesophageal anastomotic leak**
    - ❖ Leak rates of 10–30%. Major leaks present in first 5 d.
    - ❖ **Chest and abdominal pain,** tachycardia, discoloured or bilious fluid from the chest drain. New pleural effusions.
    - ❖ Suspect leak if patient develops shock within the first 48 h of surgery.
    - ❖ **Diagnosis:** CT chest/abdomen with oral contrast or endoscopy if intubated and ventilated.
    - ❖ Conservative initially with drainage, *nutrition optimization* (parenteral), and *antibiotics.* Endoscopic stenting has been increasingly used instead of re-exploration.
    - ❖ **Endoluminal vacuum therapy (EVT)** is being increasingly used. Endo-SPONGE is inserted endoscopically, and a vacuum is applied to the sponge. Sponge is replaced every 3–5 d until the leak is closed.
  - **Delayed gastric emptying:** Motility agents are first-line agents. Endoscopic balloon dilation may be needed if intact pylorus is there.
  - **Chylothorax**
    - ❖ Drain of large-volume straw- or cream-coloured fluid or **milky fluid after initiation of enteral nutrition**.
    - ❖ Drain fluid triglyceride levels >110 mg/dL or 1.2 mmol/L.
    - ❖ Pleural collection if drain removed.
    - ❖ Lymphangiography may be needed to diagnose and assess the degree of thoracic duct leak.
    - ❖ **Conservative management:** Initially adequate pleural drainage, reduced fat diet, long-chain triglycerides substitution with medium-chain triglycerides, parenteral nutrition. Consider octreotide subcutaneously.
    - ❖ **Surgical management:** Ligation of the thoracic duct or chemical pleurodesis may be needed.

- **Anastomotic stricture:** Post-operative dysphagia. Upper endoscopy clinches the diagnosis.
- **Jejunostomy complications**
  - ❖ Look for intra-abdominal feed leak, small bowel obstruction, small bowel ischaemia.
  - ❖ Stop NJ feed, and flush tube with normal saline.
  - ❖ Contrast study vis-à-vis the jejunostomy tube.
- **Dumping syndrome**
  - ❖ Rapid gastric emptying occurs when undigested food moves quickly from the stomach to the small intestine, causing diarrhoea and bloating.
  - ❖ **Diet modification:** Six small meals a day, monosaccharide substitution with polysaccharides, avoidance of fatty products, and limitation of excessive fluid intake after meals.
- **Recurrent laryngeal nerve palsy**
  - ❖ Can lead to pulmonary aspiration.
  - ❖ Diagnosis by bedside laryngoscopy.
  - ❖ Vocal cord injection may improve glottic closure.
  - ❖ Surgery may be needed ultimately to accomplish vocal cord medialization.

Boerhaave Syndrome

- ✓ **Boerhaave Syndrome**
  - Spontaneous rupture of the oesophagus that occurs during intense straining.
  - Rare yet critical condition characterized by *transmural oesophageal perforation.* Typically occurs after forceful vomiting or retching. It is an emergency and can be fatal without treatment.
- ✓ **Mallory–Weiss Syndrome**
  - *Non-transmural oesophageal tear* also associated with vomiting.
  - Other causes of oesophageal perforation are iatrogenic and foreign body.
- ✓ **Clinical Features of Boerhaave Syndrome**
  - **Risk factors:** Alcoholism and overindulgence in food.
  - **Mackler's triad^Q:** Vomiting, chest pain, and subcutaneous emphysema.
  - Fever, hypotension, tachycardia, cyanosis, decreased breath sounds, abdominal pain, abdominal rigidity, empyema.

- **Hamman's sign:** Mediastinal crunching sounds synchronized with each heartbeat in the left lateral decubitus position.
- ✓ **Investigations**
  - **Chest X-ray:** Subcutaneous emphysema, mediastinal emphysema, mediastinal widening, and pleural effusion.
  - **Gastrografin oesophagogram:** Contrast leak if perforation (barium swallow^Q is unsuitable as leak can cause fibrosis).
  - **CT scan:** Perioesophageal and mediastinal gas, mediastinal fluid collections, oesophageal wall thickening, pleural effusion, pneumothorax, and hydrothorax.
  - **Endoscopy:** For those patients where perforation location is unclear and who are appropriate candidates for endoscopic treatment.
- ✓ **Treatment**
  - Referral to tertiary care centre.
  - Stop oral intake for at least 7 d.
  - Broad-spectrum antibiotic coverage.
  - Parenteral nutritional support.
  - **Source control:** Interventional radiology or VATS with fundic reinforcement^Q (gold standard).
- ✓ **Prognosis**
  - Early diagnosis and treatment (12–24 h) have a good prognosis with survival rate of 75%.
  - Mortality rate of 90% if left untreated.
  - Prolonged rehabilitation may be required.

GASTRIC RESECTION

- ✓ **Gastric Resection**
  - Done for gastric cancers.
  - **Total gastrectomy (TG):** All the stomach is removed, and patients need ITU/HDU cover.
  - **Partial gastrectomy:** Only part of stomach is removed, and ITU/HDU cover is not needed usually.
- ✓ **Intraoperative Care**
  - Incision for total gastrectomy is either an upper midline or left thoraco-abdominal incision.
  - Thoracic epidural is used for analgesia to prevent post-operative complications.
- ✓ **Post-Operative Care**
  - **Early ambulation.**
  - **Pulmonary secretion clearance.**

- **Judicious fluid management:** To avoid oedema around anastomosis.
- **Multimodal pain management:** Epidural to be taken out on POD4/5. Regular paracetamol and tramadol.
- **Early diet initiation:** Start feeding jejunostomy with 30 mL/h water on POD1 and standard enteral feed through jejunostomy tube at 30 mL/h on POD2.

✓ **Complications**
- **Cardiopulmonary complications:** Postoperative pneumonia, ARDS, and atrial fibrillation.
- **Oesophagojejunal anastomotic leak**
  ❖ Around 1–13% leak rates after TG.
  ❖ Gastrografin upper GI swallow study can confirm the leak of an area of extravasation.
  ❖ Patients with a small leak are treated conservatively with parenteral nutrition.
  ❖ Oesophageal stents are being used in high-risk patients.
  ❖ Surgical reoperation may be needed in haemodynamically unstable patients.
- **Duodenal stump leak**
  ❖ Uncommon but severe complication.
  ❖ Bile from abdominal drain, abdominal distension.
  ❖ CT scan or ultrasound for visualizing leak.
  ❖ Managed conservatively, and re-exploration if surgically unstable.
- **Feeding jejunostomy problems**
  ❖ Look for intra-abdominal feed leak, small bowel obstruction, small bowel ischaemia.
  ❖ Stop NJ feed and flush tube with normal saline.
  ❖ Contrast study vis-à-vis the jejunostomy tube.
- **Dumping syndrome**
  ❖ Rapid gastric emptying occurs when undigested food moves quickly from the stomach into the small intestine, causing diarrhoea and bloating.
  ❖ **Diet modification:** Six small meals a day, monosaccharides substitution with polysaccharides, avoidance of fatty products, and limitation of excessive fluid intake after meals.

✓ **Prognosis**
- **Morbidity: 40%**
- **Mortality: 11%**

Additional Questions

✓ **HIPEC (Hyperthermic Intraperitoneal Chemotherapy)**
- Used for peritoneal spread of gastric, colorectal, ovarian cancer.
- Warmed anti-cancer drugs (>40°C) are infused and circulated in the peritoneal cavity for a short period of time along with cytoreductive surgery (CRS).
- **Complications** are pancreatitis and inflammatory reactions.

FREE FLAP SURGERY

✓ **Flap Surgery**
- Used for trauma, post–tumour resection (breast/oral tumours), congenital defects, or chronic wounds.

✓ **Two Types**
- **Free flap surgery**
  ❖ Transfer of a patient's own tissue from a donor site to a recipient site with a new arterial and venous supply.
  ❖ Used for large defects, defects requiring multiple tissue types, or areas with no local options for flap.
  ❖ The free flaps are devoid of sympathetic supply and lymphatics and at increased risk of failure.
  ❖ Examples are transverse rectus abdominis myocutaneous (**TRAM**) and deep inferior epigastric perforator (**DIEP**).
- **Pedicled flap**
  ❖ Transfer of a patient's own tissue from a donor site to a recipient site with the same arterial and venous supply.
  ❖ Example is latissimus dorsi flap.

✓ **Stages of Flap Insults Intraoperatively**
- **Primary ischaemia:** Interruption of blood flow during flap transfer.
- **Reperfusion:** Begins with reconnecting of vessels. Reperfusion injury due to influx of inflammatory substances.
- **Secondary ischaemia:** Due to oedema and clots.

✓ **Physiological Goals for Survival of Free Flaps**
- **Hagen–Poiseuille equation**

$$\text{Flow} = \frac{\pi \times \mathbf{\Delta P} \times \mathbf{r}^4}{8 \times L \times \eta}$$

where π = Pi = 3.14, ΔP = change in pressure, r = radius, L = length of tube, and η = viscosity.

- **Radius of vessel:** Avoid vasoconstriction, and ensure euvolaemia with good pain relief.
  - ❖ **Pressure gradient:** Low systemic vascular resistance and adequate venous drainage.
  - ❖ **Viscosity:** Haematocrit between 30 and 35%.

✓ **Causes of Free Flap Failure**
- **Surgical**
  - ❖ **Arterial:** Vasospasm, thrombosis, anastomotic leak
  - ❖ **Venous:** Kinking of anastomosis, thrombus
  - ❖ **Reperfusion injury**
- **Non-surgical**
  - ❖ **Oedema**
  - ❖ **Hypercoagulable state**

✓ **Management of Free Flap**
- **Close monitoring** of the patient and flap in ICU for first 24–48 h:
  - ❖ **Colour change:** Blue/purple means venous compromise. Pale/white means compromised arterial supply.
  - ❖ **Capillary refill:** >4 s means compromised arterial supply, and no refill means venous compromise.
  - ❖ **Temperature:** Cold means inadequate blood supply, and increased warmth means inflammatory response.
  - ❖ **Skin turgor:** Flaccid flap means compromised arterial supply, and swollen flap means venous compromise.
  - ❖ **Doppler sounds:** Handheld Doppler probe on the site of new anastomosis. However, a Doppler can give false-positive readings.
- **Anticoagulation:** Should be started as early as possible as helps maintain flap vessel patency.
- **Fluid resuscitation:** Ensure fluid to maintain urine output of 0.5–1 mL/kg/h.

SPINE SURGERY

Epidemiology

✓ **Indications**
- Congenital deformity (kyphoscoliosis), trauma, myelopathy.

Intraoperative Challenges

✓ **Long Duration of Surgery**
- Total intravenous anaesthesia used for controlling haemodynamics using remifentanil.

✓ **Positioning (Prone)**
- Periodic position checks during surgery.

✓ **Intraoperative Neurophysiological Monitoring**
- Somatosensory evoked potentials.
- Motor evoked potentials.
- Use of wake-up test.

✓ **Major Blood Loss**
- Red cell salvage and blood transfusion may be needed.

Post-Operative Analgesia

✓ **Simple Analgesia**
- Paracetamol (NSAIDs avoided)
- Tramadol
- Gabapentin
- Morphine/oxycodone PCA

✓ **Regional**
- Epidural infusion
- Paravertebral catheter
- Intercostal block

✓ **Infusions**
- Ketamine
- Lidocaine

Post-Operative Complications

✓ **Airway Compromise**
- Supraglottic oedema
- Anterior neck haematoma

✓ **Post-Operative Visual Loss**
- Central retinal artery occlusion
- Ischaemic optic atrophy

✓ **CSF Leak**
- Dural tear

✓ **Spinal Cord Compromise**
- Haematoma
- Oedema
- Nerve transection
- Ischaemia

✓ **Abdominal Organ Ischaemia**
- Raised liver enzymes
- Lactic acidosis

2

Infectious Diseases

MICROBIOLOGY

✓ **Gram-Positive**
- Organisms with thick peptidoglycan wall that retains the **violet stain**^{Q} after washing.
- **Gram-positive cocci**^{Q}
  - ❖ *Staphylococcus aureus* (coagulase-positive)^Q: Septicaemia, endocarditis, pneumonia, skin sepsis, toxic shock syndrome.
  - ❖ *Staphylococcus epidermidis* (coagulase-negative): Device-related sepsis, sternal wound osteomyelitis.
  - ❖ *Staphylococcus hominis* (coagulase-negative): Device-related sepsis, sternal wound osteomyelitis.
  - ❖ *Staphylococcus saprophyticus* (coagulase-negative): UTIs.
  - ❖ *Streptococcus pneumoniae* (*Pneumococcus*) (α-haemolytic): Community-acquired pneumonia, meningitis, sinusitis.
  - ❖ *Streptococcus viridans* (α-haemolytic): Endocarditis.
  - ❖ *Streptococcus pyogenes* (**group A Streptococcus**) (β-haemolytic): Scarlet fever, rheumatic fever, post-streptococcal glomerulonephritis, **puerperal sepsis**, necrotizing fasciitis, toxic shock syndrome.
  - ❖ *Streptococcus agalactiae* (group B *Streptococcus*) (β-haemolytic): **Neonatal pneumonia and meningitis.**^{Q}
  - ❖ *Streptococcus* (*Enterococcus faecium*) (γ-haemolytic): Endocarditis, UTIs, intra-abdominal infections, wound infection.
  - ❖ *Streptococcus* (*Enterococcus faecalis*) (γ-haemolytic): Endocarditis, UTIs, intra-abdominal infections, wound infection.

- **Gram-positive bacilli**
  - ❖ *Corynebacterium diphtheriae*: Diphtheria.
  - ❖ *Bacillus anthracis* (spore-forming): Cutaneous anthrax, pulmonary anthrax, and gastrointestinal anthrax.
  - ❖ *Bacillus cereus* (spore-forming): Gastrointestinal poisoning which self-terminates in 24 h.
  - ❖ *Clostridium perfringens* (spore-forming anaerobes): Gas gangrene.
  - ❖ *Clostridium difficile* (spore-forming anaerobes): Pseudomembranous colitis.
  - ❖ *Clostridium botulinum* (spore-forming anaerobes): Botulism.
  - ❖ *Clostridium tetani* (spore-forming anaerobes): Tetanus.
  - ❖ *Listeria monocytogenes*: Meningitis in neonates and elderly.
  - ❖ *Propionibacterium*: Skin problems, such as acne vulgaris.

✓ **Gram-Negative**^{Q}
- Organisms with thin peptidoglycan wall and are unable to retain crystal violet stain. They appear **pink-red**^{Q} on Gram staining. Contain lipopolysaccharide (LPS) that causes septic shock.
- **Gram-negative cocci**
  - ❖ *Neisseria meningitidis* (**meningococcus**): Meningitis, pharyngitis
  - ❖ *Neisseria gonorrhoeae*: Gonorrhoea, blennorrhoea neonatorum
  - ❖ *Moraxella catarrhalis*: Pneumonia, meningitis, otitis media
- **Gram-negative bacilli**
  - ❖ *Escherichia coli*: UTIs, pneumonia, neonatal meningitis, septicaemia
  - ❖ *Klebsiella pneumoniae*: Nosocomial pneumonia, UTIs
  - ❖ *Proetus mirabilis*: UTIs, bacteraemia

DOI: 10.1201/9781003476214-2

❖ *Enterobacter cloacae*: UTIs, pneumonia, endocarditis, osteomyelitis

❖ **Pseudomonas aeruginosa (non-fermenting)**: UTIs, pneumonia, septicaemia

❖ **Stenotrophomonas maltophilia (non-fermenting)**: Pneumonia, bacteraemias

❖ **Acinetobacter baumannii (non-fermenting)**: Pneumonia, UTIs, bacteraemias

❖ *Salmonella typhi*: Typhoid

❖ *Shigella flexneri*: Dysentery

❖ *Vibrio cholerae*: Cholera

❖ *Campylobacter jejuni*: Diarrhoea

❖ *Brucella*: Brucellosis

❖ *Bordetella pertussis*: Pertussis

❖ **Haemophilus influenzae**: Meningitis, epiglottitis, sinusitis

❖ *Helicobacter pylori*: Peptic ulcer

❖ **Legionella pneumophila**: Atypical pneumonia

❖ *Chlamydia pneumoniae*: Atypical pneumonia

❖ *Rickettsia rickettsii*: Rocky Mountain spotted fever

❖ **Mycoplasma pneumoniae**: Atypical pneumonia

❖ *Yersinia pestis*: Bubonic plague, pulmonary plague

❖ **Leptospira interrogans:** Leptospirosis

❖ *Treponema pallidum*: Syphilis

❖ *Bacteroides fragilis* (anaerobic): Abdominal infections

✓ **Bacteraemia: Three Types**

❖ **Transient:** Tooth extraction, urinary catheterization. No need for culture or antibiotics.

❖ **Intermittent:** Pneumonia or intra-abdominal abscess. Culture as soon as pyrexia is there.

❖ **Continuous:** Infective endocarditis. Random blood cultures will show organism.

Diagnostics Timeline for Tests Commonly Used in ITU

✓ **Time 0–2 h**
- **Gram staining**
    ❖ Tracheal secretions: Gram-positive/negative and rods/cocci.
    ❖ CSF: Diplococci/meningococci from pneumococci.

❖ Ascitic fluid: Detects GNBs for suspected spontaneous bacterial peritonitis.

❖ Pleural fluid: Detects pneumococci as they can cause pleural empyema.

✓ **Time 2–8 h**
- **Antigen testing**
    ❖ **Blood/BAL:** *Galactomannan* for aspergillosis
    ❖ **Urine:** *Legionella* (*pneumophila* only)[Q] and pneumococcal (not so sensitive)
    ❖ **CSF:** Cryptococcus and pneumococcal antigen in meningitis
    ❖ **Pharyngeal secretions:** Rapid diagnostic tests highly specific, but low sensitivity for influenza and RSV
- **PCR**
    ❖ BioFire[Q]
    ❖ CSF panel
    ❖ Sputum panel
    ❖ Bloodstream infection panel

✓ **Time 24–48 h**
- Gram stain on culture: Differentiate GNBs from GPCs
- MALDI-TOF on culture: Species identification
- PCR on culture: Species identification

✓ **Time >48 h**
- Culture antibiotic sensitivity: Escalation or de-escalation of antibiotics
- Serology: For difficult-to-grow organisms
- Broad-range PCR: For culture negative results

✓ **Culture of Specimens**
- Still the gold standard[Q] for identifying the organisms and antimicrobial susceptibility testing.
- Matrix-assisted laser desorption ionization time of flight mass spectrometry (**MALDI-TOF**) is a new technique that can identify a pathogen in 10–30 min as soon as it starts growing in a culture using ionization and analysis of its protein mass spectrum. They can give an antibiogram in 24 h. They can be done directly on the blood samples as well.
- **Any positive culture in the absence of clinical symptoms is usually colonization or contamination**.
- **Blood cultures:** Number of samples to be taken.
    ❖ **Sepsis:** Two sets of blood cultures from two different sites. One set means paired samples of both aerobic and anaerobic bottles. Each bottle should have 10 mL of blood. Aerobic bottle

should always be inoculated first. Second set should be taken 10 min apart.

❖ **Infective endocarditis:** Three different sets of blood cultures[Q] from different sites as these patients have low bacterial load.

- Clinical factors that can influence the result of blood cultures
  - ❖ Timing of sample to clinical signs
  - ❖ Number of samples taken during septic episode
  - ❖ Volume of blood obtained

Timing of Antibiotics

✓ **Kind of Antimicrobial Therapies**
- **Prophylactic:** Risk is present, organism not present.
- **Empirical:** Organism is present – we don't know which one.
- **Definitive:** Organism is known.

✓ **Initiation of Antibiotics**
- Surviving Sepsis Campaign (SSC) 2021 recommends the administration of IV antibiotics within 1 h of recognition of septic shock.
- **Empirical broad-spectrum antibiotics** should be used. Risk factors for MDR pathogens should be assessed in community-acquired infections.
- **Multidrug antibiotic therapy** can be used to broaden the spectrum, achieve synergistic effect, and prevent resistance in patients with septic shock.
- SSC 2016 recommends the optimization of antibiotics based on PK/PD properties.
- Higher initial doses in critically ill patients, especially when using hydrophilic antibiotics.
- **Loading doses** may be used in antibiotics like vancomycin, colistin, and beta-lactams.
- Antibiotics like colistin, fosfomycin, and tigecycline should be used in **combination therapy** to prevent emergence of resistance.
- *Source control optimally within 12 h of sepsis recognition.*

✓ **Watchful Waiting for Initiation of Antibiotics**[Q]
- **(To start or not to . . .junior doctor) in cases of**
  - ❖ Undifferentiated fever in non-hypotensive patient
  - ❖ Patient with ventilator-associated condition
  - ❖ Identification of catheter colonization with low-virulence organism

✓ **De-Escalation of Therapy**
- Empirical therapy to narrow spectrum when stabilization happens (decrease in vasopressor doses, decrease in leucocytes, CRP, and procalcitonin).
- **Duration of therapy**
  - ❖ Longer duration may be needed in immunosuppressed patients.
  - ❖ **5–7 d:** Pneumonias, uncomplicated UTIs, intra-abdominal infections after source control.
  - ❖ **7–14 d:** Meningitis, complicated UTIs, complicated soft tissue infections, intra-abdominal infections with protracted source control, bacteraemia with *S. aureus*, candidemia.
  - ❖ **>14 d:** Endocarditis, bone and joint infections, brain abscesses, kidney abscesses, lung abscesses, complicated intra-abdominal infections with repeated source control attempts.

✓ **Clinical Failure of Antimicrobial Therapy**
- Wrong antibiotic for the pathogen.
- Resistance: Suspect if secondary deterioration.
- Localized complications: Abscess formation/collections. Imaging followed by interventional drainage or surgical exploration.

FEVER IN ICU

✓ **Incidence**
- Around 30% of patients in ICU will have fever. Up to 90% of patients with sepsis will experience fever.

✓ **Pathophysiology**
- Society of Critical Care Medicine (SCCM) definition of *fever* is core temperature of greater than 38.3°C.
- Core temperature shows diurnal variation, with a low of 36.2°C in the morning and a peak of 37.7°C in the afternoon.
- Endogenous pyrogens: IL-1, IL-6, and TNF.
- Uremic, immunosuppressed patients and those on steroids may not be able to manifest a febrile response to bacteria.

✓ **Classification of Aetiology**
- **Infectious causes**
  - ❖ **Respiratory causes:** Pneumonia, **sinusitis,** tracheobronchitis, empyema
  - ❖ **Cardiovascular causes:** Pericarditis, endocarditis, mediastinitis

- ❖ **Urinary tract infections:** Cystitis, pyelonephritis, prostatitis, perinephric abscess
- ❖ **Surgical site infections:** Wound infections, **deep-seated abscesses**
- ❖ **Device-related:** CVC line infection, cardiac valve endocarditis, peritoneal dialysis catheter causing peritonitis
- ❖ **Gastrointestinal infections:** *Clostridium difficile* colitis, acalculous cholecystitis, intra-abdominal abscess, cholangitis, hepatic abscess
- ❖ **Skin and soft tissues:** Cellulitis, necrotizing fasciitis, decubitus ulcers
- ❖ **Neurological:** Meningitis, encephalitis, ventriculitis
- ❖ **Bone and joint infection:** Septic arthritis, osteomyelitis, discitis

- **Non-infectious causes**
  - ❖ Half of all fevers in ICU caused by them
  - ❖ **Inflammatory conditions:** ARDS, drug-induced fever, drug withdrawal fever, vasculitis, pancreatitis, transfusion reactions
  - ❖ **Metabolic conditions:** Hyperthyroidism, **adrenal insufficiency**, seizures, delirium tremens
  - ❖ **Vascular conditions:** Subarachnoid haemorrhage, *mesenteric ischaemia*, gastrointestinal haemorrhage, pulmonary embolism, deep vein thrombosis, myocardial infarction, aortic dissection, large haematomas
  - ❖ **Neoplastic conditions:** Lymphomas, colon cancer, renal cell carcinoma, hepatocellular carcinoma

- **Hyperthermic causes**
  - ❖ **Unregulated** rise of body temperature
  - ❖ Heat stroke, **malignant hyperthermia**, serotonin syndrome, neuroleptic malignant syndrome

✓ **Clinical Features**
- Hospital-associated pneumonia (HAP) is the most common **hospital-acquired infection in the ICU** and occurs among non-ventilated patients.
- Ventilator-associated pneumonia (VAP) is the most common **infection acquired in the ICU. VAP, catheter-related sepsis, and sinusitis are the three major causes of ICU fever of recent onset.**
- Fever in healthy individuals is considered to be of viral origin, whereas it is of bacterial-fungal origin in a hospitalized patient.
- Fever above 38.9°C is more likely to be infective in origin, whereas fever above 41.1°C is more likely to be non-infectious.
- Physical examination: Check sites of any catheter or surgical incision, abdomen for distension, and sputum quality and volume.

- **Drug fever**
  - ❖ Temperature range between 38.8 and 40°C, relative bradycardia, maculopapular rash in 5–10% of cases, peripheral eosinophilia, or a moderate elevation of serum transaminases.
  - ❖ β-lactams, procainamide, quinidine, antiepileptic drugs like phenytoin, diuretics, α-methyldopa, and stool softeners.
  - ❖ Time between drug initiation and fever appearance is a median of 8 d, while fever resolves usually within 72 h after removing the drug.

- **Posterior fossa syndrome:** Blood leakage in CSF due to SAH can mimic meningitis. Differentiated by negative CSF cultures and improvement as number of RBCs decrease with time.

- **Febrile patient with hepatomegaly:** Haematolymphoid malignancy or HLH (diagnosis by risk stratification)

- **Diagnosis**
  - ❖ Two sets of blood, urine, and sputum cultures should be sent immediately, and empirical antibiotic therapy started if infectious origin is suspected.
  - ❖ One set of blood culture has two bottles, and at least two sets of cultures from different venipuncture sites should be sent with at least one peripheral culture.
  - ❖ If fever persists after 48 h, consider removing CVCs that are >48 h old and nasogastric tubes. Send CVC tip for culture. Start empirical antibiotic therapy, and send stool cultures if diarrhoea present.
  - ❖ If fever still persists after 48 h of previous step, consider antifungal therapy and imaging for abdominal infections.
  - ❖ CT scan is one of the most useful imaging techniques in assessing intra-abdominal infections.
  - ❖ 1,3-β-D-glucan, and *Aspergillus*

galactomannan for detection of invasive fungal infections.

❖ **Sinusitis** can be diagnosed by fluid-air levels/opacification on CT scan, followed by needle aspiration, microscopy, and culture (>10³ CFU/mL).

❖ **Acute acalculous cholecystitis:** Wall thickness of >3 mm, distended gall bladder, intramural lucencies or sludge, and pericholecystic fluid are some of the radiological findings.

✓ **Treatment**

- The febrile ICU patient should be considered bacteraemic until proven otherwise.
- Intravenous route of drugs is preferred initially as gastrointestinal absorption can be unreliable.
- Antimicrobial administration within first hour has mortality benefit in patients with septic shock (Surviving Sepsis Campaign 2021).
- Inappropriate and delayed antibiotic

treatment is associated with increased mortality.

- **Antipyretic use in patients with non-neurological patients with fever does not affect mortality but just reduces temperature.**
- **Cooling devices:** Water-circulating external cooling methods, air-circulating external cooling methods, water-circulating external cooling device using self-adhesive gel–coated pads, and intravascular heat exchange system.
- Treatment of sinusitis includes needle aspiration, lavage, antibiotics, and sometimes surgical exploration.
- Treatment of acalculous cholecystitis involves radiological percutaneous drainage (cholecystostomy) or surgical cholecystectomy.
- Presumptive antibiotic therapy in ICU patients.

Site of Infection	Potential Causes	Initial Therapy
Lungs: Pneumonia	Gram-negative rods (GNR), *Haemophilus influenzae*, *Streptococcus pneumoniae*	Piperacillin/tazobactam or third-generation cephalosporin
	Anaerobes suspected	Add metronidazole
	Staphylococcus aureus	Vancomycin or linezolid until MRSA excluded
	Legionella pneumophila	Azithromycin/fluoroquinolones
Urinary tract infections: Pyelonephritis	GNR, *Enterococcus*	Piperacillin/tazobactam or third-generation cephalosporin or fluoroquinolones
Abdominal infections: Peritonitis/abscess/ pelvic infection/ biliary tract	GNR, *Enterococcus*, anaerobes (less common in biliary tract)	Piperacillin/tazobactam or fluoroquinolones + metronidazole
Vascular: Line-associated bacteraemia	*S. aureus*, GNR, coagulase-negative staphylococci	Vancomycin + third-generation cephalosporin or piperacillin/tazobactam
CNS: Meningitis	Community-acquired: • *S. pneumoniae, Neisseria meningitidis*	Ceftriaxone + vancomycin
	Nosocomial: • *S. aureus*, GNR, coagulase-negative staphylococci	Ceftazidime + vancomycin
	Elderly: • *S. pneumoniae, Listeria monocytogenes*, GNR	Third-generation cephalosporin + vancomycin + **ampicillin**
CNS abscess	*S. aureus*, GNR, anaerobes	Third-generation cephalosporin + **metronidazole** + vancomycin if MRSA suspected
Septic shock	*S. aureus*, GNR	Piperacillin/tazobactam + vancomycin

✓ **Prognosis**
- Fever is an independent indicator of mortality for patients admitted to ITU.

SEPSIS

Epidemiology and Aetiology

✓ **Burden of Disease**
- One-third of all ICU admissions worldwide are due to sepsis.
- About 50% of patients with sepsis will have evidence of bloodstream infections.
- Organism isolated in 30–35% of patients only.

✓ **Systemic Inflammation Response Syndrome (SIRS)**
- >2 of the following variables
  - ❖ Temperature >38°C or <36°C
  - ❖ Tachycardia >90 bpm
  - ❖ Tachypnoea >20/min
  - ❖ WBCs >12 × 10^9/L or <4 × 10^9/L or >10% immature neutrophils

✓ **Sepsis (Old Definition)**
- SIRS + documented/suspected infection.

✓ **Sepsis (New Definition)[Q]**
- Syndrome characterized by a life-threatening organ dysfunction caused by a dysregulated host response to infection that may be amplified by host factors.
- Organ dysfunction = ↑ SOFA score by 2 points, >10% in hospital mortality.

✓ **Severe Sepsis (Redundant Now)**
- Sepsis with organ dysfunction, hypoperfusion, and hypotension (adequate fluid resuscitation not completed yet).

✓ **Septic Shock[Q]**
- *Persistent hypotension* despite *adequate fluid resuscitation* requiring **vasopressors** to maintain a **MAP >65 mmHg** and the presence of lactate levels ≥2 mmol/L.

SOFA Score

Organ System	0	1	2	3	4
PaO$_2$/FiO$_2$ (kPa)	Normal	<53.3	<40	<26.7 (respiratory support)	<13.3 (respiratory support)
Hypotension (mcg/kg/min)	Normal	MAP <70 mmHg	Dopamine ≤5 or dobutamine (any dose)	Dopamine >5 or epinephrine ≤0.1 or norepinephrine ≤0.1	Dopamine >15 or epinephrine >0.1 or norepinephrine >0.1
GCS	Normal	13–14	10–12	6–9	<6
Creatinine (mmol/L) or Urine output	Normal	110–170	171–299	300–440 or <500 mL/day	>440 or <200 mL/day
Platelets × 10³/mm³	Normal	<150	<100	<50	<20
Bilirubin (mmol/L)	Normal	20–32	33–101	102–204	<204

✓ **Pathophysiological Changes**
- Microorganism's endotoxin and exotoxins engage with host's immunity.
- Pathogen-associated molecular patterns (**PAMPs**) and damage-associated molecular patterns (**DAMPs**) are detected by immune system.
- Imbalance between **pro-inflammatory cytokines** IL-1, IL-6, and TNF-α and **anti-inflammatory cytokines** IL-4, IL-10.
- Vasodilation, glycocalyx dysfunction, occlusion of capillaries, impaired myocardial contractility, and mitochondrial dysfunction.

Clinical Features and Diagnosis

✓ **qSOFA (Sepsis-Related Organ Failure Assessment)**
- For suspected sepsis in a non-ICU setting. AUROC of 0.81.

- If two-thirds of criteria are positive, qSOFA is positive
  - ❖ Altered mental status (GCS <15)
  - ❖ Tachypnoea >22/min
  - ❖ Systolic blood pressure <100 mmHg
- A positive qSOFA in a patient with infection should urge the clinician to the possibility of sepsis.
- *Shouldn't be used as a lone screening tool.*
- Other scores available are Modified Early Warning Score (MEWS), National Early Warning Score (NEWS), and Mortality in Emergency Department Sepsis (MEDS) score.

✓ **Skin Mottling**
- **Skin mottling is seen.**
- **Grading of mottling**
  - ❖ Score 0: No mottling.
  - ❖ **Score 1:** Small area of mottling in the **centre of the knee.**
  - ❖ Score 2: Modest mottling area confined to the superior border of kneecap.
  - ❖ **Score 3:** Mild mottling area, not going beyond **mid-thigh**.
  - ❖ Score 4: Severe mottling area, not going beyond groin fold.
  - ❖ **Score 5:** Extremely severe mottling area, extending beyond **groin fold.**

✓ **Complications**
- Acute respiratory distress syndrome (ARDS), acute kidney injury (AKI), intrahepatic cholestasis, disseminated intravascular coagulation (DIC), critical illness neuropathy, and critical illness myopathy can develop.
- Increased cardiac output initially, followed by decrease in cardiac output later on.
- **Multiorgan dysfunction (MODS):** Condition in which two or more organ systems have altered function during an acute illness and homeostasis can't be maintained without intervention.
- *Ruminococcus*, a Gram-positive anaerobe like *Clostridium*, in blood should raise suspicions about gut perforation, and a CT scan should be sought[Q].

✓ **Septic Arthritis**[Q]
- Turbid or purulent synovial fluid. WBCs >50,000/mm³ (>90% neutrophils)

✓ **Biomarkers**
- Procalcitonin, C-reactive protein

✓ **Risk Factors for Drug-Resistant Pathogen**
- Current hospitalization >2 d
- Hospitalization >2 d in previous 90 d
- Antibiotics in previous 90 d
- Infection or colonization by MRSA in last 90 d
- Acid-suppressive medication
- Immunocompromised status
- Patients receiving tube feeding
- Chronic haemodialysis in last 30 d

Treatment

✓ **Early Goal-Directed Therapy (EGDT)**
- **Rivers et al. (2001):** Early goal-directed therapy for severe sepsis and septic shock reduced mortality.
  - ❖ **Goals:** CVP 8–12 mmHg, *MAP ≥65 mmHg*, urine output ≥0.5 mL/kg/h, $ScvO_2$ >70% or SvO_2 >65%, haematocrit ≥30%.
- **ProCESS Trial (2014)** in the USA, **ARISE Trial (2014)** in Australia and New Zealand, and **ProMISE Trial** in UK (2015) didn't show much mortality benefit of EGDT over usual care.
- *Recent sepsis guidelines have moved away from strict adherence to EGDT protocols*[Q].

✓ **Fluids**[Q]
- >30 mL/kg[Q] fluid resuscitation within first 3 h is based on retrospective study.
- **CLOVERS Trial (2023):** In patients with sepsis-induced hypotension refractory to 1–3 L of intravenous fluids, early use of vasopressor had no mortality benefit compared to a strategy of liberally giving IV fluids.
- Balanced crystalloids are used first, and albumin can be added if patients require substantial amounts of fluids.
- Starches and gelatines are not recommended.
- Check Chapter 7 on fluids for details of **trials** on crystalloids, colloids, and albumin.

✓ **Fluid Responsiveness**
- Fluid responsiveness is the first step in the resuscitation process of the septic shock patients.
- **Dynamic assessment (PPV, SVV, and PLR test) is recommended to guide fluid therapy but doesn't show mortality benefit.**

- Lactate-guided resuscitation is recommended, with capillary refill time as an adjunct.
  - ❖ **ANDROMEDA-SHOCK Trial (2019):** In patients with septic shock patients, no mortality benefit of using lactate-based strategy vs capillary refill strategy.
- Admission to ITU within 6 h is recommended.

✓ **Ventilation**
- No recommendation on the use of conservative oxygen targets (88–92%) in adults with sepsis-induced hypoxaemic respiratory failure.
- High-flow nasal oxygen is recommended over non-invasive ventilation in sepsis-induced hypoxaemic respiratory failure.
- For patients with ARDS, low TV 6 mL/kg, plateau pressure of <30 cm H_2O, high PEEP, prone ventilation for >12 h daily, intermittent NMBA boluses, traditional recruitment manoeuvres, and VV ECMO if needed.

✓ **Vasopressors**
- MAP of 65 mmHg is recommended, with higher MAP goals associated with greater vasopressor use and arrhythmias.
- *SEPSISPAM Trial (2014)*
  - ❖ High MAP 80–85 mmHg didn't show any mortality benefit over MAP 65–70 mmHg.
  - ❖ Targeting higher MAP with vasopressors was associated with a higher risk of atrial fibrillation.
  - ❖ *Higher MAP targets in patients with chronic hypertension demonstrated a 10.5% reduction in RRT.*
- **Noradrenaline**[Q] (0.1–0.2 mcg/kg/min)
  - ❖ First-choice vasopressor, with vasopressin (0.04 U/min) added at noradrenaline dose of >0.2 mcg/kg/min. After these two, adrenaline (0.05–1 mcg/kg/min) should be added.
  - ❖ For patients with septic shock and cardiac dysfunction, addition of dobutamine to noradrenaline or using epinephrine alone is recommended.
  - ❖ Levosimendan is not recommended for patients with septic shock and cardiac dysfunction.
  - ❖ Vasopressors can be started peripherally if needed initially rather than delaying them.

- **Vasopressin/ADH:** Levels are high in cardiogenic shock but low in septic shock[Q].

✓ **Steroids**
- **Steroids**[Q] **should be used if two vasopressors are being used: IV hydrocortisone 200 mg daily.**
- **CORTICUS Trial (2008):** In patients with septic shock, use of hydrocortisone didn't reduce the mortality, although it did shorten the duration of vasopressor dependence.
- **APROCCHSS Trial (2018):** In mechanically ventilated patients with septic shock, the use of hydrocortisone and fludrocortisone reduced mortality.
- **ADRENAL Trial (2018):** In mechanically ventilated patients with septic shock, use of hydrocortisone didn't reduce mortality, although it did reduce vasopressor requirements.
- Methylene blue has been used for refractory septic shock.

✓ **Antimicrobial Administration**
- At least two sets of blood cultures should be taken.
- Empirical antibiotic therapy for 3–5 d, and then narrow down.
- Mortality benefit associated with early administration of antimicrobials.
- **Administration**
  - ❖ Sepsis with shock: Within 1 h
  - ❖ Sepsis without shock: Within 1 h
- Using **two antimicrobials with Gram-negative coverage** for empirical treatment in adults with sepsis or septic shock and high risk of MDR organisms.
- *Empirical antifungals for those at high risk of fungal infection.*
- PK/PD of antibiotics should be used, and beta-lactams should be used as prolonged infusions after an initial bolus.
- Daily assessment for de-escalation of antibiotics should be done.
- **Procalcitonin is not recommended for initiation of antibiotics. Used for discontinuing antibiotics.**
- **PRORATA Trial (2010):** In ICU patients, use of a procalcitonin-guided algorithm for suspected bacterial infections reduced exposure but had no mortality benefit.

✓ **Blood Transfusions**
- Hb transfusion <70 g/L calls for RBC transfusion.

- **TRISS Trial (2014):** In patients with septic shock, similar 90 d mortality among both restrictive (7 g/dL) and liberal (9 g/dL) groups.
- Liberal strategy favoured more in patients who have oncological background.
- **Platelets:** Transfuse if counts <10 × 10⁹/L in absence of bleeding or <20 × 10⁹/L if the patient has bleeding risk factors, and <50 × 10⁹/L if patient is bleeding, requiring any procedure or surgery.
- **Transfusion of FFP only in documented deficiency in a bleeding patient.**

✓ **Nutrition**
- Early nutrition (within 72 h) is recommended.
- Glucose control between 8 and 10 mmol/L.
- **Trials** for glucose control in ICU patients have been given in the chapter on hypoglycaemic agents.

✓ **Thromboprophylaxis**
- LMWH for all patients if creatinine clearance is >30 mL/min as there is reduction of heparin-induced thrombocytopaenia (HIT) and ease of administering LMWH.

✓ **Stress Ulcer Prophylaxis**
- Only patients with bleeding risk should receive stress ulcer prophylaxis.

✓ **SSC Guidelines 2021**
- SSC Guidelines 2021 advise against the use of polymyxin B haemoperfusion for adults with sepsis or septic shock.
- **Bicarbonate** only for pH <7.2 and patient having AKI 2 or 3.

✓ **Vitamin C**
- Cofactor for synthesis of vasopressin and increases the sensitivity of catecholamines. Direct free radical scavenger.
- **LOVIT Trial (2022):** No mortality benefits of using vitamin C.
- SSC Guidelines 2021 advise against the use of vitamin C^Q.

✓ **Activated Protein C**
- Substance that promoted fibrinolysis and inhibits thrombosis. Marketed as a product that will improve microcirculatory function. The product was withdrawn later on due to reports of bleeding.
- **PROWESS Trial (2001)** showed improvement in mortality.
- **PROWESS SHOCK Trial (2012)** showed no improvement in mortality.

✓ **Unproved Strategy**^Q
- Low-dose steroids in the absence of refractory shock, hydroxyethyl starch, selenium, immunoglobins, renal-dose dopamine.

✓ **Source Control**
- Mainstay of treatment along with antibiotics.
  - ❖ **Septic shock:** Immediately
  - ❖ **Severe sepsis:** Within 6 h, with resuscitation beforehand
  - ❖ **Sepsis:** Within 18 h (not between 10:00 p.m. and 7:00 a.m.)
- **Methods:** Drainage, decompression, debridement, and restoration of anatomy and function.

Prognosis

✓ **Septic Shock**
- Hospital mortality is 25%. A 12 h delay in source control in septic shock can increase this to mortality of 60% and higher.

✓ **P-POSSUM Score**
- Predicted mortality score of >5% means high-risk surgical patients.
- A patient with predicted mortality of >10% should get post-operative care in HDU and ICU.

ANTIMICROBIAL THERAPY

✓ **Bactericidal**
- Beta-lactams, metronidazole, rifampicin, aminoglycosides, fluoroquinolones, glycopeptides

✓ **Bacteriostatic**
- Macrolides, tetracyclines, lincosamides (clindamycin), chloramphenicol

Beta-Lactams^Q

✓ **Penicillin**
- Bind to penicillin-binding proteins (PBP) and, hence, disrupts bacterial cell wall^Q.
- **Metabolized mostly by kidneys.**
- *Time-dependent antimicrobial activity.*
- No mortality benefit shown by use of continuous infusions, but clinical cure rates have improved.
- **Side effects**
  - ❖ Hypersensitivity reactions.
  - ❖ **Penicillin G:** Active against *S. pneumoniae* **pneumonia**^Q and bacteraemia,

necrotizing fasciitis,[Q] and scarlet fever[Q] caused by group A streptococci.

- ❖ **Semisynthetic penicillins (antistaphylococcal):** Nafcillin (neutropaenia) and oxacillin (hepatitis) metabolized by liver.
- ❖ **Anti-Gram-negative penicillins**
  - Piperacillin/tazobactam.
  - Nosocomial pneumonia, intra-abdominal infections, skin soft tissue infections.
  - Against *P. aeruginosa*, consider higher doses, continuous infusions, along with or without aminoglycosides.
- ❖ **Penicillin β-lactamase inhibitor combinations**
  - Clavulanic acid, sulbactam, tazobactam.
  - Clearance is renal, like **β-lactams**.
  - **Sulbactam** alone can cover *Acinetobacter*.

✓ **Cephalosporins**
- Bind to penicillin-binding proteins (PBP) and, hence, disrupts bacterial cell wall[Q].
- Most are not active against MRSA and *Enterococcus*.
- **Side effects:** Hypersensitivity reactions. *Penicillins have 1% cross-reactivity with first-generation and 0% with third- or fourth-generation cephalosporins[Q].*
- **Dosage of all cephalosporins except ceftriaxone should be adjusted for renal impairment.**
- Bacteria producing extended-spectrum β-lactamases (ESBLs) and carbapenemases producing enterobacteriaceae (CPE) are generally resistant to cephalosporins[Q].
  - ❖ **First-generation cephalosporins** (cefazolin): Active against β-lactam-sensitive *Staphylococcus*, community-acquired strains of *E. coli*, *Proetus*, *Klebsiella*.
  - ❖ **Second-generation cephalosporins** (cefuroxime): Limited activity against hospital-acquired Gram-negative bacilli (GNB).
  - ❖ **Third-generation cephalosporins:** Increased potency against Gram-negative bacilli.
    - **Ceftriaxone:** Active against *S. pneumoniae*. Recommended for treatment of severe community-acquired pneumonia (CAP), bacterial meningitis, and bacterial endocarditis.
    - **Ceftazidime**[Q]: Less active against Gram-positive cocci (GPC). *Active against most strains of P. aeruginosa.*
- ❖ **Fourth-generation cephalosporins**
  - **Cefepime:** GPCs and *P. aeruginosa* can be dosed using continuous infusions.
- ❖ **Fifth-generation cephalosporins**
  - **Ceftaroline:** Active against acute bacterial skin and skin structure infections caused by **MRSA and VRE**. Not active against *Pseudomonas*.
  - **Ceftobiprole:** Active against MRSA and Gram-negative bacilli, including *P. aeruginosa*, that do not produce ESBLs.
- ❖ **Fifth- to fourth-generation cephalosporins**
  - **Cefiderocol:** Injectable siderophore cephalosporin. **This structure gives it activity against carbapenemases and ampC.**
  - Poor activity against GPCs and anaerobes.
  - Active against both lactose fermenting and non-fermenting Gram-negative bacteria including *carbapenem-resistant Enterobacteriaceae (CRE)*.
  - More potent than meropenem and ceftazidime + avibactam against MDR *Acinetobacter*, MDR *Pseudomonas*, and *Stenotrophomonas maltophilia*.
  - Complicated UTIs and VAPs. Renal-dose adjustment is required.
- ❖ **Cephalosporin β-lactamase inhibitor combinations**
  - **Ceftazidime/avibactam:** Active against CREs producing *K. pneumoniae carbapenemase (KPC)*, *OXA*, or *AmpC*.
    - **No MRSA, CRAB (carbapenem-resistant *Acinetobacter baumannii*), and metallo-beta-lactamases activity.**
  - Complicated UTIs and abdominal infections.

- **Ceftolozane/tazobactam: Active against CRPA (carbapenem-resistant *P. aeruginosa*) but doesn't cover CRAB.**
  - Complicated UTIs, VAPs, and abdominal infections.

✓ **Carbapenems**
- Bind to penicillin-binding proteins (PBP) and hence disrupts bacterial cell wall.
- *ESBL organisms, even if sensitive to beta-lactam/beta-lactamase inhibitors, should be treated by carbapenem[Q].*
- Carbapenems have no activity against MRSA, VRE, *Nocardia*, *Listeria*, *C. difficile*.
- Cover *Stenotrophomonas maltophilia* but shouldn't be used against them for serious infections.
- Nebulized carbapenems haven't been used, and there are no oral carbapenems.
  - ❖ **Imipenem/cilastatin:** Cilastatin is inhibitor of renal tubular dipeptidase, thus preventing hydrolysis of imipenem.
    - Imipenem is the broadest carbapenem with activity against GNBs, including *P. aeruginosa, GPCs, and anaerobic bacteria.*
    - Not active against MRSA and *Enterococci faecium.*
    - Seizures[Q] reported in around 16% of patients with renal failure.
  - ❖ **Doripenem:** Covers GNBs, including *P. aeruginosa, GPCs,* and anaerobic bacteria, and is better than imipenem against *Pseudomonas.*
  - ❖ **Meropenem:** *Slightly greater in vitro activity against Gram-negative and anaerobes.*
    - Active against non-fermenting Gram-negative bacilli like *P. aeruginosa.*
    - No activity against MRSA and *Enterococcus faecium.*
    - Cross-reactivity with penicillin allergy. Can be given in patients with rash as reaction to penicillin[Q].
    - Dose reduced in patients with reduced GFR or patients on RRT.
  - ❖ **Ertapenem:** No activity against *Pseudomonas, Acinetobacter,* and *Enterococcus.*
    - One-day dosing and can be given intramuscularly.

- ❖ **Meropenem/vaborbactam:** Active against CRE-producing KPCs.
  - Not active against Ambler class B metallo-β-lactamases (MBLs) producing *Enterobacteriaceae* and *Acinetobacter baumannii* producing Amber class D β-lactamase.
  - Approved for complicated UTIs.
- ❖ **Imipenem/cilastatin/relebactam:** Active against CRE and MDR *Pseudomonas* due to TEM (Temoneira), CTX-M (cefotaximase-Munich), KPCs, AmpC.
  - Not active against Amber class B metallo-β-lactamases (MBLs) producing *Enterobacteriaceae* and *Acinetobacter baumannii* producing Amber class D β-lactamase.

✓ **Aztreonam**
- It's a monobactam. Monocyclic ring compared to bicyclic nucleus of penicillins.
- No activity against GPCs and anaerobes. Active against GNBs, including *Pseudomonas.*
- Dose reduced in patients with reduced GFR or patients on RRT.
- Safe in severe penicillin allergies.

Non-Beta-Lactams

✓ **Aminoglycosides**
- Bind to ribosomal 30s unit[Q] and inhibit protein synthesis.
- **Concentration-dependent bactericidal killing.**
- *Intravenous or intramuscular routes only.*
- **Poor CSF, lung,** bile, and prostate penetration, and activity is reduced in purulent fluids.
- **Minimal protein binding.**
- Active against **MDR Gram-negative bacilli bacteraemia and MRSA.** Streptomycin[Q] active against *Mycobacterium tuberculosis.*
- *No activity against anaerobic bacteria[Q].*
- Resistance growing in *Enterococcus* species.
- Once-daily dosing is preferred to reduce nephrotoxicity.
- Therapeutic drug monitoring (TDM) is done.
- **Post-antibiotic effect** seen.
- **Side effects:** Neuromuscular blockade; ototoxicity, which correlates with duration of therapy and is irreversible; nephrotoxicity,

which correlates with serum concentrations and may be reversible.

❖ **Gentamicin:** Resistance is emerging. Used in combination with vancomycin for endocarditis due to *Enterococcus* or *Viridans* group streptococci. Used in combination with vancomycin for endocarditis due to coagulase-negative staphylococci. Target peak serum concentration 4–8 μg/mL. Target trough serum concentration 1–1.5 μg/mL.

❖ **Tobramycin:** More potent that gentamicin against *P. aeruginosa*. Less active than gentamicin for *Serratia* and *Acinetobacter*.

❖ **Amikacin:** Active against gentamicin-resistant Gram-negative bacilli, such as MDR ESBL–producing *Klebsiella*.

❖ **Plazomicin:** Effective against resistant bacteria producing aminoglycoside-modifying enzymes. Less toxic and better pharmacokinetics.

✓ **Fluoroquinolones**
- Broad-spectrum antibiotic works by binding to DNA gyrase^Q and topoisomerase enzymes.
- **Concentration-dependent killing.**
- Bactericidal against Gram-negative bacilli, such as *Salmonella, Shigella*.
- **Active against MSSA and coagulase-negative staphylococci.**
- Useful against pneumococcal pneumonia, complicated UTIs, prostatitis, intra-abdominal, infections and invasive external otitis *as they have good penetration in tissues.*
- **Active against *Mycobacterium tuberculosis* as well**^{Q}.
- Resistance increasing among *P. aeruginosa, Acinetobacter,* and *S. maltophilia*.
- **Side effects:** *C. difficile* infection, CNS symptoms like headache, restlessness, tendon rupture, QT prolongation. All fluoroquinolones except delafloxacin cause phototoxicity^Q.
  ❖ **Ciprofloxacin:** Has greatest activity against *P. aeruginosa* amongst fluoroquinolones.
  ❖ **Levofloxacin:** Active against *Mycoplasma, Chlamydophila, Ureaplasma,* and *Legionella pneumophila*. Requires dose adjustment in kidney impairment.
  ❖ **Moxifloxacin:** Requires dose adjustment in liver impairment.
  ❖ **Delafloxacin:** Active against MRSA.

✓ **Macrolides**
- Bacteriostatic antibiotics that act on 50s^Q ribosome unit.
- Active against atypical pneumonia due to *Mycoplasma pneumoniae, Chlamydia,* or *Legionella*.
- Useful for pharyngitis caused by *S. pyogenes*. Poor activity against staphylococci, enterococci, and anaerobes.
- **Side effects:** Hepatoxicity, mostly with erythromycin, in pregnant females and QT prolongation^Q.
  ❖ **Azithromycin:** Less active against GPCs. Active against *Mycobacterium avium* and *M. intracellulare*.
  ❖ **Clarithromycin:** More active against GPCs. Active against *Mycobacterium avium* and *M. intracellulare*.
  ❖ **Fidaxomicin:** Superior to vancomycin for *C. difficile* recurrences. No dose adjustment needed with renal or hepatic impairment.

✓ **Glycopeptides**
- Inhibit bacterial cell wall synthesis^Q.
- **Vancomycin**^{Q}: Bactericidal against MRSA, coagulase-negative staphylococci, *S. pneumoniae*, viridans *Streptococcus, Clostridium,* and *Diphtheroid* species. Resistance increasing against *Enterococcus faecium*.
  ❖ Poor GI absorption; hence, it is given IV for systemic infections.
  ❖ **Oral vancomycin for *C. difficile*.**
  ❖ Poor penetration in tissues if concentrations are too low. Trough levels of 15–20 μg/mL for MRSA pneumonia and meningitis, 10–15 μg/mL for endocarditis. Loading dose of 25–30 mg/kg should be considered in critically ill patients to rapidly achieve target concentrations.
  ❖ **Red man syndrome**^{Q}: Rapid IV administration of vancomycin causes histamine release and can cause rash over face and upper trunk, flushing, tachycardia, and hypotension.
  ❖ Neutropaenia, occasional reversible ototoxicity, and rarely, nephrotoxicity. TDM and continuous infusion done to avoid nephrotoxicity.
- **Teicoplanin:** Active against MRSA and streptococcal infections. Used for bone and joint infections^Q. Less adverse effects compared to vancomycin.

- ✓ **Polymyxins**
  - Disrupt the outer cell membrane of bacteria[Q]. Bactericidal against MDR Gram-negative infections.
  - **Polymyxin E (colistin):** Prodrug. Max dosage is 12 MU in a day. Resistance developing because of altered lipid A component in cell membrane. Neuro- and nephrotoxicity.
  - **Polymyxin B:** Not a prodrug. Not a good penetrator in kidney. Can cause hypotension if given fast.
- ✓ **Lipoglycopeptides**
  - Interfere with bacterial cell wall synthesis and disrupt the cell membrane.
  - **First-generation (telavancin)**
    - ❖ Active against GPCs like MRSA, VRSA, and VRE with vanB phenotype. Inactive against VRE species with vanA phenotype.
    - ❖ Approved for skin infections and VAPs. Dose adjustments are required in renal impairment, and it is potentially teratogenic.
  - **Long-acting lipoglycopeptides (oritavancin** and **dalbavancin)**
    - ❖ Approved for skin infections caused by MRSA.
    - ❖ Dose adjustments are required in renal impairment.
- ✓ **Oxazolidinones**
  - **First-generation oxazolidinones (linezolid)**[Q]
    - ❖ Inhibit 23s component of 50s RNA. Bacteriostatic against MRSA, VRSA, and VRE, but bactericidal against *Streptococcus pneumoniae*, *Bacteroides*, and *C. difficile*.
    - ❖ No need to adjust dosage with renal failure; 100% oral bioavailability. Good lung penetration and, hence, better survival rates than vancomycin for MRSA pneumonia.
    - ❖ **Side effects:** Reversible **thrombocytopaenia** with longer duration (>2 wk), **serotonin syndrome**, anaemia, ocular and peripheral neuropathy, and **lactic acidosis**.
  - **Second-generation oxazolidinones (tedizolid)**
    - ❖ Skin infections caused by MRSA and *E. faecalis*.
    - ❖ No dose adjustment required for renal or hepatic impairment.
    - ❖ Lower risk of thrombocytopaenia, anaemia, and serotonin syndrome.
- ✓ **Streptogramins**
  - **Quinupristin/dalfopristin**
    - ❖ Dalfopristin binds to 23s ribosomal subunit of the 50s ribosomal subunit and enhances the binding of quinupristin. Quinupristin binds to 50s subunit of ribosome and prevents elongation of the polypeptide.
    - ❖ Active against VRE, *faecium*, and MRSA. However, no activity against *E. faecalis*.
    - ❖ Can cause phlebitis, hence given by CVC. Myalgias and arthralgia are prominent side effects.
- ✓ **Cyclic Lipopeptides**
  - **Daptomycin**[Q]
    - ❖ Daptomycin kills bacteria by disrupting the cell membranes.
    - ❖ MDR skin infections caused by MRSA, *S. pyogenes*, and *Enterococcus*. Recommended for bacteraemia and right-sided endocarditis caused by MRSA. Not effective in pneumonia as it binds to the surfactant.
    - ❖ **Side effects:** Sickle cell crisis, eosinophilic pneumonitis, creatine kinase elevations, myalgias.
    - ❖ Dose should be adjusted in kidney impairment.
- ✓ **Tetracyclines**
  - They bind to 30s ribosomal subunit.
  - **Tigecycline**
    - ❖ Active against GNBs, including MDR *Acinetobacter*. No activity against *P. aeruginosa* and *Proteus*. Active against MRSA, VRE, anaerobes, and atypical mycobacteria.
    - ❖ *Approved for treatment of skin infections and complicated abdominal infections.*
    - ❖ IV administration only. Dose adjustment required for severe hepatic impairment.
  - **Omadacycline**
    - ❖ Active against GNBs, including *Acinetobacter*. No activity against *P. aeruginosa* and *Proteus*. Active against MRSA, VRE, and anaerobes.
    - ❖ Approved for treatment of skin infections and community-acquired pneumonia.
    - ❖ Both IV and oral prescription available. No dose adjustment required in renal and hepatic impairment.
  - **Eravacycline**
    - ❖ Active against CREs, MRSA, VRE. Covers CRAB. Approved for treatment of complicated abdominal infections.
    - ❖ IV administration only. Dose adjustment required for severe hepatic impairment.

✓ **Metronidazole**
- Disrupts the DNA of the bacteria and inhibits the protein synthesis.
- Active against obligate anaerobes. Most potent agent against *B. fragilis*.
- About 90% oral absorption. Metabolized by liver. No dose adjustment in kidney disease.
- **Side effects:** Metallic taste, neutropaenia, peripheral neuropathy, pancreatitis, and hepatitis.

✓ **Clindamycin**
- Binds to 50s ribosomal subunit, preventing polypeptide formation.
- Covers anaerobic bacteria, β-haemolytic *streptococcus*, Viridans group streptococci, *S. pneumoniae*, and staphylococci. Resistance against *B. fragilis* growing.
- Dose adjustment not recommended in liver and kidney disease. Used in necrotizing fasciitis.
- **Side effects:** *C. difficile* infection.

✓ **Cotrimoxazole**[Q]**: Trimethoprim/Sulfamethoxazole (1:5 Ratio)**
- Inhibits bacterial folate synthesis. Separately, they are bacteriostatic, but combination is bactericidal.
- Active against MRSA, GNBs, *Nocardia*, atypical mycobacteria. **Drug of choice for *Pneumocystis jirovecii*.**
- Side effects: Leucopaenia, thrombocytopaenia, hepatotoxicity, nephrotoxicity.

✓ **Rifampicin**
- Inhibits DNA-dependent RNA polymerase.
- Active against MRSA and *streptococcus*. Used against *Mycobacterium tuberculosis* as well.
- Can be used for post-exposure prophylaxis in *Neisseria/Haemophilus* meningitis.

✓ **Fosfomycin**
- Cell wall inhibitor by inhibiting the **MurA enzyme**.
- Has been used as oral antibiotic, so resistance is there in community.
- It doesn't work against *Acinetobacter*. Used as combination therapy. Used against MRSA and VRE.

✓ **Coverage**
- **Gram-positive coverage:** Flucloxacillin, vancomycin, meropenem, teicoplanin, linezolid, clindamycin
- **Anti-pseudomonal:** Quinolones, ceftazidime, piperacillin/tazobactam, meropenem, aztreonam (*but not ertapenem*), aminoglycosides
- **Anaerobic bacteria:** Carbapenems, metronidazole, clindamycin, quinolones
- **Atypical coverage:** Macrolides and quinolones (*Legionella, Mycoplasma*, and *Chlamydia*), tetracyclines (*Rickettsia, Chlamydia*), ampicillin (*Listeria*)
- **MRSA:** Vancomycin, linezolid, cotrimoxazole, clindamycin, rifampicin, daptomycin, quinupristin/dalfopristin, telavancin, tigecycline
- **VRE:** Linezolid and quinupristin/dalfopristin FDA-approved; daptomycin, tigecycline, telavancin used otherwise
- **CPE:** Fosfomycin plus colistin, gentamicin, tigecycline

✓ **Special Circumstances**
- **Coagulase-negative *Staphylococci*:** Treat only in immunocompromised and if positive on repeated cultures. No treatment needed if only one out of many blood cultures positive.
- BAL fluid showing mixed pathogens: Repeat sample and don't treat straight away.
- If only one of two blood cultures is positive with bacteria, it might be contamination.
- Anaphylaxis with one group of beta-lactam; avoid other groups of beta-lactams.
- UTI: Trimethoprim/sulfamethoxazole can be given if organism is susceptible.
- **Late-onset VAP:** Multidrug-resistant bacteria. Combination therapy should be used.
- Due to high prevalence of MRSA, vancomycin should be used for empiric therapy of suspected staphylococcal infection pending results of cultures.

ANTIMICROBIAL PK AND PD

✓ **Definitions**
- **Pharmacokinetics (PK):** How the body deals with the drug.
- **Pharmacodynamics (PD):** What drug does to the body.

✓ **Antibiotic PK/PD**
- Antibiotics' effect against bacteria is influenced by
  - ❖ Concentration
  - ❖ Time of exposure
  - ❖ Combination of both (area under the curve)
- **Minimum inhibitory concentration (MIC)**[Q]
  - ❖ Lowest concentration of an antimicrobial needed to inhibit the visible growth

of a microorganism after overnight incubation.

❖ Generally, drug concentrations need to be 4–5 times[Q] greater than the MIC to ensure that an antimicrobial is effective.

- **Cmax:** Peak concentration of antimicrobial drug. Optimal is 8–10 times above MIC for antibiotics dependent on Cmax.
- **T > mic:** The time for which the microbial concentration stays above the level of MIC. Should be >50% of the time for antibiotics dependent on T > mic. *It is 100% of the time for critically sick patients, encouraging use of infusions.*
- **AUC:** Area under the serum concentration curve.
- **Breakpoint concentration:** Chosen concentration of an antibiotic, which decides if a species of bacteria is susceptible or resistant to the antimicrobial.
  ❖ If MIC ≤ breakpoint concentration, organism is susceptible.
  ❖ If MIC > breakpoint concentration, organism is resistant.

✓ **Kill Characteristics of Antimicrobials**
- Yes, there is an overlap in some antibiotics.

Concentration-Dependent Killing (Cmax/MIC)	Time-Dependent Killing (T > mic)	Concentration-and Time-Dependent Killing (AUC/MIC)
• *Aminoglycosides*[Q] • Colistin • **Quinolones**[Q] • Metronidazole	• *All beta-lactams*[Q] • *Vancomycin* • Macrolides (erythromycin and clarithromycin) • Linezolid • Clindamycin	• Quinolones • **Vancomycin** • Azithromycin • Tigecycline • Daptomycin • *Linezolid* • *Clindamycin*

✓ **Physiological Changes in Critically Ill Patients**[Q]
- Increased volume of distribution (Vd): ↓ plasma concentration
- Hyperdynamic circulation: Increased clearance →↓ plasma concentration
- Renal or hepatic dysfunction: Decreased clearance →↑ plasma concentration
- **Augmented renal clearance**[Q]: Seen in YOUNG patients. Renal clearance is

actually enhanced in young patients and leads to ↓ plasma concentration of drug.

✓ **Therapeutic Drug Monitoring (TDM)**
- Used to monitor drug levels and avoid toxicity. Used for drugs with narrow therapeutic index, like vancomycin and gentamicin[Q]. Azoles require TDM because of unpredictable PK/PD.
- **Peak concentration** denoted efficacy. Measured 1 h after the dose.
- **Trough concentration** to prevent accumulation. Measured 1 h before next dose.
- It takes **five half-lives**[Q] of the drug to achieve the targeted steady state (most common MCQ asked from this topic).
- **Post-antibiotic effect (PAE):** Suppression of bacterial growth that continues after exposure of antimicrobials (e.g. gentamicin[Q], quinolones, rifampicin, quinupristin/dalfopristin). Non-antimicrobial agents, like glucocorticoids,[Q] also show this effect. No post-antibiotic effect in meropenem.

✓ **Hydrophilic Drugs**
- Hydrophilic drugs have a smaller Vd, have lower protein binding, and mostly are excreted unchanged by the kidney.
- Creatinine clearance changes and increased volume of distribution in critically sick patients can affect the pharmacokinetics of hydrophilic antibiotics, like β-lactams, glycopeptides, and aminoglycosides.
- For β-lactams, a loading dose (1.5–2 times the standard dose) may be needed in septic patients with high volume of distribution.
- Increase the first dosage of water-soluble agents when patient is sick. Monitor trough levels for water-soluble agents (vancomycin), hence front loading in initial stage of distributive shock.
  ❖ Consider renal function when adjusting dosage subsequently when they are on CRRT.
- Antibiotics are administered every three to four half-lives[Q].

✓ **Lipophilic Drugs**
- Lipophilic drugs have much larger Vd, have higher degree of protein binding, and are metabolized mostly by the liver.
- Lipophilic drugs enter intracellularly as well.

Hydrophilic Drugs				Lipophilic Drugs			
Drugs	Protein Binding	Vd	Clearance	Drugs	Protein Binding	Vd	Clearance
Beta-lactams[Q]	Moderate	Low	Renal	Macrolides[Q]	Variable	High	Hepatic
Vancomycin	Moderate	Low	Renal	Quinolones[Q]	Moderate	Moderate	Hepatic metabolism and renal clearance
Aminoglycosides[Q]	Low	Low	Renal	Clindamycin	High	High	Hepatic
Metronidazole	Low	High	Renal				

✓ **Drug Penetration in Tissues**
- Tissues like CNS and lungs have significant barrier to drug penetration, whereas the bloodstream and the urinary tract are easily reached.
  - ❖ The **lungs** have alveolar–blood barrier, as alveolar wall has no fenestration. Linezolid has good lung penetration, whereas colistin and aminoglycosides have poor lung penetration (consider nebulized drugs).
  - ❖ **Urinary tract:** β-lactams, quinolones, and aminoglycosides have good penetration.
  - ❖ **CNS:** Inflammation of meninges increases penetration, whereas acidosis reduces penetration. β-lactams and rifampicin have good penetration. Aminoglycosides have poor CNS penetration (consider intrathecal drugs).
  - ❖ **Bloodstream:** Easy to reach for all antibiotics.
  - ❖ **Abdomen:** β-lactams, quinolones, tigecyclines, and aminoglycosides have good penetration.
  - ❖ **Soft tissues and bones:** Good penetration for most antibiotics. β-lactams, daptomycin, and linezolid have good penetration.
- Quinolones are lipophilic and reach high concentrations in all tissues, whereas aminoglycosides are hydrophilic and have low penetration in lungs, CNS, and eye.
- β-lactams are exceptions as they are hydrophilic but still achieve high tissue concentrations.

✓ **Dose Reduction on the Basis of Creatinine Clearance**
- Dose reduction on basis of creatinine clearance shouldn't be routinely applied in ITU, and full antimicrobial dose should be provided to patients with septic shock at least for the first 24–48 h.
- Increased dosage may be needed for those undergoing renal replacement therapy.
- Loading dose should be given independent of renal function.
- Obese patients based on lean body mass.

✓ **Renal Dysfunction**
- Irrespective of renal dysfunction, **first dose should be full dosage**[Q].
- Clindamycin, linezolid, and tigecycline do not require renal dose adjustment.
- Beta-lactams: We decrease dose amount rather than frequency as time-based killing.
  - ❖ Beta-lactams, being small hydrophilic molecules, are likely to be cleared by CRRT. An additional loading dose may be required when CRRT is initiated.
  - ❖ From second onward, drug concentration depends on estimated drug clearance than the volume of distribution.
  - ❖ Meropenem reduced as excreted through the kidney.
- On RRT, with aminoglycosides, we increase dose interval but keep same dosage.
- Clindamycin, linezolid, and tigecycline do not require renal-dose adjustment.
- Teicoplanin has similar PK/PD in critically ill patients, but vancomycin does not.

- Voriconazole has varied PK/PD in critically ill patients.
- Colistin has varied PK/PD in critically ill patients.

ANTIMICROBIAL RESISTANCE

✓ **Antibiotic Resistance**
- When an organism will not be killed or inhibited by an antimicrobial agent at concentrations of the drug achievable in the body after a normal dose.
- **Intrinsic (natural)**
  - ❖ Intrinsic lack of activity of an antibiotic beyond its spectrum of activity.
  - ❖ Organisms with intrinsic resistance are often of low virulence but invade when host becomes immunosuppressed – e.g. *Pseudomonas, Acinetobacter* species.
- **Acquired:** Organisms previously sensitive to an antibiotic become resistant.

✓ **Acquired Resistance**
- Mutation or intercell transfer:
  - ❖ **Mutation:** Occasional way of resistance.
  - ❖ **Intercell transfer:** Most important way of resistance.
    - **Transformation:** *Naked DNA* released by killing of a bacterium is taken up by another bacteria. Commonest way of resistance.
    - **Transduction:** *Bacteriophage* (viral vector) helps to transfer genetic material.
    - **Plasmid conjugation:** *Self-replicating extra chromosomal* circles of DNA transferred in bacteria-to-bacteria contact.
    - **Transposons:** DNA sequences that can move from one location to another in genome.

Mechanisms by Which Bacteria Acquire Resistance[Q]

Method	Mode	Action	Examples
Drug inactivation	Enzyme production by bacteria	β-lactamases	*Staphylococci, Pseudomonas* produce β-lactamases
Target site modification	Structural changes to bacterial ribosomes, cell wall precursors, enzymes	1. **Reduced affinity of penicillin-binding protein (PBP)** 2. Reduced affinity to ribosomes 3. **Resistance to degradation of cell wall peptidoglycan**	1. **MRSA- and coagulase-negative** *Staphylococcus* **produce low-affinity PBP** 2. Aminoglycosides, macrolides 3. **Vancomycin-resistant enterococci (VRE)**
Active expulsion	Modification of naturally occurring **efflux pumps**	Throwing out of antibiotics from bacteria	*Pseudomonas with pumps for beta-lactams, tetracyclines and quinolones*
Decreased entry of bacteria	Structural changes to cell wall components	1. Reduced permeability of cell wall 2. **Blocked porins** 3. Reduced active uptake by transporters	1. Pseudomonas 2. **Imipenem-resistant** *Pseudomonas* 3. Tetracyclines
Metabolic	Alternate pathway development in bacteria	1. Resistant dihydrofolate reductase 2. **Alternate pathway of developing peptidoglycan**	1. Cotrimoxazole 2. **MRSA**

✓ **Multidrug Resistance (MDR)**
  - Acquired non-susceptibility to at least one agent in three or more antimicrobial categories.
  - **Extensively drug-resistant (XDR):** Non-susceptibility to at least one agent in all but two or fewer antimicrobials categories.
  - **Pan-drug-resistant (PDR):** Non-susceptibility to all agents in all antimicrobials categories.
  - **ESKAPE pathogens:** These six bacteria frequently show multidrug resistance: *Enterococcus faecium, Staphylococcus aureus, Klebsiella pneumoniae, Acinetobacter baumannii, Pseudomonas aeruginosa,* and *Enterobacter* species.
    - ❖ T2 magnetic resonance techniques (e.g. T2Bacteria and T2Resistance assays) can detect amplified DNA of these six ESKAPE pathogens and different resistance determinants from whole-blood specimens.
    - ❖ *Enterobacteriaceae* mainly produce carbapenemases for resistance to β-lactams, whereas *Pseudomonas and Acinetobacter* use a variety of mechanisms, like efflux pumps, porin expression, drug inactivating enzymes, and antibiotic target mutations.
    - ❖ MRSA acquires its resistance from expression of **mecA gene** that produces a penicillin-binding protein (**PBP2a**) that has low affinity for β-lactams. *S. aureus* may also acquire **vanA gene** from **VRE** and become **VRSA.**

Common Pathogens

✓ **Methicillin-Resistant *Staphylococcus aureus* (MRSA)**
  - Patients often have comorbidities and previous history of antibiotic treatments.
  - **Risk factors:** Gastrostomy, femoral catheter, long ICU stay, quinolones/glycopeptide use, and MRSA nasal colonization.
  - Staphylococcal cassette chromosome **mec** (SCCmec) gene is responsible for this resistance to both beta-lactams and non-beta-lactams.
  - No significant excess mortality adjusted for comorbidity in patients with MRSA compared to MSSA.

- **Universal decolonization** with *mupirocin* and *chlorhexidine* is as effective as screening and isolation of MRSA-positive patients.
  - ❖ **QacA** and **QacB efflux pumps** can cause chlorhexidine resistance in MRSA isolates.
  - ❖ Isolation and alcohol gel handwashing should be done.
- **Treatment options[Q]:** Vancomycin, teicoplanin, linezolid, rifampicin, daptomycin, ceftaroline, telavancin, ceftobiprole.

✓ **Coagulase-Negative *Staphylococci***
  - **Most of them are resistant to methicillin and aminoglycosides.**
  - Sensitivity to vancomycin remains high.

✓ **Vancomycin-Resistant *Enterococcus* (VRE)**
  - *E. faecalis* and *E. faecium* are normal bowel commensals in humans.
  - Low virulence but invade when host becomes immunosuppressed, with little risk to health population.
  - *Infections are associated with longer hospital stay and increased mortality* (previously it was thought that the comorbidity-adjusted mortality is the same).
  - Gene clusters of **vanA** and **vanB** are responsible for resistance.
  - **Infection cause:** UTIs, abdominal infections, endocarditis, surgical wound infections.
  - *E. faecalis* is more common, but *E. faecium* is more likely to be vancomycin-resistant.
  - **Treatment:** Linezolid, **tigecycline,** or **quinupristin/dalfopristin[Q].** Antibiotic restriction on vancomycin and third-generation cephalosporins.

✓ *Pseudomonas*
  - Low natural virulence and opportunistic infection in immunocompromised patients. Leading cause of nosocomial pneumonia[Q].
  - Resistance due to multidrug efflux pumps, impermeable membrane in its cell wall, and production of β-lactamase.
  - High chances of clinical failure. Strict isolation and hygiene required.
  - *Start with combination therapy:* Aminoglycoside + piperacillin and tazobactam/quinolone/carbapenem. *Little supporting evidence for combination therapy currently.*
  - Difficult-to-treat *Pseudomonas* may be susceptible to ceftolozane/tazobactam,

ceftazidime/avibactam, or imipenem/cilastatin/relebactam.

- *Pseudomonas producing **metallo-β-lactamases** may respond only to **colistin** or **cefiderocol**.*

✓ ***Klebsiella* spp.**

- Opportunistic nosocomial infection. Colonizes respiratory tract and skin and causes VAPs.
- Likeliest of all the *Enterobacteriaceae* family to develop extended-spectrum β-lactamases **(ESBLs).**
- **Treatment of choice:** Carbapenems. Aminoglycosides may also be helpful.

✓ ***Enterobacter* spp.**

- Opportunistic nosocomial infection. Can cause VAPs, surgical site infection (SSIs), UTI, and CRBSI.
- They have an inducible β-lactamases called **AmpC.**
- **Treatment of choice:** Carbapenems.

✓ ***Stenotrophomonas maltophilia***

- Previously classified as *Pseudomonas.*
- Low virulence but invade when host becomes immunosuppressed.
- Involved in VAP, SSIs, or CRBSI.
- Multiple-drug resistance inherently to beta-lactams, aminoglycosides, and quinolones. Strict isolation and hygiene required.
- **Trimethoprim/sulfamethoxazole (TMP-SMZ)** is drug of choice.

✓ ***Acinetobacter baumannii***

- Omnipresent and part of normal flora of the skin, especially moist areas, like the groin, and is of low virulence but can invade healthy populations as well.
- Resistance is due to plasmid-mediated β-lactamases, chromosomal cephalosporinases, altered penicillin-binding proteins, and membrane impermeability.
- Intrinsically resistant to vancomycin, clindamycin, macrolides, and quinupristin/dalfopristin. Frequently resistant to carbapenems as well.
- **Combination therapy** initially with at least two active agents: colistin + ampicillin/sulbactam.
- Carbapenem-resistant *Acinetobacter baumannii* (CRAB) are often susceptible only to **colistin** or **cefiderocol.**

Enzymes

✓ **Ambler Classification of β-Lactamases**

- Based on amino acid homology.
  - ❖ **Class A:** Extended-spectrum β-lactamases (ESBLs), *Klebsiella pneumoniae* carbapenemase (KPC).
  - ❖ **Class B:** Metallo-β-lactamases (MBLs) like NDM.
  - ❖ **Class C:** AmpC.
  - ❖ **Class D:** Oxacillinases (OXA).
- Ambler classes A, C, and D act by serine ester hydrolysis mechanism, whereas class B enzymes have a zinc ion participating in catalysis.

✓ **Extended-Spectrum β-Lactamases (ESBLs)**

- ESBLs are **plasmid**-mediated form of resistance in Gram-negative bacteria against β-lactam antibiotic.
- Examples: Cefotaxime-Munich **(CTX-M) gene** found in at least 26 bacterial species.
- ESBL-carrying bacteria can also have other resistance mechanisms (e.g. membrane protein deficiencies) and resistance to other antibiotics (aminoglycosides, quinolones, cotrimoxazole).
- **Resistance:** ESBL-producing *Enterobacteriaceae* are resistant to third-generation cephalosporins.
- Treatment options are carbapenems,[Q] or resistance can be overcome by using β-lactams/β-lactamase inhibitors (BLBLI), like ceftazidime/avibactam, meropenem/vaborbactam, or imipenem/relebactam.
- **Tigecycline can also be given, but it is ineffective in urosepsis.**

✓ **Carbapenemases**

- They are a group of enzymes that run across Ambler class A, B, and D. Examples are KPC (class A), NDM (class B), and OXA (class D).
- **Class A: *Klebsiella pneumoniae* carbapenemase (KPC)**
  - ❖ Resistant to all β-lactams, including carbapenems.
  - ❖ Treatment options: β-lactams/β-lactamase inhibitors (BLBLI), like ceftazidime/avibactam, meropenem/vaborbactam, fosfomycin + colistin.
  - ❖ It is easier to treat KPCs than NDMs, though normally.

- **Class B: Metallo-β-lactamases (MBLs), like NDM, VIM**
  - ❖ Resistant to all β-lactams, including carbapenems, including new β-lactams/β-lactamase inhibitors (BLBLI), like ceftazidime/avibactam, meropenem/vaborbactam, or imipenem/relebactam.
  - ❖ Sensitive to aztreonam, but these bacteria are usually also producing ESBL, and hence, resistance to aztreonam might be there.
  - ❖ Still susceptible to **cefiderocol and colistin**^{Q}.
- **Class D: Oxacillinases (OXA)**
  - ❖ Resistance to cephalosporins, carbapenems, and **vaborbactam/relebactam**.
  - ❖ CTXM and OXA strains can co-exist in *Acinetobacter* species.
  - ❖ Treatment options: Resistance can be overcome by using β-lactams/β-lactamase inhibitors (BLBLI), like ceftazidime/**avibactam**.

✓ **AmpC β-Lactamase**
- Resistant to all the cephalosporins
- They are sensitive to carbapenems and ceftolozane/tazobactam.

Trials and Guidelines

✓ **EPIC III Study**
- Mortality is higher in ICU-acquired infections and in cases caused by antibiotic-resistant microorganisms (VRE, *Klebsiella* resistant to carbapenems, or carbapenem-resistant *Acinetobacter*) compared to community-acquired infections.

✓ **Surviving Sepsis Campaign (SSC) 2021**
- Empirical **antimicrobials with MRSA coverage** in adults with sepsis or septic shock at high risk of MRSA but against their use in case of low risk.
- Using **two antimicrobials with Gram-negative coverage** for empirical treatment in adults with sepsis or septic shock and high risk of MDR organisms, but against their use in case of low risk or when susceptibilities are known.
- **High-risk factors:** Recent hospitalization or antibiotic use, exposure to medical devices, immunocompromised conditions, chronic illnesses, and history of MRSA infection.

ANTIBIOTIC STEWARDSHIP

✓ **Antibiotic Stewardship**
- Hospital-wide practice that links infection control measures with judicious antibiotic management.
- Key aspects of antibiotic stewardship
  - ❖ Audit and feedback
  - ❖ Formulary restriction
  - ❖ Evidence-based guidelines
  - ❖ Antibiotic optimization
  - ❖ Dose optimization
  - ❖ Education and training
  - ❖ Information technology
  - ❖ Computer-assisted support
  - ❖ Microbiology laboratories
  - ❖ Leadership and teamwork

✓ **Start Smart, Then Focus**
- Antibiotic stewardship campaign by the Department of Health and Public Health England.
- **Start smart**
  - ❖ Do not start antibiotics in the absence of clinical evidence of bacterial infection.
  - ❖ Take drug allergy history thoroughly.
  - ❖ Start antibiotics within 1 h of diagnosis in patients with sepsis.
  - ❖ Use local antimicrobial prescribing guidelines.
  - ❖ Document clinical indication, dose, and route on drug chart.
  - ❖ Include stop date or duration.
  - ❖ Obtain culture prior to starting therapy.
- **Then focus**
  - ❖ Clinical review and decision at 48–72 h.
  - ❖ Stop antibiotic/switch to oral/change antibiotic/continue the same antibiotic/outpatient parenteral antibiotic therapy.

✓ **Advantages of Antibiotic Stewardship**
- Improved patient safety
- Reduced antimicrobial resistance
- Reduced healthcare costs
- Improved public health

✓ **Colonization vs. Infection**
- **Colonization**
  - ❖ Presence of multiplying pathogens on a host, but without interaction between host and organism. No overt host response or clinical symptoms.

❖ Treatment can lead to selection of resistant strains of colonizing pathogens.

- **Infection**
  ❖ Process of invading body tissues by the microbe to cause the symptoms of disease, like pyrexia, leucocytosis, tachycardia, or raised inflammatory markers (CRP).
  ❖ Most nosocomial infections are endogenous in origin and may be preceded by colonization with endogenous MDR pathogens.
  ❖ Breaching natural defence mechanisms (tubes, catheters, surgery) or impairing host defences by immunosuppression predisposes to infection.

INFECTION CONTROL POLICIES

✓ **Epidemiology**
- **Extended Prevalence of Infection in Intensive Care (EPIC) III Study** in 2017 showed that the prevalence of suspected or proven infection amongst patients sampled across ICUs from 88 countries was reported to be 54%, out of which 22% were ICU-acquired.
  ❖ Amongst sites, **respiratory tract infections (60%)**[Q] were followed by abdominal (18%), bloodstream (15%), and genitourinary tract infections (14%) in the same study in critically ill patients.
  ❖ The same study showed **Gram-negative organisms** were the leading isolated microbes (67%), followed by Gram-positive (37%) and fungal infections (16%).
  ❖ *Klebsiella* **was most common (18.5%)** amongst Gram-negative bacteria. *Staphylococcus aureus* was most common (14.8%) amongst Gram-positive cases.

✓ **Risk Factors**
- Length of stay is the leading risk factor for nosocomial infection, followed by use of medical devices.
  ❖ Even stay of more than 1 d put the patient at greater risk compared to stay less than 1 d.
- **Other risk factors** include male sex, comorbid conditions (like COPD, diabetes mellitus, chronic kidney disease, cancer, HIV infection), and hyperglycaemia.

Prevention and Control Measures

✓ **Infection Control Precautions**
- **Isolation:** *Standard* precautions (masks, gloves, gowns) are for all patients and reduce risk of transmission of blood-borne pathogens.
- **Transmission**-based precautions based on pathogens
  ❖ **Airborne (<5 μ size) precautions**
    - Negative pressure isolation with closed doors. Pulmonary **tuberculosis, measles,** varicella, Covid-19.
    - Isolation for ≥2 wk[Q] from starting treatment in patients with rifampicin-sensitive active pulmonary tuberculosis.
  ❖ **Droplet (>5 μ size) precautions**
    - Droplets generated by sneezing and coughing are prevented from transmission. Maximum up to a meter spread, so can have open doors.
    - **Influenza A or B**, RSV, *Neisseria meningitidis, Haemophilus, Diphtheria*, pertussis, *Mycoplasma*, chlamydia, mumps, rubella.
  ❖ **Contact transmission**
    - Prevent transmission through direct or indirect contact.
    - Private room and patient care items should be dedicated to a single patient.
    - Glove and gown, five moments of handwashing should be observed.
    - **MRSA**, VRE, *C. difficile*, ESBL, scabies.
- **Hand hygiene:** Five moments of hand hygiene (before and after patient contact, after touching a patient's surroundings, after contact with blood and body fluids, and before clean/aseptic procedures). Most doctors fail to comply after touching patient's surroundings. *Single most important factor in reducing the rate of HCAIs (reduces by 40%[Q]).*
  ❖ Wash hands with soap and water if soiled or visibly dirty.
  ❖ Wet your hands, apply soap, and scrub them for at least 15–20 s.
  ❖ An alcohol-based hand rub (0.5% chlorhexidine with 70% w/v ethanol) if hands are not visibly dirty. Alcohol gels are virucidal.

- ❖ *Clostridium difficile* is resistant to alcohol; hence, use soap and water for them[Q].
- ❖ Air dryers are not recommended in ICUs, and single-use towels are used.
- **Antimicrobial bathing**
  - ❖ Decreasing the reservoir of MDR organisms can lead to a risk of nosocomial transmission.
  - ❖ Use of chlorhexidine for daily bath in patients aged more than 2 months has shown to reduce the incidence of hospital-acquired BSIs and contribute to reduce transmission of MDR organisms.
- **Environmental cleaning:** "No touch" automated room–disinfection methods using hydrogen peroxide vapour or ultraviolet light have been shown to reduce rates of pathogen transmission of MRSA, VRE, and *C. difficile* infections among patients.

✓ **Architectural Design**
- Single-patient rooms with negative and positive pressure ventilation
- Individual patient sinks
- Alcohol gel dispensers at entry, exits, every bed space, and every workstation
- Adequate room ventilation with filtered air
- At least six air changes per hour

✓ **Selected Pathogens**
- **Methicillin-resistant *Staphylococcus aureus* (MRSA)**
  - ❖ Around 30% of *S. aureus* infections are resistant.
  - ❖ *Contact precautions recommended. Use is controversial as studies have reported no increase in MRSA infections after use of contact precautions were discontinued.*
  - ❖ Horizontal measures active against multiple organisms, such as universal decolonization and daily chlorhexidine bathing, were more effective.
  - ❖ Netherlands has near zero incidence of MRSA due to intensive screening and isolation policy.
- **Vancomycin-resistant *Enterococci***
  - ❖ Contact precautions recommended.
  - ❖ *Use is controversial as studies have reported no increase in VRE infections after use of contact precautions was discontinued.*

- ❖ Horizontal measures were more effective, like MRSA.
- ***Clostridium difficile***
  - ❖ Contact precautions recommended.
  - ❖ *Clostridium difficile* is resistant to alcohol; hence, use soap and water for them.
  - ❖ Use of 10% sodium hypochlorite solution is effective for decreasing *C. difficile* spores and is associated with decreasing *C. difficile* infection rates.
- **MDR Gram-negative bacilli**
  - ❖ Contact precautions for MDR organisms.
  - ❖ Active surveillance for asymptomatic rectal CRE colonization is not routinely recommended.

✓ **Biomedical Waste**
- Lacks in 30–35% of health providers.
- Mixing of 15% infectious waste happens with non-infectious waste.
- **Blue-coloured bins:** Unbroken glassware.
- **Black bin:** Non-infected waste.
- *Yellow-coloured bins: Body parts and human tissues.*

✓ **Spill Management**
- A **1% sodium hypochlorite solution** is used to clean urine, blood, and body spillage.
- Clean cytotoxic spill on eye with 0.9% saline or water. Major spill is >30 mL.
- Soiled linens in yellow bags.

✓ **CVC Maintenance**
- Chlorhexidine skin preparation is necessary.
- **Transparent dressings should be changed every 7 d**, and chlorhexidine should be applied while changing it. If it gets dampened with blood or moisture, change it immediately.
- **Gauze dressing should be changed within 48 h.**
- Transparent dressing is better than gauze dressing.
- Blood or lipid tubing should be changed within 24 h.

✓ **Other Precautions**
- Arterial transducers should be changed at 96 h intervals.
- **Burns in neutropenic patient:** Positive air pressure isolation room.
- **Patient with diarrhoea:** Containment isolation.

- **Aseptic non-touch technique (ANTT):** Handling CVC, PVC, and endotracheal suctioning.

✓ **Decontamination**[Q]
- Process of removing matter so that it cannot cause infection or inflammation.
- **Cleaning**
  - ❖ Physical removal of foreign material from equipment without destroying infectious agents.
  - ❖ It lowers the bioburden before they are subjected to disinfection or sterilization.
- **Disinfection**
  - ❖ *Elimination of all pathogenic organisms, except bacterial spores.*
  - ❖ Chemicals used to disinfect inanimate physical objects are known as **disinfectants**.
  - ❖ Chemicals used to disinfect human body surfaces are known as **antiseptics**.
  - ❖ Chemical methods, like 2% glutaraldehyde for 20 min or 6–7.5% H_2O_2 for 30 min.
  - ❖ *Thermal methods, like pasteurization, where an object is heated 60–100°C for up to 30 min.*
- **Sterilization**
  - ❖ *Elimination of all pathogenic organisms except prions.*
  - ❖ Autoclaving (moist heat), dry heat, gamma irradiation, and ethylene oxide gas[Q].

✓ **Spaulding Classification**
- **Critical:** Items that enter sterile tissue or the vascular system of body (e.g. surgical instruments, needles). Items should be sterilized.
- **Semi-critical:** Items that contact mucous membranes and non-intact skin but do not break the blood barrier (e.g. laryngoscopes, endoscopes). Sterilization or high-level disinfection.
- **Non-critical:** Items that come into contact with healthy skin but not mucous membranes (e.g. pulse oximeter). Low-level disinfection or cleaning.

✓ **CRBSI**
- The highest in dialysis catheters, and rare in arterial or peripheral cannulas.
- Both 0.5% and 2% chlorhexidine provide a MIC for most nosocomial bacteria and yeasts and hence are recommended for CVC insertion.
- **A 2% chlorhexidine in 70% alcohol is better than povidone-iodine solutions; however, due to reports of arachnoiditis, use of 0.5% chlorhexidine is recommended for central neuraxial procedures.**

✓ **Notifiable Diseases**
- Responsibility of patient's treating physician.
- Notification can be done if suspecting disease; no need to wait for laboratory diagnosis.
- Huge list, but for exam purposes, acute infectious hepatitis and acute meningitis of any cause are also notifiable.

✓ **Selective Digestive Decontamination (SDD)**[Q]
- Prophylactic strategy to minimize nosocomial endogenous and exogenous infections.
- Targeted microorganisms: MSSA, MRSA, *Streptococcus pneumoniae, Haemophilus influenzae, Moraxella catarrhalis, E. coli, C. albicans, Klebsiella, Enterobacter, Serratia, Proteus, Morganella, Pseudomonas,* and *Acinetobacter.*
- Short course of 4 d of IV antibiotics.
  - ❖ Previously healthy patient: Cefotaxime[Q] 80–100 mg/day.
  - ❖ Chronic underlying disease: Ceftazidime.
  - ❖ Enteral antimicrobials given to control oropharyngeal and intestinal carriage. Polymyxin[Q], tobramycin,[Q] and amphotericin B[Q].
  - ❖ A 2% gel or paste of amphotericin B is applied in oropharyngeal cavity four times a day.
  - ❖ Suspension of 10 mL with 100 mg of polymyxin E, tobramycin 80 mg, and 500 mg of amphotericin B, given through NG tube four times a day.
  - ❖ Add vancomycin[Q] to intestinal solution in case of MRSA.
- High level of hygiene to prevent exogenous infection.
- Surveillance cultures of throat and rectum, on admission and twice weekly.
- Suggestion that selective oral decontamination is as good as SDD and IV cephalosporins are not needed.
- Not used in the UK due to fear of resistance but has been shown to reduce incidence of VAP and mortality.

COMMUNITY-ACQUIRED PNEUMONIA

Epidemiology and Aetiology

✓ **Community-Acquired Pneumonia (CAP)**
  • Pneumonia developing in the outpatient setting or within 48 h after hospitalization.
  • Less than 20% of patients with CAP will be hospitalized, and 1 out of the 5 hospitalized patients will require ICU.

✓ **Causes**
  • Influenza virus is the most common cause of CAP along[Q] with *Streptococcus pneumoniae*, the most common bacterial cause of CAP. Incidence decreasing due to pneumococcal vaccination and herd immunity.
  • *Legionella* can cause atypical pneumonia. *Hyponatraemia*, abdominal pain, diarrhoea. Atypical pathogen without cell wall. Urinary antigen positive[Q].
  • *Staphylococcus aureus* pneumonia can occur as a complication of influenza.
  • *Haemophilus influenza* and *Moraxella catarrhalis* are common among patients with chronic bronchitis.
  • *Pseudomonas* in corticosteroids and chronic lung disease like cystic fibrosis.
  • *Mycoplasma pneumoniae*: Walking pneumonia. Diagnosed by **PCR.**
  • *Klebsiella* and anaerobes in patients suffering with alcoholism.

✓ **Mixed Viral-Bacterial Infection**
  • Observed in 20% of adult cases of CAP.
  • One-third of cases admitted to ITU have no causative organism.

Clinical Features and Diagnosis

✓ **Presenting Symptoms**
  • Fever, cough, sputum, dyspnoea, and pleuritic chest pain.
  • Patients who have altered immune function have less dramatic symptoms.
  • Elderly present with non-respiratory presentation, like symptoms of confusion and failure to thrive.

✓ **Diagnostic Testing**
  • Sputum Gram staining. Sputum, blood, and urine culture in critically ill patient.
  • **Urine sample** used to diagnose *Pneumococcus* or *Legionella* antigen.

❖ Yield for urinary[Q] sample for Legionella is 50% and is specific for group I infection.
  • **Rapid diagnostic antigenic and molecular tests** are being increasingly used.
    ❖ PCR[Q] for influenza-19, RSV, *Mycoplasma*.
  • **Chest X-ray** may not show findings clearly, and CT scan has a higher sensitivity in diagnosing occult pneumonia.
  • **Procalcitonin (PCT)** can help diagnose bacterial CAP from viral ones.

✓ **Pleural Effusion**
  • Seen more commonly in infections with *Haemophilus*, *S. pneumoniae*, group A *Streptococci*, and *Aspergillus*.

✓ **Haemoptysis**
  • Seen in pyogenic streptococcal pneumonia, anaerobic lung abscess, staph aureus, necrotizing Gram-negative organisms and invasive aspergillosis.

✓ *Legionella*
  • Affects the young and smoker and has greater multisystem involvement with disease of greater severity.

✓ **Panton–Valentine leucocidin (PVL)**
  • A cytotoxin[Q] that is secreted by both MSSA and MRSA and forms pores in the cell membranes of neutrophils and macrophages.
  • Associated with community outbreaks of cellulitis, necrotizing skin infections, and necrotizing pneumonia in healthy children and young adults.
  • Presents with influenza-like prodrome and progresses rapidly to septic shock and respiratory failure.
  • A 40–60% mortality with **leucopaenia**, thrombocytopaenia, airway haemorrhage, and pleural effusions as complications.
  • **Treatment**[Q] is vancomycin, clindamycin/ linezolid (toxin clearance), rifampicin (intracellular clearance), and IVIg.

Treatment (ATS/IDSA 2019 Guidelines)

✓ **Antibiotic Therapy (ATS/IDSA 2019 Guidelines)**
  • Initial empirical cover.
  • Rule out **risk factors for *Pseudomonas* infection** (broad-spectrum antibiotic >7 d in the last month, corticosteroids >10 mg of prednisone daily, malnutrition, HIV, or prior colonization of *P. aeruginosa*).

- Early administering of the antibiotic dose has got mortality benefit.
- For **severe CAP** requiring admission in ICU: Empirical cover with **beta-lactam** other than penicillin and **macrolide/quinolone** for treatment.
- **Add beta-lactam/beta-lactamase inhibitor (BL-BLI) anti-*Pseudomonas* cover** if fever not improving, and send blood cultures.
- *For patients with risk factors for pseudomonas, start with anti-pseudomonal beta-lactam (piperacillin/tazobactam, meropenem) with anti-pseudomonal quinolone.*
- Influenza, treat with antivirals (oseltamivir) as well as cover for MRSA.
  - ❖ **RSV:** Ribavirin.
- **Cavitating lesions:** *Staphylococcus*, *Streptococcus*, and *Klebsiella*. Add Gram-positive cover.
- **PVL-MRSA** can be treated with vancomycin (more soft tissue penetration compared to lung), linezolid.

✓ **NIV/CPAP**
- Not recommended in CAP routinely.
- Use of HFNO also shouldn't delay intubation if needed.

✓ **Duration of Treatment**
- Around 5–7 d for pneumococcal pneumonia. *Legionella* may require therapy for 14 d.
- Switch to oral therapy when patient is a febrile on at least two occasions 8 h apart, able to take food by mouth, or other clinical signs of improvement.
- Biomarkers, like PCT, can be used along with other data to shorten the duration of antibiotics.

✓ **Steroids**
- Showed mortality benefit in bacterial severe CAP, as seen in **CAPE-COD Trial (2023).**
- Steroids not useful in H1N1 pneumonia.

✓ **Notification**
- *Legionella* is a notifiable disease and health professionals must inform local health protection teams of suspected cases.

✓ **Prophylaxis**
- **Pneumococcal and influenza vaccines** are recommended in elderly population above 65 yr of age.

Prognosis

✓ **Pneumonia Severity Index (PSI)Q**
- Complex system and includes measurement of both chronic and acute disease factors.

- Lactates not a part. **Predicts mortality.**
- American Thoracic Society (ATS) support PSI over CURB-65 for determining hospitalization.

✓ **CURB-65 ScoreQ**
- 1 point for each finding
- Confusion, not long-standing (mini–mental test score ≤8/10)
- **Urea** >7 mmol/L
- **Respiratory rate** ≥30/min
- **Blood pressure (SBP <90 mmHg or DBP <60 mmHg)**
- Age ≥65 yr
  - ❖ Score 0–1: <3% mortality, 2: 9% mortality, 3–5:15–40% mortality.
  - ❖ Score 0–1: Care in community.
  - ❖ Score 2–3: Hospital admission.
  - ❖ Score 4–5: Admission to critical care.

✓ **CAP Risk Factors**
- **For mortality in patients with CAP.** (At the end of the day, they are all the same for all the diseases, but you can use this classification.)
- **History:** Advanced age, serious comorbidity, poor functional status, recent hospitalization, immunosuppression, delayed or inappropriate therapy, prolonged mechanical ventilation.
- **Physical findings:** RR > 30/min, tachycardia > 120/min, hypotension, high fever > 38°C, or altered mental status.
- **Laboratory findings:** Multi-lobar infiltrates, positive blood cultures, multiple organ failure, hypoalbuminaemia, renal insufficiency, thrombocytopaenia.

✓ **Mortality**
- Mortality in patients admitted to ICU is almost 35%.

VENTILATOR-ASSOCIATED PNEUMONIA

Epidemiology and Aetiology
✓ **Healthcare Associated Infection (HCAI)**
- HCAI is an infection occurring due to contact with healthcare facilities or from medical interventions. Respiratory tract infection is the commonest HCAI. UTIs form the second most common infections.

- About 6.4% of all inpatients in hospital are suffering from HCAI at any time.
- Around 23.4% of all ITU patients are suffering from HCAI at any time.

✓ **Hospital-Acquired Pneumonia (HAP)**[Q]
- Pneumonia that develops >48 h post-admission.
- It may present up to 14 d post-discharge from hospital.

✓ **Ventilator-Associated Pneumonia (VAP)**[Q]
- Pneumonia occurring 48 h or more after intubation.
- VAP is the commonest nosocomial infection in ventilated patients, seen in 10–25% of them.
- **Disease onset ≤4 d (early VAP)**[Q]: Community-acquired pathogens, like *Haemophilus*, *Streptococcus pneumoniae*, MSSA.
- **Disease onset ≥5 d (late VAP)**[Q]: Hospital-acquired pathogens, like MRSA, *Pseudomonas*.
- **Patients on steroids:** *Pseudomonas*, *Legionella*, and *Aspergillus*.

✓ **Pathophysiology**
- Biofilm formation within the endotracheal tube and microaspiration of secretions. Lung host defence impairments due to malnutrition.

✓ **Ventilator-Associated Tracheobronchitis (VAT)**
- Fever, purulent sputum, and pathogens in the sputum, but no invasive parenchymal lung infection. Considered precursor of VAP.
- About 15% prevalence in mechanically ventilated patients. Limited impact on overall mortality as compared to VAP.
- Increased patient costs, length of stay, antibiotic use, and duration of mechanical ventilation.

Clinical Features and Diagnosis

✓ Presence of VAP in patients is always a clinical dilemma as evidence has showed that up to two-thirds of patients diagnosed based on clinical criteria alone don't have truly a pneumonia.
✓ No universally agreed diagnostic criteria, with a lot of subjectivity in making a diagnosis.
✓ **Clinical Pulmonary Infection Score (CPIS Criteria)**
✓ Has 93% sensitivity and 96% specificity. Seven parameters (2 points each) are **used to define VAP**. *Score >6 is accepted as pneumonia*[Q].

- **Fever (°C):** 36.5 – 38.4 = 0; 38.5 – 38.9 = 1; ≥39 or <36.5 = 2.
- **White blood cell counts:** 4,000–11,000 = 0; <4,000 or >11,000 = 1, rod form ≥50% = add 1 point.
- **Sputum purulence:** No secretion = 0; tracheal secretion with less purulence = 1; tracheal secretion with abundant purulence = 2.
- **Oxygenation changes:** PaO2/FiO2 (mmHg) >240 or signs of ARDS = 0; PaO2/FiO2 (mmHg) ≤240 or no signs of ARDS = 2.
- **Radiologic patterns:** No infiltrates on chest X-ray = 0, diffuse infiltration = 1, add 1 for localized infiltration.
- **Progression of radiological infiltrates:** No progression = 0; progression (after exclusion of HF and ARDS) = 2.
- **Pathogenic bacteria in tracheal aspirate:** No bacteria = 0; moderate or high levels of pathogenic bacteria = 1; pathogenic bacteria seen on Gram staining = add 1 point.

✓ **Johannson Criteria**
- Another criterion used for diagnosis of VAP and has sensitivity of 69% and specificity of 75%.

✓ **Centers for Disease Control and Prevention (CDC) Surveillance Criteria**
- Highly sensitive but not specific. Has interobserver variability.
- **Radiological criteria:** Two or more serial chest imaging results showing new, progressive, persistent infiltrate, consolidation, or cavitation.
- **Clinical criteria**
  ❖ At least one out of the following three signs: **Fever (>38°C)**, **WBC ≥12 × 10⁹/L** or ≤4 × 10⁹/L, or **altered mental status in adults ≥70 yr old.**
  ❖ And at least one of the following four signs: new or change in purulent sputum, dyspnoea or tachypnoea, bronchial breath sounds, and worsening gas exchange.
- **Microbiological criteria:** At least one of the following:
  ❖ Organism identified in blood.
  ❖ Organism identified in pleural fluid.
  ❖ Positive quantitative culture of endotracheal aspirate ≥10⁵ CFU/mL, BAL ≥10⁴ CFU/mL, or PSB ≥10³ CFU/mL[Q].

❖ Around 5% or more of cells with intra-cellular bacteria on direct microscopy examination of stained BAL fluid.

❖ Positive quantitative culture of lung tissue ≥10⁴ CFU/g tissue.

❖ Histopathologic exam showing either abscess formation or invasion of lung parenchyma by fungal hyphae.

✓ **Hospitals in Europe Link for Infection through Surveillance (HELICS)**

- Surveillance criteria in Europe and divides pneumonia into PN1 to PN5 based on microbiological method used for diagnosis.

✓ **Sampling for Microbiological Culture**

- **Quantitative culture:** Differentiates pathogen (heavy growth) from colonizer (low growth).

- **Qualitative culture:** Pathogen present or absent (can't differentiate a colonizer).

- **Semi-quantitative culture:** Light, moderate, or heavy growth.

- **Non-invasive technique**

  ❖ Respiratory samples may be obtained by endotracheal aspirate.

  ❖ **Invasive technique** (BAL, blind BAL, and protected specimen brush, or PSB). No technique is superior to another technique.

  ❖ No superiority between quantitative and qualitative culture as well.

- **European guidelines:** For VAP, take a lower respiratory tract sample (distal quantitative or proximal quantitative/qualitative culture).

- **American guidelines:** For VAP, non-invasive respiratory sampling (endotracheal aspiration) with semi-quantitative cultures is taken.

✓ **Ventilator-Associated Events**[Q]

- CDC surveillance definition in those cases where diagnosis of VAP is difficult to make.

- **Ventilator-associated condition (VAC):** At least one of the following indicators of worsening oxygenation:

  ❖ Minimum daily FiO2 value increase of ≥0.20 from baseline, remaining like that for ≥2 d.

  ❖ Minimum daily PEEP value increase of ≥3 cm H_2O from baseline, remaining like that for ≥2 d.

- **Infection-related ventilator-associated complication (IVAC):** Patient has VAC plus 2 of the following criteria:

  ❖ Temperature >38°C or a WBC ≥12 × 10⁹/L or ≤4 × 10⁹/L.

  ❖ A new antimicrobial agent is started and continued for >4 d.

- **Possible VAP**

  ❖ On or after 3 d of mechanical ventilation and within 2 d before or after the onset of worsening oxygenation, one of the following criteria.

  ❖ Presence of purulent respiratory secretions (≥25 neutrophils and ≤ 10 squamous epithelial cells per low-power field).

  ❖ A positive culture from respiratory secretions (qualitative, quantitative, or semi-quantitative culture).

- **Probable VAP:** On or after 3 d of mechanical ventilation and within 2 d before or after the onset of worsening oxygenation, one of the following criteria:

  ❖ Purulent respiratory secretions and positive quantitative or semi-quantitative culture.

  ❖ Positive pleural fluid culture, positive lung histopathology, positive diagnostic test for *Legionella*, or positive diagnostic test for influenza, parainfluenza, respiratory syncytial virus, adenovirus.

✓ **CRP Increases in Both VAP and VAT**

- **Procalcitonin (PCT)** increases in severe VAP and helps differentiates VAP from VAT.

- CRP and PCT higher in VAP patients compared to VAT.

✓ **Lung Ultrasound**

- Tissue sign and dynamic air bronchograms are seen with pulmonary consolidation.

Treatment

✓ **VAP Care Bundle**[Q]

- Daily sedation hold, bed head elevation 30–45°, gastric ulcer prophylaxis, oral hygiene care, and ETT with subglottic aspiration.

✓ **Supportive Therapy**

- Enteral nutrition is preferred using a continuous infusion.

- Chest physiotherapy in the patients with inadequate cough.

- Good lung down^Q can improve V/Q by increasing perfusion in the healthy lung.
- *Bronchodilators have not shown any improved outcome in the absence of bronchospasm and are best used in patients with COPD and pneumonia.*

✓ **Antibiotic Treatment**
  - Initial empirical therapy. Access the risk factors for MDR pathogens.
  - **Risk factors for MDR pathogens for VAP** IV antibiotic use within 90 d, septic shock, RRT, ARDS, >5 d of hospitalization.
    - ❖ Cover MRSA and MDR *Pseudomonas* in these cases.
    - ❖ In ICUs with >10–20% of *S. Aureus* isolates as MRSA, consider coverage for it.
    - ❖ In ICUs with >10% of Gram-negative isolates are MDR, consider using two antipseudomonal antibiotics.
  - **Risk factors for MDR HAP:** IV antibiotic use within 90 d.
  - **In those without risk factors for MDR pathogens/early-onset VAP:** Start with piperacillin/tazobactam or third-generation cephalosporin or fluoroquinolone or ertapenem.
  - **In those with risk factors for MDR pathogens/late-onset VAP/septic shock**
    - ❖ Two different class antipseudomonal antibiotics are used (anti-pseudomonal beta-lactam plus anti-pseudomonal quinolone/aminoglycoside).
    - ❖ Add linezolid if suspected MRSA as it penetrates the lung better.
  - *Candida* in sputum, urine, stool, or skin is a commensal. No need to treat isolated samples in each.
  - *Aspergillus* is treated by voriconazole.

✓ **Tailoring of Antibiotics**
  - Narrow down from initial combination therapy to single agent as per culture report.
  - Continue combination therapy in patients with extensively drug-resistant (**XDR:** susceptible to only one or two classes of antibiotics) or pan-drug-resistant (**PDR:** not susceptible to any antibiotic) or carbapenem-resistant *Enterobacteriaceae* (**CRE**) isolates or non-fermenting Gram-negative bacteria.
  - Avoid aminoglycoside/polymyxins if alternate agents with Gram-negative activity are available.

- If patient is on right antibiotic and deteriorating, add polymyxin for XDR bacteria.
- **Inhaled antibiotic therapy**
  - ❖ Not indicated in all cases of VAP. Can be used in some patients with VAT but can cause *bronchospasm* in hyper-reactive airway disease, so use nebulized lignocaine before nebulized colistin. It reduces drug resistance.
  - ❖ Consider both inhaled and systemic aminoglycosides or polymyxins for patients that are susceptible to just these agents.

✓ **Duration of Antibiotics**
  - Stable patient with HAP: 3 d.
  - VAP, including non-fermenting, Gram-negative *Acinetobacter* and MRSA: 7–8 d.

✓ **VAT with COPD, CF, Haematolymphoid Malignancy, and Uncontrolled Diabetes**
  - Requires antibiotics.
  - Antibiotics should not be used for ventilator-associated tracheobronchitis otherwise.

Aspiration Pneumonia

✓ **Definition**
  - **Aspiration pneumonia:** Infection due to colonized orogastric contents.
  - **Aspiration pneumonitis:** Chemical injury due to ingested orogastric contents (Mendelson syndrome).

✓ **Risk Factors**
  - Full stomach, obesity, hiatal hernia, diabetes mellitus, supine position, sedation.

✓ **Management: ABCDE Approach**
  - **Recovery position** if own airway.
  - Decompress stomach (can further cause vomiting if airway not secured).
  - Suction through endotracheal tube.
  - Antimicrobials covering anaerobic bacteria if pneumonia; avoid in pneumonitis.
  - Chest physiotherapy.

URINARY TRACT INFECTIONS

Aetiology

✓ **Urinary Tract Infections (UTIs)**
  - It is a broader term that encompasses a spectrum of infections from urethra to kidneys.

- It accounts for up to one-quarter of all the infections in ICU.
- Around 71% of UTIs are caused by Gram-negative bacilli, with **E. coli** as the most common organism.
- **Long-term (>30 d) catheterization** is associated with bacteria like *Proteus, Providencia, Morganella*, and *Pseudomonas*.

✓ **CA-UTI**
- Catheter-associated urinary tract infection surveillance (**definition by Centers for Disease Control and Prevention (CDC) guidelines**). All three conditions must be met:
  ❖ Patient had an indwelling catheter for >2 d.
  ❖ Patient has one of the following signs or symptoms: fever (>38°C), suprapubic tenderness, costovertebral angle tenderness, urinary urgency, urinary frequency, or dysuria.
  ❖ A positive urine culture with no more than two species of organisms identified, at least one of which is a bacterium ≥10⁵ CFU/mL.

✓ **CA-UTI**
- Catheter-associated urinary tract infection (definition by Infectious Disease Society of America [IDSA]).
- Presence of symptoms and signs compatible with UTI, with no other identified source of infection along with ≥10³ CFU/mL of ≥1 bacterial species in a single-catheter urine specimen.

✓ **CA-ASB**
- Catheter-associated asymptomatic bacteriuria: Presence of >10⁵ CFU/mL of ≥1 bacterial species in a single-catheter urine sample without symptoms and signs compatible with UTI.

Clinical Features and Diagnosis

Urinary tract infections may be divided into lower urinary tract infections (**e.g. cystitis**) or upper urinary tract infections (**e.g. pyelonephritis**).

✓ **Cystitis**
- Infections limited to the bladder and urethra.
- Local symptoms, like frequency, dysuria, but rarely systemic symptoms, like fever.
- **Urinalysis for pyuria**
  ❖ Pyuria ≥10 WBCs/μL.

- ❖ Absence of pyuria has a great negative predictive effect, and its absence suggests against a diagnosis of CAUTI unless the patient is neutropenic.
- ❖ Presence of pyuria is non-specific, as this can be caused by the urinary catheter itself or CAUTI.
- **Urine dipstick test**
  ❖ Urine shows positive dipstick results for **leucocyte esterase**, which is an enzyme released by lysed WBCs and **nitrites**^Q in the urine are due to ability of Gram-negative bacteria (*E. coli*) to convert nitrates into nitrites. Around 10% of bacteria (*Enterococci* and *Pseudomonas*) can't produce nitrites and, hence, won't be positive by this method.
- Cystitis is very rarely a cause of septic shock, and other causes of shock should be evaluated in patients with haemodynamic instability.

✓ **Acute Pyelonephritis**
- Costovertebral angle tenderness, bacteraemia, and septic shock.
- In contrast to cystitis, urinalysis, and urine cultures, it is recommended for all cases of suspected pyelonephritis.
- If the Foley catheter is dysfunctional and not draining smoothly, or finding a distended bladder, there is a high risk of pyelonephritis.
- The Foley catheter should be replaced prior to obtaining a urine culture as bacterial growth within the Foley catheter can contaminate it.
- **Complications of pyelonephritis** are acute renal failure, renal or perinephric abscess, psoas abscess, kidney stones, and emphysematous pyelonephritis.

✓ **Candiduria**
- Quantitative cultures with >10³ CFU/mL in a catheterized patient or >10⁴ CFU/mL in a non-catheterized patient is considered clinically significant.
- Fungus ball within urinary collecting system, papillary necrosis, fungal casts in the urine, or renal abscess in the presence of candiduria are considered clinically significant.
- In medically stable patients without major immunocompromised states, simple removal of an indwelling catheter without

specific antifungal therapy may be an acceptable therapy.
- For multisite colonization, candidemia, or upper urinary tract involvement by ultrasound, antifungal treatment is warranted.

✓ **Renal Ultrasonography**
- Rapid method of detecting hydronephrosis.

✓ **CT Scan**
- Contrast-enhanced CT scan gives better anatomic definition of the kidney and perirenal tissues and is the preferred imaging method for complicated UTIs.

✓ **MRI Scan**
- Best for psoas abscess[Q].

Prevention and Treatment

✓ **Prevention**
- Catheter-associated asymptomatic bacteriuria isn't associated with increased mortality in critically ill patients and hence shouldn't be treated whether an indwelling catheter is present or not.
- However, asymptomatic bacteriuria should be treated in pregnant women, patients undergoing endourological procedures with mucosal trauma, and immunocompromised patients.
- **Isolated pyuria with asymptomatic bacteriuria is also not an indication for antimicrobial treatment.**
- Urinary collection bag should not be allowed to be elevated above the urinary bladder.
- Bladder irrigation and washouts should not be used to prevent catheter-associated infection.
- *Intermittent catheterization and condom catheters as compared to indwelling urinary catheters have no mortality benefit.*

✓ **Medical Treatment**
- **Septic shock: Empirical antibiotic treatment should be started with monotherapy** with a third-generation cephalosporin, or carbapenem or β-lactam/β-lactamase inhibitor should be started for 5–7 d.
- Replace the indwelling catheter if signs of UTI are there.
- Fever alone shouldn't be treated with antibiotics pending additional investigations.

✓ **Surgical Treatment**
- Urgent percutaneous nephrostomy tube placement for urinary drainage for severely septic patients with obstructed urinary collecting systems.
- **Prognosis:** Mortality is 15–25% in patients CAUTI.

NECROTIZING FASCIITIS

Epidemiology and Aetiology: 500 Cases per Year

✓ **Description**
- Severe, rapidly progressive, necrotizing soft tissue infection that involves the fascial planes and the tissues surrounding them. **True surgical emergency[Q].**

✓ **Classification[Q]**
- **Type 1: Polymicrobial (50–70%)**
  - ❖ *Clostridium* bacteria is a common finding.
  - ❖ Seen in elderly and those with comorbidities.
  - ❖ Fournier gangrene is a subtype of type 1 NF.
- **Type 2: Streptococcal group A beta-haemolytic (*Streptococcus pyogenes*/*S. aureus*)**
  - ❖ *Streptococcus*: Pairs or chain.
  - ❖ Staphylococcus: Clusters.
- **Type 3: *Vibrio vulnificus***
  - ❖ Seen in upper-extremity trauma in patients with hepatic, renal, or adrenal failure. High mortality.
- **Type 4: Fungal** with *Candida* species.
  - ❖ Rare.

✓ **Pathophysiology**
- Enzymes released by bacteria necrose the hypodermis, thrombose the nutrient vessels. Ischaemia of the nerves leads to hyperesthesia.

Clinical Features and Diagnosis

✓ **Risk Factors**
- Diabetes; age >50 yr; obesity; immunosuppression; chronic liver, renal, or pulmonary disease; malignancy; intravenous drug abuse (IVDA); and *tissue trauma*.

✓ **Fever and Pain**
- Initial features. Pain presents before any physical finding and is disproportionate to clinical findings.
- Lower extremities, perineum, and genitalia are most commonly involved.
- Bullae, crepitus, and skin necrosis develop over time.

- Spread at the level of subcutaneous fat and deep fascia compared to cellulitis, where infection is between dermis and superficial fascia.
- Can quickly progress to septic shock[Q] and multiorgan failure.

✓ **Leucocytosis, Coagulopathy, Thrombocytopaenia, Hypocalcaemia**
- Sequestration in fat necrosis.

✓ **Plain X-ray**
- May show air within subcutaneous tissue and musculature with oedema.
- **CT scan** can help in diagnosis but shouldn't delay it. **MRI** is the most sensitive imaging modality, but it is often the most efficient.

✓ **Laboratory Risk Indicator for Necrotizing Fasciitis (LRINEC)[Q]**
- Scoring system that has been used, and a score ≥6 is very suggestive of necrotizing fasciitis and differentiates it from cellulitis.
- Includes Hb, WBCs, CRP, glucose, sodium, and creatinine.

Treatment[Q]

✓ **Aggressive Resuscitation Using ABCDE Approach**

✓ **Wide Surgical Excision**
- Most important treatment. Debridement later than 24 h is considered to be delayed surgical intervention.
- Multiple visits are often needed. Skin grafts may be needed later on.

✓ **Empirical Antibiotic Treatment**
- *Piperacillin/tazobactam* plus *clindamycin or linezolid* **(both reduce toxin production)**[Q] plus *vancomycin* (MRSA coverage) is the initial treatment.
- IVIG[Q] has been used to neutralize the exotoxins by *Clostridium* and beta-haemolytic *Streptococcus* but is not a widely accepted option.

✓ **Negative Pressure Wound Therapy**
- Has been used to decrease time to complete wound healing.
- **Hyperbaric oxygen:** No mortality benefit. Helpful for anaerobic infections.

Prognosis: Mortality rate of up to 40%

Ludwig's Angina

✓ **Ludwig's Angina**
- Rare and life-threatening, rapidly progressive, gangrenous cellulitis of the floor of the mouth, jaw, and neck.

✓ **Causes**
- Dental abscess, mandibular fracture, submandibular sialadenitis.
- **Bacteria involved:** *Streptococcus pyogenes, Staphylococcus aureus, Prevotella, Fusobacterium.*

✓ **Risk Factors**
- Diabetes mellitus, chronic alcohol abuse, IV drug abuse, HIV/AIDS, malnutrition, recent dental procedures, poor oral hygiene.

✓ **Clinical Features**
- Throat pain, trismus, hot potato voice, dysphagia, fever, tachycardia.

✓ **Complications**
- Airway compromise (laryngeal oedema, secretions), mediastinitis, septic shock.

✓ **Investigations**
- CT neck and face to assess spread of disease.

✓ **Management**
- ENT standby for tracheostomy as distortion of normal anatomy.
- Sit upright.
- Elective awake fibre-optic intubation may be needed.
- Nebulized adrenaline and dexamethasone to decreased oedema.
- Broad-spectrum antibiotics.
- Vasopressors for septic shock if present.
- Surgical decompression by maxillofacial surgical team.
- ITU referral for post-operative ventilation.

MENINGITIS

Aetiology

✓ **Meningitis**
- Inflammation of the meninges and subarachnoid space. Acute bacterial meningitis is a **medical emergency**.
- [Q] *Streptococcus pneumoniae* **(Gram-positive diplococci)** is one of the commonest organisms involved in adults.
- *N. meningitidis* type B **(Gram-negative diplococci)** is the most common type in Europe.
- *Haemophilus influenzae infection* has come down due to vaccination and is seen in patients with defects in humoral immunity[Q].
- *Listeria monocytogenes* at extremes of ages[Q], malignancy, alcoholism, and immunocompromised.
- *Staphylococcus epidermidis* and *S. aureus* should be considered in neurosurgical patients[Q].

<3 months[Q]	Group B streptococci • E. coli • Klebsiella • Listeria monocytogenes	Cefotaxime and ampicillin
Children[Q]	Neisseria meningitidis • Haemophilus influenzae • Streptococcus pneumoniae	Ceftriaxone
Adults[Q]	Streptococcus pneumoniae • N. meningitidis (Gram-negative) • S. aureus • Listeria monocytogenes (>50 yr) E. coli (post-trauma or post-neurosurgery)	Ceftriaxone
Overall incidence	• N. meningitidis (22%) • S. pneumoniae (18%) • S. aureus (10%) • Group B streptococci (5%) • E. coli (5%)	Ceftriaxone and ampicillin

✓ **Listeria monocytogenes[Q]**
- Gram-positive bacilli; in elderly, immuno-compromised, or pregnant patients.
- Diarrhoea can be a presenting symptom. Blood cultures positive in 30–35% of cases.
- Flagellar-driven tumbling motility pattern[Q] in mounts of CSF.

✓ **Nosocomial Meningitis**
- Around 0.4% of all hospital infections. Gram-negative organisms, coagulase-negative staphylococcal, *Staphylococcus aureus.*

✓ **Aseptic Meningitis[Q]**
- When bacteria can't be isolated. Most commonly *enterovirus and coxsackievirus.*
- HSV-1, HSV-2 (20–40 yr), HIV, measles, mumps, and influenza are other viruses involved.
- Viral disease is mostly acute and less severe and resolves spontaneously.

✓ **Other Infectious Causes**
- **Fungal:** *Cryptococcus, Coccidioides, Histoplasma.*
- **Parasite:** Malaria, trypanosomiasis, schistosomiasis.

Clinical Features and Diagnosis

✓ **Risk Factors**
- **Inadequate level of antibodies** (extremes of ages and acquired immunodeficiencies).

- **Opsonophagocytic deficiencies** (asplenia, diabetes, or alcoholism) are the most common risk factors for meningitis.

✓ **Signs and Symptoms**
- **Triad:** Fever, meningism (headache, stiff neck), altered mental status.
- Seizures, focal neurological deficits (sensorineural deafness), *SIADH[Q]* are also seen.
- A thorough ear, nose, and throat examination can reveal possible foci, seen commonly with **streptococcal aetiology.**
- **Petechiae and purpura suggest meningococcal disease.**

✓ **Complications of Bacterial Meningitis[Q]**
- Cerebral venous sinus thrombosis and hydrocephalus.

✓ **Waterhouse Friedrichsen Syndrome**
- Haemorrhagic adrenalitis in fulminant meningococcaemia.
- More common in paediatric age group. DIC is common and is a predictor of high risk along with rapidly progressive rash.
- Can happen with *Streptococcus pneumoniae* as well.

✓ **Lumbar Puncture**
- CT scan isn't essential to rule out raised ICP, and raised ICP can be excluded clinically (focal neurological deficits, seizures, papilloedema, low GCS)[Q].

✓ **CSF Analysis in Meningitis**
- CSF glucose, protein, cell count with differential, Gram stain, and bacterial culture.
- **CSF PCR**
  ❖ Pneumococcus, meningococcus, HSV, VZV, EBV, CMV.
  ❖ HSV PCR[Q] may be repeated after 3–7 d if negative.
- Autoimmune encephalitis panel, oligoclonal bands, cytology.
- Some typical scenarios seen in meningitis:
  ❖ **Basal exudate/hydrocephalus:** TB meningitis. A normal CSF may be seen.
  ❖ **Raised CSF lactate:** Bacterial meningitis.
  ❖ **Fungal meningitis:** Moderately elevated CSF lymphocyte count of 200 cells/μL, raised protein, and low glucose. Commonest cause is crypto-coccal[Q] and occurs in immunocompromised patients.

Finding	Normal	Bacterial	Viral	TB	Fungal
Opening pressure	<20 cm H_2O	High	Normal/high	High	Very high
Colour	Clear	Cloudy/turbid	Clear	Yellow/cloudy	Clear/cloudy
Glucose mmol/L	2.5–3.5, 2/3 blood glucose	<40% of blood glucose	Normal	<30% of blood glucose	Low-normal
Protein (g/L)	0.18–0.45	>1	<1	>1	>0.5
WBCs/microlitre	0–5	100–50,000	<1,000	25–500	0–1,000
Type of WBCs	N/A	Neutrophils	Lymphocytes	Lymphocytes	Lymphocytes

✓ **Blood Cultures**
- About 60–90% of patients will have an organism isolated by culture. Gram stain positivity in 50–75% of patients.

✓ **Blood Investigations**
- PCR for pneumococcus, meningococcus, and HIV screen.
- **Cryptococcal antigen assay** in both serum and CSF should be done in immunocompromised and cirrhotic patients[Q].

✓ **Urine**
- For pneumococcus antigen.

✓ **CT and MRI Brain**
- Mainly to evaluate complications of meningitis. Rapid deterioration should lead to consideration of subdural empyema[Q].

Prevention and Treatment

✓ **Prevention**
- Babies in the UK receive a meningitis B and C vaccine.
- Teenagers get a **meningococcal ACWY vaccine**.

✓ **ABCDE Approach**
- Up to 50% of patients with meningitis will require intubation because of altered mental status.
- Other causes of ICU admission are septic shock, seizures, and management of raised intracranial pressure.
- *Lumbar puncture and blood cultures* within 1 h if safe to do so.

✓ **Antibiotics**
- Ceftriaxone/cefotaxime 2 g QDS with ampicillin[Q] for suspected *Listeria* plus acyclovir for covering HSV encephalitis.
- **Vancomycin plus** ceftazidime to provide adequate coverage for MRSA and pseudomonas in post-neurosurgical patients[Q].

Vancomycin is added for resistant pneumococcal meningitis[Q]. Meropenem is a good alternative as well.
- **Nosocomial meningitis:** Empiric treatment of vancomycin and Gram-negative cover. If MDR GNBs, duration of therapy from 2 to 3 wk.
- *Intrathecal colistin, if used, has to be used along with systemic therapy.*
- *S. pneumoniae* is treated for 10–14 d, while *Haemophilus* or *Meningococci* are treated for 7–10 d, *Listeria* for 21 d, and Gramnegative bacilli for 21 d.
- **Repeat LP if clinical instability persists after 48 h.**

✓ **Dexamethasone[Q]**
- Helps in reduction of long-term neurological sequelae and hearing loss[Q] in *S. pneumoniae* and not meningococcal meningitis. Mortality benefit as well. At **0.15 mg/kg** (max 10 mg) QDS in patients over 3 months of age for **4 d.**
- Start steroids in all suspected pneumococcal meningitis patients (IDSA Guidelines), and stop if a pathogen other than **pneumococcus or tuberculosis (along with antitubercular therapy only)**[Q] is isolated.
- Give before the dose of antibiotics to prevent inflammation due to bacterial degradation products.
- Not recommended for children <3 months of age and in meningococcal sepsis[Q].

✓ **Infection Control**
- Respiratory isolation and barrier nursing until diagnosis excluded or the patient has received 24 h of treatment.

✓ **Chemoprophylaxis: Rifampicin**
- Prophylaxis for close contacts of *Haemophilus*; otherwise, **ciprofloxacin** or

ceftriaxone or rifampicin for meningococcal meningitidis.
- Staff members during aerosol generation procedure should also get prophylaxis.
✓ **Prognosis**
- Case fatality rate in pneumococcal meningitis is 20–30%.

Additional Questions

✓ **Raised CSF Protein Causes**[Q]
- Infections
- Guillain–Barré syndrome
- Haemorrhage
- Tumours
- Seizures
- Multiple myeloma
- Multiple sclerosis

ENCEPHALITIS

Aetiology

✓ **Encephalitis**
- *Infection or inflammation of the brain parenchyma.* Aetiology is not identified in over 50% of the cases.
- Encephalopathy[Q]: Non-inflammatory diffuse brain dysfunction – e.g. metabolic causes.

✓ **Causes of Encephalitis**
- **Infection: Viral** (HSV, VZV, HIV, measles, rubella, West Nile virus, Japanese encephalitis, dengue, rabies, zika), **bacterial** (*Mycoplasma*, *Listeria*), **fungal** (*Candida*, *Cryptococcus*), and **parasites** (malaria, toxoplasma).
- **Autoimmune:** Anti-N-methyl-D-aspartate (anti-NMDA) receptor antibody, anti-voltage-gated potassium channel (anti-VKGC) antibody, acute disseminated encephalomyelitis (ADEM), paraneoplastic encephalitis.

✓ **HSV Encephalitis**
- **Commonest cause.** Young children, older people >50 yr, focal neurological deficits, focal seizures, **temporo-frontal** involvement.
- **HSV-1 in 90% cases**[Q], and HSV-2 in 10% cases. HSV persists in the trigeminal region.

✓ **Autoimmune Encephalitis**
- **Anti-N-methyl-D-aspartate receptor (NMDAR) encephalitis**
  ❖ Presents similar to infectious encephalitis and is seen mostly in young women.
  ❖ Half of the patients will have a tumour, most commonly ovarian teratoma.
  ❖ Diagnosis is by detection of anti-NMDAR IgG antibodies in CSF. Tumour should be ruled out[Q].
- **Leucine-rich glioma-inactivated 1 (LG1) antibodies** in people above 50 yr of age.
- CNS vasculitis or sarcoidosis may manifest as acute or subacute encephalitis.
- **Acute disseminated encephalomyelitis (ADEM):** Also known as post-infectious encephalomyelitis. Seen after respiratory illness or vaccination.

Clinical Features and Diagnosis

✓ **Symptoms**
- Febrile illness with **altered cognition behaviour**, personality, or conscious level.
- New seizures or focal neurological deficits, like cranial nerve palsies and hemiparesis.
- *Autoimmune processes present, with more predominance of psychiatric disturbances or movement disorders*[Q].

✓ **Diagnostic Criteria**[Q]
- **Major:** Any patient with **altered mental status** lasting over 24 h with no alternative cause identified.
- **Minor: At least two of the following**
  ❖ Temperature >38°C within 72 h of before and after presentation
  ❖ Seizure not related to previous seizure disorder
  ❖ New focal neurological signs
  ❖ CSF pleocytosis
  ❖ New neuroimaging findings suggestive of encephalitis
  ❖ Abnormal EEG findings

✓ **Diagnosis**
- **Lumbar puncture**
  ❖ Normal or raised opening pressure, clear CSF with slightly raised white cell count (lymphocytes)[Q], normal glucose, and normal or raised protein.
  ❖ **HSV-1/2 PCR** on CSF in all cases. Repeat HSV PCR in 3–7 d if the diagnosis is suspected but first sample is negative.
  ❖ **Enteroviral and VZV PCR of CSF should also be sent in all cases.**
  ❖ CSF EBV, CMV, and HHV-6 can also be sent, but then additional serological testing may be required.

❖ *Oligoclonal bands and abnormal IgG index in CSF are sent in patients with non-infectious aetiologies.*

❖ *Autoimmune antibodies:* Anti-NMDA, anti-VKGC, LG-1, CASPR-2, anti-GABA$_{A/B}$, anti-GAD65, anti-AMPAR.

- **Serological testing**
  ❖ HIV
  ❖ Arboviral encephalitis
- **MRI** *is recommended for all patients with encephalitis (hyperintensity of frontal/temporal areas on T2/FLAIR).*
- **EEG:** Non-convulsive status epilepticus, lateralized periodic discharges, or spikes in temporal regions.

Treatment

✓ **Cover Meningoencephalitis Initially**
- Give acyclovir if suspicion of HSV encephalitis, as untreated HSV encephalitis has mortality of up to 70% compared to properly treated one (30% mortality).
- **Acyclovir dose 10 mg/kg TDS for 14 d.** Acyclovir can cause renal dysfunction, and renal function should be monitored.
- **Foscarnet** is active against HSV if resistance against acyclovir.
- **Ganciclovir or valganciclovir** for CMV infections.
- **Zanamivir** is active against **influenza A and B.**
- Ribavirin to treat RSV infections and hepatitis C.

✓ **Treatment of Immune-Mediated Encephalitis**[Q]
- Steroids.
- Treatment of underlying malignancy.
- *Plasmapheresis and IVIg have been used in such cases.*
- *Rituximab, cyclophosphamide.*

✓ **Supportive Management**
- *Management of cerebral oedema*
  ❖ *3% hypertonic saline: 2–3 mL/kg over 20–30 min*
  ❖ *20% mannitol: 0.5 g/kg*
- *Seizures, including status epilepticus.*

Additional Questions

✓ **Wernicke Encephalopathy**[Q]
- Ophthalmoplegia, ataxia, and confusion due to vitamin B12 deficiency and not due to infections.

CATHETER-RELATED BLOODSTREAM INFECTIONS

Epidemiology and Aetiology

✓ **Healthcare-Associated Infection**[Q]
- Problem which develops as a direct result of medical and surgical interventions.
- Pneumonia (22.8%), catheter-related bloodstream infections (CRBSI), catheter-associated urinary tract infections (CAUTI), surgical site infections (SSI), gastrointestinal infections.

✓ **Central Line**
- CDC (Centers for Disease Control and Prevention) defines it as an intravascular catheter that terminates at close to the heart or in one of the great vessels that is used for infusion, withdrawal of blood, or haemodynamic monitoring.
- Arterial lines, IABP devices are not considered a central line as per CDC.
- Arterial lines are considered central lines as per ECDC (European Centre for Disease Prevention and Control).

✓ **Coagulase-Negative *Staphylococci***[Q]
- Most common organism causing CRBSI.

✓ **Catheter-Related Bloodstream Infections (CRBSI)**
- Seen in 16% of patients with CVC inserted.
- Dialysis catheters have the highest chance of infections, and femoral vein site forms the sites with the highest chance.

✓ **Short-Term Catheter (<30 d)**
- Organisms gain entry from the insertion sites.

✓ **Long-Term Catheter (>30 d)**
- Organisms gain entry after contamination of the catheter hub and, ultimately, the internal lumen of the catheter.

✓ **Central Line–Associated Bloodstream Infections (CLABSI)**
- It's a definition used by CDC for surveillance purposes. Bloodstream infections (BSI) occurring in an inpatient who has a central line present for more than 2 d without an alternative source are known as CLABSI. Some BSI may be due to other sources, like pancreatitis, and hence might not be easily identified. Therefore, CLABSI overestimates the true incidence of CRBSI.

Clinical Features and Diagnosis

✓ **Criteria for Diagnosis of a CRBSI[Q]**
  - Clinical signs (at least one out of fever >38°C, chills, or hypotension).
  - No other apparent source of infection.
  - Positive peripheral blood culture.
  - At least one of the following:
    ❖ **Positive culture from the *CVC tip*** with the same organism as peripheral culture and signs of infection at the line site (semi-quantitative >15 CFU/catheter segment or quantitative >10³ CFU/catheter segment).
    ❖ Simultaneous **quantitative cultures of blood samples** with a ratio of ≥3:1 (*CVC hub* vs peripheral), ≥5:1 as per ECDC.
    ❖ **Differential time to positivity[Q]:** When blood from the CVC shows microbiological growth at least 2 h earlier than growth in blood collected simultaneously from a peripheral vein.
    ❖ Positive culture with the **same organism from pus** from the insertion site.

✓ **Paired Quantitative Blood Culture**
  - Has greater sensitivity and specificity than differential time to positivity[Q].

✓ **Local CVC-Related Infection**
  - No positive peripheral blood culture; semi-quantitative >15 CFU/catheter segment or quantitative >10³ CFU/catheter segment AND pus/inflammation at the insertion site.
  - **Local signs** at site of insertion are warmth, erythema, and pain at the site.
  - Isolating microorganisms from a catheter tip culture in an asymptomatic patient is not indicative of infection, and sometimes, local findings might just be signs of phlebitis.

✓ **General CVC-Related Infection**
  - No positive peripheral blood culture; semi-quantitative >15 CFU/catheter segment or quantitative >10³ CFU/catheter segment AND **clinical signs** that improve within 48 h after catheter removal.

✓ **2D Ultrasound Imaging for CVC Insertion into IJV**
  - Recommended by NICE for all elective conditions. The landmark technique can still be used in emergency.

  - In adults, use of femoral CVC has greatest risk of infection and deep vein thrombosis. Subclavian lines have lowest risk.
  - In children, risk of infection with femoral route is as much as other routes and, hence, is the preferred route.

✓ **Peripherally Inserted Central Venous Catheter (PICC) Line[Q]**
  - Less risk of CRBSI in outpatients, but infection risk is similar for hospitalized patients.
  - Avoids pneumothorax, haemothorax, arterial bleeding.
  - Basilic vein is used. It runs on the medial side of the arm closer to the median nerve. Basilic vein becomes axillary vein as it moves up in the arm and is joined by cephalic vein at an acute angle, making cannulation of cephalic vein difficult for PICC line insertion.
  - Complications include venous thrombosis, tip migration.

✓ **Arterial Catheters**
  - Indwelling arterial catheters have rates of complications like that of venous catheters.
  - Distal embolic lesions and haemorrhage are highly suggestive of arterial catheter–associated bloodstream infection.

Treatment

✓ **Start Empirical Treatment**
  - In a patient with fever in whom CRBSI is suspected.
  - Gram-positive cocci should be covered (**vancomycin**), and Gram-negative bacilli may be covered based on local epidemiology.
  - In patient with risk factors for candidemia, an antifungal, preferably an echinocandin, should be used.
  - **Antibiotics duration:** 1 wk once catheter removed, 2 wk if uncomplicated *S. aureus* or fungus.

✓ **Before CVC Removal**
  - Even if fever is there, exclude other causes of fever before removing CVC.
  - *S. aureus* can cause aortic valve or mitral valve endocarditis, and *Candida* can cause endophthalmitis.
    ❖ **Transthoracic echocardiography** is recommended in all cases of catheter-associated *S. aureus* bacteraemia.

❖ **Antifungal treatment** should be used to treat all patients with catheter-associated fungemia, and retinal examination should be done by an ophthalmologist.

- Blood culture results with coagulase-negative *Staphylococcus* are considered clinically significant if present in **more than one bottle** and are rapidly growing in culture. Cultures should be repeated again to establish bloodstream infection if single blood sample is positive with coagulase-negative staphylococcus.

✓ **Catheter Removal**
- Catheters in which insertion site is erythematous, is painful, has gross purulence, or is indurated should be removed as soon as possible.
- In patients presenting with fever and who are clinically stable, without the localizing signs of infections, catheter should be removed only after sending microbial cultures.
- **Removal of non-tunnelled catheters** in **all complicated infections** (thrombosis, endocarditis, and osteomyelitis) **and** in infections caused by *S. aureus*, enterococcus, Gram-negative bacilli, and *Candida* species is highly recommended.

✓ **Catheter Salvage**
- **Catheter may be retained if infection with coagulase-negative *Staphylococcus*** is there, provided systemic antibiotics are given along with antibiotic lock therapy. Lock therapy involves instilling 2–5 mL of antibiotics in a catheter until the catheter is used.
- In case of tunnelled catheters or for patients with limited vascular access, treatment of catheter-associated infection with antibiotics without catheter removal may be tried.
- **Catheter salvage is not recommended** for patients with complicated infections, infection in tunnel of tunnelled line, severe sepsis, or an implanted intravascular device.
  ❖ In patients with *S. aureus*, *Pseudomonas*, or *Candida* infection, risk associated with salvage is very high, and catheter removal is highly recommended.

✓ **CVC Placement**
- New CVC placement should be delayed until at least 48 h after the first negative blood culture unless there is an urgent need for it.

✓ **Impregnated Catheters**
- Catheters impregnated with antimicrobials[Q] (chlorhexidine/silver sulfadiazine) or antibiotics (minocycline/rifampicin) are associated with a decrease in catheter-related bacteraemia and are recommended by CDC for patients requiring catheters for >5 d.

✓ **CVC with Minimum Number of Ports**
- CVC with minimum number of ports required should be used.

Additional Questions

✓ **Thoracic Duct Injury**
- Associated with left subclavian CVC insertion[Q].
- Subclavian vein: Avoid in dialysis patients due to chances of stenosis. But it has got least chances of infection.

✓ **IJV**
- A continuation of sagittal sinus and has a valve just before its junction with the subclavian vein in the root of the neck.

✓ **Persistent Left-Sided Superior Vena Cava (PLSVC)[Q]**
- Occurs in 1 in 200 healthy individuals. The right side should ideally be used, but the left could still be used.
- Utmost care must be taken during insertion because the risk of arrhythmias is high due to proximity of the coronary sinus. It is a low-flow site and is unsuitable for use for haemofiltration.
- Most of the left-sided SVCs empty into the coronary sinus, but left-sided SVCs can drain directly into the left atrium, bypassing the pulmonary circulation.

✓ **Lemierre's Disease[Q]**
- Caused by *Fusobacterium necrophorum* (Gram-negative anaerobe). Thrombophlebitis of IJV. Antibiotics for 2–6 wk + anticoagulation.

FEBRILE NEUTROPAENIA

Epidemiology and Aetiology

✓ **Febrile Neutropaenia[Q]**
- Fever >38°C in a patient with neutrophil count <500 cells/μL or expected to drop

<500 cells/µL in the next 48 h. It's a **medical emergency**[Q].

- Prolonged neutropaenia: >7 d, bad prognosis.
- Neutropaenia: Absolute neutrophil count <1,500 cells/µL.
- Severe neutropaenia: Absolute neutrophil count <500 cells/µL.
- Profound neutropaenia: <100 cell/µL, bad prognosis.
- Lymphopaenia: Less than 600 cells/µL.

✓ **Microorganisms**
- About 80% of infections are due to endogenous source of infection (gut and skin) (e.g. aerobic Gram-positive and Gram-negative bacteria that live on the skin and within gut).
- *Staphylococcus epidermidis* is the most common pathogen.
- Fungal infections like *Candida* and *Aspergillus* are common when the duration of neutropaenia increases.

Clinical Features

✓ **Fever in Neutropaenia**
- Seen in 5–10% of solid tumour patients receiving **cytotoxic therapy**, 20–25% of non-leukemic haematological malignancy, and up to 95% of acute leukaemic patients.

✓ **Risk Factors**
- **High risk of infection:** *Mucositis*, unstable haemodynamics, gastrointestinal symptoms, intravascular catheter.
- **Low risk of infection:** Solid organ transplantation, <500 cells/µL for <7 d.

✓ **Respiratory Failure**
- Most common cause of admission to ITU. **Bacterial pneumonia** is the most common cause.
- Fever and shortness of breath tend to be common symptoms. Cough and sputum production are often absent.

✓ **Mucositis**
- Increases the risk of infections of the sinuses, oropharynx, and gastrointestinal tract.
- **Invasive fungal sinusitis** has high morbidity and mortality.
- GIT: Typhlitis[Q] (neutropenic enterocolitis affecting ileocaecum and ascending colon), anorectal cellulitis, fasciitis, abscess, necrotizing colitis, and *C. difficile*–associated colitis.

✓ **Fungal Infections**
- Disseminated candidiasis presents as bloodstream infection.
- Hepatosplenic candida abscesses may be subtle and diffuse and difficult to detect.

Diagnosis

✓ **Microbiological Cultures**
- Positive for bacteria in less than 40% of febrile episodes.
- **BAL *Galactomannan*** has a positive predictive value near 100% for invasive pulmonary aspergillosis.
- **β-D-glucan** has been shown to be more sensitive than blood culture for diagnosis of deep *Candida* infections and *Pneumocystis jirovecii*.

✓ **Specimen**
- BAL fluid: Bacterial/fungal/mycobacterial/*Nocardia*/*Legionella* **culture**; **PCR** for *Nocardia*/CMV/*Mycoplasma*/SARS-CoV-2/*Pneumocystis jirovecii*; **cytology**; **and** *Galactomannan*.
- **Urine:** Antigen for *Legionella*, *Histoplasma*, *Blastomyces*.
- **Blood:** *Galactomannan*, β-D-glucan, bacterial cultures, CMV PCR.
- **Nasal swab:** PCR for MRSA/MSSA.

Treatment

✓ **Empirical Broad-Spectrum Antibiotics**
- For all patients with fever >38°C and absolute neutrophil count less than 500/µL or less than 500/µL and falling even in the absence of documented infections.

✓ **Neutropenic Patient with Stable Haemodynamics**
- Single anti-pseudomonal therapy (piperacillin/tazobactam) should be enough.
- For patients with septic shock, a second agent against Gram-negative (**aminoglycoside** or fluoroquinolone) and an agent against MRSA (**vancomycin**) may be added.
- Consider adding **metronidazole** for suspected intra-abdominal source or *Clostridium difficile* infection.
- **Mucositis, previous trimethoprim/sulfamethoxazole use, fever >40°C, or skin infections:** Add Gram-positive-coverage antibiotic (vancomycin).

- **Antifungal therapy (voriconazole vs liposomal amphotericin B)** is added if no improvement in first 5 d.
- Antiviral agent if skin lesions suggestive of HSV or VZV or active influenza or Covid-19 are identified in the community.

✓ **Tunnelled Lines**
- Can be left initially as source of infection is mostly gut. In cases not responsive to initial therapy, with high suspicion of line infection, known line colonization, or tunnel infection, then indwelling lines should be removed.

✓ **Granulocyte Colony-Stimulating Factor**
- Can be used. However, they may not help in overcoming infection developing during neutropaenia in the critically ill patient.

Prognosis

✓ **Mechanical Ventilation**
- Need of mechanical ventilation for respiratory failure: Poor prognosis.

✓ **Immunocompromised Patients**
- Immunocompromised patients requiring intensive care unit have high mortality rates between 44 and 74%.

FUNGAL INFECTIONS

Epidemiology

✓ **Fungi**
- Slow-growing eukaryotes. **Cell walls** contain chitin, mannan, and glucan. **Cell membranes** contain ergosterol instead of cholesterol.
- *Candida* and *Aspergillus* are the commonest fungal infections in ICU.
- *Candida albicans* is the most common cause of fungal disease.

✓ **Classification of Fungi**
- **Moulds (hyphae):** *Aspergillus, Zygomycetes*
- **Yeasts (round cells):** *Candida, Cryptococcus*
- **Dimorphic:** *Histoplasma, Blastomyces, Coccidioides*

✓ **Risk Factors for Fungal Infections**[Q]
- Trauma, burns, malignancy, parenteral nutrition, central venous catheters, renal replacement therapy, peritoneal dialysis, upper GI surgery, PPIs, broad-spectrum antibiotics, cystic fibrosis, IV drug abuser, heart valves, immunosuppression.

Candida

✓ *Candida albicans, Candida parapsilosis, Candida glabrata, Candida krusei.*

✓ **Candidiasis**
- **Superficial candidiasis:** Mucous membranes or skin.
- **Invasive candidiasis:** Haematogenous spread (candidemia) to heart (endocarditis), liver, spleen, brain, and eyes (endophthalmitis). It can cause intra-abdominal abscesses.
  - ❖ Non-*albicans* species are associated with worse outcomes.
  - ❖ *Candida parapsilosis:* CVC catheter. Azoles are drug of choice.

✓ **Diagnosis**
- *Candida* in sputum and urine is mostly colonizer.
- **Candiduria:** >10^5 CFU/mL in two urine specimens taken before and after change of a urinary catheter in a patient with signs of sepsis may indicate *Candida* as the aetiology.
- Recovery of *Candida* from two or more otherwise-sterile sites (excluding urine and sputum) along with leucocytosis may indicate towards *Candida* sepsis.
- **Serum 1,3 beta-D-glucan:** Cell wall polysaccharide biomarker for both infective candidiasis and aspergillosis.
- **Serum mannan/anti-mannan assays** can also be used.

Aspergillus

✓ **Aspergillosis**
- *Aspergillus fumigatus, Aspergillus niger, Aspergillus flavus.*
- **Allergic bronchopulmonary aspergillosis (ABPA)**
  - ❖ In long-standing *asthma*, bronchiectasis, or cystic fibrosis.
  - ❖ Steroids used for acute exacerbations.
- **Aspergilloma**
  - ❖ Fungus ball affecting patients with *pre-existing cavities.*
  - ❖ Surgical debridement in high-risk patients with life-threatening haemoptysis.

- **Chronic necrotizing aspergillosis:** Affects patients with history of *chronic lung disease*, like COPD, sarcoidosis, tuberculosis.
- **Invasive pulmonary aspergillosis**
  - ❖ Seen in *immunocompromised patients*. Dense, well-circumscribed lesion with or without **halo sign, air-crescent sign**, cavity in CT scan. Sinusitis can be seen.
  - ❖ Antifungal drugs form the mainstay of treatment.

✓ **Presentation**
- Fever, cough, dyspnoea, haemoptysis, pseudoaneurysms.

✓ **Diagnosis**
- Presence of *Aspergillus* in respiratory washings alone cannot distinguish between colonization and true infection. Results should be interpreted in context of clinical picture.
- Chest CT scan can help in diagnosis.
- **Serum/BAL *Galactomannan*:**
  - ❖ Highly sensitive for neutropenic patient with **invasive aspergillosis**.
  - ❖ Low sensitivity in solid organ transplant patients. Helps in follow-up of fungal therapy.

Cryptococcus neoformans

✓ Infection in immunocompromised.

✓ **Pulmonary Cryptococcosis**
- Nodules, hilar lymphadenopathy, pleural effusions.

✓ **Cryptococcal Meningoencephalitis**
- Develops slowly over weeks and presents with non-specific neurological symptoms, like headache, cranial nerve palsies, meningeal irritation, and reduced consciousness.
- Diagnosed by microscopy/culture of CSF.

Zygomycetes

✓ Mucormycosis in uncontrolled diabetic patients. Affects sinuses, skin, brain, lungs, and gastrointestinal tract.

✓ **Angio-Invasion and Disseminated Infection**
- Cornerstone of the disease.
- Treatment is prompt surgical debridement with antifungal therapy.

Blastomyces

✓ Thermally dimorphic fungi and causes self-limiting pneumonia and haematogenous spread to liver, bones, joints, brain, or skin in immuno-compromised individuals.

Histoplasma

✓ Thermally dimorphic fungi that can cause **cavitating pulmonary disease** similar to tuberculosis.

Pneumocystis jirovecii

✓ Explained in section on HIV.

Treatment

✓ **Antifungal Prophylaxis**[Q]
- Acute liver failure, upper GI perforation/surgery, neutropaenia, immunosuppression following solid organ transplant and HIV with low CD4 count.

✓ **Invasive Candida in Blood with *Unstable Haemodynamics/Neutropaenic Patients*[Q]**
- **Echinocandins are treatment of choice.** Start antifungals immediately even if patient is having stable haemodynamics. In uncomplicated patients[Q] and in patients with no azole exposure, fluconazole can be used.
- Indwelling catheter should be removed in non-neutropaenic patients. Neutropaenic patients may have a different source, so decide on a case-to-case basis in them.
- **Ophthalmology review**[Q] (**fundoscopy will show cotton wool ball changes**) for endophthalmitis, **echocardiography**[Q] for fungal endocarditis.
- Renal ultrasound[Q] only if concomitant candiduria.

✓ **Candida in Sputum (Yeasts)**
- Colonization, so antibiotic only in specific cases, like immunosuppressed, multifocal colonization.

✓ **Candiduria**
- Take out Foley's catheter. Start antifungal only in specific cases (neutropenic, recurrent multifocal).

✓ **Invasive Aspergillosis (Septate Hyphae)**
- Voriconazole is treatment of choice[Q]. If contraindicated, liposomal amphotericin B is second line of drug. Posaconazole can be given for prophylaxis for at-risk patients.

✓ **Cryptococcal Infection**
- A 2 wk treatment of amphotericin B plus flucytosine (acts intracellularly) followed by 8 wk on fluconazole.

✓ **Histoplasmosis**
- Amphotericin B for severe cases, and itraconazole in mild cases.

✓ **Unspecified Invasive Filamentous Fungal Infection**
- Amphotericin B (renal dysfunction).

✓ **Amphotericin B + Flucytosine**
- For endocarditis and meningitis.

✓ **Zygomycosis (Mucor)**
- Amphotericin B + posaconazole.

✓ **Blastomycosis**
- Fluconazole.

Antifungal Drugs[Q]

✓ **Triazoles**
- Inhibits lanosterol 14-alpha demethylase and, hence, ergosterol synthesis[Q] and therefore inhibits cell membrane.
- **Fluconazole**
  - ❖ Active against most *Candida* species, but not *Aspergillus*.
  - ❖ Oral fluconazole has 90% bioavailability. Good CSF penetration.
  - ❖ Dose adjustment needed in renal impairment.
  - ❖ **Side effects:** Liver dysfunction, QT prolongation, and cytochrome P450 inhibition[Q].
- **Itraconazole**
  - ❖ Broad-spectrum antifungal active against both *Candida* and *Aspergillus*. Available for oral use and can be used for treatment of sporotrichosis, blastomycosis, and histoplasmosis.
  - ❖ Poor CSF penetration. No dose adjustment required in renal and hepatic impairment.
  - ❖ Itraconazole has a steroid-sparing effect in ABPA[Q].
  - ❖ **Side effects:** Mineralocorticoid excess effect[Q], liver dysfunction, and QT prolongation.
- **Voriconazole:**
  - ❖ Treatment of choice against *Aspergillus*[Q]. Active against *C. krusei* and *C. glabrata*.
  - ❖ Available as oral and IV formulation. Dose adjustment needed in hepatic disease.
  - ❖ **Side effects:** Hepatotoxicity, QT prolongation, transient ocular toxicity, visual and auditory hallucinations.

- ❖ IV voriconazole is a cyclodextrin and can cause nephrotoxicity, but dose adjustment is not required.
- **Posaconazole**
  - ❖ Oropharyngeal candidiasis resistant to itraconazole and fluconazole. Approved for prophylaxis for invasive *Aspergillus* and *Candida* infections in patients at risk of fungal infections, like stem cell transplant recipients and neutropaenic patients with haematologic malignancies.
  - ❖ Available as delayed-release oral and IV formulation.
  - ❖ IV posaconazole is a cyclodextrin and can cause nephrotoxicity, but dose adjustment is not required in both hepatic and renal impairment.
  - ❖ **Side effects:** Liver dysfunction, QT prolongation, and cytochrome P450 inhibition, like fluconazole.
- **Isavuconazole**
  - ❖ Treatment of invasive aspergillosis and mucormycosis.
  - ❖ Available as oral and IV formulation (non-cyclodextrin).
  - ❖ Dose adjustment is not required in both hepatic and renal impairment.
  - ❖ Causes QT shortening.

✓ **Polyenes (amphotericin B)**
- Binds ergosterol in the fungal cell membrane and makes the wall porous.
- Effective against most species of fungi pathogenic to humans.
- Drug of choice for empiric therapy of life-threatening invasive fungal infections, like mucormycosis, cryptococcosis, histoplasmosis, and coccidioidomycosis.
- Non-*albicans Candida* are less susceptible to it.
- Poor CSF penetration, so intrathecal injection or use of triazoles may be necessary.
- Liposomal formulations have reduced incidence of nephrotoxicity.
- **Side effects**
  - ❖ Infusions may cause fever, chills, and rigors. Pretreatment with acetaminophen, hydrocortisone, diphenhydrinate can be done.
  - ❖ Bone marrow suppression. Amphotericin B exhibits dose-limiting

nephrotoxicity, which is usually reversible.

✓ **Echinocandins**
  - *Acts on cell walls. Inhibits glucan cell wall synthesis* by non-competitive inhibition of beta-1,3 d glucan synthesis.
  - Fungicidal against *Candida* but fungistatic against *Aspergillus.*
  - *Empiric therapy for candidemia in ICU.*
  - Only IV formulations are available. Good side effect tolerability.
  - **Caspofungin** is contraindicated in liver dysfunction and should be used with care in pregnancy.
  - **Anidulafungin** requires loading dose and causes liver dysfunction. Can be used for *antifungal prophylaxis in neutropaenic children.*
  - **Micafungin** doesn't require loading dose and can be used for antifungal prophylaxis for patients undergoing stem cell transplant.
✓ **Flucytosine**
  - *Inhibits DNA/RNA synthesis.* Oral drug generally used in combination with amphotericin for *Cryptococcus* and *Candida* meningitis.
  - Dose adjustment needed in renal impairment. Leucopaenia is most serious side effect.
✓ **Griseofulvin**
  - Inhibits cell mitosis.
✓ **Terbinafine**Q
  - Inhibits squalene epoxidase. Blocks the biosynthesis of ergosterol, causing fungal cell membrane damage and cell death.

Prognosis

✓ Invasive candidemia can have mortality of 20–40%.
✓ *C. glabrata* can become resistant to azoles. *C. krusei* is always resistant to azoles and polyenes.

VIRAL INFECTIONS

Classification of Human Viruses

✓ **DNA**
  - **Icosahedral:** *Herpesviridae*, hepadnavirus (hepatitis B), adenovirus.
  - **Complex:** Pox virus.
✓ **RNA**
  - **Icosahedral:** Picorna (hepatitis A), flavi (dengue, Zika).
  - **Helical:** Orthomyxovirus, paramyxovirus, coronavirus.
  - **Complex:** Retroviruses.

Opportunistic Infections

✓ These viruses establish a latent infection but can reactivate from latency to produce an infectious virus periodically.
✓ Virus replication is controlled in immunocompetent individuals by the *cell-mediated (T cell) immune response.*
✓ **Herpes Simplex Virus (HSV)**
  - *dsDNA.* Herpesviridae family.
  - Alphaherpesviruses (HSV-1 and 2 and varicella-zoster virus) cause **ballooning of the cells and formation of multinucleated giant cells**, leading to cell death.
  - These viruses can invade and replicate in the nerves and establish latency in **dorsal root ganglia**.
  - Vast majority of primary infections with HSV-1 are **subclinical**. Infections in immunocompetent can present as gingivostomatitis, genital herpes, conjunctivitis, keratitis, encephalitis, and disseminated neonatal HSV infection.
  - In immunocompromised, patients will present with pneumonia, encephalitis, hepatitis, and colitis.
  - **PCR of CSF/lower respiratory tract specimen for HSV will confirm the diagnosis.**
  - Contact precautions are recommended.
  - **Treatment** is with acyclovir.
✓ *Varicella-Zoster Virus (VZV)*
  - dsDNA. Family Herpesviridae. Aerosol transmission.
  - Incubation period is 10–20 d.
  - **Pneumonia** presents 1–6 d after onset of typical rash of **chickenpox**. Encephalitis is a sequela as well.
  - Infection is serious in the *fetus, neonates, adults,* and *immunocompromised.*
  - VZV pneumonia is considered a life-threatening emergency.
  - Diagnosis is by blood, CSF, or BAL **PCR**.
  - Contact precautions are recommended.
  - **Acyclovir** is used for treatment. *Varicella-zoster immunoglobin (VZIG) is*

recommended for susceptible women exposed in the first 20 wk of pregnancy and neonates.

✓ **Epstein–Barr Virus (EBV)**
  - dsDNA virus. Herpesviridae family.
  - These cells are lymphotropic and **infect B cells** and have oncogenic potential.
  - They cause a self-limiting illness called **infectious mononucleosis**[Q] characterized by fever, pharyngitis, headache, malaise, and lethargy.
  - Risk of splenic rupture, and patients should avoid contact sports.
  - Mononuclear spot (heterophile antibody test) is used.
  - Circulating activated cells known as Downey cells[Q].
  - It predisposes patients to the development of **Burkitt's lymphoma and nasopharyngeal carcinoma.**
  - Causes **post-transplant lymphoproliferative disease (PTLD)** in post-transplant population.
  - Diagnosis is by identifying atypical mononuclear in peripheral blood film. **EBV-PCR, IgM, and IgG can be used for diagnosis as well.**
  - Standard universal precautions are recommended.
  - **Corticosteroids** are used in significant neurological involvement, haemolysis, or thrombocytopaenia.

✓ **Cytomegalovirus (CMV)**
  - dsDNA virus. Herpesviridae family.
  - Usually causes an asymptomatic infection (80% of patients have antibodies) and remains latent till reactivation (disease)[Q].
  - **Quantitative PCR detecting viral load**[Q] is done to distinguish between infection and disease.
  - However, cutoff values can be arbitrary, and viral load doesn't correlate with clinical findings[Q].
  - They have an affinity for lymphocytes and monocytes and cause infected cells to become enlarged.
  - Incidence of seropositivity[Q] increases with age, and 90% of people above 80 yr old are positive.
  - Clinically significant CMV disease mostly occurs in immunocompromised patients but can happen in immunocompetent patients as well.

- It can present as pneumonia, hepatitis, colitis, retinitis, meningitis, encephalitis, nephritis, and graft-versus-host disease[Q].
- *Reactivation in the immunocompromised patient is the commonest reason for ICU admission*[Q].
  - ❖ **MC presentation is retinitis in HIV** patients,[Q] whereas donor-positive and recipient-negative transplants have highest incidence of solid organ transplant CMV disease[Q].
  - ❖ **Leucopaenia, lymphocytosis, and thrombocytopaenia are seen.**
- Placental transfer of CMV in 40% of patients after primary CMV infection and congenital CMV can lead to severe brain damage or sensorineural deafness.
- **CMV-PCR and IgG and IgM can be used for diagnosis of infection.** Detection of CMV in damaged tissue is required to confirm CMV end-organ disease.
- Standard universal precautions are recommended.
- Treatment is ganciclovir, valganciclovir, and foscarnet[Q] (resistant cases).

Respiratory Infections

✓ **Patients with Viral Pneumonia**
  - Prone to rapid deterioration. Influenza A and B are most commonly detected organisms.
  - Up to 23% of severe nosocomial pneumonia in adults can be attributed to viral infections. Possibility of viral infections should be considered in immunocompromised patients.
  - **Droplet transmission** occurs with particles >5 μm in diameter and travel less than 3 to 6 ft. Droplet transmission is the most common mode of transmission in respiratory viruses.
    - ❖ **Aerosols** are <5 μm in diameter and travel further. Viruses transmitting by aerosols have high rates of transmissions.
  - Most respiratory viruses start with "influenza-like illness," that is, acute onset of headache, chills, and myalgias, followed by upper respiratory symptoms, like sore throat.
    - ❖ Progression to lower respiratory tract disease happen with cough and

sputum and, ultimately, dyspnoea and tachypnoea.

- Viruses that produce influenza-like illness include respiratory syncytial virus (RSV), **parainfluenza**, adenovirus, and **human metapneumovirus**.
- *Most respiratory viral pneumonias except measles present with lymphopaenia and normal neutrophil counts.*
- PCR on throat, nasal, and tracheal aspirates is recommended for diagnosis.
- Contact and droplet precautions, including single room, is recommended.

✓ **Respiratory Syncytial Virus (RSV)**
- (−) ssRNA. Paramyxoviridae family. Droplet transmission.
- RSV is the most common cause of pneumonia and bronchiolitis in infants. **Older patients >75 yr and immunocompromised patients** are at increased risk.
- **Patients most often have underlying chronic lung disease.**
- Prevention measures include handwashing, barrier methods, isolation or cohorting patients, and rapid RSV screening.
- Diagnosis is by reverse transcription polymerase chain reaction (RT-PCR) test.
- **Palivizumab** has been used in NICUs, and aerosolized **ribavirin**[Q] in immunocompromised patients.

✓ **Influenza Viruses**
- Segmented (−) ssRNA virus. Orthomyxoviridae family. Droplet transmission.
- Four types: A (more severe and pandemic)[Q], B, C (mild disease), and D.
- **Influenza type A virus is further divided based on hemagglutinin (HA) and neuraminidase (NA).**
- **Seasonal**[Q]: Antigenic drift.
- **Pandemic**[Q]: Antigenic shift.
- Fever, headache, dry cough, sore throat, myalgia. Vomiting and diarrhoea are more common in pandemic flu.
- Viral shedding starts before symptoms are apparent. Incubation period is 24–48 h. Viral shedding is for 5 d.
- **Risk factors**[Q]: Age >65 yr, DM, pregnancy, morbid obesity, immunosuppression, chronic disease.
- **Lymphopaenia**, thrombocytopaenia, elevated LDH, creatinine phosphokinase, and creatinine are adverse prognostic factors.

- Chest X-ray shows bilateral infiltrates in lower zones and at least three out of four quadrants involved once the patient is intubated. Consolidation suggests superimposed bacterial pneumonia.
- Secondary bacterial pneumonia is common. *Transthoracic echocardiography is required to rule out myocarditis.*
- **Diagnosis**
  - ❖ RT-PCR test is the preferred diagnostic test. BAL and endotracheal aspirates have better yield than sputum swabs. Nasopharyngeal aspirates in non-intubated patients.
  - ❖ **RT-PCR** and viral cultures are used for diagnosis with high sensitivity (>95%) and specificity (>98–100%). RT-PCR is fastest, with turnover of 4–6 h.
  - ❖ **Immunofluorescence assays (IFAs)** and **rapid antigen testing** are used for screening of infection with >90% specificity. Rapid antigen testing has sensitivity between 20 and 70% compared to 70 and 90% of IFAs, and results of rapid diagnostic tests are available in 30 min.
- **Isolation** in a single room with negative airway pressure and use of PPE for aerosol-generating procedures are highly recommended. All healthcare workers should be vaccinated against the latest strain.
- Surgical masks during routine care and N95 during aerosol-generating procedures.
- **Pandemic flu – Neuraminidase inhibitors**
  - ❖ Oseltamivir, zanamivir. They block release of progeny virus from infected host cells.
  - ❖ **Oral oseltamivir**[Q] is the first-line treatment for pandemic flu. Given in pregnant females as well. Seasonal flu is resistant to oseltamivir.
  - ❖ **Zanamivir**[Q] is available as inhaled and IV form. *Inhaled form is not given in intubated patients because of risk of ventilator dysfunction and death.*
  - ❖ **Peramivir:** IV formulation. Can cause liver dysfunction.
- **Seasonal flu** – adamantanes: *Amantadine and rimantadine (block the M2 ion channel and prevent virion uncoating) are effective*

for seasonal H1N1 influenza strains. They are not effective against pandemic flu (influenza A).

- Symptomatic high-risk patients and patients with respiratory failure should be treated with oseltamivir[Q] to reduce the **length of symptoms** and **death; hence, all hospitalized patients with suspected or documented influenza virus infection should be started as soon as possible on antiviral therapy.**
- Empirical antibiotics should be started, and beta-lactams are the initial choice.
- **Complications:** Encephalitis, Guillain–Barré syndrome, myocarditis, and superimposed bacterial infections. Older patients are more likely to develop complications and require ICU care.

✓ **Adenovirus**
- dsDNA. Family Adenoviridae. Droplet transmission.
- Severe pneumonia, diarrhoea, **haemorrhagic cystitis**, and kerato-conjunctivitis.
- Droplet and contact precautions along with isolation are highly recommended.
- **PCR** on throat, nasal, tracheal aspirate is diagnostic.
- **Cidofovir** is used along with probenecid for treatment.

✓ **Avian Influenza (H5N1)**
- Segmented (−) ssRNA. Orthomyxoviridae family. Origin: Poultry. Droplet transmission and direct contact with birds.
- Incubation period: 2–5 d. **Younger patients (18 yr)** are affected more.
- Pneumonia, watery diarrhoea, and multiorgan failure. High rates of pneumothorax.
- RT-PCR is used for diagnosis.
- Mortality rate is 60%.

✓ **MERS-CoV**
- (+) ssRNA. Coronaviridae family. Origin: Camels. Droplet transmission.
- Incubation period: 5–14 d. **Older males** are affected more. Most patients have comorbidities.
- Presents with fever, myalgias, and cough and deteriorates rapidly into ARDS and septic shock.
- Pneumomediastinum without preceding intubation is a characteristic sign.
- RT-PCR or antigen tests are used for diagnosis.

- **Recombinant interferon β1b and lopinavir/ritonavir** have been associated with reduced mortality.
- Mortality rate is 40%.

Gastrointestinal Infections

✓ **Norovirus**
- (+) ssRNA (positive sense). Caliciviridae group.
- Faecal and vomitus-oral route and causes gastrointestinal infections.
- Low infectious doses, rapid spread, very short incubation period, and survival in human excreta demand rapid control strategies.
- Highly resistant to standard disinfections, and bleach solutions of hydrogen peroxide-based disinfections should be used.
- WHO recommends hand disinfection with an alcohol-based rub with minimum of 60% concentration.
- Diagnosis is usually based on symptoms, and a stool sample can also be used to identify the virus using RT-PCR test.
- No specific treatment. Rehydration therapy.

✓ **Rotavirus**
- (+) dsRNA. Member of Reoviridae group.
- Gastroenteritis in infants and young children.
- Low infectious doses and survival for extensively long periods.
- Contact precautions are advocated and disinfected with >40% alcohols.
- Diagnosis is usually based on symptoms, and a stool sample can also be used to identify the virus using RT-PCR test.
- No specific treatment. Rehydration therapy.

Viral Haemorrhagic Fever

✓ **Zoonotic Infections**
- Life-threatening zoonotic infections. Dengue is the most common infection. Bleeding is an uncommon feature, and they mostly present with **inflammatory multisystem disease**.
- Lassa virus, Lujo virus, hantavirus, Rift Valley fever, yellow fever, Marburg virus, and Ebola virus are other common examples. **Ebola and Marburg viruses present in an identical way.**
- Blood samples of all suspected patients must be considered as highly infectious

and marked as biohazard. **Patients should be isolated.** PPE for healthcare workers is recommended.

- Co-infections with other bacteria are a common finding. Bloodstream infections from bacterial translocation are common.
- Supportive care forms the cornerstone of therapy.

✓ **Ebola Virus**

- (−) ssRNA. Filoviridae family. Host are bats and primates. High virulence. Transmitted by contact of broken skin or mucosal membrane to infected blood or secretions. It persists in semen for years, making Ebola virus disease a sexually transmitted disease.
- **Incubation period:** 2–21 d. Four principal strains known to cause disease to humans: Zaire, Sudan, Bundibugyo, and Tai Forest.
- **Presentation** is with fever and conjunctivitis and progresses to abdominal pain, maculopapular rash, bleeding, and seizures.
  - ❖ Massive fluid losses of up to 10 L/day happen in the form of diarrhoea and vomiting.
  - ❖ Shock and multiorgan failure with hypovolaemia develops between day 7 and 12.
  - ❖ Leucopaenia, thrombocytopaenia, and elevated liver enzymes (AST > ALT).
  - ❖ Liver, kidney, and coagulation system (DIC) are the most commonly affected organs.
  - ❖ Hypokalaemia, hypocalcaemia, and hyponatraemia due to diarrhoea are common features and cause arrhythmias in 50% of patients.
  - ❖ **Rhabdomyolysis is seen, and CK levels are high.**
  - ❖ Despite being classified under haemorrhagic fever, it doesn't present with frank haemorrhage.
- **RT-PCR tests during initial few days.** Lateral flow or loop-mediated isothermal amplification rapid antigen tests are recommended during Ebola outbreaks as screening tests. High sensitivity and specificity. IgM or IgG during later stages.
- **Biosafety level 4 protocols** are used while dealing with patients. Testing is minimized due to infectivity of samples, and point-of-care testing is used as much as possible.

- **Supportive ICU treatment mainly.** Empirical antibiotic and antimalarial therapy are recommended. Fluid resuscitation to prevent rhabdomyolysis-induced acute kidney injury.
- In paediatrics cases <6 yr, crystalloids with 5% dextrose should be given. Overzealous fluid loading should be avoided.
- **FDA-approved therapeutics** are available in market. One is a mixture of three monoclonal antibodies (atoltivimab, maftivimab, and odesivimab-ebgn), and second is a monoclonal antibody (ansuvimab-zykl).
- FDA-approved vaccine (rVSV-ZEBOV) is available in the market.
- Mortality of 40–90% with Zaire and Sudan strain; 25% mortality with Bundibugyo strain.

✓ **Dengue**

- (+) ssRNA. *Flaviviridae* genus. Vector-borne illness caused by four serotypes (DENV-1 to 4). Transmitted by *Aedes aegypti.*
- Infection by one specific subtype gives life-long immunity against that subtype, but not against the rest of the subtypes.
- **Incubation period:** 3–14 d. WHO classifies it in two types:
  - ❖ Dengue fever with or without warning symptoms
  - ❖ Severe dengue
- **Dengue without warning signs:** High fever, chills, severe frontal headache, arthralgia, maculopapular rash over the face, trunk, and flexor sites. Self-limiting.
- **Dengue with warning signs:** Abdominal pain, mucosal bleeding, platelet count <100^Q.
- **Severe dengue:** *Severe plasma leakage,* severe haemorrhagic shock, and severe organ impairment with one of the following: renal failure, hepatic failure, cardiomyopathy, and encephalopathy.
  - ❖ **Leucopaenia^Q and neutropaenia are seen.**
  - ❖ Inflammatory markers are not elevated in proportion to the disease. Mortality of >20%.
  - ❖ Bacterial co-infection is common in severe dengue. They present as bloodstream infections.

- ❖ DEN-2 and DEN-3 are viral subtypes responsible for dengue encephalitis.
- Substantial number of infections are asymptomatic. **Atypical manifestations** are encephalitis, Guillain–Barré syndrome, optic neuritis, hepatitis, pancreatitis, myocarditis, and pericarditis.
- Plasma leakage typically lasts for 24–48 h and resolves spontaneously.
  - ❖ Bleeding may be there, but no coagulopathy (INR is normal).
  - ❖ Transaminitis^Q is seen in 90% of cases.
- **Diagnosis:** RT-PCR has highest sensitivity and specificity in first few days after symptom onset.
  - ❖ NS-1 is non-structural antigen and will appear at day 1–5. NS-1 antigen has sensitivity of 90% for diagnosing primary infection.
  - ❖ IgM antibodies appear around day 6 and stay for up to 3 months. IgG appear after 7–10 d and lasts for months.
  - ❖ In the later phase, during defervescence, IgM and IgG are the diagnostic tests of choice.
- **Treatment:** Supportive treatment forms the pillar of dengue management.
  - ❖ **Fluid resuscitation:** Less systemic inflammation compared to bacterial sepsis, and hence overall lower cumulative fluid requirement. Plasma leakage causes increase in haematocrit. Haemorrhage causes decrease in haematocrit. A narrow pulse pressure may indicate further fluid resuscitation. Hence, haematocrit-guided fluids are given.
  - ❖ **Haemorrhagic complications management:** Most common cause of haemodynamic instability is gastrointestinal haemorrhage. Current recommendations are not to prophylactically transfuse platelets in patients with severe dengue.
- **Paediatrics:** They progress to severe dengue more often. Epistaxis, seizures, oliguria, and hepatomegaly are more common. Children typically require higher amounts of resuscitation fluids.

- Increase mortality in well-nourished patient. No benefit of previous IgG antibodies. Admission platelets have correlations with prognosis.

✓ **Hantavirus**
- (−) ssRNA. Bunyaviridae family. Hosts are rodents. Low virulence. Transmitted by rodent bite.
- Incubation period: 2–3 wk. Can produce both haemorrhagic manifestations and pneumonias.
- Presents with fever, cough, diarrhoea and can have a non-cardiogenic pulmonary syndrome known as **hantavirus cardiopulmonary syndrome (HCPS)**.
- *Haemorrhagic fever with renal syndrome.*
- **ELISA-based anti-hantavirus IgM** helps in diagnosis of HCPS.
- Supportive treatment and **ribavirin.**

Other Viruses

✓ **Measles Virus (Rubeola)**
- (−) ssRNA. Paramyxoviridae. Aerosol and contact transmission.
- Incubation period of 10–14 d.
- Presents with fever, cough, coryza, morbilliform rash, and grey-white lesions on the buccal mucosa (**Koplik's spot**).
- Primary viral pneumonia, secondary bacterial pneumonia, **myocarditis**, and encephalitis can be the sequelae.
- Leucopaenia is seen. Diagnosis is by RT-PCR from throat, urine, and CSF specimen. Serological testing (IgG and IgM) can be used for diagnosis.
- Vitamin A and **ribavirin** are used for treatment.
- Human normal immunoglobin can be given to immunocompetent infants and pregnant females ideally within 72 h of symptoms.

✓ **Mumps Virus**
- (−) ssRNA. Paramyxoviridae family. Droplet transmission.
- Virus replicates in upper respiratory tract and then can disseminate to more distant organs.
- Parotid and testicular swelling can happen. Meningitis and encephalitis are the reasons for ITU admission. **Pancreatitis,**

myocarditis, and **hepatitis** are other notable complications.

- Diagnosis is by RT-PCR of saliva. Serological testing (IgG and IgM) can be used for diagnosis.
- *Treatment is supportive.*

✓ **Chikungunya**
- (+) ssRNA. Togaviridae family. Chikungunya virus causes this mosquito-borne disease. *Aedes aegypti* and *Aedes albopictus* are the vectors.
- **Incubation period is 2–4 d.** Self-limiting. Fever, back pain, symmetrical joint pains, and transient maculopapular rash on trunks and extremities.
- **Neurological manifestations**, like seizures, delirium, and paraplegia, are seen in up to 30% of cases.
- **Myocarditis (10%),** hepatitis, and AKI are seen in few cases.
- **Leucopaenia with lymphocyte predominance is seen. Thrombocytopaenia is rare.**
- PCR tests during initial few days. ELISA-based IgG and IgM during later stages.
- *Supportive treatment is needed.*

Antiviral Drugs

✓ **Acyclovir**
- Nucleoside analogue of guanosine. Prodrug itself.
- Active against HSV and *varicella*-zoster virus, but poor against CMV.
- Drug of choice for HSV encephalitis.
- Dose reduced in impaired renal function.
- **Side effects:** Reversible renal impairment, neurologic reactions like hallucinations.

✓ **Valacyclovir**
- Prodrug of acyclovir. Better oral absorption.
- Used prophylactically in patients undergoing bone marrow or solid organ transplant.
- Dose adjustment needed for renal impairment.
- **Side effects:** Thrombocytopaenia and other side effects of acyclovir.

✓ **Ganciclovir**[Q]
- *Nucleoside analogue of guanosine.* Inhibits viral DNA synthesis. Active against CMV.
- Dose adjustment needed for renal impairment.
- **Side effects:** Myelosuppression like neutropaenia.

✓ **Valganciclovir**
- Prodrug for ganciclovir. More complete absorption.
- Used as prophylaxis for CMV in transplanted patients.
- Dose adjustment needed for renal impairment.

✓ **Cidofovir**
- Inhibits **viral DNA polymerase**. Active against CMV, HSV, and VZV.
- Used for ganciclovir-resistant CMV. Side effect is nephrotoxicity.

✓ **Foscarnet**
- Inhibits viral DNA polymerase of CMV and reverse transcriptase of HIV-1.
- Used for CMV retinitis in AIDS patients. Side effects are nephrotoxicity and metabolic disturbances.

✓ **Oseltamivir**
- *Neuraminidase inhibitor* that inhibits both influenza A and B viruses.
- First line of drug for influenza A. Given by oral route.
- When started within 48 h of onset of symptoms, it can reduce the intensity of influenza infection.
- **Side effects:** Neuropsychiatric events.

✓ **Zanamivir**
- Neuraminidase inhibitor.
- Active against influenza A and B. Can be given inhaled, nebulized, or intravenously. Can cause bronchospasm.

✓ **Baloxavir Marboxil**
- *Polymerase inhibitor.* Third category of anti-influenza drugs apart from neuraminidase inhibitors and adamantanes. It inhibits endonuclease function of viral polymerase.
- Inhibits both influenza A and B viruses. Given by oral route.
- Monotherapy is not recommended for fears of resistance.

Additional Questions

✓ **High-Consequence Infectious Diseases (HICDs)**
- Acute infectious disease characterized by aggressive ability to spread in the community and healthcare settings, difficulty in rapid detection, absence of effective treatment, and high case fatality rate.
- **Contact HCID:** Ebola, Lassa, Marburg virus.
- **Airborne HCID:** MERS, SARS.

CLOSTRIDIUM DIFFICILE

Epidemiology

✓ **Incidence**
- About 20–30% cases of antibiotic-associated diarrhoea. Leading cause of hospital-associated infectious diarrhoea.
- Anaerobic, Gram-positive, spore-forming bacillus. *Most patients are asymptomatic.*
- Faecal-oral transmission.
- Toxin A (enterotoxin): Increases intestinal permeability and fluid secretion.
- Toxin B (cytotoxin): Colonic cell inflammation and death.
- Non-toxigenic strains are non-pathogenic.
- Asymptomatic colonization in 7–26% of acute care facilities and 5–7% of long-term care facilities.

Clinical Features and Diagnosis

✓ *Clostridium difficile* **Infection (CDI)**
- Only diarrhoea with occult blood or mucus in milder cases.
- Clinical diagnosis with laboratory confirmation.
- Pseudomembranes are present in only 50% of cases and are seen in ischaemic colitis and CMV colitis as well.

✓ **Risk Factors**
- Long-term antibiotics (clindamycin/quinolones/penicillin/cephalosporins)[Q], elderly, immunocompromised, gastric acid suppression.
- Even a single dose of broad-spectrum antibiotic can cause CDI in susceptible patients.

✓ **ESCMID (European Society of Clinical Microbiology and Infectious Diseases)**
- Suggests that at least all unformed stool samples (formed stool in case of paralytic ileus) from patients should be tested for CDI.

✓ **Diagnosis**
- Two-step algorithm used for diagnosis.
- **Step 1:** Highly sensitive **NAAT** (nucleic acid amplification test) using polymerase chain reaction (PCR) or **glucose dehydrogenase (GDH)** antigen enzyme immunoassays:
  - ❖ **GDH assay** is a rapid screening test which has high sensitivity but can't differentiate between a toxigenic and a non-toxigenic strain.
  - ❖ "Toxin gene" testing by NAAT; hence, they do not detect the presence of biologically active toxin in stool specimen.
- **Step 2: Highly specific test toxin A/B enzyme immunoassays (toxin EIAs)**
  - ❖ **Toxin EIAs** are specific but not sensitive (33–65%). High-negative predictive value of >95%.
- The most sensitive method for diagnosis is *C. difficile* culture in anaerobic media but has a high 72–96 h turnaround time.

✓ **Toxic Megacolon**
- Seen in ascending or hepatic part of colon, >6 cm in size.
- CT findings are peri-colonic fat stranding, mucosal hyperaemia, oedema, and thickening of haustral folds (**accordion sign**).
- Surgery needed in 80% of patients.

✓ **Recurrence**
- Around 20% of patients with an initial episode will have a recurrence.
- At least 45% of patients with one recurrence will have another recurrence.
- More than 60% with at least two recurrences will have another recurrence.

Prevention and Treatment

✓ **Prevention**
- Early isolation of patient and use of PPE (gloves and aprons). **Handwashing with soap and water and not alcohol gel is beneficial**[Q] (an MCQ repeated so frequently I will get it tattooed).
- Probiotics may reduce rate of *Clostridium difficile*–positive cases but haven't shown any mortality benefit.
- Stop unnecessary antibiotics or proton pump inhibitors.

✓ **Treatment**
- Fluid and electrolyte repletion in case of shock.
- Empirical CDI treatment only in the presence of fulminant infection characterized by shock, ileus, or toxic megacolon.
- Early surgical consultation in severe, complicated *Clostridium difficile* infection and decompression if signs of peritonism or toxic megacolon.

Treatment Classification According to Disease Classification[Q]: NICE Guidelines

Disease Severity	Clinical Symptoms	Treatment
Mild disease	• WBCs normal • <3 stools/day	• **Oral vancomycin 125 mg QDS for 10 d** • Oral fidaxomicin 200 mg BD for 10 d
Moderate disease	• WBCs ↑, but <15 × 10⁹/L • 3–5 stools/day	• **Oral vancomycin 125 mg QDS for 10 d** • Oral fidaxomicin 200 mg BD for 10 d
Severe disease	• WBCs ↑↑ and >15 × 10⁹/L • Temperature >38.5°C • Severe colitis • Acute rising serum creatinine (>50% increase above baseline)	• **Oral vancomycin 125 mg QDS for 10–14 d** • Oral fidaxomicin 200 mg BD for 10 d
Life-threatening disease	• Hypotension • Ileus • Toxic megacolon • CT evidence of severe disease	• **Oral vancomycin 500 QDS for 10–14 d + IV metronidazole 500 mg TDS**

- **Relapse:** Further episode of CDI within 12 wk of symptoms resolution. Oral Fidaxomicin 200 mg BD for 10 d.
- **Recurrence:** Further episode of CDI after 12 wk of symptoms resolution. Oral vancomycin 125 mg QDS for 10 d or oral fidaxomicin 200 mg BD for 10 d.
  - ❖ **Faecal microbiota transplant** in adults who have had two or more previous confirmed episode.
- ✓ **Antibiotic Profile**
  - **Metronidazole**
    - ❖ It is absorbed from upper GI, with 6–15% of drug excreted in stool.

- ❖ **Oral/IV metronidazole** dose is 400–500 mg TDS for 10–14 d.
- ❖ However, due to high frequency of recurrences, it has been abandoned as first line of treatment by many countries.
- **Oral vancomycin**
  - ❖ Can be given in CKD and septic patients.
  - ❖ Tapered oral vancomycin has also been given for recurrent disease, where it is given four times a day for first 14 d and then one dose withdrawn per day for one week at a time, until patient is taking one dose every 2–3 d.
- **IV vancomycin[Q]:** Ineffective as it does not penetrate the large bowel in sufficient doses.
- **Vancomycin enemas:** For patients in ileus. Dose is 250 mg in 250 mL of water 4 times a day.
- **Fidaxomicin** is a macrolide that is minimally absorbed and highly excreted in stool.
- Consider oral fidaxomicin for patients at high risk of recurrence (elderly, multiple comorbidities, with concomitant antibiotics).
- **Rifampicin and IV immunoglobins:** Have been used for severe CDI.

Prognosis

✓ Mortality of cases with colitis is 20%.

HUMAN IMMUNODEFICIENCY VIRUS (HIV)

✓ **Retrovirus: HIV-1 (More Common) and HIV-2**
- Reverse transcriptase[Q] enzyme that converts viral RNA into viral DNA.

✓ **Diagnosis and Ethics**
- Antigen testing positive from 18th day and antibody testing from 30th day.
- HIV p24 antigen testing.
- HIV-1/2 antibody testing immunoassay.
- Consent should be sought from awake patient, and any patient unable to consent should be tested in best interest.
- If HIV contributed to a patient's death, it should be included in a patient's death.
- No patient should be refused admission in ITU based on HIV status.

Classification for HIV

Stage	HIV Class	CD4+ Count (× 10⁶/L)	CD4+ Cells (%)
1	Acute HIV infection	≥500	≥26
2	Chronic HIV infection	200–499	14–25
3	AIDS	≤200 or opportunistic illnesses	<14

AIDS-Defining Illnesses

Cause	Specific Types
Neoplasm	• **Kaposi's sarcoma** • Invasive cervical cancer • **Lymphomas: Burkitt's,** immunoblastic, or brain • Wasted syndrome attributed to HIV
Bacterial	• ***Mycobacterium: Tuberculosis,*** avium complex, *kansasii* • Pneumonia: Recurrent (>1 episode in 12 months) • Recurrent *Salmonella septicaemia*
Viral	• **Cytomegalovirus: Retinitis;** diseases other than liver, spleen, and glands • Herpes simplex: Ulcers >1 month, oesophagitis, pneumonitis, bronchitis • **JC: Progressive multifocal leucoencephalopathy** • Encephalopathy: HIV-related
Fungal	• ***Pneumocystis jirovecii*** pneumonia • ***Candida*: Bronchi,** trachea, lungs, or oesophagus • Coccidioidomycosis: Disseminated or extrapulmonary • Cryptococcosis: Extrapulmonary • **Histoplasmosis**
Parasitic	• Cryptosporidiosis: Chronic intestinal (>1 month's duration) • **Toxoplasma of brain** • Isosporiasis: Chronic intestinal

✓ **Respiratory Failure**
- Commonest reason for ITU admission in HIV patients is respiratory failure (35–40%)[Q].

- Common respiratory causes[Q] are bacterial pneumonia, *Pneumocystis jirovecii* pneumonia, tuberculosis, and Kaposi's sarcoma (late presentation with perihilar streaks).
- Most common cause of respiratory failure in HIV patients now is bacterial pneumonia (*Streptococcus pneumoniae*).
- Sepsis is also a leading cause of ICU admission (15–20%).
- Decreased consciousness and seizures as a result of HIV are the most common causes of admission to ITU due to neurological reasons and are most commonly due to *Tuberculous meningitis*[Q].
- Toxic effects of antiretroviral treatment (ART) can also lead to ITU admission.
- Accelerated inflammatory response related to immune reconstitution syndrome (IRIS) related to use of ART.

✓ **Pneumocystis Pneumonia (PCP)**
- Caused by *Pneumocystis jirovecii*, a fungus.
- Seen in patients with CD4 count <200 cells/μL.
- Also seen in transplant recipients, long-term steroids, and chemotherapy.
- Fever, dry cough, dyspnoea, weight loss with profound oxygen desaturation on exertion.
- Chest X-ray and CT scan show bilateral perihilar interstitial "ground-glass" infiltrates. Normal chest X-ray in one-fourth of cases.
- Increased risk of pneumothorax with poor prognosis[Q].
- **Diagnosis is from histopathological specimen, BAL, or induced sputum**[Q].
  ❖ Identification of organism on **methenamine silver stains** of respiratory secretions or **immunofluorescent monoclonal antibody** technique can help in establishing the diagnosis.
  ❖ **Targeted BAL may be better than blind BAL** specifically in the context of PCP.
  ❖ **PCR**[Q]**: High sensitivity but poor specificity as colonization in 70% of cases.**
  ❖ **Plasma β-D-glucan** is an indicator of PCP as well, and **high values**, along with findings on the chest X-ray, have high positive predictive value.
- **Trimethoprim/sulfamethoxazole (TMP-SMX)** is antibiotic of choice. Side effects are rash, fever, nausea, leucopaenia, and methaemoglobinaemia[Q].

❖ Clindamycin/primaquine[Q] can also be given as second line of treatment. Patients should be screened for G-6-PD deficiency.

❖ Dapsone or pentamidine is another alternative.

- **Corticosteroids** if patient is **severely hypoxic (PaO$_2$ <9.2 kPa)** and started within 72 h of treatment.

  ❖ Prednisolone 40 mg BD for 5 d.

- Intubation is a poor prognostic indicator.
- HAART during an acute illness is risky and shouldn't be started immediately. *Start it within 2 wk of the diagnosis of PCP.*

✓ **Central Nervous System Involvement**

- *Cryptococcus neoformans[Q]*

  ❖ Subacute meningitis. Headache and altered mental status.

  ❖ ICP is high, so CT scan is suggested before lumbar puncture for diagnosis.

  ❖ **Lumbar puncture:** CSF for **cryptococcal antigen**. Mononuclear cells, mildly elevated protein, and low glucose.

  ❖ **Indian ink staining tests[Q].**

  ❖ Therapeutic lumbar punctures may be needed for raised ICP.

  ❖ **Treatment, induction: Amphotericin B + flucytosine** for 1 wk. Consolidation with high-dose fluconazole for 8 wk. Maintenance with lower-dose fluconazole for 2 yr.

  ❖ *ART is delayed for 4–10 wk.*

- *Toxoplasma gondii*

  ❖ Focal encephalitis presents with headache, altered mental status, seizures, and focal neurological signs. Most common opportunistic CNS infection in AIDS[Q].

  ❖ MRI plus CSF sampling (**PCR for toxoplasma**) helps in diagnosis.

  ❖ MRI alone can't distinguish between toxoplasmosis, CNS lymphoma, and abscess.

  ❖ **Treatment:** *Pyrimethamine* and *sulfadiazine* with *leucovorin*.

  ❖ **Adjunctive corticosteroids or anticonvulsants may be needed.**

- **AIDS-related lymphoma (ARL):** 90% of cases of ARL are extranodal sites, like CNS, skin, and gut.

✓ **Antiretroviral Therapy (ART) Classification**

- **Nucleoside reverse transcriptase inhibitors (NRTIs):** Zidovudine, stavudine, didanosine, lamivudine, abacavir, tenofovir, emtricitabine.
- **Non-nucleoside reverse transcriptase inhibitors (NNRTIs):** Nevirapine, efavirenz.
- **Integrase inhibitors:** Raltegravir, dolutegravir.
- **Fu**sion inhibitors: En**fu**virtide.
- **Protease inhibitors:** Lo**pi**navir, atazanavir, darunavir, fosamprenavir.
- **CCR-5 inhibitors:** Maraviroc.

✓ **Toxicities of ART**

- Didanosine: **Pancreatitis**, peripheral neuropathy, lactic acidosis, Stevens–Johnson syndrome.
- Zidovudine: **Bone marrow suppression**, Stevens–Johnson syndrome, **lactic acidosis.**
- Abacavir: Hypersensitivity syndrome.
- Emtricitabine: Neutropaenia.
- Tenofovir: **Fanconi syndrome**, lactic acidosis, toxic epidermal necrolysis.
- Nevirapine: Hepatic **n**ecrosis, toxic epidermal necrolysis.
- Efavirenz: **Psychosis**, depression.
- Raltegravir: Rhabdomyolysis.
- Lopinavir: Pancreatitis.

✓ **HAART Therapy in ICU[Q]**

- In ICU gastrointestinal dysfunction is common, and these drugs can be stopped for a few days. However, an HIV specialist should be contacted if ART interruption is for more than a few days.
- **For patients with non-AIDS-related illness or CD4+ >200 × 10^6/L, HAART should be delayed.**
- HAART should be considered in patients with AIDS-related illness or CD4 counts less than 200/μL.

  ❖ For patients with **CNS TB and cryptococcosis**: HAART started after disease control or >4 wk[Q].

  ❖ For patients with **extra-CNS TB and PCP**: Start after 2 wk.

  ❖ For **HIV encephalitis**: Start immediately.

- Patients already on HAART and with suppression of viral multiplication should continue with it.

- **Immune reconstitution inflammatory syndrome (IRIS)**
  - ❖ Develops weeks or months after HAART therapy and is characterized by worsening of respiratory, neurological, and systemic symptoms due to opportunistic infections.
  - ❖ Continue HAART therapy and start prednisone unless caused by cryptococcal meningitis or Kaposi's sarcoma[Q].
- ✓ **Antimicrobial Prophylaxis**
  - Depends on level of CD4+ cell count.
  - *Pneumocystis jirovecii* pneumonia: CD4 <200 cells/μL: TMP-SMX.
  - Toxoplasmosis: CD4 <100 cells/μL: TMP-SMX.
  - *Mycobacterium avium* complex: CD4 <50 cells/μL – azithromycin or clarithromycin.
- ✓ **Risk to Healthcare Worker**
  - About 1 in 10,000 for mucous membrane exposure, 1 in 300 for needlestick injury.
  - Zidovudine prophylaxis reduces the risk of infection by 81%.
  - Three or more drugs prophylaxis for high-risk exposures from a known HIV-positive source.
- ✓ **Prognosis**
  - Critically ill patients with HIV infection have similar short-term outcomes as other patients with comparable severity of illness.

COVID-19

Epidemiology

- ✓ **Coronavirus Epidemics**
  - **SARS-CoV:** 2002, 8,000 cases. Fatality rate of 10%.
  - **MERS-CoV:** 2012, 2,500 cases. Fatality rate of 35%.
  - **SARS-CoV-2:** 2019, Covid-19. More than 800 million cases.
- ✓ **Coronavirus**
  - Single positive strand RNA.
  - About 90% nucleotides similarity to viruses found in bats.
  - **Spike protein** on virus attaches to host cell protein **angiotensin-converting enzyme 2 (ACE-2) receptor**.
  - Most patients generate good T cell and B cell response to the virus.

- ❖ People with defects in interferon production (drug-induced or genetic) are predisposed to severe infection.
- ❖ **Microangiopathic occlusion of smaller vessels is significant.**
- **Variant of concerns:** Variant that shows increase in transmissibility, virulence, or decrease in effectiveness of public health measures. Some previous variants of concerns were:
  - ❖ **Delta:** Originated in India first in December 2020. High transmission and severity of disease.
  - ❖ **Omicron:** Detected in South Africa first in November 2021. High transmission but low severity of disease.
- ✓ **Clinical Features and Diagnosis**
  - **Incubation period:** 2–14 d, with mean time of 5 d.
  - **Transmission:** Respiratory droplets.
  - **Presentation:** Majority of cases are asymptomatic. Fever and cough. Diarrhoea seen in some cases. New loss of smell or taste. Lymphopaenia and thrombocytopaenia.
  - **Disease course:** Early upper respiratory infection, followed by a second phase of lower respiratory disease in those who develop severe disease.
    - ❖ **Second phase** presents with hypoxia, hypotension that may progress to multiorgan failure.
      - Exaggerated inflammatory response seen.
      - Disseminated intravascular coagulation, pulmonary emboli, venous thromboembolism, ischaemic stroke, and myocarditis are known complications.
      - Secondary bacterial infections lower compared to other respiratory viruses, like influenza, although increased risk of **pulmonary aspergillosis**.
  - **Chest X-ray/CT Scan:**
    - ❖ Bilateral infiltrates with ground-glass appearance in severe disease.
    - ❖ PCR test remains positive for weeks after infection and hence not useful for checking disease resolution.

- **Multisystem Inflammatory Syndrome – Adults (MIS-A)**
  - ❖ Rare but serious condition that presents 4 wk after acute COVID-19.
  - ❖ Extrapulmonary multiorgan dysfunction is the hallmark of MIS-A.
  - ❖ Fever, rash, conjunctivitis, neurological signs, shock, gastrointestinal symptoms, and thrombocytopaenia.
  - ❖ Steroid IVIG is the treatment.
- **Multisystem Inflammatory Syndrome – Children (MIS-A)/Paediatric Multisystem Inflammatory Syndrome (PIMS)**
  - ❖ A child presenting with persistent fever, inflammation (neutrophilia, elevated CRP, lymphopaenia), and evidence of single- or multiorgan dysfunction.
  - ❖ Exclusion of any other microbial causes.
  - ❖ SARS-CoV-2 PCR testing may be positive or negative.
  - ❖ Rash, lymph node swelling, hypotension, and increased oxygen requirement.
  - ❖ High fibrinogen, CRP, D-dimer, and ferritin.
  - ❖ **CXR:** Infiltrates and effusion.
  - ❖ **Echo^Q:** Myocarditis, coronary artery dilatation, LV dysfunction, mitral regurgitation.
  - ❖ **Abdominal USG:** Colitis, lymphadenopathy, hepatosplenomegaly.
  - ❖ **Differential diagnosis:** Kawasaki disease, streptococcal and staphylococcal toxic shock syndromes (TSS), bacterial sepsis, and macrophage activation syndrome.
  - ❖ **Treatment:** Empirical antibiotics, anticoagulation, early involvement of critical care, infectious disease, immunology, and rheumatology.
  - ❖ Consider IVIg if criteria of Kawasaki disease or TSS fulfilled.
  - ❖ Respiratory failure is uncommon, and ITU admission is for cardiovascular indications.
  - ❖ Good prognosis, with stay in paediatric ICU of around 3–4 d.

Prevention

- ✓ **Vaccination**
  - **mRNA-based:** Pfizer and Moderna. Viral mRNA translated by host cells to produce spike protein, against which immune response is generated.
  - **Inactivated killed virus:** Sinopharm, Covaxin.
  - **Viral vector vaccine:** AstraZeneca. Adenovirus used as a carrier to deliver SARS-CoV-2 RNA.
  - **Viral protein:** Novavax.
- ✓ **Aerosol-Generating Procedures**
  - PPE, including N-95 mask, for intubation.
  - Staff with greatest airway experience to attempt intubation.
  - Minimizing ventilation during apnoeic time.
  - Inflation of cuff prior to starting ventilation.

Treatment

- ✓ **Non-hospitalized patients:** Three FDA approved drugs to reduce the risk of hospitalization in patients with mild to moderate COVID-19
  - **Remdesivir:** Inhibitor of viral RNA–dependent RNA polymerase.
    - ❖ **Nirmatrelvir/ritonavir:** Protease inhibitors
    - ❖ **Molnupiravir:** Nucleoside analogue
  - It is advised not to use antiplatelet and anticoagulant therapy.
- ✓ **Airway: NIV/HFNO If FiO$_2$ above 40%**
  - **RECOVERY-RS Trial (2021):** In patients with AHRF and Covid-19, there was no difference in tracheal intubations or mortality within 30 d in HFNO-treated patients or COT.
  - Significantly less tracheal intubations or mortality within 30 d in CPAP treated patients compared to patients on COT.
  - Awake prone position can be given, but it shouldn't be used as a rescue therapy to avoid intubation.
  - Even pregnant females can do it. Failure rate is as high as 60%.
- ✓ **Breathing**
  - Lung protective ventilation. Tidal volume: 6–8 mL/kg PBW. Plateau pressure <30 cm H$_2$O.
  - VV-ECMO in selective cases with severe ARDS.
- ✓ **Cardiovascular**
  - Give balanced crystalloids for resuscitation. Aim MAP of 60–65 mmHg rather than big MAP values. Norepinephrine is the vasopressor of choice.

✓ **Immunomodulators**
- **Steroids** showed reduction in mortality in patients **requiring oxygen**. Dexamethasone and methylprednisolone (may be better) can both be used.
  - ❖ **REMAP-CAP (2020):** In critically ill patients, treatment with a 7 d fixed-dose course of hydrocortisone or shock-dependent dosing of hydrocortisone resulted in 93% and 80% probabilities of superiority with regard to odds of improvement in organ support-free days within 21 d.
  - ❖ **RECOVERY Trial (2021):** Use of dexa-methasone for hospitalized patients requiring oxygen or mechanical ventila-tion showed mortality benefit.
- **IL-6 inhibitors**[Q] (tocilizumab/sarilumab): Used as an adjunct to dexamethasone in rapidly progressive disease and started within 48 h of starting respiratory support.
  - ❖ **REMAP-CAP IL-6 (2021):** In critically ill patients, requiring organ support in ITU, tocilizumab and sarilumab had mortality benefit.
- **Convalescent plasma and IVIG:** No ben-efit in patients.
- **Neutralizing monoclonal antibodies:** They bind to spike protein and prevent entry in the host cell.
  - ❖ **RECOVERY Trial (2022):** *Casirivimab/ imdevimab* prevented progression to severe Covid-19 and prevented mor-tality in seronegative patients, but not seropositive patients (those who pro-duced anti-spike antibody).
  - ❖ Bamlanivimab, bamlanivimab/etesevimab, and *sotrovimab* may reduce hospitalization.
- **Janus kinase inhibitor (JAK):** Baricitinib acts on JAK1 and JAK2 enzymes involved in cytokine mediation.
  - ❖ **RECOVERY Trial (2022):** Baricitinib has shown mortality benefit.

✓ **Therapies Not Recommended**
- Hydroxychloroquine, doxycycline, ivermec-tin, azithromycin.

✓ **Hospitalized Patients on Oxygen Requirement**
- Give therapeutic anticoagulation only if D-dimer is high. Otherwise, give prophy-lactic dose.
- Therapeutic anticoagulation is to continue for 14 d or till hospital discharge.
- In non-hospitalized patient, it is advised not to use antiplatelet and anticoagulant therapy.

Prognosis

✓ Severity of disease and mortality increase with age.
✓ Elevated levels of IL-6, CRP, procalcitonin, and ferritin are associated with more severe disease.
✓ **Long Covid:** Chronic condition that occurs after SARS-CoV-2 infections and is present for at least 3 months (CDC definition).
- **Symptoms:** Extreme fatigue, breathlessness, muscle weakness, anxiety, and depression.
- **Risk factors:** Women, age >65 yr, severe disease, non-vaccinated patients.

TUBERCULOSIS

Epidemiology and Aetiology

✓ **Tuberculosis**
- Caused by aerobic, slow-growing, acid-fast *Mycobacterium tuberculosis*[Q].
- **Pathogenesis:** Airborne inhalation of *M. tuberculosis* can have the following outcomes:
  - ❖ Failure to register the infection.
  - ❖ Becoming infected but then clearing the infection.
  - ❖ Successfully containing the infection but then continuing to harbour bacilli in the absence of symptomatic disease **(latent TB infection)**.
  - ❖ Developing primary progressive TB disease (more common in children).
- **Reactivation:** Progression from latent TB infection to active TB in patients with low immunity, stress, poor nutrition.
- Acute respiratory failure, septic shock, and multiorgan dysfunction are the reasons for admission to ITU.

Clinical Features and Diagnosis

✓ **Risk Factors**[Q]
- HIV, immunosuppression, illicit drug use, institutional living, close contact with a TB patient, immigration from high-TB-prevalence areas.

✓ **Pulmonary TB**
  - Most common form and is responsible for roughly two-thirds of cases. Presents with fever, night sweats, weight loss, cough, and haemoptysis (due to erosion of a bronchial artery[Q], seen in 20% of patients).
  - **Rasmussen aneurysm** is a pseudo-aneurysmal dilation of pulmonary artery branch.

✓ **CNS TB**
  - TB meningitis or tuberculomas. Seen more commonly in people with miliary TB, in children, and in HIV.
  - Headache, seizures (more common in children), and focal neurological deficits due to cranial nerve palsies.
  - **Prominent leptomeningeal and basal cistern enhancement**, along with hydrocephalus (blockage by gelatinous exudates),[Q] seen in contrast-enhanced CT scan.
  - Stroke is seen in up to two-thirds of cases.

Grading of Tuberculous meningitis by the British Medical Research Council

Grade	Characteristics
I	GCS 15 without focal neurological deficits
II	GCS 10–14 with or without focal neurological deficit, or GCS 15 with focal neurological deficit
III	GCS < 10 with or without focal neurological deficit

✓ **Disseminated TB**
  - Multiorgan involvement. Seeding to liver, spleen, kidney, and meninges.
  - Haematological spread seen in immunosuppressed patients.
  - ARDS, shock, multiorgan dysfunction, DIC, and adrenal insufficiency.

✓ **Pericardial or Pleural TB**
  - Pain, fever, and night sweats.
  - **Pericardial TB** can present with hypotension or cardiogenic shock.
  - **Pleural TB** may present as tuberculous pleuritis, which may be asymptomatic, or *tubercular empyema*, which results from rupture of an adjacent cavity into pleural space.

✓ **Abdominal TB**
  - Can present as **gastrointestinal TB** or **peritoneal TB**. Abdominal complicates one-third of cases of pulmonary TB.

- **Gastrointestinal TB:** Ingestion of infected sputum and involves terminal ileum and ileocaecal region.
- **Peritoneal TB:** Due to haematogenous spread and can present with ascites and may mimic presentation as a gastrointestinal cancer.

✓ **Other Forms**
  - Haematogenous spread to liver, spleen, and kidneys can happen.
  - Involvement of lower thoracic spine is known as **Pott's disease**.
  - **TB lymphadenitis** may present with lymphocutaneous fistulas.
  - **Conjunctivitis** and **erythema nodosum** are due to hypersensitivity reactions to bacillary antigens.

✓ **Diagnosis**
  - *Five components:* History, physical examination, TB blood tests, chest radiographs, and bacteriologic examination.
  - **History:** Exposure to a person with TB, risk factors for TB, comorbidities like HIV, DM.
  - **Examination:** Lymph nodes.
  - **Blood tests: Interferon gamma** release assay or **Mantoux** tuberculin skin test.
    ❖ A positive test signifies TB infection[Q] and not disease.
    ❖ These tests can't rule in or rule out TB in a suspected patient.
  - **Chest radiograph:** Upper lobe fibrotic nodules and cavities suggest TB disease and cannot definitively diagnose TB disease.
    ❖ Primary progressive TB after recent infection or immunocompromised patient present with CD4 cell count <100/mm^3 as lower lobe infiltrate compared to reactivation.
    ❖ Children mostly have hilar lymphadenopathy without infiltrates.
  - **Bacteriological examination:** Examinations of clinical specimens:
    ❖ At least three consecutive sputum specimens[Q], 8 h apart, with at least one collected early in the morning. AFB detected by Ziehl–Neelsen staining. Induced sputum with nebulized hypertonic saline in patients who cannot produce sputum.
    ❖ **Nucleic acid amplification tests (NAAT)**[Q]/PCR to detect *M. tuberculosis*

DNA in specimens. They also give information about drug resistance.

❖ **Culture:** A positive culture is gold standard[Q] for laboratory confirmation of TB disease.

❖ **Biopsies can be sent for histology.**

- A negative AFB smear, PCR, or culture does not rule out tuberculosis disease[Q].
- AFB in a sputum sample can be due to non-tuberculous mycobacteria and is not diagnostic and should be clinically correlated.
- Extrapulmonary TB usually has lower burden of bacteria compared to pulmonary disease, and granulomas with or without caseous necrosis in tissues sampled are seen.
- **Adenosine deaminase (ADA)**[Q] levels in fluids have been used for diagnosing extrapulmonary TB, like tuberculous pleuritis.
- Serial sputum sampling from expectorating patients provides yields like that form bronchoscopic sampling[Q].
- TB PCR test can be used if diagnosis is in doubt[Q].

✓ **NAAT**

- WHO recommends[Q] NAAT, such as **Xpert MTB/RIF**, as the initial diagnostic method to detect *M. tuberculosis* bacilli in respiratory samples; CSF; lymph node biopsy; pleural, pericardial, or peritoneal fluid; or urine.

  ❖ Sensitivity of 98% in patients with smear- and culture-positive TB and specificity of 99–100%.

  ❖ Sensitivity is lower for other samples, like CSF, pericardial fluid, urine, or pleural or ascitic fluid.

  ❖ Low-complexity NAATs are recommended over culture-based drug sensitivity testing for the detection of resistance to anti-TB drugs.

  ❖ WHO recommends **lateral flow lipoarabinomannan**[Q] assay as a screening test to detect TB in hospitalized HIV-positive adults and children with CD4 cell count <100/mm³.

  ❖ All patients in whom TB is diagnosed should have testing for HIV[Q]. Testing for hepatitis depends on individual risk profile.

  ❖ CT scan is indicated in patients with extensive pathologies on chest X-ray, patients where abdominal disease or tuberculoma is suspected.

Prevention and Treatment

✓ **BCG Vaccine**

- Has an overall efficacy of approximately 50%. Inefficient in preventing primary infection and reactivation. It decreases the risk of TB meningitis and disseminated TB, though.
- Aerosol precautions with isolation and PPE should be taken. Reporting to local authorities has to be done.

✓ **Treatment**

- Should not be delayed while waiting for bacteriologic results if TB disease is the presumptive diagnosis and no alternative diagnosis is considered, as early treatment is associated with better outcomes[Q].

✓ **Characteristics**

- TB bacteria have two characteristics: High frequency of mutations (hence multidrug therapy) and slow-growth cycle (hence long treatment).
- Only 8.4% of TB isolates are resistant to any first-line drug, and 1.6% are multidrug-resistant.

✓ **Standard Treatment**[Q]

- **Intensive therapy** (2 months): Isoniazid, rifampicin, pyrazinamide, ethambutol.
- **Continuation phase** (4 months): Isoniazid + rifampicin.

  ❖ Continuation phase is longer for CNS (12 months) or bone and joint disease (9 months).

✓ **Enteral Absorption**

- Critically ill patients will have unreliable enteral absorption. So parenteral route should be preferred, and therapeutic drug monitoring should be done.
- Only isoniazid, rifampicin, and ethambutol are available as IV formulation.

✓ **MDR and Extreme Drug-Resistant TB**[Q]

- Resistance to isoniazid and rifampicin for the former; resistance to isoniazid, rifampicin, quinolones, and one second-line injectable for the latter.
- *MDR should be treated with at least four second-line drugs over 18 months.* **Core drugs:** *Bedaquiline,* **delamanid,** amikacin, kanamycin, linezolid, quinolones like moxifloxacin and levofloxacin, clofazimine, ethionamide, cycloserine. **Non-core drugs:**

Para-aminosalicyclic acid, meropenem/clavulanate, imipenem/cilastatin, amoxycillin/clavulanate, thioacetazone.

✓ **Adjuvant Therapy**
- Steroids should be given for meningeal disease in HIV-negative patients and who have shown mortality benefit[Q].
- Recommendations regarding use of steroids in pericarditis are controversial, and some authors recommend use only in patients with recurrent large effusions who do not respond to anti-TB drugs and drainage.
- Steroids also reduce the incidence of IRIS in HIV patients in whom CD4 count is <100 cells/mm³.
- Aspirin 150 mg daily has been shown to prevent stroke and mortality in patients with TB meningitis.

✓ **Adverse Drug Reactions[Q]**
- TB treatment should be changed or held if transaminases are three times the upper limit and patients have symptoms of toxicity, like nausea and vomiting, or five times the upper limit in asymptomatic patient. Therapy when held in patients with hepatotoxicity can be resumed cautiously with one drug at a time. In severe TB where therapy can't be held, a liver-safe regimen should be started.
  - ❖ **Isoniazid:** P450 enzyme inhibitor[Q]. Liver dysfunction, peripheral neuropathy[Q] (given with pyridoxine), lupus-like syndrome. Good CNS penetration (100%).
  - ❖ **Rifampicin:** P450 enzyme inducer[Q]. Liver dysfunction, hypersensitivity, haemolytic anaemia, leucopaenia, thrombocytopaenia, orange discolouration of urine[Q]. Low CNS penetration (20%).
  - ❖ **Ethambutol:** Optic nerve toxicity[Q] (red-green discolouration progressing to blindness), pericarditis, myocarditis. Moderate CNS penetration (20–50%).
  - ❖ **Pyrazinamide:** Most frequent cause of **drug-induced liver injury[Q]**, rashes, rhabdomyolysis. Good CNS penetration (100%).

✓ **Immune Reconstitution Inflammatory Syndrome (IRIS)**
- Worsening of symptoms despite effective chemotherapy. Usually seen 2 wk after starting anti-TB drugs. Severe form is rare, and treatment is steroids plus continuation of anti-TB drugs.

✓ **Special Situations**
- **HIV**
  - ❖ **Leading cause of death in HIV-positive persons.** Start TB treatment before ART in patients with CD4 counts <50 cells/µL; associated with lower mortality if ART is started within 2 wk of TB regimen.
  - ❖ In patients with CD4 >50 cells/µL, ART is often recommended at 2 months of starting anti-TB treatment.
  - ❖ In patients with TB meningitis, ART should be started only 8 wk after starting anti-TB drugs.
  - ❖ Patients with TB and HIV should get cotrimoxazole prophylaxis for PCP.
- **Liver failure:** Levofloxacin, ethambutol (rifampicin if not fulminant failure), amikacin, linezolid, or a carbapenem with clavulanate. Avoid isoniazid and pyrazinamide[Q].
- **Renal failure:** No adjustment in dosing of isoniazid, rifampicin, linezolid, and moxifloxacin, and adjust dose for ethambutol, pyrazinamide, aminoglycosides, and levofloxacin.
- **Pregnancy:** Isoniazid, rifampicin, and ethambutol can be given. Pyrazinamide in patients who have severe disease or are immunocompromised.

✓ **Prognosis**
- Increase in hospital mortality (50%) for TB patients requiring mechanical ventilation.

BACTERIAL AND PARASITIC INFECTIONS

✓ **Meningococcal Disease**
- **Meningococcal disease:** Includes meningitis, meningococcal septicaemia, or a combination of both.
- **Causative agent:** *Neisseria meningitidis*, encapsulated Gram-negative cocci. Five serogroups: A, B, C, Y, and W-135.
- Median age of patients now is 42 yr.
- *Neisseria meningitidis* normally colonizes the nasopharynx. Deficiency of **complement system** can lead to invasive disease.
- **Clinical symptoms**
  - ❖ Fever, signs of meningism, rash starting as erythema and progresses to petechiae and purpura.
  - ❖ Septic shock with hypotension, renal failure, and thrombocytopaenia happens.

❖ Purpura fulminans is characteristic of meningococcaemia.

❖ Waterhouse–Friderichsen syndrome (adrenal haemorrhage) is a less common complication.

• **Diagnosis** is done by isolation of *N. meningitidis* from cultures of blood.

• **Treatment:** Droplet and contact isolation. Third-generation cephalosporins. Steroids may be needed in adrenal failure.

• **Chemoprophylaxis** for close contacts (personnel who managed an airway or those exposed to respiratory secretions) is recommended by CDC.

❖ **Rifampicin**[Q] 600 mg BD for 2 d or one dose of ceftriaxone[Q] 250 mg IM can be given.

• **High mortality** (20–50%) in children with meningococcal septic shock.

✓ **Typhoid/Enteric Fever**

• **Causative organism:** *Salmonella typhi* and *Salmonella paratyphi*.

• Incubation period is 7–14 d.

• Faecal-oral transmission.

• **Presentation:** Fever, bradycardia, abdominal pain, and rose spots (2–3 mm) on the trunk.

❖ Perforation peritonitis in young patients after day 14.

❖ Myocarditis, meningitis, encephalitis, and hepatitis are some of the complications.

• **Diagnosis:** Blood or stool cultures are sent for diagnosis.

❖ Widal test is sensitive but not specific for typhoid.

❖ Typhidot test is a qualitative assessment of antibodies and can be used for diagnosis.

• **Treatment:** IV ceftriaxone and azithromycin – Drugs of choice.

❖ **MDR typhoid** is resistant to the three first-line recommended antibiotics (chloramphenicol, ampicillin, and cotrimoxazole).

❖ Chloramphenicol can cause aplastic anaemia[Q] and is not used nowadays.

✓ **Cholera**

• **Causative organism:** *Vibrio cholerae*.

• Incubation period is 12 h to 5 d.

• Toxin stimulates cAMP in gut.

• O1 and O139 cause epidemic cholera.

• **Presentation:**

❖ Patients develop painless diarrhoea of up to 1 L per hour.

❖ Diarrhoea is often most severe within the first 2 d.

❖ Acute renal failure is seen in 30% of cases.

• **Diagnosis:** Stool cultures for isolation of *V. cholera*. Rapid diagnostic tests are also available.

• **Treatment**

❖ Aggressive IV fluid therapy should be done with at least 200 mL/h of fluid for the first 24 h.

❖ Azithromycin and doxycycline single doses are used for treatment. Antibiotics shorten the volume and duration of diarrhoea.

✓ **Enterohaemorrhagic *Escherichia coli* (EHEC)**

• **Causative organism:** *E. coli* O157:H7 is the most common organism involved.

• Incubation period is 1–8 d.

• It produces Shiga toxins 1 and 2. Haemolytic uraemic syndrome (HUS) is seen in 10–15% of patients with *E. coli* O157.

• **Presentation:** Acute watery diarrhoea initially which turns into bloody diarrhoea later.

• **Diagnosis:** Stool culture confirms the diagnosis of *E. coli* O157 initially. Later, testing for Shiga toxin is done as it triggers HUS.

• **Treatment**

❖ Supportive management.

❖ Antibiotics and antimotility drugs should be withheld as they increase the risk of developing HUS.

❖ Platelet transfusions are discouraged in HUS. Renal replacement therapy is often needed in HUS.

✓ **Leptospirosis**

• **Causative organism:** Spirochete *Leptospira*.

• Spirochete is seen in standing water and contaminated soil. They are found in the urine of rats.

• **Presentation**

❖ Conjunctival suffusion is seen, not pathognomonic.

❖ Fever, hepatorenal dysfunction with pulmonary haemorrhage, called Weil's syndrome, develops within 1 wk of illness.

- Proteinuria, pyuria, granular casts, and microscopic haematuria.
  - **Diagnosis**
    - The organism can be grown in blood and CSF in first 2 weeks of illness and urine from third week onwards but is difficult to culture.
    - Leptospira IgM on day 10 of illness has good yield.
  - **Treatment:** Penicillin or ceftriaxone is the recommended antibiotic.

✓ **Lyme Disease**[Q]
- **Causative organism:** *Borrelia burgdorferi.*
- **Early infection:** A rash, looking like a bull's-eye target (erythema migrans), appears at the site of the tick bite.
- **Disseminated disease**
  - Neurological: Meningitis, cranial nerve palsies.
  - Cardiac: Heart block and arrhythmia.
  - Joints: Migratory arthralgia.
  - Muscle weakness and spread of erythema.
- **Late disease:** Peripheral neuropathy develops months to years later after the initial infection.
- **Diagnosis:** History plus antibodies in the blood.
- **Treatment:** Antibiotics like doxycycline, amoxicillin, and cefuroxime.

✓ **Rocky Mountain Spotted Fever**
- **Causative organism:** *Rickettsia rickettsii.*
- Infects endothelial cells and vascular smooth vessels.
- **Presentation**
  - Appears after 3–12 d of tick bite. Fever, myalgia, and headaches along with rash are seen.
  - Severe infection presents with shock, cutaneous necrosis, ARDS, and seizures.
  - Thrombocytopaenia and increased hepatic transaminases.
- **Diagnosis:** Organisms can't be cultured in most laboratories.
- **Treatment**
  - Empirical treatment is started based on history and symptoms.
  - Doxycycline is treatment of choice, including pregnancy near term, due to teratogenic risk.

- Chloramphenicol is treatment of choice in first or second trimesters.

✓ **Scrub Typhus**
- **Causative organism:** Bacteria, *Orientia tsutsugamushi.*
- **Presentation**
  - Fever, headache, GI symptoms are initial symptoms.
  - Patients can present with severe encephalopathy, aseptic meningitis, and myocarditis in later stages.
- **Diagnosis**
  - Immunofluorescence, rapid diagnostic kits, and serological tests are used for diagnosis.
  - Weil Felix reaction isn't used because of lack of specificity.
- **Treatment**
  - Azithromycin is drug of choice.
  - Chloramphenicol and injection doxycycline are treatment options.

✓ **Babesiosis**
- **Causative organism:** Intracellular parasite *Babesia.*
- Tickborne disease.
- **Presentation**
  - Infects red blood cells and causes their destruction to cause haemolytic anaemia.
  - Maltese cross is seen on peripheral blood smear.
  - Severe disease in immunocompromised patients.
  - ARDS, heart failure, liver failure, and renal failure.
  - Thrombocytopaenia and increased hepatic transaminases.
- **Diagnosis:** Organisms can't be cultured in most laboratories.
- **Treatment**
  - Empirical treatment is started based on history and symptoms.
  - Atovaquone and azithromycin.

TETANUS

Aetiology

✓ *Clostridium tetani*[Q]
- Anaerobic, spore-forming, Gram-positive bacillus.

- Spores distributed in soil and dust as well as in the intestines and faeces of animals.

Clinical Features and Diagnosis

✓ **Incubation Period**
  - Typically 3–21 d. The shorter the incubation period, the worse the prognosis.
✓ **Two Types of Toxins: Tetanospasmin and Tetanolysin**
  - **Tetanospasmin:** *Exotoxin that binds to neuromuscular junction and* **prevents the release of GABA and glycine** *from presynaptic inhibitory neurons.*
    ❖ It cleaves **synaptobrevin,** a protein which is essential for the release of neurotransmitters.
    ❖ *Inhibitory pathways are abolished, causing* **increased muscle tone, rigidity,** *sudden extreme muscle spasms.*
    ❖ Irreversible binding; recovery takes 4–6 wk.
✓ **Clinical Tetanus Forms**
  - Present in **three forms:** Local, cephalic, and generalized.
✓ **Generalized Tetanus**
  - About 80% of cases. Tetanus occurs in those with a penetrating wound or necrotic tissue.
  - Starts with skeletal muscle rigidity and spasms that classically involve the muscles of the face (masseter rigidity: **lockjaw; risus sardonicus:** fixed contraction of the facial muscles leading to a peculiar, distorted grin) and moves down to the rest of the body.
  - Spasms may resemble seizures with flexion of arms and extension of legs (**opisthotonos**) and is accompanied by severe pain.
  - Neck stiffness, sore throat, dysphagia, trismus.
  - Rhabdomyolysis and AKI.
  - Spasms are followed by **autonomic disturbances,** like haemodynamic instability.
  - Death is because of **laryngospasm,** diaphragmatic paralysis.
✓ **Diagnosis**
  - Diagnosis of exclusion[Q] and should be considered in presentation of meningitis with a history of a contaminated wound.

Treatment

✓ **Critical Care Setting**
  - Patients should be managed in **critical care setting**. Supportive management includes ventilatory support and decrease of stimuli to prevent spasms.
  - **Wound debridement** to reduce the bacterial and toxin load.
✓ **Metronidazole/Benzyl Penicillin**
  - Antibiotics to treat the tetanus bacterium.
  - **Human tetanus immunoglobin (HTIG)** to neutralize free-circulating toxin only.
✓ **Muscle Spasms**
  - Treated with **benzodiazepines** usually, and neuromuscular blocking agents are added for refractory spasms.
  - Autonomic instability is usually treated with beta-blockers, like labetalol.
✓ **Vaccination**
  - Patient will require **vaccination** after recovery.
  - Total three doses: at diagnosis, at 4–6 wk, and at 1 yr.
✓ **Notifiable Disease under Public Health**

Prognosis

✓ Most patients will require 4–6 wk of supportive care.
✓ In the developing world, neonatal tetanus accounts for mortality in 50% of cases.
✓ In developed nations, case fatality rate is highest (>30%) in patients above 65 yr of age.

BOTULISM

Aetiology

✓ **Acute Descending Motor Paralysis**[Q]
  - Affecting cranial, respiratory, and **autonomic nerves**.
✓ **Exotoxin**
  - Released by anaerobic,[Q] spore-forming, Gram-positive bacilli *Clostridium botulinum*, which causes it.
  - Toxin binds irreversibly to cholinergic neurotransmitter ends and prevents the release of acetylcholine from the presynaptic terminal by binding to SNARE proteins (docks vesicles containing Ach to presynaptic membrane.)
  - Large-size toxin and hence can't cross blood–brain barrier, preventing CNS effect.
✓ **Seven Different Forms of Neurotoxins**
  - Produced by *C. botulinum* (A to G), but only **A, B, E, and F affect humans.**

✓ **Heat Resistance**
- Spores are heat-resistant to boiling and grow well in canned food.
- **Neurotoxin** itself gets readily inactivated by heat at >85°C for 5 min.

✓ **Botulinum Toxin**
- The most dangerous poison, with 1 g of toxin able to kill 1 million people. **It's a category A biological agent**[Q].

✓ **Clinical Features and Diagnosis**
- Three most common syndromes are **foodborne**, **wound**, and **infant** botulism. No human-to-human transmission or through intact skin of toxin has been reported.
- **Foodborne botulism** starts around 24–48 h after ingestion of infected food.
  - ❖ Features include nausea, vomiting, and abdominal distension. Fever is an uncommon feature. Patients have **clear sensorium** and **sensory nerves**, and adrenergic synapses are spared[Q].
  - ❖ Cranial nerve palsies and descending flaccid paralysis (dysarthria, diplopia, dysphonia, and dysphagia) start after this symmetry of symptoms:
    - Proximal muscles are involved before distal muscles.
    - Ocular findings like dilated, fixed pupils, ptosis, nystagmus, and sixth cranial nerve dysfunction are common.
    - Paralysis correlates with the amount of toxin ingested and length of affected nerve, with short cranial nerves affected first and long lower-limb nerves last.
  - ❖ Type 2 respiratory failure due to involvement of respiratory muscles.
  - ❖ **Autonomic involvement** may lead to hypotension, urinary retention, constipation, and fixed dilated pupil.
  - ❖ **Nerve conduction studies**[Q] show normal nerve conduction velocity, reduced muscle action potentials with post-tetanic enhancement, and no post-tetanic exhaustion.
    - Repetitive nerve stimulation shows incremental responses[Q].
- **Wound botulism** shows same features without gastrointestinal symptoms. Seen in IVDU who present with cranial nerve palsies in the setting of abscesses.

- **Infant botulism** causes most cases. It occurs after intestinal colonization by *C. botulinum*. There is a history of constipation and feeding difficulties.
- Confirmation of the diagnosis requires identification of toxin in serum, stool, gastric samples, or the food eaten by symptomatic individual.

Prevention and Treatment

✓ **Supportive Management**
- Often needed with elective intubation and ventilatory support.
- Several months of supportive care needed; hence, tracheostomy may be needed.
- **Antibiotics are ineffective.**

✓ **Trivalent (A, B, E) Botulinum Equine Antitoxin (BAT)**
- Given on clinical grounds as soon as possible. Repeated after 24 h if no improvement.
- Antitoxin is ineffective once the toxin has bound to the receptors. Antitoxin can lead to anaphylaxis.

✓ **Notifiable Disease under Public Health**

Prognosis

✓ Recovery in 95% cases but may be protracted and may take up to 6 months.
✓ Ventilatory strength returns to normal by 1 yr, but exercise capacity is reduced.

MALARIA

Epidemiology and Aetiology

✓ **Malaria**
- Most common tropical infection to present in the UK. Among returning travellers having fever, the most common cause is malaria.

✓ **Protozoa Species *Plasmodium***
- Transmitted by female mosquitoes. Serious disease caused by *Plasmodium falciparum*.
- Other species are *Plasmodium vivax*, *P. ovale*, *P. malariae*.

Clinical Features and Diagnosis

✓ **Stages of Malaria**
- **Human liver stage (7 d)**
  - ❖ Human entry of ***Plasmodium* sporozoite** by mosquito bite.

- ❖ Sporozoites reach liver and enter hepatocytes and mature as schizonts.
- ❖ Each schizont of malaria has 6–12 merozoites, which are released in the blood again after rupture of hepatocytes.
- **Human blood stage (48 h)**
  - ❖ **Merozoites** infect RBCs and multiply into **trophozoites** and then again change into schizonts.
  - ❖ Some plasmodia differentiate into **gametes**, which are taken by another mosquito by another bite.
- **Mosquito stage**
  - ❖ Gametes in mosquito undergo reproduction and produce eggs.
  - ❖ These eggs release sporozoites, which reach mosquito saliva.
- ✓ **Risk factors:** Travel to endemic area, poor compliance with chemoprophylaxis and mosquito bites (obviously).
- ✓ **Signs and symptoms**
  - **Incubation period:** 1–3 wk.
  - **Cerebral malaria is the most common manifestation of severe malaria** and presents with high-grade fever (with parasite release from schizont), chills, altered mental state, tachypnoea, malaise, arthralgia.
  - **Complications:** ARDS (25% of severe cases), hepatomegaly, **splenomegaly**, **jaundice (haemolysis)**, anaemia, **thrombocytopaenia**, and **renal failure**.
  - Hypoglycaemia and lactic acidosis are seen more frequently in pregnant females.
  - Convulsions occur more commonly in children (80%) as compared to 15% in adults.
  - Severe malaria predisposes to bacterial co-infections like pneumonia by *S. pneumoniae* and enteric pathogens like *Salmonella*.
- ✓ **Diagnosis**
  - Peripheral blood smear is used for diagnosis.
  - **Thick films** are used for detecting the parasite.
  - **Thin films** are used for identifying species, quantifying parasitaemia, and prognosis.
  - **Rapid diagnosing tests** (detection of parasitic proteins by monoclonal antibodies) and **real-time PCR** can also be used to confirm the diagnosis.

- ✓ **Severe Malaria by WHO Definition**[Q]
  - **Pulmonary oedema:** Radiologically confirmed; saturation <92% with RR >30/min.
  - **Circulatory shock:** CRT >3 s, temperature gradient in leg, SBP <80 mmHg.
  - **Impaired consciousness/coma:** GCS <11 in adults, >2 seizures in 24 h, prostration.
  - **Hypoglycaemia:** Glucose <2.2 mmol/L.
  - **Acute kidney injury:** Creatinine >265 mmol/L or blood urea >20 mmol/L.
  - **Acidosis:** Base deficit >8 mEq/L or bicarbonate <15 mmol/L or lactate >5 mmol/L.
  - **Anaemia: Haemoglobin** <70 g/L in adults, with parasitaemia >10,000/μL.
  - **Jaundice:** Bilirubin >50 mmol/L, with a parasite count of >100,000/μL.
  - **DIC:** Significant bleeding from gut, nose, gums, or venipuncture sites.
  - **Parasite density >10%.**
- ✓ **Algid Malaria**
  - Severe malaria with circulatory collapse. Gram-negative septicaemia, splenic rupture, and GI bleed are the most common causes.

Prevention and Treatment

- ✓ **Uncomplicated Malaria**
  - Artemisinin combination therapy (ATC) with *artemether* and *lumefantrine* is the drug of choice. Quinine with doxycycline or clindamycin/atovaquone with proguanil if ATC not available.
- ✓ **Complicated Malaria**
  - Management in ITU is recommended. **IV artesunate** should be started. Dose is 2.4 mg/kg IV at 0, 12, and 24 h, and then every 24 h. Higher doses in children < 20 yr (3 mg/kg)
  - Parenteral treatment is also recommended for parasitaemia >2% or jaundice.
  - Monitoring of treatment is done by doing thin smears every 12 to 24 h till resolution of parasitaemia.
  - Once patient has improved and **parasitaemia is <1%**, ATC should follow IV artesunate.
  - Quinine if artesunate is not available.
  - Delayed haemolysis occurs after 10–14 d of artesunate therapy, and repeated blood counts should be taken 2 wk after therapy.

✓ **Pregnancy**
- Uncomplicated malaria in second and third trimester is treated with artemether with lumefantrine.
- IV artesunate is treatment of choice in severe malaria in all trimesters.
- *Quinine with clindamycin can be used in all trimesters.* Quinine increases the risk of prolonged QT syndrome and hypoglycaemia. Doxycycline is contraindicated in pregnancy.

✓ **Supportive Management**
- **Judicious fluid management**, as excess fluid can lead to non-cardiogenic pulmonary oedema and ARDS, especially in infants and young children.
- Hypoglycaemia should be treated aggressively using enteral feed or 10% glucose.
- *Empirical antibiotic therapy is recommended in children but, in adults, should be started only if suspected of co-infection.*

- Levetiracetam or phenytoin should be used for seizure prophylaxis.
- Transfusion thresholds are lower in children compared to adults. Red blood cells are required if haemoglobin falls below 40 g/L. Blood is required if haemoglobin is between 40 and 60 g/L and patient has severe symptoms, like respiratory distress and altered sensorium.
- *Renal replacement therapy might be needed and is generally required for longer period (2–3 wk) compared to other patients of sepsis, leading to AKI.*

Prognosis

✓ Case fatality of severe malaria is between 5 and 50%, depending upon the degree of organ involvement. Cerebral malaria has a mortality of 30%.

✓ *Secondary bacterial sepsis is the major cause of death after 7 d in patients with severe malaria.*

Cardiovascular Problems

NON–ST-ELEVATION ACUTE CORONARY SYNDROME

Epidemiology

✓ **Acute Coronary Syndrome (ACS):** Pain occurring at rest and usually lasting more than 20 min, severe and of new onset (within 1 month), and occurring with a crescendo pattern.
- **ACS** includes unstable angina (UA), non–ST-elevation myocardial infarction (NSTEMI), and ST-elevation myocardial infarction (STEMI).
- **Unstable angina** and **NSTEMI** are usually associated with non-occlusive lesion of the coronary artery and are characterized by absence of ST-segment elevations^Q. Together they are called **non–ST-elevation acute coronary syndrome (NSTE-ACS).**
  - ❖ Raised markers of myocardial necrosis are seen in NSTEMI patients, which differentiate them from patients with unstable angina.
- **NSTE-ACS:** Platelet-rich thrombi are seen in 35–75% of patients, and they partially occlude the vessel.
  - ❖ Other causes seen are coronary vasospasm, coronary artery dissection, imbalances between oxygen demand and supply, and restenosis after percutaneous coronary intervention (PCI).

Clinical Features and Diagnosis

✓ Chest pain, epigastric pain, nausea, vomiting, dyspnoea, and diaphoresis. Prodromal symptoms seen in 20–60% of patients.

✓ **ECG:** 12-lead ECG should be done to check the location of the block.
- ST-segment depression and T-wave changes are seen in up to 50% of patients with NSTE-ACS.
- A normal ECG doesn't rule out ACS and should be repeated at regular intervals.
- About 50% of patients with non–ST-segment elevation ACS will have raised biomarkers, and remaining 50% will be classified as **unstable angina.**

✓ **Cardiac Biomarkers**
- **Raised markers** defined as rise or fall (>20%) in cardiac troponin with at least one value greater than the 99th percentile of the upper reference range.
- **Cardiac-specific troponins T or I** rise in 4–6 h, peak in 12–24 h, and get normal within 7–14 d.
- **CK-MB** starts rising in 4–6 h, peaks within 18–24 h, and remains elevated in 48–72 h.
- The American Heart Association (AHA) recommends **cardiac troponins T or I** at 0 h and between 3 and 6 h.
- The **European Society of Cardiology (ESC)** recommends **high-sensitivity cardiac troponin I** at 0 h/1 h (best option) or 0 h/2 h (second best option).
  - ❖ Patients who do not meet these criteria should have levels checked at 3 h ± echocardiography done.
- **Raised troponins** are seen in pulmonary embolism, patients on vasoconstrictors, sepsis, and patients with renal dysfunction as well.

✓ **Cardiac Imaging**
- **Echocardiography:** Can be done in cases with suspected ACS with uncertainty but should not delay cardiac catheterization.
  - ❖ All patients with haemodynamic instability should undergo transthoracic echocardiography to identify for the cause, LV, or RV failure.
  - ❖ Regional wall motion abnormality is seen when >20% transmural thickness is affected.
- **CT angiogram (CTA):** Effective in ruling out coronary artery disease in patients with low-risk chest pain, non-diagnostic ECG, and negative biomarkers.
- **Cardiovascular magnetic resonance (CMR):** Useful for late-presentation MI as it can detect subendocardial scarring and differentiate ischaemic cardiomyopathy from non-ischaemic cardiomyopathy.
- **Coronary angiography:** Helps in establishing the diagnosis and is gold standard for defining the extent of coronary disease and as a prelude to revascularization.

✓ **Risk Stratification:** Two concurrent processes of prediction of morbidity/mortality and deciding between early invasive or early conservative approach.
- **Individual risk factors:** Pain at rest, increasing frequency of symptoms, tachycardia, hypotension, signs of heart failure, and ST-segment deviation.
- There is a linear relationship between the **levels of cardiac troponin** in the blood and subsequent risk of death.
  - ❖ Evidence shows that troponins can help in assessing the risk and in determining which patients will derive the most benefit from abciximab and invasive cardiac therapy.
- Current AHA and ESC guidelines recommend the use of **risk scores** to facilitate risk stratification.
- **Thrombolysis in Myocardial Infarction (TIMI) risk score:** Uses **seven** risk factors – age >65 yr, >3 risk factors for coronary artery disease, ST-segment elevation of 0.5 mm, greater than two episodes of angina in 24 h, aspirin use within the prior week, elevated cardiac biomarkers, and previous documented coronary artery disease at

catheterization (≥50% stenosis); 1 point is assigned to each variable.
  - ❖ 0–2: **Low risk**, 3–5: **Intermediate risk**, 6–7: **High risk**
  - ❖ Patient with score >3 have a 13.2% risk of mortality or MI within 14 d compared to >40.9% risk with score of 6/7.
  - ❖ **TACTICS-TIMI 18 Trial (2001):** It showed that patients with intermediate or high risk had mortality benefit from early invasive cardiac intervention compared to medical therapy.
- **Global Registry of Acute Coronary Events (GRACE) risk score:** It includes age, heart rate, systolic blood pressure, creatinine, cardiac arrest at admission, ST deviation, elevated cardiac markers, and **Killip** class of heart failure for calculating the score and identifies patient at risk of in-hospital and mortality in 6 months.
  - ❖ **TIMACS Trial (2009):** It showed that patients with a GRACE risk score of greater than 140 had a 35% reduction in mortality with early angiography compared to delayed intervention.

Treatment

✓ **Treatment Goals:** Stabilizing the acute coronary lesion, treatment of residual ischaemia, and long-term secondary prevention.
- All patients, irrespective of the risk, get **aspirin, P2Y12 inhibitor**, and **an anticoagulant**. Timing of intervention depends upon the level of risk.

✓ **Antiplatelet Therapy:** Cornerstone of therapy, as thrombus is predominantly made of platelets.
- Dual antiplatelet therapy (aspirin and P2Y12 inhibitor) is recommended for 12 months.
- **Aspirin:** *Irreversible inhibitor of cyclooxygenase* and, hence, inhibitory effect of platelets for 7–10 d.
  - ❖ **ISIS-2 Trial (1988):** It leads to a significant reduction in the risk of death or MI.
  - ❖ A loading dose of 325 mg followed by 75–81 mg daily has shown mortality benefit and is given in all patients presenting with NSTE-ACS.
  - ❖ Aspirin may be discontinued (7–10 d preoperatively) in patients deemed at

low risk of cardiovascular events and patients at high risk of bleeding (intracranial, epidural, or ocular spaces)

❖ Aspirin should be continued in patients having moderate to high risk of cardiovascular events and requiring non-cardiac surgery.

- **P2Y12 ADP receptor blockers** (clopidogrel, prasugrel, ticagrelor): Inhibits the binding of ADP to the P2Y12 receptor.

    ❖ ESC does not recommend immediate pre-angiography administration of P2Y12 inhibitors in patients with unknown anatomy as they can increase bleeding in patients requiring CABG after angiography.

    ❖ *In patients having a non-invasive strategy, clopidogrel or ticagrelor is recommended as soon as diagnosis of NSTE-ACS is made.*

    ❖ ***Addition of a P2Y12 to aspirin further reduces risk by 20%.***

    ❖ They should be stopped 7 d before an elective surgery.

    ❖ **Clopidogrel:** Prodrug that undergoes hepatic metabolism by CYP2C19 to become an active metabolite. Around 25–30% of population have a reduced functioning variant of this allele and, hence, have a higher rate of ischaemic events. Proton pump inhibitors (PPIs) inhibit CYP2C19 and should be used with caution in these patients.

    ❖ **Prasugrel:** New-generation drug. Prodrug. Faster onset (30 mins) and more predictable and more potent inhibition than clopidogrel. **TRITON-TIMI Trial (2007)** showed, with the use of prasugrel, a 19% reduction of the rate of cardiovascular death as well as a 52% reduction in stent thrombosis as compared to clopidogrel. However, there was a significant increase in rate of **major bleeding**. Hence, *prasugrel is preferred over clopidogrel in patients treated with PCI who are not at risk for bleeding.*

    ❖ **Ticagrelor:** Reversible inhibitor, unlike clopidogrel or prasugrel. Active drug. Like prasugrel, faster onset (30 mins) and more predictable and more potent inhibition than clopidogrel. *Ticagrelor is preferred over clopidogrel for patients treated with medical therapy or with PCI.* Like prasugrel, it has also shown mortality benefit over clopidogrel.

    ❖ **Cangrelor:** Reversible drug that can be used intravenously, with fast onset of action (2 mins), and platelet function is restored within 60 min of stopping the drug. Can be used as a bridge for patients planned for surgery.

- **GP IIb–IIIa inhibitors**[Q] (abciximab, eptifibatide, and tirofiban): They block the fibrinogen-mediated cross-linking of platelets. Given intravenously.

    ❖ They have been shown to **increase risk of bleeding** without significant reductions in ischaemic events.

    ❖ Hence, the *ESC recommends against the use of GP IIb–IIIa inhibitors for patients in whom coronary anatomy is not known and gives a class IIa recommendation for use during PCI in bailout situations or thrombotic complications.*

    ❖ *They can be considered in high-risk troponin-positive patients.*

✓ **Anticoagulation Therapy:** *Given along with antiplatelet therapy as they reduce the risk of events. Choice depends upon local protocols and patient specifics.*

- **Unfractionated heparin (UFH):** Inhibits both thrombin and factor Xa.

    ❖ A 60 U/kg bolus is given, followed by 12 U/kg/h infusion.

    ❖ It should be continued for 48 h or until PCI is performed.

- **Low-molecular-weight heparin:** Inhibits factor Xa.

    ❖ Recent meta-analysis has shown that enoxaparin reduced ischaemic events without a significant increase in major bleeding.

    ❖ Recommended dose is 1 mg/kg every 12 h.

- **Fondaparinux:** Inhibits factor Xa.
- ESC recommends the standard dose UFH to be used during PCI for patients treated with fondaparinux beforehand, as fondaparinux is associated with increased risk of catheter-related thrombi.

- **Bivalirudin:** Directly inhibits thrombin.
  - ❖ AHA recommends that bivalirudin is only for patients managed with early invasive strategy, whereas ESC recommends bivalirudin as an alternative to UFH-GP IIb–IIIa inhibitor during PCI.
- **Oral anticoagulants:** At the time of presentation, in patients on chronic oral anticoagulation for AF or DVT, UFH should be deferred until the patient is subtherapeutic or next dose in case of direct oral anticoagulants (DOAC).
  - ❖ After PCI, a short course of triple therapy with aspirin, clopidogrel, and a DOAC should be transitioned to clopidogrel and DOAC after approximately 1 wk.

✓ **Anti-Ischaemic Therapy:** Supplemental oxygen for saturation >90%^{Q}.
- **Pain relief: Nitrates** for symptom relief and have no mortality benefit.
  - ❖ Intravenous nitroglycerine is recommended for refractory pain or hypertension.
  - ❖ Consider **intravenous morphine** if pain is not sufficiently controlled by nitroglycerine.
- *Beta-blockers: Start oral beta-blockers within first 24 h for patients who are not in heart failure or at risk of it. Early initiation was associated with mortality benefit.*
  - ❖ In the presence of contraindications, beta-blockers should be considered once the patient is stable.
  - ❖ Beta-blockers should be given orally (not IV) within first 24 h of onset of symptoms.
- **Calcium channel blockers:** Non-dihydropyridine **calcium channel blockers**, like diltiazem and verapamil, should be used only for patients with preserved LV function and resistant ischaemia to nitrates and beta-blockers or for patients in which beta-blockers are contraindicated.
- **Angiotensin-converting enzyme inhibitors (ACE inhibitors):** *Shown to reduce mortality in patients with LVEF <40% and heart failure and recommended in these*

patients along with patients with hypertension, diabetes, or stable CKD.
  - ❖ Angiotensin receptor blockers (ARBs) can be used as alternatives for patients who are intolerant to ACE inhibitors.
- **Mineralocorticoid receptor antagonism:** *Aldosterone blockers, like **eplerenone**, have shown mortality benefit in patients with LVEF <40% and are recommended in these patients along with beta-blockers and ACE inhibitors.* Not recommended in patients with renal dysfunction.
- **Lipid-lowering therapy:** *Statins have been shown to have mortality benefit and are recommended.* **Ezetimibe** is recommended as additional lipid-lowering agent for patients in which LDL cholesterol is not controlled by a maximum statin therapy.

✓ **Interventional Therapy**
- **Invasive strategy:** Within first 72 h, angiography and revascularization with PCI or bypass surgery as needed.
  - ❖ Invasive therapy has been associated to have 25% lower rates of death and 17% lower rates of MI over 2 yr compared to ischaemia-guided strategy.
  - ❖ **Urgent invasive (within 2 h): Very high risk.** Haemodynamic instability, refractory ischaemia, acute heart failure, mechanical complications, and recurrent malignant VT or VF.
  - ❖ **Early invasive (within 24 h): High risk.** GRACE risk score >140, elevated troponin compatible with MI.
  - ❖ **Delayed invasive (within 72 h): Intermediate risk.** GRACE risk score 109–140, TIMI score >2, prior PCI or CABG, reduced LVEF <40%, diabetes or renal insufficiency (eGFR <60 mL/min/1.73 m^2).
- **Ischaemia-guided strategy:** More conservative approach with initial medical therapy and angiography and revascularization only for recurrent ischaemia.
  - ❖ **Ischaemia-guided: Low risk.** GRACE risk score <109, TIMI score <2, low-risk troponin-negative female patients.

Complications: 2–3% of patients with NSTEMI will develop cardiogenic shock 4–5 d later.

Prognosis

✓ 10% of patients with a NSTEMI will die or have myocardial infarction at 6 months.

ST-ELEVATION ACUTE CORONARY SYNDROME

Pathophysiology and Definition

✓ The characteristic feature of **ST-elevation acute coronary syndrome (STE-ACS) or ST-elevation MI (STEMI)** is complete occlusion of coronary artery, leading to transmural myocardial injury.

✓ Initiating event is rupture of a lipid-rich atherosclerotic plaque.
- Platelets adhere to the subendothelial collagen and aggregate to form a **white thrombus**.
- This is followed by activation of coagulation cascade and cross-linking of fibrin with red cells enmeshed.
- This is called a **red thrombus**, and it totally blocks the artery.

✓ Reperfusion therapy will limit the necrosis to the subendocardial regions only and prevent development of Q waves.

✓ **Myocardial infarction (MI) can be classified into five types[Q] based on aetiology and circumstances**
- **Type 1:** Spontaneous MI caused by ischaemia due to a primary coronary event (e.g. plaque rupture, erosion, coronary dissection).
- **Type 2:** Ischaemia due to ischaemic imbalance (i.e. increased oxygen demand) (e.g. hypertension) or decreased supply (e.g. coronary artery spasm, embolism).
- **Type 3:** Related to sudden unexpected cardiac death.
- **Type 4a:** Associated with PCI.
- **Type 4b:** Associated with documented stent thrombosis.
- **Type 5:** Associated with CABG.

✓ Myocardial infarction seen in ICU patients is mostly type 2, with imbalance between oxygen supply and demand.
- In patients with ECG changes and raised troponin levels, consider the use of echocardiography to identify regional wall motion abnormality for diagnosis of acute myocardial infarction in ITU.

✓ **Fourth Universal Definition for Types 1, 2, and 3 MI**
- Rise and/or fall of troponin levels, with at least one value above the 99th percentile of upper reference limit and at least one of the following:
  - ❖ Symptoms of myocardial ischaemia
  - ❖ New ischaemic ECG changes
  - ❖ Development of pathological Q waves
  - ❖ Imaging evidence of new loss of viable myocardium or new regional wall abnormality in a pattern consistent with an ischaemic aetiology
  - ❖ Identification of a coronary thrombus by angiography or autopsy (not for type 2 or 3 MIs).

✓ **Myocardial Infarction with Normal Coronary Arteries (MINOCA):** Patients with troponin elevation and ST-segment elevation may have normal coronary arteries. It is seen in 5% of patients.

Clinical Features and Diagnosis

✓ Severe, constant pressure-type chest pain radiating to the left arm, neck, or jaw. Duration >20 min.
- Females and patients with diabetes often have atypical pain.
- Cool extremities may suggest accompanying heart failure.

✓ **ECG Changes:** Target is within 10 min in patient suspected with ACS. ECG should be repeated in 15 to 30 min if initial study is non-diagnostic.
- **The diagnostic criteria of ST elevation are**
  - ❖ *>0.1 mV in two contiguous leads in all leads other than V2–V3.*
  - ❖ In lead V2–V3, >0.2 mV in men >40 yr, >0.25 mV in men <40 yr, and >0.15 mV in women.
- A new LBBB lacks specificity and is no longer considered a STEMI equivalent in isolation. However, the development of a bundle branch block indicates extensive anterior wall infarction.
- **Additional leads, such as V7 to V9, can be used to look for posterior MI[Q] seen in left circumflex occlusion.** In these cases, leads V1–V3 may show reciprocal ST-segment depression.

- Bradycardia/complete heart block[Q] is seen if right coronary artery is affected in **inferior myocardial infarction**[Q] as it affects a branch to the SA node in roughly 60% and AV node in approximately 80–90%.
  - ❖ **V3R and V4R leads should be used to identify right ventricular infarction.**
- ST-segment elevation will typically have a convex configuration compared to concave segment seen in pericarditis[Q].
- **ECG changes**[Q] **in acute MI are as follows**
  - ❖ **Hyperacute (0–20 min):** Tall, peaking T waves
  - ❖ **Acute (minutes to hours):** Upward-coving and elevation of ST segment
  - ❖ **Early (hours to days):** Loss of R wave, return of ST segment to baseline, with T wave inversion
  - ❖ **Indeterminate (days to weeks):** Q wave with T wave inversion
  - ❖ **Old (weeks to months):** Q wave with normal ST segment and T wave

Artery Occluded[Q]	Infarcted Territory	ECG Leads[Q]
LCA/proximal LAD	Anterolateral	V1–V6, I, aV$_L$
LAD	Septum	V1–V3
LAD	Anterior	V2–V5
Circumflex	Lateral	V5, V6, I, aV$_L$
Circumflex	Inferolateral	II, III, aV$_F$, V5, V6, I, aV$_L$
RCA proximal	Right ventricle	V1, V$_4$R, II, III, aV$_F$
RCA	Inferior	II, III, aV$_F$
RCA dominant	Infero-posterior	II, III, aV$_F$, V7, V8

- ✓ **Cardiac Biomarkers:** More important for initial diagnosis of NSTEMI compared to STEMI.
  - For patients with STEMI, cardiac markers are used to confirm the diagnosis in patients with equivocal ECG changes.
  - Peak levels of troponin provide an estimation of infarct size.
- ✓ **Risk Stratification:** GRACE score[Q] is same across the whole spectrum of ACS. A separate TIMI risk score predicts 30 d adverse events in patients with STEMI is available. Score > 8/15 is associated with 36% risk of mortality. The variables for TIMI risk score are:
  - Age >75 yr: 3 points
  - Age 65 to 74 yr: 2 points

- History of diabetes, hypertension, or angina: 1 point
- Systolic blood pressure < 100 mmHg: 3 points
- Heart rate > 100/min: 2 points
- Killip class II to IV: 2 points
- Weight <67 kg: 1 point
- Anterior ST elevation or LBBB: 1 point
- Time to reperfusion therapy > 4 hr: 1 point

Prevention and Treatment

- ✓ **Rapid reperfusion therapy** is the cornerstone of STEMI management.
  - Early successful coronary reperfusion limits infarct size and improve LV dysfunction and survival.
  - Benefits of reperfusion therapy are time-dependent. It can be either percutaneous coronary intervention (PCI) or medical fibrinolytic therapy.
  - **Primary PCI:** Normal epicardial blood flow is achieved in >90% of STEMI patients.
    - ❖ Tissue perfusion may still be inadequate in around one-third of patients who achieve normal epicardial blood flow and can be assessed by degree of resolution of ST-segment elevation.
    - ❖ Patients with ST elevation even after reperfusion therapy have higher incidence of heart failure and death.
    - ❖ *Indication*[Q]: *A primary PCI is recommended for presentation within 12 h of symptoms onset, and the time of first medical contact (FMC) to device in a PCI-capable patient should be <90 min. Time for FMC to device in a non-PCI-capable patient should be <120 min.*
    - ❖ *In patients with cardiogenic chock, presentation after > 12 h of symptoms onset, contraindication to fibrinolysis, evidence of failed fibrinolysis, transfer to a PCI centre for PCI is preferred even if delay times are longer.*
    - ❖ *Drug-eluting stents (DES) are preferred as lower chances of in-stent restenosis compared to bare metal stents. They should be continued for 1 yr*[Q].
    - ❖ *Bare metal stents are given only if patient can't comply with >1 month of DAPT or has a non-cardiac surgery in 4 to 6 wk.*

❖ Radial artery is preferred for access compared to femoral artery as it has fewer bleeding complications.

❖ **In patients with multivessel disease, multivessel PCI over culprit vessel–only PCI has a IIB recommendation (may be considered). However, in patients with cardiogenic shock, culprit vessel–only revascularization is preferred.**

- **Fibrinolytic therapy** (streptokinase, alteplase, tenecteplase, reteplase): Normal epicardial blood flow is achieved in 50% of STEMI patients.

  ❖ Compared to placebo, fibrinolytic therapy has shown mortality benefit.

  ❖ *Indication:* **AHA** recommends that fibrinolysis should be used in patients with STEMI and ischaemic symptom onset <12 h when it is apparent that PCI won't be performed within 120 min of first medical contact.

  ❖ *Give fibrinolytic therapy within <30 min of arrival.*

  ❖ Bleeding is the most common complication, and major haemorrhage happens in 5–15% of patients.

  ❖ **Tenecteplase** is most fibrin-selective and has slightly better safety profile compared to others and is the preferred agent for fibrinolytic therapy.

  ❖ **Alteplase:** Only fibrinolytic approved for acute stroke as well.

  ❖ **Rescue PCI:** Urgent PCI is indicated for all patients with persistent ST elevation and ongoing chest pain 90 min after the administration of fibrinolytic therapy. In patients who are pain-free but still unresolved ST-segment elevation, PCI should be strongly considered,Q especially in patient with high-risk profile, like advanced age, anterior location of infarct, or diabetes.

  ❖ **AHA gives a class IIa recommendation for coronary angiography in STEMI after fibrinolysis therapy, either as rescue PCI if needed or between 3 and 24 h after successful reperfusion with fibrinolytic therapy.**

Contraindications to Fibrinolytic Therapy

Absolute Contraindications	Relative Contraindications
Known brain tumour	Proliferative diabetic retinopathy
Prior intracranial haemorrhage	Known bleeding diathesis
Ischaemic stroke within last 3 months	Ischaemic stroke >3 months old
Head trauma within last 3 months	Pregnancy
Aortic dissection	Prolonged CPR >10 min
Active internal bleeding	Active peptic ulcer or recent internal bleeding.
Intracranial or intraspinal surgery within 2 months	Major surgery <3 wk
Severe uncontrolled hypertension	Blood pressure > 180/110 mmHg

✓ **Pharmacological Treatment**

Antiplatelet therapy: Limits the white thrombus.

✓ **Aspirin**Q**:** Decreases mortality by 25% in patients with STEMI. Loading dose of 325 mg followed by lifelong daily 75 mg is the regimen.

✓ **P2Y12 inhibitors** (clopidogrel, prasugrel, or ticagrelor): It should be added to aspirin for a minimum of 12 months in a patient receiving a stentQ. *Stopped 7 d before a lumbar puncture*Q.

  - **Clopidogrel** addition to aspirin had shown further mortality benefit, but newer P2Y12 agents are more predictable with more potency and are thus preferred over clopidogrel.

  - **Prasugrel:** Newer P2Y12 inhibitor. It shouldn't be used for patients with a history of CVA/TIA, age >75 yr/weight <60 kgs, and moderate to severe hepatic dysfunction.

  - **Ticagrelor:** Newer P2Y12 inhibitor. It can cause transient dyspnoea in 10–15% of patients. It can cause ventricular pauses as well.

    ❖ Contraindicated in patients with history of haemorrhagic stroke, active bleeding, or moderate to severe hepatic dysfunction.

✓ **GP IIb/IIIa inhibitors:** Recommended for selected patients who are receiving unfractionated heparin during PCI.

Anticoagulation therapy: Limits the red thrombus.

✓ AHA recommends administration of an anticoagulant (UFH, enoxaparin, or fondaparinux) for all patients receiving fibrinolytic therapy.
  • Fibrinolytic therapy can lead to progression of thrombin activation; hence, anti-thrombin agents like heparin are used along with it.
  • LMWH given up to 8 d or until PCI has been shown to be superior to short-term use of UFH in patients undergoing fibrinolysis.
  • **Fondaparinux** is the antithrombin therapy of choice, unless PCI is being done in 24 h or in patients with renal disease or bleeding disorders, in whom unfractionated heparin should be used.
  • **IV UFH** with or without GP IIb/IIIa receptor antagonist is recommended in **patients undergoing PCI.**
  • **Oral anticoagulation:** Newer oral anticoagulants (NOAC) + P2Y12 inhibitor without aspirin are preferred in patients with PCI and AF.
    ❖ After PCI, a short course of triple therapy with aspirin, clopidogrel, and a NOAC should be transitioned to clopidogrel and DOAC after approximately 1 wk.

Anti-ischaemic therapy: Oxygen for keeping saturation above 90%.

✓ **Pain Relief**
  • **Nitrates:** Dilate vein and coronary arteries. Sublingual nitroglycerine 0.4 mg every 5 min for a total of three doses is recommended.
  • Intravenous nitroglycerine is suggested for refractory pain or hypertension. They have not shown any mortality benefit.
  • They should be avoided in patients with right ventricular infarction and patients on phosphodiesterase-5 inhibitors.
  • Consider intravenous morphine if pain is not sufficiently controlled by nitroglycerine.
✓ **Beta-Blockers**[Q]
  • They exert their beneficial effect by reducing the frequency and severity of arrhythmias.
  • AHA recommends that beta-blockers be initiated orally within the first 24 h once the patient is stable, with no signs of heart failure.
  • In the presence of contraindications, beta-blockers should be considered once the patient is stable.

• Long-term beta-blockers should be continued for at least 3 yr in patients without heart failure after MI.
✓ **Calcium Channel Blockers:** Not given routinely and are given if patient can't tolerate a beta-blocker, given no heart failure and resistant hypertension.
✓ **ACE Inhibitors/Angiotensin Receptor Blockers (ARBs)**[Q]: ACE inhibitors prevent cardiac remodelling, and the benefit was greater in patients with Killip class II or III heart failure, those with LV dysfunction, and those with anterior MI. ARBs are alternative to ACE inhibitors.
✓ **Aldosterone Antagonists:** Mortality benefit in patients with LVEF <40%.
✓ **Statins**[Q]: Statins have shown mortality benefit as well.

Secondary Prevention Summary

✓ **Non-pharmacological interventions**, like smoking cessation, healthy diet, decreased alcohol consumption, weight loss, and exercise.
✓ **Pharmacological interventions:**[Q]
  • Low-dose aspirin, **DAPT** up to 1-yr post-STEMI
  • PPI for those on DAPT
  • **Beta-blockers** for all patients post-STEMI
  • **ACEIs** for all patients post-STEMI; ARBs if intolerant to ACEIs
  • **Eplerenone (aldosterone antagonist)** if evidence of heart failure with LV impairment
  • **Statins**

Complications: 7–10% of patients with STEMI will develop cardiogenic shock in the range of 6 h.

✓ Other complications are ventricular septal rupture, free wall rupture, malignant arrhythmias, RV dysfunction, and mitral valve regurgitation due to papillary muscle necrosis.
✓ Infranodal conduction pathways[Q] are affected in anterior MI due to blockage of left anterior descending artery. Hence, atropine may be ineffective in managing complete heart block in these cases.

MECHANICAL COMPLICATIONS OF MI[Q]

Left Ventricle Free Wall Rupture

✓ **Aetiology:** Ischaemic necrosis of LV free wall
✓ **Predisposing Factors:** Late reperfusion, elderly women

✓ **Timing Post-MI:** Within first 5 d in half of the patients (first 48 h with reperfusion).

✓ **Presentation:** Complete rupture is usually a catastrophic event. Those with incomplete rupture present with sudden chest pain after coughing, progressing to cardiogenic shock, tamponade, PEA, sudden cardiac death. **Beck's triad of tamponade** (hypotension, raised JVP, and muffled heart sounds), pulsus paradoxus.

✓ **Microbubble Echocardiography[Q]:** New signs of tamponade, pericardial effusion, pseudoaneurysm.

✓ **Right Heart Catheterization (Pulmonary Artery Catheter):** Equalization of diastolic pressure.

✓ **Treatment:** Initially treat tamponade with IV fluids, inotropes, and emergent pericardiocentesis. Definitive emergency surgery would be needed.

✓ **Prognosis:** 5–24% of in-hospital mortality of MI.

Ventricular Septal Rupture

✓ **Aetiology:** Ischaemic necrosis of interventricular septum.

✓ **Predisposing Factors:** Incomplete reperfusion, large MI, elderly women.

✓ **Timing Post-MI:** First day and 3–5 d after an acute MI in those without reperfusion (first 24 h with reperfusion).

✓ **Presentation:** Chest pain, cardiogenic shock, dyspnoea. New loud, harsh holosystolic murmur[Q], pulmonary congestion.

✓ **Echocardiography:** Left to right shunt through VSD.

✓ **Right Heart Catheterization (Pulmonary Artery Catheter):** Shows step-up in oxygen saturation at level of right ventricle.

✓ **Treatment:** Vasodilators, inotropic agents, diuretics, and **IABP.** Urgent surgical intervention even in haemodynamically stable patients.

✓ **Prognosis:** Around 90% medical mortality, 50% surgical mortality.

Acute Mitral Regurgitation

✓ **Aetiology:** Due to papillary muscle rupture[Q]. Posteromedial muscle is more prone to rupture due to single blood supply compared to dual blood supply of anterolateral.

✓ **Predisposing Factors:** Inferior wall MI.[Q]

✓ **Timing Post-MI:** 2–7 d after inferior MI.

✓ **Presentation:** Sudden onset of chest pain, dyspnoea, progressing to cardiogenic shock. Elevated JVP, pulmonary congestion, holosystolic murmur.

✓ **Echocardiography:** Flail segment of mitral valve, ruptured papillary muscle, hyperdynamic LV function.

✓ **Right Heart Catheterization (Pulmonary Artery Catheter):** Prominent c–v wave.

✓ **Treatment:** Afterload reduction by vasodilators and IABP.

✓ Cardiac surgery: MV repair or replacement may be needed. Simultaneous CABG.

✓ **Prognosis:** 90% medical mortality, 40–90% surgical mortality.

Right Ventricle Infarction

✓ **Aetiology:** RV infarction is a common complication (50%) of inferior transmural MI. RCA occlusion proximal to origin of acute marginals causes it.

✓ **Predisposing Factors:** RCA occlusion.

✓ **Timing Post-MI:** First few hours.

✓ **Presentation:** Hypotension/shock, elevated JVP, clear lungs. The presence of 1 mm ST elevation in lead V1 and in right precordial lead V4R is the most sensitive ECG marker of right ventricular myocardial infarction.

✓ **Echocardiography:** RV enlargement, septum bowing towards LV, elevated RA pressure (>10 mmHg).

✓ **Treatment:** IV fluids, inotropes, early reperfusion, pacing (if AV block), cardioversion (if AF). Avoid diuretics and nitrates.
  • **Cardiac surgery:** If CABG is required and more than 6 h have elapsed since presentation, delaying CABG may be a better option to allow for recovery of RF function.

Left Ventricular Aneurysm

✓ **Aetiology:** Majority of LV aneurysms are located in the anterior apical walls due to occlusion of the left anterior descending coronary artery.

✓ **Presentation:** Congestive heart failure, thromboembolism, and malignant ventricular tachyarrhythmias.
  • Suspected in patients with large anterior MI with persistent ST-segment elevation on ECG.

✓ **Diagnosis:** Confirmed by echocardiography, CT, or cardiac MRI.

✓ **Treatment:** Long-term anticoagulation and ICD[Q] implantation.
- Surgical aneurysmectomy may be considered when there are refractory ventricular arrhythmias, heart failure, or recurrent thromboembolism.

Dynamic LV Outflow Obstruction (DLVOTO)

✓ **Aetiology:** Occurs due to compensatory hyperdynamic contraction of the basal inferior and inferolateral segments in the setting of a mid-anterior MI and LV apical akinesis.
- Hyperkinesis of the basal segments may result in reduction of the LVOT cross-sectional area, acceleration of blood flow across the LVOT, systolic anterior motion of the mitral valve, and ultimately, DLVOTO, similar to what is seen in hypertrophic cardiomyopathy.
✓ **Presentation:** They present as an acute anterior MI with a new systolic murmur and unstable haemodynamics.
- Posteriorly directed mitral valve regurgitation that can lead to acute pulmonary oedema.
- Always suspect LVOT in an anterior MI patient in whom cardiogenic shock is not responding to usual treatment with inotropes, IABP support, and afterload reduction.
✓ **Diagnosis:** Transthoracic echocardiography is the diagnostic modality of choice.
- Apical akinesis with hyperdynamic function of the inferobasal segment and systolic anterior motion of the mitral valve.
✓ **Treatment:** IV fluids, beta-blockers, phenylephrine, and discontinuation of vasodilators and inotropic agents.

Dressler Syndrome (Post–Myocardial Infarction Syndrome)

✓ **Aetiology:** Rare form of pericarditis that can happen after a myocardial infarction.
- Fibrinohaemorrhagic secondary pericarditis that occurs as a result of injury to the heart or pericardium.
✓ **Presentation:** Patient presents with fever, malaise, chest pain, dyspnoea around 1–6 wk post-event.
- Should be suspected in all patients presenting with persistent malaise or fatigue following a myocardial infarction.
✓ **Diagnosis:** ECG shows global ST-segment elevation and T wave inversion.

- **Echocardiography** is the most sensitive imaging study that will allow for evaluation of the pericardial fluid.
✓ **Treatment:** NSAIDs[Q] tapered over 4 to 6 wk as the accumulated pericardial fluid diminishes.
- Corticosteroids may be given in patients who do not respond to the treatment.
- Colchicine is the other option.

PULMONARY EMBOLISM

Epidemiology and Aetiology

✓ **Pulmonary Embolism:** Blood vessels in lungs blocked by blood clots.
- Incidence of pulmonary embolism in post-mortem studies is 27%.
✓ **Risk Factors:** Malignancy, trauma, burns, prolonged immobilization, major abdominal surgery, hip replacement, knee replacement, haemodialysis, thrombophilia-like factor V Leiden mutation, inflammatory conditions like rheumatoid arthritis.

Clinical Features

✓ **Hypoxaemia** with increased P (A-a) O2 gradient, dyspnoea, **pleuritic chest pain**, haemoptysis, sudden hypotension, **sinus tachycardia[Q] (most common feature)**, and **S1Q3T3 pattern** (10% patients) on ECG.
- **Proximal lower extremity DVT** is the most frequent source of PE. Other sources are pelvic, renal, or upper extremity veins.
- **Pulsus paradoxus[Q]** is seen, which is an increase in systolic drop of >10 mmHg during inhalation. Also seen in cardiac tamponade and tension pneumothorax.

Clinical Prediction Models[Q]: Pretesting probability models to assess a patient's risk for VTE.

✓ **Revised Geneva Score:** Objective criteria to assess risk for VTE. **Score 0–3** indicates low probability, 4–10 intermediate probability, and ≥ *11 high probabilities of PE*.
✓ **Wells Score:** Subjective clinical judgement involved. **Score 0–1** indicates low probability, 2–6 intermediate probability, and *>6 high probabilities of PE[Q]*. (Trainees with medical background wouldn't mind this table; feel sorry for trainees with anaesthetic background. No need to learn it by heart.)

Wells Score for PE Diagnosis	Score
Clinical signs of DVT (pain and swelling)	3
Alternative diagnosis less likely than pulmonary embolism	3
Tachycardia >100 bpm	1.5
Immobile for 3 d, or major surgery within previous 4 wk	1.5
Previous VTE	1.5
Haemoptysis	1
Active cancer (within 6 months)	1

Diagnosis

✓ **D-Dimer:** D-dimers, along with clinical pre-dictability models, have been used to rule out DVT and PE for **outpatients**.
  - D-dimer is non-specific and elevated in cancer, infection, pregnancy, and recent surgery and, **hence**, **less useful for hospitalized patients**.
  - D-Dimer (<500) is useful in excluding PE in **low- and intermediate-risk cases** only.
  - Abnormal D-dimer in **low- to intermediate-risk cases** warrants CT pulmonary angiography.

✓ **CT Pulmonary Angiography (CTPA):** In **high-risk cases**, CTPA is investigation of choice straight away, unless patient is unstable when echocardiography is used.
  - CTPA can reveal emboli up to subsegmental pulmonary arteries as well.

✓ **Echocardiography^Q:** RV dysfunction (RV/LV diameter >1), presence of RV thrombus, flattened interventricular septum, tricuspid annular plane systolic excursion (TAPSE) <16 mm.
  - **McConnell's sign:** 40% of cases. Reduced RV free wall contractility with sparing of apex. High positive predictive value.

  - RV dilation in 20–30% of cases.
  - *Pulmonary artery pressure above 55–60 mmHg means chronic pulmonary disease rather than acute pulmonary embolism.*

✓ **V/Q Scan:** Used in pregnant patients, patients with contrast allergies, and those at risk of contrast-induced nephrotoxicity.
  - It can't detect subsegmental PE.

✓ **Pregnancy:** *Non-invasive test, like lower limb duplex ultrasound, is done first, and if negative, a chest radiograph is done to rule out alternative diagnosis.*
  - In case of a normal chest X-ray, V/Q scan or CTPA is done, in which V/Q scan is more likely to conclusively diagnose or rule out PE.

Risk Stratification^Q: Essential for appropriate treatment strategy.

✓ **American Heart Association (AHA) PE classification:**
  - **Massive/high risk^Q:** SBP <90 mmHg or drop of ≥40 mmHg for 15 min or cardiac arrest. Requiring vasopressor support; 30 d mortality risk ~30%.
  - **Sub-massive/intermediate risk:** Presence of RV strain, dilation, or dysfunction; 90 d mortality risk 3–15%.
  - **Low risk:** None of the above; 30 d mortality risk ~1%.

✓ **PE Severity Index Score:** Validated score to predict mortality. Original score had five classes.
  - **Simplified PESI (sPESI) score** ≥1 point signifies a 30 d mortality of 10.9%.

✓ **ESC Classification:** Classification of patients with acute PE based on early (30 d) mortality.

Early Mortality Risk		Indicators of Risk			
		Haemodynamic Instability (Cardiac Arrest or SBP < 90 mmHg)	sPESI ≥ 1	RV Dysfunction on TTE or CTPA	Elevated Cardiac Troponin Levels (cTnI > 0.05)
High		+	+	+	+
Intermediate^Q	Intermediate high	–	+	+	+
	Intermediate low	–	+	One or none positive	
Low		–	–	–	Assessment optional; if assessed, negative

Prevention and Treatment

✓ **Resuscitation:** Cautious IV fluids challenge (500 mL over 15–30 min) to augment pre-load. Dobutamine and norepinephrine for hypotension.

✓ **Systemic Thrombolysis: Used in massive PE[Q].** Bleeding risk of 20%, haemorrhagic stroke risk 5%.

- *No benefit of thrombolysis in sub-massive pulmonary embolism.* Alteplase (fibrin-specific agents) better than streptokinase as less antigenic.
- Systemic thrombolysis is as good as catheter intervention in PE in massive PE.
- **Alteplase dose for thrombolysis is 100 mg[Q] over 2 h (fixed dose).**
  - ❖ **A 50 mg bolus alteplase can be given in peri-arrest situation[Q]** in patients suspected of having PE.
- In a patient with recent PE on anticoagulation, presence of haemodynamic instability or worsening oxygenation calls for consideration of thrombolysis.
- In patients with massive PE and contraindication to systemic thrombolysis, reduced-dose systemic thrombolysis, catheter-directed thrombolysis, or surgical embolectomy can also be tried.

✓ **Anticoagulation: In sub-massive PE, give therapeutic LMWH/fondaparinux as treatment.** *Can be started while diagnostic workup is going on.*

- UFH if patient has renal failure according to ESC guidelines. LMWH with anti-Xa monitoring can be used in renal failure (eGFR <30 mL/min/1.73 m^2) as well according to NICE guidelines. UFH suggested by both NICE and ESC guidelines for patients with increased chance of bleeding.
- Enoxaparin 1 mg/kg BD or 1.5 mg/kg OD.
- **Duration of anticoagulation treatment:** Lifelong for unprovoked PE and 3–6 months for post-surgery cases.

✓ **IVC Filter:** If a patient has a contraindication to anticoagulation[Q], use of IVC filter is recommended.

- They should be removed as soon as anticoagulation can be resumed, as they can cause IVC thrombosis.
- They are also used post-recurrence of emboli despite anticoagulation therapy

and when temporary cessation of anticoagulation is anticipated within 1 month – e.g. pregnant females within a month of expected date of delivery.

- No long-term mortality benefit.

✓ **Surgical pulmonary embolectomy is recommended for patients in whom thrombolysis is contraindicated or failed.**

✓ **ECMO has been used in refractory cases as well.**

Prognosis

✓ *Severity of PE doesn't depend on the size and location. Saddle embolus is not associated with increased mortality.*

✓ ECG changes associated with poor prognosis[Q].

- Tachycardia (>100 bpm)
- New and complete right bundle branch block
- Atrial arrhythmias (AF)
- ST elevation in aVR
- S1Q3T3 pattern
- Anterior ST-segment changes and T wave inversion

STRESS CARDIOMYOPATHY

✓ **Aetiology**

- **Stress cardiomyopathy:** Also known as **Takotsubo cardiomyopathy**, or **broken heart syndrome[Q]**, or apical ballooning syndrome; a condition where the pumping ability of the heart weakens due to intense physical or emotional stress.
  - ❖ Also seen in pheochromocytoma, subarachnoid haemorrhage, and seizures due to catecholamine surge, physical triggers like pregnancy, and drug abuse like amphetamines.

✓ **Clinical Features and Diagnosis**

- Seen in elderly women, precipitated by **emotional distress**.
  - ❖ About 90% of patients are post-menopausal.
- Chest pain is associated with antero-apical ST elevation and T wave inversions.
  - ❖ Gigantic T wave inversion and prolonged QT are seen 2–3 d later.
- ECHO shows **regional dysfunction** with LV hypokinesia/akinesia along with **apical ballooning** and reduced LV ejection fraction, but angiography is negative.

- Cardiac troponins are elevated in >90% of the patients.
  - ❖ BNP are raised as well, reaching its peak in 24–48 h after symptoms onset.
- High risk of arrhythmias, treated with beta-blockers.

✓ **Treatment**
- In patients with heart failure (pulmonary congestion), treat as systolic heart failure and give diuretics, nitroglycerine, low-dose beta-blockers, and ACE inhibitors.
- For patients with heart failure going in cardiogenic shock:
  - ❖ Consider non-adrenergic inotropic drugs, like levosimendan/milrinone, and vasopressors, like phenylephrine, if needed.
  - ❖ Mechanical support with a left ventricular assist device (IABP or impella) may be needed as bridge to recovery.
- Identify **LVOT obstruction** and start beta-blockers. **Avoid inotropes. Give IV fluids.**
  - ❖ Peripherally acting vasopressors like phenylephrine or vasopressin if concomitant shock.
  - ❖ Mechanical support with a left ventricular assist device (ECMO) may be needed as bridge to recovery.
- Initiate anticoagulation to reduce thromboembolic risk (in patients with large areas of akinesis).

✓ **Prognosis**
- Resolves within days to weeks. In hospital, mortality of 5%.
- Recurrences are common with up to 20% in 10 yr.

Sepsis-Induced Cardiomyopathy (SIC)

✓ **Epidemiology**
- Seen in up to 20% of sepsis cases at 6 h and 60% cases at 48 h.
- Body's response to severe infection, leading to widespread inflammation and heart muscle weakness.
  - ❖ Mitochondrial dysfunction is one of the mechanisms. Cytokine-mediated impaired contractility. Coronary perfusion is maintained (no occlusion).

✓ **Clinical Features and Diagnosis**
- **Rapid onset:** Chest pain, shortness of breath, and rapid heartbeat.

- Echocardiography is the best method of diagnosis.
  - ❖ Biventricular dysfunction. Systolic > diastolic dysfunction.
  - ❖ **LV global hypokinesia**[Q] with dilatation of the heart and normal or low LV filling pressure.
  - ❖ **Absence of regional dysfunction.**

✓ **Treatment**
- Reversible. Treat sepsis. Around 10–20% of patients will need inotropes.
- **Dobutamine** is used when cardiac output is low. Dobutamine has no effect on pulmonary pressure but decreases systemic vascular resistance. Can cause tachycardia.
  - ❖ Noradrenaline can be used. It won't cause ischaemia in a well-resuscitated patient.
  - ❖ Levosimendan may avoid catecholamine-related toxicity.

✓ **Prognosis**
- SIC normally resolves within 7–10 d in survivors.

ACUTE DECOMPENSATED HEART FAILURE

Epidemiology and Aetiology

✓ **Acute Decompensated Heart Failure:** Rapid onset or worsening of heart failure symptoms and signs that requires hospitalization.
- Causes of acute heart failure: **Ischaemic heart disease** is the commonest cause.
  - ❖ **Other causes** are non-compliance to medications, critical aortic stenosis, viral myocarditis, pulmonary embolism, cardiomyopathy, sepsis, arrhythmias, severe anaemia, thyroid storm, phaeochromocytoma, bilateral renal artery stenosis.

✓ **Stages of Heart Failure According to AHA/ACC**
- **Stage A (at risk of heart failure):** At risk but no symptoms yet. Risk factors like hypertension, coronary artery disease, obesity.
- **Stage B (pre–heart failure):** Patients with structural heart disease or increased filling pressures in the heart but without current or previous symptoms.
- **Stage C (symptomatic heart failure):** Patients with current or previous symptoms of heart failure.

- **Stage D (advanced heart failure):** Severe symptoms that interfere with daily life or require hospitalization.
✓ **NYHA Classification of Heart Failure According to Patient Symptoms**
  - **Class I:** No limitation of physical activity. No symptoms from ordinary daily physical activity.
  - **Class II:** Slight limitation of physical activity. Symptoms from ordinary daily physical activity.
  - **Class III:** Market limitation of physical activity. Symptoms from lighter than ordinary daily physical activity.
  - **Class IV:** Symptoms at rest.
✓ **Classification of Heart Failure Based on Ejection Fraction (NICE Guidelines)**
  - Heart failure with reduced ejection fraction **(HFrEF): LVEF ≤ 40%.** Systolic heart failure.
  - Heart failure with mildly reduced ejection fraction **(HFmrEF): LVEF 41–49%.** Evidence of spontaneous LV filling pressures
  - Heart failure with preserved ejection fraction **(HFpEF): LVEF ≥ 50%.** Diastolic heart failure.
✓ **Haemodynamic Classification of Patients with Acute Decompensated Heart Failure**
  - **Classification:**
    ❖ **Warm and dry**
    ❖ Warm and wet
    ❖ **Cold and dry**
    ❖ *Cold and wet*
  - Two principle-presenting features are:
    ❖ Signs of **low perfusion/cardiogenic shock (cold):** Cold forearms and legs, sleepy and drowsy, narrow pulse pressure, pulsus alternans, worsening renal function.
    ❖ Signs of **congestion/pulmonary oedema (wet):** Oedema, ascites, orthopnoea, high JVP.
    ❖ Around *95% of all patients of acute heart failure will present with congestion without shock and respond to diuretics ± vasodilators.*
✓ About 50% of patients at admission will have preserved ejection fraction. Most common pathophysiological problem is systolic dysfunction, leading to compensatory sympathetic overactivity.
  - Most common reasons for patients with acute heart failure requiring ICU

management are pulmonary oedema and cardiogenic shock.
- Around 30% of weaning failures are due to cardiac origin and will require a diuretic.

Clinical Features and Diagnosis

✓ **Symptoms:** Dyspnoea, peripheral oedema, abdominal swelling.
  - Crepitation and pulmonary oedema may be absent despite heart failure due to increased lymphatic drainage with chronic heart failure.
✓ **BNP:** Peptides synthesized in heart in response to myocardial stretch. BNP half-life is 20 min, whereas NT-proBNP half-life is 60–90 min.
  - Useful for identifying patients at increased risk of death and readmission.
  - NT-proBNP test for heart failure (NICE 2025 guidelines)
    ❖ >2,000 ng/L: Urgent echo in 2 wk.
    ❖ 400–2,000 ng/L: Echo in 5 wk.
    ❖ <400 ng/L: Heart failure unlikely.
  - A ≥ 30% decrease in BNP has been used as a guide for therapy but has not shown any mortality benefit.
  - Increases in systolic heart failure, diastolic heart failure, kidney dysfunction, pulmonary embolism, sepsis.
  - Decreased in obesity[Q].
✓ **Troponin:** Seen in 30–70% of patients of decompensated heart failure. Elevation is related with increased post-discharge mortality and rehospitalization.
✓ **ABG:** Metabolic and respiratory acidosis may be seen.
✓ **Chest X-ray:** LV failure will present as prominent upper lobe veins (earliest sign), Kerley B lines, prominent fissures, and cardiomegaly. Cardiomegaly indicates a chronic problem.
✓ **Echocardiography:** Useful modality for determining chamber size, wall thickness, ventricle function, valve function, and presence of pulmonary hypertension.
✓ **Cardiac Catheterization:** Done in patients with ongoing signs of ischaemia and patient undergoing valve surgery.
✓ **Killip–Kimball Classification for Prognostication:** Used in acute heart failure after ACS.

Class	Signs	30 d Mortality
I	No signs of heart failure	<6%
II	Signs of congestion, like bibasilar crepitations	<11%
III	Severe heart failure with florid pulmonary oedema	38
IV	Cardiogenic shock	81

✓ **Haemodynamic Monitoring:** *Recommended in certain situations only, like worsening heart failure, unclear haemodynamic profile, and to guide IV vasodilator or inotropic therapy.*

- Goals are right atrial pressure < 8 mmHg, PCWP < 15 mmHg, SVR between 1,000 and 1,200 dynes-sec/cm^5, and cardiac index < 2.2 L/min/m^2.
- Do not target a specific heart rate as it is a compensatory tachycardia in many cases.
- Restoration of sinus rhythm should be attempted only in cases of acute arrhythmias as patients with chronic arrhythmias may throw emboli.
- Target SBP < 110 mmHg in these patients to facilitate forward flow.

Treatment[Q]

✓ **Respiratory Support:** Maintain SpO$_2$ >90%. **Continuous positive airway pressure (CPAP)**[Q] will benefit dyspnoeic patients with tachypnoea and improve oxygenation and has shown mortality benefit.

- Intubation is high risk and may precipitate cardiovascular collapse.

✓ **Fluid Restriction:** Sodium <2–3 g per day, and fluid <2 L/day. Sometimes, a patient with resistance to decongestive therapy may benefit from increased salt intake when combined with diuretics.

✓ **Diuretics:** *Congestion* is the most common cause of admission for decompensated heart failure and should be treated with **intravenous diuretic** irrespective of aetiology or ejection fraction. No mortality benefits.

- **Furosemide or bumetanide** is first-line diuretic. IV furosemide dose of 40–80 mg or 5 mg/h is often needed to achieve natriuresis. Maximum bolus dose of 500 mg or 80 mg/h.
- IV dose of **bumetanide** is 1 mg, and maximum single dose is 12.5 mg. **Bumetanide**

causes less ototoxicity at higher doses but more severe myalgia.

- **DOSE-HF Trial (2011)** showed that IV dose 2.5 times the oral dose improves fluid and weight loss in patients with chronic heart failure. Bolus or infusion are both acceptable.
- Urinary sodium <50 mmol/L collected 2 h after diuretic dose suggests poor diuretic response to current dose, whereas urinary sodium >100 mmol/L suggests good diuretic response. Urinary sodium <100 mmol/L suggests doubling the dose of diuretic.
- Diuretic response by urine output should be assessed within 6 h as their action hardly exceeds 6 h. UOP <150 mL/h suggests doubling the dose of diuretic.
- Common goals are a fluid loss of 3–5 L/day and/or urinary sodium excretion of 230–500 mmol/day.
- Diuretic resistance shows worst prognosis. Most common causes are intrarenal causes rather than prerenal. Therefore, inotropic and vasodilator action have limited role in diuretic resistance.
- Escalate loop diuretics first to maximum dose, as combination with thiazides is associated with electrolytes abnormalities and worst outcomes.
- When used as combination therapy, commonly used thiazides are IV chlorothiazide and oral metolazone.
- **Ultrafiltration** using dialysis machine is not used routine because of need for systemic anticoagulation and increased adverse effects but may be needed in patient with diuretic resistance or anuric renal failure.

✓ **Vasodilator Therapy:** Use differs in patients with reduced vs preserved ejection fraction.

- Arterial vasodilators are helpful in heart failure in reduced ejection fraction primarily, whereas venodilators decrease preload and help in heart failure, with preserved ejection fraction and reduced ejection fraction both.
- They have not shown any mortality benefit and do not improve diuretic response.
- *They may benefit decompensated heart failure due to hypertensive crisis and dyspnoea with impending respiratory failure.*
- **Nitrates:** Venodilators at low dose, arterial dilators at higher dose. Tolerance can develop,

which can be broken by a nitrate-free interval of 8 h a day or use of hydralazine.

- **Sodium nitroprusside:** Arterial and venodilator and used in hypertensive emergencies or mitral regurgitation causing dyspnoea.
- Opiates like morphine as they reduce anxiolysis and have a venodilator effect.

✓ **Inotropic Agents:** Salvage therapy in cardiogenic shock. **Inodilators are preferred.**

- **Dobutamine**[Q] (decreases systemic vascular resistance), **levosimendan** (decreases systemic and pulmonary vascular resistance), and **milrinone** (decreases systemic and pulmonary vascular resistance) have been used to improve cardiac contractility.
  - ❖ Trials have shown increased adverse effects and mortality with positive inotropic drugs.
  - ❖ *Reserved only for patients with advanced HFrEF complicated by cardiogenic shock.*
  - ❖ Beta-blockers should be discontinued during inotropic use.
- **A cut-off systolic pressure of 90 mmHg** is often chosen when deciding to follow a diuretic/CPAP, as opposed to an inotropic/mechanical support strategy.
- Vasopressors like noradrenaline may be needed to offset the systemic vasodilatory effect of inodilators.

✓ **Mechanical Circulatory Support**

- For patients not responding to medical management of cardiogenic shock, temporary mechanical support devices can be used for stabilizing haemodynamics.
  - ❖ Patients with reversible causes or requiring bridging to heart transplant are appropriate candidates.
  - ❖ **Contraindications** are advanced age, significant comorbidities, established organ failure, inability to use anticoagulation, severe peripheral vascular disease, incompetence of aortic or mitral valve, and presence of a metallic aortic valve.

✓ **Guideline-Directed Medical Therapies:** Discontinued during acute unstable phase of decompensated heart failure. Restarted and optimized after patient becomes stable.

- **Drug therapy based on class of heart failure**
  - ❖ **HFrEF:** ACE inhibitors (ACEI), or angiotensin receptor–neprilysin inhibitors (ARNIs) if not tolerated, beta-blockers, mineralocorticoid antagonists

(MRA), sodium glucose transport protein 2 (SGLT-2) inhibitors.
  - • Add-on therapy: IV iron, ivabradine, digoxin.
- ❖ **HRmrEF:** ACEI/angiotensin receptor blocker (ARBs), beta-blockers, MRA, SGLT-2 inhibitors.
  - • Specialist adjustment based on symptoms.
- ❖ **HFpEF:** MRA, SGLT-2 inhibitors, and diuretics for symptoms.
  - • Specialist adjustment based on symptoms.
- **ACE inhibitors, angiotensin receptor blockers (ARBs):**
  - ❖ ACE inhibitors in a patient with bilateral renal stenosis[Q] can cause pulmonary oedema and refractory hypertension.
  - ❖ ACE inhibitors in pregnant females during the second and third trimesters can cause serious malformations,[Q] like oligohydramnios, fetal and neonatal renal failure, pulmonary hypoplasia.
- **Sacubitril/valsartan (angiotensin receptor–neprilysin inhibitor/ARNIs)**[Q]
  - ❖ **Sacubitril**[Q], a neprilysin inhibitor, is a prodrug that prevents the breakdown of BNP. This process increases the levels of angiotensin II, which are blocked by concomitantly giving **valsartan**. They have shown mortality benefits.
- **Beta-blockers:** Mortality benefit[Q] in patients with HFrEF and NYHA class II to IV symptoms. Used in patients with HOCM as well.
  - ❖ Can cause decompensation in acute disease.
- **Mineralocorticoid antagonist** (spironolactone and eplerenone): Spironolactone causes reduction in mortality in HFrEF and reduction in hospitalizations in HFpEF independent of the diuretic action.
  - ❖ Eplerenone is equally efficacious and doesn't cause gynecomastia.
- **Sodium glucose transport protein 2 (SGLT-2) inhibitors** (dapagliflozin and empagliflozin): Reduced mortality in patients with or without type 2 diabetes.
  - ❖ Current indications of SGLT-2 inhibitors: Type 2 diabetes, heart failure, chronic kidney disease, and atherosclerotic cardiovascular disease (ASCVD) risk reduction.
  - ❖ They can cause euglycaemic ketoacidosis.

- **Digoxin:** Causes mild inotropy and reduces activation of the sympathetic and renin–angiotensin system.
  - ❖ Current role is in advance HFrEF and heart failure with atrial fibrillation.
  - ❖ Not associated with mortality benefit, but it decreases symptoms and hospitalizations and improves LVEF and exercise tolerance.
  - ❖ Measure serum levels in renal dysfunction (toxicity above 2 ng/mL).
- **Ivabradine:** Blocks SA node by inhibiting funny channel current.
  - ❖ Used along with beta-blockers in heart failure in patients in whom heart rate is not coming less than 70/min.
  - ❖ No mortality benefits, however, in heart failure.
  - ❖ Contraindicated in severe liver dysfunction.
- **Vericiguat:** Soluble guanylate cyclase inhibitor (sGC) stimulator.
  - ❖ Used for recent worsening of symptoms despite standard therapy.
- **Intravenous iron therapy:** Current recommendations call for screening for iron deficiency and treating iron deficiency with iron.

Prognosis

✓ Mortality among those with heart failure is around 10%.

✓ Hypotension and renal dysfunction are the greatest risk factors for predicting in-hospital outcomes.
  - Mild to moderate increase of serum creatinine should not stop use of loop diuretics.

MECHANICAL CIRCULATORY SUPPORT DEVICES

Cardiogenic Shock (CS)

✓ **Incidence:** 2–3% among NSTEMI and 7–10% among STEMI (commonest cause).
  - About 1 in 5 patients in a cardiac ICU. High mortality with hypotension, 60–90%; without hypotension, 40%
  - A loss of >40% of myocardium is required to cause cardiogenic shock, and patient may present 6 h post-STEMI with confusion, oliguria, skin mottling.
  - Early revascularization[Q] has shown mortality benefit in infarct-related cardiogenic shock.

✓ **Criteria for Diagnosis[Q]:** State of inadequate tissue perfusion due to cardiac dysfunction.
  - Hypotension (SBP <90 mmHg)
  - Pulmonary oedema
  - Signs of impaired tissue perfusion (e.g. high lactates).
  - Cardiac index <2.2 L/min/m², with a wedge pressure of >18 mmHg.

Classification of Cardiogenic Shock

Stage	Characteristics	Profile	Haemodynamics
A	**At risk**, due to underlying acute decompensated HF	**Normotensive** with baseline end organ function	• Normal
B	**Beginning of cardiogenic shock**, subclinical hypoperfusion	• **Warm and wet patient** • **SBP <90 mmHg** • HR >100 bpm • Mild kidney dysfunction	• CI >2.2 mL/min/m²
C	**Classic cardiogenic shock** requiring inotropic support	• **Cold and wet** • SBP <90 mmHg • **Lactate >2 mmol/L** • UOP <30 mL/h or >200% increase in serum creatinine	• CI <2.2 mL/min/m² • PCWP >15 mmHg • RAP/PCWP >0.8
D	**Deteriorating cardiogenic shock**	Stage C features and deteriorating	• CI <2.2 mL/min/m² • PCWP >15 mmHg • RAP/PCWP >0.8
E	**Extremis**	Near pulseless	• CI <2.2 mL/min/m² • PCWP >15 mmHg • RAP/PCWP >0.8

Mechanical Circulatory Support (MCS) Devices

✓ Cardiogenic shock is treated with vasopressors and inotropes, and the *patient's refractory-to-medical management* (diuretics, vasoactive agents, revascularization, if ACS) is supported with MCS devices.
  - *Early use of MCS is recommended by some experts to avoid the potential adverse effects of high doses of catecholamines.*
  - MCS devices increase cardiac output, improve coronary perfusion, reduce cardiac filling pressures, and reduce ventricular afterload.

✓ **Indications for Temporary MCS**[Q]
  - **Bridge to decision:** Short-term MCS for patients with uncertain suitability for transplantation or long-term MCS.
  - **Bridge to bridge/support:** Short-term MCS for patients with a provisional plan to transition to long-term MCS.
  - **Bridge to transplant:** Short-term MCS for patients for cardiac transplantation.
  - **Bridge to recovery:** Short-term MCS due to potentially reversible myocardial dysfunction, like myocarditis or post-extracorporeal cardiopulmonary resuscitation (eCPR).

✓ **Contraindications for Temporary MCS**
  - **Absolute contraindications**
    ❖ Established liver, kidney, or neurological disease
    ❖ Medical non-compliance
    ❖ Severe psychosocial issues
  - **Relative contraindications**
    ❖ Advanced age >80 yr
    ❖ Significant musculoskeletal comorbidities that will hamper rehabilitation
    ❖ Severe peripheral vascular disease
    ❖ Untreated cancer
    ❖ Active substance abuse
    ❖ Lack of social support

Left Ventricular Support Devices (Short Term)

✓ **Intra-Aortic Balloon Pump (IABP)**
  - **Current status:** The European Society of Cardiology (ESC) recommends that it should be considered in patients with *acute MI with cardiogenic shock due to mechanical complications only*, and routine use is not recommended.
    ❖ The **American Heart Association (AHA)** recommends continuous flow

pump devices, like Impella CP and tandem heart, in cases with profound cardiogenic shock, as IABP is less likely to provide benefit.

- **Device:** Dual-lumen device inserted via **femoral artery/axillary artery**[Q] and positioned about 2 to 3 cm **distal to the origin of the left subclavian artery**[Q] **and distal extent above renal arteries**[Q].
  ❖ Outer polyurethane balloon is inflated with **20 to 50 cc of helium** and partially occludes the descending aorta **(80–90%) of its diameter**[Q].
  ❖ Inner portion of the IABP cannula with a central lumen that helps in placement and arterial pressure monitoring.
  ❖ *Inflation is timed with diastole with the middle of T wave or dicrotic notch on arterial wave*[Q].
  ❖ Inflation increases diastolic blood pressure (DBP) as it aims to improve coronary perfusion[Q]. The augmented DBP should be higher than systolic blood pressure.
  ❖ Deflation[Q] occurs on the R wave on the ECG or just before the upstroke of the systole on the arterial pressure.
  ❖ Deflation reduces afterload[Q] and increases cardiac output[Q] by up to 20% or ~0.5–1 L/min.
  ❖ IABP helps in giving thrombolysis as it facilitates drug delivery to coronaries.
  ❖ Balloon should not be left in situ once it is turned off because of a high risk of thrombus formation.
  ❖ **IABP-SHOCK II Trial (2012)**[Q]: It didn't show any mortality benefit with IABP. Study was done in population with acute MI and cardiogenic shock. Hence, its use in this clinical setting has declined.
- **Specific indications**[Q]
  ❖ Acute myocardial infarction (AMI) with cardiogenic shock, including complications like VSD and acute mitral regurgitation[Q].
  ❖ Non-acute myocardial infarction (non-AMI) conditions with cardiogenic shock, like myocarditis, post–cardiac arrest.
  ❖ Periprocedural support for high-risk PCI, high-risk EP procedures, and high-risk percutaneous valve procedures.

- **Contraindications**[Q]
  - ❖ Aortic regurgitation[Q]
  - ❖ Aortic dissection
  - ❖ Severe peripheral artery disease
  - ❖ Contraindication to systemic anticoagulation
- **Troubleshooting**[Q]
  - ❖ **Early inflation:** Inflation prior to the dicrotic notch. **Immediate second peak after the systole seen on the trace.** Can cause premature closure of aortic valve or aortic regurgitation.
  - ❖ **Late inflation:** Inflation after the dicrotic notch. **Second peak seen after the dicrotic notch on the trace.** Can cause decreased coronary perfusion.
  - ❖ **Early deflation:** Deflation is seen as a sharp drop (perpendicular drop rather than slope) following diastolic augmentation. Can cause decreased coronary perfusion. Can cause retrograde coronary and carotid blood flow.
  - ❖ **Diastolic deflation:** Diastolic augmentation appears widened. Rate of rise of assisted systole is prolonged. Can impede left ventricular ejection fraction and increase afterload.
  - ❖ **Multiple tracings:** Due to irregular R wave in ECG.
- ✓ **Impella 2.5/CP/LD/5/5.5**
  - Impellas are catheter-based ventricular-assist devices. Left-sided Impella devices are non-pulsatile, microaxial flow pumps which use an Archimedes screw design to propel blood from inlet cannula in the **LV to the ascending aorta**.
    - ❖ Inlet should be 3.5 cm caudal to the aortic valve, and inlet region should be away from the mitral apparatus.
    - ❖ Pressure sensing on the cannula is just below the outlet cage, and the pressure wave form seen is aortic. If the pressure waveform shows LV pressure tracing, it suggests that the outlet cage has migrated to LV.
    - ❖ They cause immediate unloading of the left ventricle and, hence, increase cardiac output.
    - ❖ Not enough statistical power in the current trials to demonstrate mortality benefit.
- **Indications**
  - ❖ Acute myocardial infarction complicated by **cardiogenic shock** and to **facilitate high-risk PCI (HRPCI)**.
  - ❖ Post-cardiotomy cardiogenic shock.
  - ❖ Cardiomyopathy with cardiogenic shock.
  - ❖ Post–off-pump cardiopulmonary bypass surgery.
  - ❖ Offload the LV in VA ECMO.
- **Contraindications** are LV thrombus and moderate to severe aortic regurgitation and stenosis. Peripheral artery disease can make insertion difficult or impossible.

Impella Device	2.5	CP (Cardiac Power)	5	LD (Left Direct)	5.5	RP
Indications	HRPCI and CS	HRPCI and CS	CS	CS	CS	Right heart failure
Access	Percutaneous femoral or axillary	Percutaneous femoral or axillary	Femoral or axillary cutdown	Direct insertion into axillary artery	Axillary cutdown or direct insertion into axillary artery	Percutaneous femoral vein
Maximum average flow (L/min)	2.5	3.7	5	5.3	5.5	4.4
Maximum duration of support	HRPCI ≤6 h, CS ≤4 d	HRPCI ≤6 h, CS ≤4 d	14 d	14 d	14 d	14 d

✓ **Tandem Heart:** It's a percutaneous transeptal ventricular assist device.

- It shifts blood from **left atrium to femoral artery**. It has a centrifugal blood pump, transseptal cannula, arterial cannula, and an external microprocessor-based controller.
- A catheter is inserted through the femoral vein and goes transeptally from the right atrium into the left atrium. It drains the blood towards the externally placed centrifugal pump, which pumps blood into femoral artery in a retrograde manner.
- Blood flows between up to 4 L/min and speed of the pump up to 7,500 rpm.
- **Indications** are cardiogenic shock and high-risk PCI.
- It differs from VA ECMO as it doesn't use an oxygenator, but it does increase LV afterload like VA ECMO.
- **Specific complications** related to transeptal puncture are air embolization, tamponade, and catheter dislodgement into right atrium or migration to pulmonary veins.

✓ **Extracorporeal Membrane Oxygenation (ECMO):** Veno-arterial ECMO (VA ECMO) provides **biventricular** support as well as **respiratory support in a patient with cardiogenic shock.**

- **A VA ECMO** shifts blood from **right atrium to femoral artery**. It has a centrifugal blood pump, venous drainage cannula, arterial cannula, and **oxygenator.**
    - ❖ Venous drainage cannula is inserted in the right atrium or SVC, and blood is transported to the oxygenator through the centrifugal pump. Blood from the pump can be pushed back in the artery through an arterial cannula.
- It can be inserted percutaneously (peripheral) or surgically (central).
    - ❖ The most common peripheral approach is femoral artery and femoral vein. IJV and subclavian artery can also be used.
    - ❖ Peripheral VA ECMO can be started rapidly at bedside during eCPR.
- Blood flows up to 6 lpm can be achieved. Oxygenation can be improved by increasing FiO_2 at the sweep, whereas carbon dioxide can be removed by increasing the countercurrent gas flow across the oxygenator.
    - ❖ Dialysis and temperature control can also be done through it.

- Increased afterload can be improved by LV venting by IABP/Impella, augmenting LV contractility, or decreasing systemic vascular resistance pharmacologically.
    - ❖ Early offloading (withing 12 h of VA ECMO deployment) is preferred. Impella 2.5 or CP is preferred over other Impellas as the low flow rates (0.5–2 lpm) unloads while minimizing the risk of haemolysis.
- Specific complication is **Harlequin syndrome**, where lung function is poor but LV function is good. The good LV throws deoxygenated blood into the proximal aorta, which can't be countered by the retrograde flow from the femoral artery below. These flows normally meet in the arch of aorta, but meeting after the left subclavian artery means that deoxygenated blood goes to the head and arms. VVA ECMO or central VA ECMO can be used.

✓ **Surgically Placed Non-Dischargeable LVADs**

- Centrally inserted MCS that can provide **left ventricular support**. Flows up to 10 L/min and facilitates patient movement. Can be used for up to 30 d.
- Continuous-flow LVADs[Q] are preferred over pulsatile ones due to increased survival, decreased stroke volume, and decreased device failure.

Right Ventricular Support Devices (Short Term)

✓ **Impella RP:** Right-sided support using femoral venous access. Pump inflow is in IVC, and outflow is in pulmonary artery.

- Used in right ventricular dysfunction during acute myocardial infarction or during LVAD placement.

✓ **TandemHeart with the ProtekDuo Cannula:** TandemHeart's configuration is used with a specially designed cannula to pump blood from right atrium into pulmonary artery.

- ProtekDuo cannula is a dual-lumen cannula that is inserted via IJV. Proximal lumen of the cannula is in the right atrium and draws blood into it. The distal lumen is in the pulmonary artery, and it returns blood.
- TandemHeart with the ProtekDuo cannula can be used with an oxygenator as well.

✓ **VV ECMO with the ProtekDuo Cannula:** VV ECMO configuration, along with ProtekDuo, gives respiratory support along with isolated RV support.

✓ **VA ECMO**: Gives biventricular support along with respiratory support.

✓ **Surgically Placed Non-Dischargeable RVADs**
  • Centrally inserted MCS that can provide **right ventricular support**. Flows up to 10 L/min and facilitates patient movement. Can be used up to 30 d.

Biventricular Support Devices (Short Term)

✓ VA ECMO, surgically placed non-dischargeable LVAD and RVAD (BiVADs), biventricular femoral Impellas, biventricular TandemHearts, or TandemHeart with ProtekDuo with a left-sided Impella.

Device Selection

✓ **Respiratory Support Required:** VA ECMO or TandemHeart with an additional oxygenator.

✓ **Severe Cardiogenic Shock:** The more severe the shock, the higher the flows needed in the device selected.

✓ **Cardiac Arrest:** VA ECMO only. Flows in the rest of the devices will be insufficient.

✓ **Candidacy for Heart Transplant:** They may require to be on long durations of MCS as it can take time for the heart to be available (2 wk on average). MCS devices that allow mobility are preferred.

✓ **Access Site Anatomy:** Severe peripheral vascular disease or difficult femoral access may dictate the choice of device.

✓ **Complications:** Haemolysis or distal limb ischaemia may necessitate transition to surgical VADs. Post-cardiotomy shock calls for a surgical VAD.

Complications[Q]

✓ **Bleeding:** Commonest complication. The larger the cannula, the higher the chances of bleeding. Risk of bleeding appears to be higher with Impella compared to IABP.
  • Upper GI bleeding[Q] in patients with LVAD is common and is due to comorbidities, anticoagulation, and AV malformations.

✓ **Haemolysis:** Mechanical breakdown of RBCs.

✓ **Thrombosis:** Absent hum on auscultation[Q] suggests thrombosis.

✓ **Thrombocytopaenia:** Mechanical breakdown and heparin-induced.

✓ **Vascular Complications:** *Limb ischaemia*, arterial dissection, embolism, and pseudoaneurysm.

✓ **Infections:** Access site infections. The longer the duration, the higher the chance of fungal infections[Q]. High mortality rates.

✓ **Stroke:** Ischaemic and haemorrhagic, both with high mortality with haemorrhagic stroke.

✓ **Arrest with LVAD[Q]:** Check for signs of life, and auscultate heart for humming sound.
  • If no humming sign, then possible LVAD failure.
  • Start ventilation, but do not start chest compressions (can lead to cannula dislodgement and anastomotic rupture[Q]).
  • Make sure all connections and components are working, including replacing controller.
  • Chest compressions may be started when all attempts to troubleshoot the LVAD fail.

Monitoring

✓ **Device function:** Monitor device flows and pressure in the systems.

✓ **Device positioning:** Done using chest X-ray or echocardiography.

✓ **Anticoagulation:** Platelet count, haemoglobin, and aPTT should be assessed at least daily.

✓ **Limb ischaemia:** Distal pulses should be checked multiple times a day to monitor for new pulse deficits. Distal perfusion catheter is used, and vasopressors are decreased.

Weaning Off MCS: Daily assessment for ability to wean.

✓ **Parameters**
  • Clinical diagnosis (acute MI, shorter time to wean vs decompensated heart failure, longer time to wean).
  • Myocardial function: Aortic pulsatility 30–40 mmHg, MAP >65 mmHg, HR <100 bpm, and minimal vasoactive support.
  • End-organ function: Stable mental status, lactates <2 mmol/L, acceptable oxygenation/ventilation, and improving LFTs and KFTs.

✓ **IABP:** By reducing the assist ratio (from 1:1 to 1: 8) or progressively decreasing the volume of inflation.

✓ **Impella:** Slow wean by gradually decreasing the pump speed by 1 to 2 P levels every 4 h to reach the minimum of P2. Rapid wean from P9 to P2 immediately can also be done.

✓ **TandemHeart:** Decrease flows by 0.5 L/min every 1 to 2 h over a 4–8 h period to a minimum of 1.5 to 2 L/min.

✓ **VA ECMO:** Pulse pressure >40 mmHg is more likely to result in a successful wean. Decrease flows by 0.5 L/min to a minimum of 1.5 to 2 L/min.

Mechanical Circulatory Support Devices (Long Term)

✓ Options for isolated RV or biventricular long-term MCS are poor. Isolated LV support devices are used more commonly.

✓ Used in patients with cardiogenic shock who are unlikely to recover ventricular function and are unexpected to wean from temporary MCS or inotropic support but are likely to have a recovery to meaningful quality of life.

✓ For patients with severe cardiogenic shock and multiorgan failure, it is recommended to optimize them first on temporary MCS before putting patients on long-term MCS.

✓ **Suitable patients** are those with contraindication to transplant (bridge to destination) or long waiting for heart transplant.

✓ **Contraindications:** Significant RV dysfunction or pulmonary hypertension, severe comorbidities, or psychosocial barriers to close follow-up.

✓ **HeartMate III** is the most used device. Device has got an inflow cannula (LV), an outflow cannula (aorta), and a single impeller that pumps blood in a continuous flow (2.5–10 L/min). It uses magnetic levitation.

  • Patients are kept on warfarin and antiplatelet agents to prevent pump thrombosis.

✓ **REMATCH Trial (2001)[Q]:** Permanent LVAD insertion vs best medical management in those not eligible for transplant. They showed decreased mortality with permanent LVAD insertion.

Additional Questions

✓ **Classification of Ventricular Assist Devices[Q]**
  • **Ventricle-supported:** LVAD, RVAD, BiVAD.
  • **Mechanism:** Pulsatile (first gen), non-pulsatile (second gen).
  • **Drivetrain:** Electrical, magnetic, pneumatic.

EXTRACORPOREAL LIFE SUPPORT

✓ **Extracorporeal Life Support (ECLS):** Lifesaving technology that temporarily replaces the function of the lungs, heart, or both to support patients with life-threatening respiratory or cardiac failure.

  • Currently, *ARDS is the most common indication for ECLS in adults.*

✓ **Indications of ECMO in Adults with Respiratory Failure[Q]**

  • **Severe hypoxaemia** due to any cause with *80% mortality risk or greater* (PaO_2/FiO_2 <100 on FiO_2 >0.9 and/or Murray score 3–4, adjusted oxygenation index (AOI) >80, or acute physiology of stoke score (APSS) 8.

  • CO_2 **retention** on mechanical ventilation despite high P plat (30 cm H_2O) with pH <7.2.

  • Bridge to lung transplantation to avoid mechanical ventilation or primary graft dysfunction post–lung transplant.

  • Severe **air leak syndromes** (large bronchopleural fistula).

✓ **Indications of ECMO in Adults with Cardiac Failure[Q]**

  • Refractory cardiogenic shock to maximal medical therapy.

  • Refractory cardiac arrest with potential for favourable neurological recovery.

✓ **Contraindications of ECMO**

  • Mechanical ventilation at high settings (FiO_2 >0.9, P plat >30 cm H_2O) for 7 d

  • *Established multiorgan failure*

  • Any significant contraindication to anticoagulation *(CNS haemorrhage)*

  • Immunosuppression

  • Significant comorbidities, like *terminal malignancy*

✓ **Types of ECMO Circuits**

  • **Venovenous ECMO (VV ECMO):** Only oxygenation support.

    ❖ Used in ARDS[Q].

    ❖ Blood is taken from one central vein (catheter tip in inferior vena cava with insertion from femoral vein or catheter tip in superior vena cava with insertion from IJV) and returned to other central vein (catheter tip in right atrium, with insertion from femoral vein/IJV).

    ❖ A dual-lumen cannula[Q] can be inserted via IJV. Cannula extends across the right atrium to the IVC. Blood is taken from ports situated in SVC and IVC and returned through the second lumen into the right atrium directed towards the tricuspid valve. They use larger-size cannula but can help patient become mobile.

- ❖ **VV ECMO** is used for ARDS, and for patients with ARDS and cor pulmonale, **VA ECMO** is used.
- ❖ ECMO has not shown much mortality benefit in ARDS compared to low-TV ventilation. No difference in mortality benefit between VA ECMO and VV ECMO. Success is if started within 7 d of mechanical ventilation.
- ❖ **EOLIA Trial** (2018): ECMO vs conventional treatment.
  - • It was stopped early because of interim results being in favour of ECMO.
  - • However, the final analysis revealed a non-statistically significant reduction in 60 d mortality with VV ECMO.
  - • Patients were allowed to cross over from conventional group to ECMO group if there was persistent severe hypoxaemia.
- ❖ **CESAR Trial** (2009) showed that in patients with ARDS, transfer of patient to a facility specializing in ARDS with ECMO *was associated with an improvement in 6-month survival compared to conventional treatment.*
  - • Patients between age 18 and 65 yr with severe respiratory failure (Murray score >3 or pH <7.20) were included.
  - • Patients with peak inspiratory pressure >30 cm H_2O or FiO_2 >80% for more than 7 d were excluded.
  - • Best survival rates are seen in patients with non-necrotizing viral pneumonia.
  - • Of all the subjects sent to Leicester for ECMO, only 76% received ECMO.
  - • Around 30% of patients did not receive lung protection ventilation in the conventional group.

- • **Venoarterial ECMO (VA ECMO):** Both oxygenation and circulatory support. Up to 80% of cardiac output can be provided.
  - ❖ *Used for cardiogenic shock[Q] and post–cardiac arrest.*
  - ❖ A cannula drains blood from one central vein (catheter tip in vena cava with insertion from femoral vein) and returns it to an artery (catheter tip in distal abdominal aorta, with insertion from femoral artery).
  - ❖ Retrograde flow in aorta can increase cardiac afterload,[Q] and that is why flows in VA ECMO are lower than in VV ECMO.
  - ❖ Systemic blood pressure lacks normal pulsatility, unless some native pump function is there.
  - ❖ *Cardiogenic shock: ECLS-Shock Trial (2023) showed no mortality benefit in early use of VA ECMO in patients with acute myocardial infarct with cardiogenic shock.* Centres with higher case volume had better outcomes.
  - ❖ **Post–cardiac arrest: ARREST Trial (2020)** showed mortality benefit in patients with out-of-hospital cardiac arrest and refractory VF, but mortality benefit couldn't be replicated in **INCEPTION Trial (2023).**
  - ❖ **Harlequin syndrome[Q]** can happen when lung function is poor but LV function is good. The good LV throws deoxygenated blood into the proximal aorta which can't be countered by the retrograde flow from the femoral artery below. These flows normally meet near the aortic valve, but meeting after the left subclavian artery means that deoxygenated blood goes to the coronaries, head, and arms. Right side is monitored for saturation and arterial pressures to capture native cardiac output. VVA ECMO or central VA ECMO can be used.
  - ❖ Severe aortic regurgitation is a **specific** contraindication to VA ECMO.
- • **Venovenous-arterial ECMO (VVA ECMO):** Drains blood from a vein (IVC through insertion from femoral vein) and **returns it back to both a vein (SVC through IJV) and an artery (contralateral femoral artery).**

❖ This ensures that oxygenated blood is delivered to pulmonary circulation and oxygenated blood passes through the normal circulation via the native cardiac output and prevents Harlequin syndrome.

- **Venovenous (VV) extracorporeal CO_2 removal (ECCO$_2$R):** Only for CO_2 removal and used in hypercapnic failure.
  - ❖ *Low-flow ECMOs with configuration same as dual-lumen VV ECMO.*
  - ❖ CO_2 clearance is more efficient than O_2 supplementation, and hence, low flows are sufficient.
  - ❖ Low flows mean that smaller cannulas can be used.
  - ❖ **May be used for treating status asthmaticus and COPD in difficult-to-wean patients. It has also been used in patients to avoid intubation.**
  - ❖ Has also been used in *ARDS to give ultraprotective lung ventilation.*
- **Arteriovenous (AV) pumpless (ECCO$_2$R):** It uses the patient's own blood pressure as a driving force for circuit flow due to use of low-resistance polymethyl pentene membranes.
  - ❖ Blood is drained from femoral vein and returned to distal aorta with insertion through the contralateral femoral artery.

✓ **Components**
- **Cannulae** can be dual-lumen or single-lumen and can be inserted percutaneously or surgically.
  - ❖ Right axillary vein can be one of the placement options for return blood.
  - ❖ Cannulas drain blood from central vein to an oxygenator and then take oxygenated blood back to central veins.
  - ❖ ECMO pipes may already be heparin-coated, so IV anticoagulation may not always be necessary.

❖ Saline can be used in emergency to prime the circuit.
❖ Unfractionated heparin (50–100 IU/kg) followed by ACT target of 160–220 s, or aPTT goal for ECMO is 50–75.

- **Oxygenator:** Semipermeable membrane that divides blood from the gases.
  - ❖ Extracorporeal blood flow is the main determinant of oxygenation, while CO_2 elimination depends on the sweep gas flow through the oxygenator[Q].
  - ❖ Diffusion of oxygen through the walls of membrane can be compromised with thrombus, but even in the presence of visible clot in the oxygenator, most contemporary oxygenators can perform for many days.
  - ❖ Fractional oxygen can be changed at the blender.
  - ❖ **CO_2 clearance is more efficient than O_2 supplementation.**
  - ❖ Pump: Blood flow up to 10–12 lpm.
- **Blood pump:** Centrifugal pumps cause less haemolysis.
- **Monitor:** Displays pump speed, blood flow rates, pressures before and after the oxygenator, and temperature.

✓ **Supportive Therapy:** Lung-protective ventilation should be continued with TV <6 mL/kg PBW, driving pressure <14 cm H_2O, adequate PEEP of 10–15 cm H_2O, low FiO$_2$, and very low respiratory rate 6–10 breaths per minute. Patient can be extubated if safe to reduce the complications like VAP.
- Patients need anticoagulation, and heparin and argatroban (in patients with HIT) have been used. Risk of VTE is less compared to VA ECMO.
- Patient can be mobilized, and hence, critical care illness and deconditioning can be avoided.

Murray Score for Referral[Q]: Four components, with each scored from 0 to 4. Total divided by four to give a final score. *Referral criteria is a score of 3 or 2.5 with rapid deterioration.*

Score	0	1	2	3	4
Chest X-ray quadrants	0	1	2	3	4
Compliance	≥80	60–79	40–59	20–39	<20
PEEP	≤5	6–8	9–11	11–14	>14
PaO$_2$/FiO$_2$		≥40	30–39.9	23.3–29.9	13.3–23.2	<13.3

✓ **Complications**[Q]
- Bleeding most common (41%), death during ECMO (40%), infection (40%).
  - ❖ Intracranial haemorrhage in 7–10% of ECLS cases.
  - ❖ ELSO recommends platelets to be above 80×10^9/L.
- **Air in circuit:** *In case of minor air, release air from oxygenator.* In case of sufficient amounts of air to cause pump failure, clamp the circuit (return line followed by drainage line) and change it.
- **Clots in the circuit**[Q]: *Clots >5 mm on the side of return cannula should be removed.* Heparin (50 IU/kg) can be given to establish a new ACT[Q] target of 220 s.
- **Chatter:** Swinging movements of venous lines. Caused by volume depletion, too high flows, cannula migration into smaller vessel.
- *In a patient with VV ECMO undergoing cardiac arrest, first start chest compressions and then put on VA ECMO.*

Outcomes

✓ Recently, survival rates of up to 70% have been shown in patients with ARDS.
✓ **Respiratory ECMO survival prediction (RESP) score:** Predicts hospital survival on initiation of ECMO. Total score from −22 to 15. A score ≤3 indicates low potential to recover, and at least two ECMO centres must agree to proceed for ECMO initiation.

INFECTIVE ENDOCARDITIS

Epidemiology and Aetiology

✓ **Infective Endocarditis (IE):** Inflammation of the endocardium as well as the valves of the heart.
- Can be classified as
  - ❖ **Native valve endocarditis (NVE)**
  - ❖ Prosthetic valve endocarditis **(PVE)**
  - ❖ IE in **IV drug abusers**
  - ❖ **N**osocomial IE
- **Risk factors:** Rheumatic heart disease in developing nations, as bicuspid valves and intracardiac devices in developed nations.
- Majority of patients are >65 yr of age.
✓ In Europe, most common cause is **_Streptococcal infection (31%)_**[Q], with *S. viridans* accounting

for half of these, followed by *S. aureus* in 28% of cases, and *Enterococcus* (10%).
- **_S. aureus_** is more common in IV drug abusers[Q], haemodialysis patients, transplant recipients, and healthcare-associated infections.
  - ❖ *S. aureus* is most common organism in first 2 months of PVE.
- **_Streptococcus bovis/gallolyticus_** endocarditis is associated with colorectal adenomas[Q].
- **Fungal endocarditis**[Q] seen commonly in IV drug abusers and prosthetic valve recipients and causes bulky vegetations, metastatic infections, and perivalvular invasion.
- **HACEK group** is *Haemophilus, Actinobacillus, Cardiobacterium, Eikenella,* and *Kingella* and accounts for 2–5% of patients and affects mostly the native valve.
- **Slow-growing organisms** like *Bartonella, chlamydia,* and *Coxiella* can cause endocarditis as well.

Clinical Features and Diagnosis

✓ Lesions **mostly affect left side of the heart,** with the aortic valve (55–60%)[Q] being the most affected.
- Patients with aortic valve involved have the worst prognosis, and tricuspid valve endocarditis is the most benign comparatively.
  - ❖ Pulmonary valve is least affected.
- Patients with **IV drug abuse history have right-sided lesions** with *Staphylococcus aureus* or fungal infections as aetiology.
- **Fever is the commonest sign,** followed by a new murmur. About 25% of the patients have already thrown emboli by the time of diagnosis.
  - ❖ *Any fever in patient with valvular heart disease, cardiovascular implantable electronic device (CIED), IV drug abuse should prompt a consideration of infective endocarditis.*
- Persistent bacteraemia is highly suggestive of endovascular infection.
- Splenomegaly is seen in nearly half of patients of subacute bacterial endocarditis.
✓ **Mucocutaneous lesions**[Q] **most commonly observed are petechiae.**
- **Janeway lesion:** Irregular, non-tender haemorrhagic macular lesions on palms and soles.

- **Osler nodes:** Slightly raised, painful red-purple nodules in fingers and toes.
- **Roth spots:** White-centred, exudative retinal haemorrhagic lesions.

✓ **Duke's Criteria**[Q] – **Definite IE:** *Clinical criteria (2 major or 1 major + 3 minor criteria or 5 minor criteria).* **Possible IE:** *1 major + 1 minor or 3 minor criteria.* **Rejected IE:** Alternate diagnosis or resolution of IE, with 80% sensitivity. Diagnosis is either by pathological or clinical criteria. *Pathological criteria require either surgery or post-mortem examination.*

- **Pathological criteria**
  - ❖ **Microorganism:** Demonstrated by culture or histology in either vegetations, embolized vegetations, or intracardiac abscess.
  - ❖ **Pathologic lesion:** Vegetation or intracardiac abscess confirmed by histology showing active endocarditis.
- **Clinical criteria**
  - ❖ **Major criteria**
    - **Positive blood cultures** for an organism typical causative of IE (*Streptococcus viridans, Streptococcus bovis, S. aureus, Enterococcus,* HACEK, *Pseudomonas*) from two sources >12 h apart or in all three cultures sent. Single positive blood culture for *Coxiella burnetii* or IgG antibody titre >1:800.
    - **Positive echocardiogram:** Oscillating intracardiac mass on valve or abscess or *new partial dehiscence of prosthetic valve* or new valvular regurgitation.
  - ❖ **Minor criteria**
    - Predisposing heart condition or IVDU.
    - Fever >38°C.
    - **Vascular phenomenon:** Major arterial emboli, Janeway lesions, conjunctival haemorrhage.
    - **Immunological phenomenon:** Glomerulonephritis, Osler's nodes, Roth spots, or rheumatoid factor.
    - **Microbiological phenomenon:** Blood culture not meeting major criteria.

✓ **Microbiological Diagnosis:** Three sets of blood cultures from separate sites should be sent before starting antimicrobial therapy.

- Blood culture–negative infective endocarditis is seen in 30% of patients.
- Serological tests for *Coxiella, Chlamydia, Bartonella, Legionella,* and some fungi.

✓ **ECG** for aortic and mitral valve endocarditis to look for invasion of interventricular septum.

✓ **A negative transthoracic echocardiography (TTE) (sensitivity 30–60%)**[Q] should be followed by a transoesophageal echocardiography (TOE) (gold standard) in those in whom IE is suspected[Q].

- TOE recommended if prosthetic valve endocarditis confirmed by TTE to rule out perivalvular complications.
- TOE has >90% sensitivity for both native and prosthetic valve endocarditis.
- *S. aureus* and *Candida* bacteraemia should prompt for looking for endocarditis.

✓ **CT scan** of the chest, abdomen, and pelvis is routinely performed to identify silent visceral embolization.

Medical Treatment

✓ **Antibiotic Prophylaxis:** Given in patients with the following pathology: Acquired valvular heart disease, hypertrophic cardiomyopathy, previous endocarditis, prosthetic valve replacement, or congenital heart disease.

- Dental extractions, subgingival instrumentation, and manipulations involving the gums, teeth, or oral mucosa are high-risk procedures which will require prophylaxis.
- No more prophylaxis for genitourinary or gastrointestinal procedures.

✓ **Antibiotic Treatment:** Repeat blood cultures every 24–48 h till bacteraemia is cleared. Duration of treatment is calculated from first day of blood culture negativity.

- **Empirical therapy:**
  - ❖ In patients with NVE or late PVE (>12 months after surgery), ampicillin + ceftriaxone/flucloxacillin + gentamicin is given (few times when two beta-lactams are given together).
  - ❖ In patients with early PVE (<12 months after surgery) or nosocomial IE: vancomycin/daptomycin + gentamicin + rifampicin.
  - ❖ In acutely ill PVE patient, IV vancomycin + meropenem is recommended (imagine the sickest patient in the ITU).

- **Streptococci**
  - ❖ In penicillin-sensitive organisms, IV co-amoxiclav/ceftriaxone is recommended; 4 wk for NVE and 6 wk of treatment for PVE. Addition of gentamicin 3 mg/kg once a day in patients with normal renal function will reduce the duration of treatment to 2-wk in case of NVE. The 2-wk treatment regimen is not recommended for PVE. Vancomycin is given in patients allergic to penicillin.
  - ❖ In patients with penicillin-resistant organisms or increased exposure to penicillin, 4 wk of IV co-amoxiclav/ceftriaxone along with 2 wk of gentamicin is recommended in cases with NVE. Then, *6 wk of IV co-amoxiclav/ceftriaxone with 2 wk of gentamicin recommended in cases with PVE.* For patients allergic to penicillin, vancomycin is recommended for NVE, and vancomycin and gentamicin for PVE.
- **Staphylococci: Rifampicin[Q] is added to PVE regimens for its biofilm activity, and gentamicin is added to PVE regimens for its synergistic bactericidal role.**
  - ❖ In patients with NVE due to MSSA, flucloxacillin/cefazolin is recommended for 4–6 wk. *In patients with PVE due to MSSA, flucloxacillin/cefazolin plus rifampicin is recommended for 6 wk, along with 2 wk of gentamicin.*
  - ❖ In patients with NVE due to MRSA, vancomycin is recommended for 4–6 wk. *In patients with PVE due to MRSA, vancomycin plus rifampicin is recommended for 6 wk, along with 2 wk of gentamicin.*
- *Enterococcus*
  - ❖ In patients with NVE ampicillin/co-amoxiclav + ceftriaxone/gentamicin for 6 wk. In patients with PVE, ampicillin/co-amoxiclav with ceftriaxone for 6 wk, or ampicillin/co-amoxiclav with gentamicin for 2 wk.
  - ❖ In patients with NVE resistant to beta-lactams (*E. faecium*), vancomycin for 6 wk combined with gentamicin for 2 wk is recommended.
  - ❖ In patients with vancomycin-resistant enterococcus, daptomycin plus

ampicillin/ertapenem/ceftaroline, or daptomycin + fosfomycin, should be used.
- **HACEK:** IV ceftriaxone/ciprofloxacin for NVE (4 wk) and PVE (6 wk).
- **Fungal endocarditis**
  - ❖ *Candida:* Caspofungin or amphotericin B and flucytosine.
  - ❖ *Aspergillus:* Voriconazole or amphotericin B and flucytosine.
- ✓ Infections of the pacemaker wires and electrodes are treated with antibiotics and by replacing the old system with a new system at a different site.

Surgery

- ✓ **Emergency surgery**, within 24 h; **urgent surgery**, within 7 d; and **elective surgery** means after at least 1 to 2 wk of antibiotic therapy.
- ✓ **Left-sided infective endocarditis:** Surgery is required in 30–35% of cases. Presence of just vegetations is not an indication of valve replacement. Patients with intracerebral haemorrhage should have their surgery delayed for 4 wk and by 2 wk for a CNS embolic event by AHA standards. EHS recommends surgery within first 72 h of embolic phenomenon if CT scan can rule out haemorrhage. Indications for surgery for left-sided lesions by the American Heart Association (AHA) and the European Heart Society (EHS) classification. (*Questions are asked on indications for surgeries in exams, so please read them.*)
  - **Heart failure[Q]: Class I indication (AHA and EHS)**
    - ❖ Severe acute regurgitation, obstruction, or fistula causing refractory pulmonary oedema or cardiogenic shock: **Emergency surgery**.
    - ❖ Severe regurgitation or obstruction causing symptoms of heart failure or echocardiography signs of poor haemodynamic tolerance: **Urgent surgery**.
  - **Uncontrolled infection[Q]: Class I indication (AHA and EHS)**
    - ❖ Locally controlled abscess, false aneurysm, fistula, enlarging vegetation, PVE complicated by heart block: **Urgent surgery**.
    - ❖ Infection caused by fungi or MDR organism: **Urgent/elective**.

❖ Persisting positive blood culture despite appropriate antibiotic therapy (>7 d), and control of septic metastatic foci: **Urgent surgery (AHA class I/EHS class IIa).**

❖ PVE caused by staphylococci or non-HACEK Gram-negative bacilli: **Urgent/elective (AHA not applicable/EHS class IIa).**

❖ Relapsing PVE: **Urgent/elective (AHA class IIa/EHS not applicable).**

- **Prevention of embolism**[Q]

❖ Persistent vegetations >10 mm after ≥1 embolic episode despite appropriate antibiotic therapy: **Urgent surgery (AHA class IIa/EHS class I).**

❖ NVE with vegetation >10 mm associated with severe valve stenosis or regurgitation and low operative risk or mobile vegetation: **Urgent surgery (AHA class IIa/EHS class IIa).**

❖ Isolated vegetation >15 mm and no other indication of surgery: **Urgent surgery (AHA not applicable/EHS class IIb).**

❖ Isolated vegetation >30 mm: **Urgent surgery (AHA not applicable/EHS class IIa).**

❖ Mobile vegetation >10 mm in PVE or NVE, especially on anterior leaflet mitral valve, with other relative indications for surgery: **Urgent surgery (AHA class IIb/EHS not applicable).**

✓ **Right-Sided Endocarditis:** Valve repair is preferred over valve replacement because of risk of reinfection from continued injection drug use. Indications for surgery by AHA and EHS guidelines are as follows
- Right-sided heart failure due to severe tricuspid regurgitation with poor response to medical diuretic treatment.
- Difficult-to-eradicate organisms.
- Clinical failure: Bacteraemia for at least 7 d despite adequate antimicrobial therapy.
- Large tricuspid vegetation (>20 mm) with recurrent pulmonary embolism.

Prognosis

✓ Short-term mortality is 10–24%.
✓ IE caused by staphylococcal or fungal infections has a higher mortality[Q] (30–40%).

✓ IVDU with right-sided lesions actually have a better prognosis (4–5% mortality). Overall mortality otherwise is 20%.
✓ **Poor prognosis**[Q]: Old age, prosthetic valve endocarditis, staphylococcal, fungal, non-HACEK Gram-negative bacilli, large vegetations, pulmonary hypertension.

CARDIOMYOPATHY[Q]

Hypertrophic Cardiomyopathy

✓ **Epidemiology:** Prevalence: 1:500.
- **Age at presentation:** 25–40 yr.
✓ **Clinical Features and Diagnosis**
- **Symptoms:** Syncope, exercise intolerance, palpitations, dyspnoea, sudden cardiac arrest.
- **Diagnosis:** Echocardiography and cardiac MRI.
  ❖ Criteria: LV wall thickness ≥15 mm, LVOTO = peak LVOT pressure gradient ≥30 mmHg.
- **Risk factors for sudden cardiac death (SCD):** Unexplained syncope, LVH ≥30 mm, non-sustained VT, LVOTO ≥50 mmHg, family history of SCD <40 yr.
✓ **Treatment:** Beta-blockers or non-DHP calcium channel blockers.
- ICD in high-risk patients.
- Septal ablation, septal myectomy.
✓ **Prognosis:** Annual mortality 3%. Annual sudden cardiac death mortality 1%.

Dilated Cardiomyopathy

✓ **Epidemiology:** Prevalence 1:250.
- **Age at presentation:** 25–50 yr.
- **Causes:** Ischaemic, post–viral infection, valve dysfunction, excess alcohol.
✓ **Clinical Features and Diagnosis:**
- **Symptoms:** Fatigue, tachycardia, dyspnoea, sudden cardiac arrest.
- **Diagnosis:** Echocardiography and cardiac MRI.
  ❖ Criteria: LVEF <50%.
- **Risk factors for sudden cardiac death (SCD):** ↓ LVEF, small age at diagnosis, T wave alternans.
✓ **Treatment** (standard therapy for HF): ACE inhibitors, diuretics, beta-blockers, digoxin.
- ICD in high-risk patients.
- Common reason for heart transplant.

✓ **Prognosis:** Annual mortality 5–6%. Annual sudden cardiac death mortality 2–3%.

Restrictive Cardiomyopathy

✓ **Epidemiology:** Rare outside tropical regions.
- **Causes:** Amyloidosis^Q, sarcoidosis^Q, haemochromatosis, and eosinophilic endocarditis.

✓ **Clinical Features and Diagnosis**
- **Symptoms:** Fatigue, tachycardia, dyspnoea, sudden cardiac arrest.
- **Diagnosis:** Echocardiography and myocardial biopsy.
  - ❖ Diastolic dysfunction in absence of left ventricular hypertrophy.

✓ **Treatment** (standard therapy for HF): ACE inhibitors, diuretics, beta-blockers.
- Digoxin is contraindicated in patients with amyloidosis.
- ICD in high-risk patients.

✓ **Prognosis:** Worst prognosis and lowest survival among all cardiomyopathies.

Arrhythmogenic Cardiomyopathy

✓ **Epidemiology:** Prevalence 1:2,000 to 1:5,000
- **Age at presentation:** 20–45 yr.
- Fatty tissue replaces heart muscle, leading to irregular heartbeats.

✓ **Clinical Features and Diagnosis**
- **Symptoms:** Syncope, palpitations, dyspnoea, and sudden cardiac arrest.
- **Diagnosis:** ECG, echocardiography, and cardiac MRI.
  - ❖ Criteria: Task force criteria.
- **Risk factors for sudden cardiac death (SCD):** Male sex, small age at diagnosis, non-sustained VT, cardiac syncope, number of leads with T wave inversions, ↑ PVC count/24 h, ↓ RVEF.

✓ **Treatment:** Beta-blockers and standard therapy for HF if indicated.
  - ❖ ICD in high-risk patients.

✓ **Prognosis:** Annual mortality 1%. Annual sudden cardiac death mortality 2–3%.

Peripartum Cardiomyopathy

✓ **Epidemiology:** Prevalence 1:3,000 to 1:10,000.
- Heart failure that presents in late pregnancy or in the post-partum period. Absence of heart disease previously.

✓ **Clinical Features and Diagnosis**
- **Symptoms:** Shortness of breath and orthopnoea are common in third trimester.
- **Diagnosis:** ECG may show SVT and AF.
  - ❖ Echocardiography: Ventricular systolic dysfunction due to a global reduction^Q in myocardial contraction. LVEF <45%.
  - ❖ Diagnosis of exclusion.
- **Risk factors for sudden cardiac death (SCD):** Maternal age >30 yr, multiparity, African descent, obesity, multiple pregnancy, pregnancy-associated hypertensive disorders.

✓ **Treatment** (standard therapy for HF): ACE inhibitors (post-partum only), vasodilators, diuresis, beta-blockers, and salt restriction.
- Prophylactic-dose, low-molecular-weight heparin.
- Mechanical circulatory support and cardiac transplant may be needed.

✓ **Prognosis:** Mortality rate of 15–50%.

VALVULAR HEART DISEASE

✓ **Aortic Stenosis (AS):** Progressive disease for which there is no medical treatment.
- Accounts for 50% of all chronic valvular heart disease.
- **Causes:** Calcified degeneration of congenital bicuspid aortic valve, rheumatic heart disease.
  - ❖ Up to 40% patients with bicuspid valves will have a root or ascending aortic aneurysm.
  - ❖ Rheumatic AS is associated with aortic regurgitation as well.
- **Symptoms:** Angina, dyspnoea, and syncope.
  - ❖ Fixed obstruction with falling cardiac output.
  - ❖ **Preload-dependent^Q.** Normally, 20% of diastolic filling is contributed by atrial kick, which can increase to 40% in atrial stenosis.
  - ❖ AS causes diastolic dysfunction due to left ventricular hypertrophy.
  - ❖ Atrial fibrillation and tachycardia^Q are poorly tolerated.
- **Diagnosis** by echocardiography and cardiac CT for evaluation:
  - ❖ **Normal** aortic valve is 2.6–3.5 cm^2. **Severe AS^Q** <1 cm^2, or a mean gradient of >40 mmHg or jet velocity >4 m/s.

- **Treatment:** Aortic valve replacement, either surgically or TAVI preferred treatment for patients with symptomatic severe AS or asymptomatic severe AS with EF <50%.
  - ❖ TAVI is an attractive proposition for ICU patients.
  - ❖ **Noradrenaline/phenylephrine**[Q] is a good option as it maintains good coronary perfusion which is a must[Q].
  - ❖ Vasodilators are used very carefully in decompensated heart failure.
  - ❖ Beta-blockers should be used cautiously in patients with AS and AF.
  - ❖ CPR is often poorly tolerated.
✓ **Aortic Regurgitation (AR)**
  - Acute severe AR is a surgical emergency and patients appear gravely ill and have tachycardia, dyspnoea, and hypotension.
    - ❖ Chronic severe AR is often asymptomatic.
  - **Causes:** Acute severe AR mostly caused by infective endocarditis. Other causes are blunt chest trauma and aortic dissection.
  - **Symptoms** (acute AR): Angina, dyspnoea, tachycardia, weakness.
    - ❖ Chronic AR: Water hammer pulse, dancing carotids.
  - **Diagnosis:** Urgent TTE for diagnosis whenever acute AR is suspected.
  - **Treatment:** Urgent surgery required, with aortic valve replacement performed.
    - ❖ Vasodilators and diuretics form mainstay of the medical management.
✓ **Mitral Stenosis (MS)**
  - Rheumatic fever is the leading cause.
  - **Symptoms:** Orthopnoea, paroxysmal nocturnal dyspnoea, atrial fibrillation[Q], and haemoptysis[Q] due to rupture of bronchial veins.
    - ❖ Peripheral oedema, ascites, elevated JVP, and congestive hepatomegaly due to right heart failure[Q].
  - **Echocardiography:** Normal is 4–6 cm². Severe MS is <1 cm², with the mean gradient being >10 mmHg.
    - ❖ Thickened mitral leaflet tips, immobility of posterior leaflet, and restricted anterior leaflet motion.
  - **Treatment:** Rate control of AF and decongestion by loop diuretics.
    - ❖ Percutaneous mitral balloon commissurotomy (PMBC) is preferred treatment

for symptomatic patients with severe rheumatic MS and favourable valve morphology (pliable mitral leaflets).
  - ❖ If the anatomy is unfavourable for PMBC, open surgical valvotomy may be performed.
  - ❖ A prosthetic mitral valve[Q] is more likely to develop a thrombotic complication compared to aortic valve.
✓ **Mitral Regurgitation (MR)**
  - **Causes:** Acute MI, infective endocarditis, myxomatous degeneration, blunt trauma can cause acute MR.
    - ❖ Dynamic MR is also a feature of HOCM.
  - **Symptoms:** Acute severe MR presents with pulmonary oedema.
  - **Echocardiography:** Regurgitant fraction ≥50% in severe MR.
  - **Treatment**[Q]: Vasodilators and increased HR. IABP as a bridge to surgery.
    - ❖ Acute severe MR requires surgery, but not as urgent as acute AR.
    - ❖ Valve replacement if papillary muscle rupture.
✓ **Tricuspid Regurgitation (TR)**
  - Secondary TR is the most common cause of acute TR, mostly seen in left heart disease, pulmonary hypertension, or coronary artery disease.
    - ❖ Most common cause of primary TR is infective endocarditis.
  - **Symptoms of right heart failure:** Fatigue, oedema, and ascites.
  - **Echocardiography:** Severe TR shows large jet area (>10 cm²) and plethoric IVC.
  - **Treatment:** Acute TR due to IE is medically managed mostly.
    - ❖ Diuretics and inotropes for RV failure.
    - ❖ TV surgery at the time of left-sided surgery is routinely performed when TR is severe.

Additional Questions
(I have deliberately not put the types of murmurs for these valvular heart diseases. If you can hear them during the noisy ICU environment, you need some genetic testing.)

✓ **Carcinoid Syndrome**[Q]: Right-sided heart valves, like tricuspid valve (regurgitation) and pulmonary valve (stenosis), are involved.

- **Carcinoid tumours** are normally located in small intestine. Symptoms are skin flushing, diarrhoea, wheezing, and abdominal cramps.

RIGHT VENTRICULAR FAILURE

Aetiology and Pathophysiology

✓ Seen in ARDS, myocardial infarction, pulmonary embolism, cardiac surgery, and decompensated chronic lung diseases.

✓ **Right ventricle** is the most anterior chamber in the normal heart and the sternum.
  - Triangular in the side profile, and crescent shape in cross section.
  - Right ventricle (RV) is thin-walled (1/6 of LV cardiac mass), with superficial circular fibres with deeper longitudinal fibres.
  - RV contracts in a peristaltic manner compared to concentric contraction of the LV free wall and septum, along with a twisting movement of the heart.

✓ RV is tolerant to **preload**; it has low muscular mass, which means that RV can dilate with excess volume. **Excess RV dilatation** is associated with tricuspid regurgitation and atrial septal defect.
  - RV is intolerant to acute changes in **afterload** due to reduced cardiac muscle mass.
    - ❖ PVR increases gradually in pulmonary hypertension, and right ventricular hypertrophy happens.
    - ❖ PVR increases acutely in acute pulmonary embolism, and RV failure happens.
  - Reduced preload and increased afterload with mechanical ventilation during IPPV can lead to deranged mechanics, which is exaggerated in hypovolaemia and shows fluid responsiveness.
    - ❖ These changes can also be seen in RV dysfunction, and caution should be taken before interpreting it as hypovolaemia.
  - In general, RV adapts to volume overload better than pressure overload.
  - RV pressure overload → decreased cardiac output → systemic hypotension → RV ischaemia → RV failure.

Clinical Features and Diagnosis

✓ **ARDS:** Hypoxia and hypercapnia cause increased afterload. RV dysfunction happens in 22–55% of patients with ARDS.

✓ **Pulmonary Embolism:** Acute increase in RV afterload occurs. Resolution of the embolus over time occurs, pulmonary artery pressures can decline, and RV function can return to normal.

✓ **Pulmonary Hypertension** (mPAP >20 mmHg at rest) is the commonest cause of RV failure. Measured by right heart catheterization.
  - Left ventricular failure is the commonest cause of pulmonary hypertension.

✓ **COPD and OSA** population should be considered at risk of RV dysfunction and less tolerant to the stresses of mechanical ventilation.

✓ **Congenital heart diseases**, like pulmonary stenosis, RV outflow tract obstruction after correction of tetralogy of Fallot (TOF), and repair of transposition of the great arteries, cause **pressure overloaded right heart failure.**
  - Atrial septal defect, ventricular septal defect, tricuspid regurgitation, and pulmonary regurgitation lead to **volume overloaded RV failure.**

✓ **Post–cardiac surgery:** Acute RV failure in up to 30% of patients having **cardiac surgery**. PVR increases post-operatively. Myocardial stunning and air emboli also cause RV dysfunction.
  - Patients undergoing surgery for mitral valve disease may already have pulmonary hypertension and RV dysfunction.
  - TR repair can increase afterload post-operatively and cause RV failure.
  - Post–LVAD insertion, when RV has to match an unloaded LV.
  - RV in heart transplant can be either primary graft dysfunction or secondary graft dysfunction due to hyperacute rejection or surgical complication.

✓ **Investigations:** Deranged LFTs, ↑ urea and creatinine, high lactates, and ScvO$_2$ <60%.
  - Deep S wave in Lead I, Q wave and inverted T wave in Lead III. (S1Q3T3) in pulmonary embolism on ECG (10%).
  - Troponin and BNP can be raised in RV dysfunction.

- Raised CVP is seen. Pulmonary artery catheter (PAC) is useful for diagnosis of pulmonary hypertension and should be used in complex cases.
- ✓ *Early use of transthoracic echocardiography (TTE) is recommended. Transoesophageal echocardiography (TOE) in mechanically ventilated patients*.
  - TTE will show flattening of the septum, an RV/LV basal diameter >1.
  - Tricuspid annular plane systolic excursion (TAPSE) <17 mm^Q is indicative of poor RV function.
- ✓ **Cardiac MRI** is gold standard nowadays for measurement of RV volumes and function.
- ✓ **Right heart catheterization** is needed for diagnosis of pulmonary artery hypertension and may also be help in the diagnosis of constrictive pericarditis.

Prevention and Treatment

- ✓ **General principles:** Treat underlying aetiology as early as possible.
  - Aim to maintain higher HR (prevents RV distension) and normal sinus rhythm. Cardiovert if new-onset AF with instability.
  - **Optimize cardiac preload^Q:** Small fluid boluses if underfilled (50–100 mL), and diuresis (furosemide, bumetanide) if overfilled and dilated. Monitor CVP.
  - **Inotropic support^Q:** Inodilators (dobutamine, milrinone) and vasopressors (noradrenaline, vasopressin).
  - **Reduce afterload^Q:** Prevent hypoxia, hypercapnia, and acidosis. Reduce pulmonary pressures and PEEP^Q. Use inhaled pulmonary vasodilators (nitric oxide or epoprostenol) and intravenous pulmonary vasodilators.
  - **Mechanical support^Q:** To completely offload the RV.
  - **RV protective mechanical ventilation:** Minimize plateau (<27 cm H_2O) and driving pressures (<17 cm H_2O), reverse pulmonary vasoconstriction, and prone position to unload the RV.
- ✓ **Thrombolysis** in pulmonary embolism returns RV function to normal.
- ✓ **Pulmonary vasodilators**
  - **Inhaled nitric oxide** reduces PVR only in areas of the lung that are well ventilated and improve V/Q matching, improving oxygenation, compared to intravenous pulmonary vasodilators (milrinone, levosimendan), which can worsen the V/Q matching.
- **Epoprostenol** is a prostacyclin and another inhaled pulmonary vasodilator.
- Other **pulmonary vasodilators** that can be used are **sildenafil** (phosphodiesterase-5 inhibitor), **bosentan** (endothelin receptor antagonist), and **riociguat** (soluble guanylate cyclase stimulator).
- ✓ **Early MCS** is effective in cases of acute RV failure refractory to medical therapy, like primary graft failure following heart transplant and is associated with improved survival.
  - **Impella RP:** Displaces blood from RV to the PA. Percutaneously placed through right femoral vein and flows up to 4 L/min can be achieved. Low-level systemic anticoagulation is maintained with ACT between 160 and 180s.
  - **RVAD:** Drains blood from RA and returns it via an extracorporeal circuit to the pulmonary artery. Can be percutaneous or surgically placed. Systemic anticoagulation is maintained with ACT between 180 and 220s.
  - **VA ECMO:** Drains blood from RA and returns it via an extracorporeal circuit to the aorta. Systemic anticoagulation is maintained with ACT between 180 and 220 s.
- ✓ **Heart transplant:** Indicated in refractory advanced heart failure in the absence of significant comorbidity.
- ✓ **Lung transplant:** Indicated in patients with end-stage lung disease.
  - Risks are higher in patients with co-existing pulmonary hypertension as prolonged RV dysfunction may lead to LV dysfunction, which may not recover immediately once the PVR is returned to normal. These patients may need ECMO initially.

HYPERTENSIVE EMERGENCIES

Epidemiology and Aetiology

- ✓ **Hypertension:** European Society of Hypertension (ESH) 2023 Guidelines: **Blood pressure (BP) >140/90** mmHg.

Classification Based on ESH 2023 Guidelines[Q]

Normal BP Ranges (mmHg)	Hypertensive BP Ranges (mmHg)
Optimal: <120/80	Grade 1: 140–159/90–99
Normal: 120–129/80–84	Grade 2: 160–179/100–109
High-normal: 130–139/85–89	Grade 3: ≥180/110

✓ **Hypertensive emergency:** Systolic blood pressure (SBP) ≥180 mmHg or diastolic blood pressure (DBP) ≥110 mmHg with ongoing or impending end-organ damage.
  • **Accelerated malignant hypertension:** Specific type of hypertensive emergency associated with signs of retinal haemorrhage and papilloedema.
  • **Hypertensive encephalopathy:** Specific type of hypertensive emergency associated with headache, irritability, and change in mental status.

✓ **Hypertensive urgency:** BP ≥180/110 without evidence of new or worsening end-organ damage.

✓ **Confusion buster[Q]:** At the bifurcation of common carotid artery, we have **chemoreceptors** sensitive for PaO_2 and $PaCO_2$.
  • The **carotid sinus** is a swelling in the **internal carotid artery** that contains **baroreceptors** and is involved in **blood pressure** control.

✓ **Renal disease** is the commonest cause of secondary malignant hypertension.
  • Other causes are OSA, endocrine disorders like pheochromocytoma, primary aldosteronism, and vascular disease like coarctation of aorta, giant cell arteritis.

Clinical Features and Diagnosis

✓ **Measurement of BP:** Arm at the level of heart. Width of the **bladder inside the cuff** should be 40% of the arm circumference, and length should be 80% of the arm circumference[Q].
  • The rate at which blood pressure increases and the prior level of BP are more important than the absolute level.

✓ **Assessment of end-organ damage**
  • **Neurological damage:** Headache, vomiting, visual disturbances, confusion, seizures, focal neurological deficits, *cotton wool exudates*, or *flame-shaped haemorrhages* on fundoscopy.
    ❖ **Non-contrast CT scan:** Bleed typically in basal ganglia, hypothalamus, or cerebellum. Cerebral oedema may be present without any bleed.
    ❖ **Posterior reversible encephalopathy syndrome (PRES)[Q]:** Clinicoradiological diagnosis characterized by hypertensive encephalopathy. White matter vasogenic oedema mostly in the occipital and posterior parietal lobe.
  • **Cardiovascular damage:** Anginal pain, breathlessness. Pulse deficits in the extremities may signify **aortic dissection**.
    ❖ **Echocardiography:** Left ventricular hypertrophy or dilation.
    ❖ **Systolic dysfunction:** Increase in diastolic blood pressure is mild, cardiomegaly on X-ray, lack of hypertensive retinopathy.
    ❖ **Diastolic dysfunction:** Increase in diastolic blood pressure is severe, left ventricular hypertrophy on ECG, presence of hypertensive retinopathy.
  • **Renal damage:** Oliguria, nocturia, haematuria.
    ❖ Urine analysis for proteinuria, haematuria, cellular casts.
  • **Hypertensive retinopathy**
    ❖ **Grade 1:** Arterial narrowing
    ❖ **Grade 2:** AV nicking
    ❖ **Grade 3:** Haemorrhages, cotton wool spots, and exudates
    ❖ **Grade 4:** All of the above + papilloedema

Treatment

✓ Goal of antihypertensive therapy is to decrease blood pressure while maintaining organ perfusion.
  • **Hypertensive emergency:** Treat in ITU and lower BP to safer levels (not normal) within minutes or hours. Use parenteral agents initially, and start oral agents at the same time to get off IV agents faster.
    ❖ *Reduce mean arterial blood pressure by 20–25% within minutes to an hour, or reduce DBP to 100–110 mmHg.*
    ❖ *Aim for a goal BP of approximately 160/110 mmHg if initial reduction is well tolerated.*
  • **Hypertensive urgency:** Treat in ward and *use oral therapy to lower BP to safer levels over several hours to 24 h.*

IV Drugs Used for Hypertensive Emergency

Drug	Dosage	Onset of Action	Features
Labetalol	0.5–2 mg/min	3–5 min	α- and β-blocker (1:7 ratio)
Sodium nitroprusside (SNP)	0.25–10 mcg/kg/min	1 min	Arteriolar and venous dilator^Q; cyanide toxicity
Nitroglycerine (GTN)	5–300 mcg/min	1–2 min	Venous and coronary artery dilator
Nicardipine	5–15 mg/h	5–10 min	Calcium channel blocker, systemic and coronary artery vasodilation
Esmolol	1 mg/kg loading dose f/b 150–300 mcg/kg/min	1–2 min	Cardio-selective β-blocker
Fenoldopam	0.1–1.6 mcg/kg/min	15 min	Dopamine-1 (D-1) receptor agonist; arterial vasodilatation, renal vasodilatation, and natriuresis
Phentolamine	5–10 mg bolus every 10 min	1–2 min	α-Adrenergic blocker
Hydralazine	5–20 mg bolus	10–30 min	Arteriolar dilator

✓ **Labetalol:** Can be used in most hypertensive emergencies. Can be used in preeclampsia and post–AAA repair. **Use carefully in heart failure.**

✓ **Nitrates, such as GTN or SNP:** SNP can be used in most emergencies. Both can cause increase in intracranial pressure (ICP), coronary steal syndrome, tachyphylaxis.
  • SNP is a prodrug and appears as a reddish-brown powder. Exposure to sunlight can lead to brown/blue discolouration, releasing cyanide and causing lactic acidosis and cyanide toxicity.
  • GTN is indicated in acute coronary syndromes and is a reasonable agent for hypertensive crisis due to cocaine overdose.

✓ **Nicardipine:** Used for perioperative hypertension and preeclampsia/eclampsia.

✓ **Esmolol:** Used for perioperative hypertension. **Avoid pure beta-blockers** in patients showing signs of left ventricular dysfunction and pulmonary oedema.

✓ **Phentolamine:** Used for phaeochromocytoma and cocaine abuse. Unopposed alpha blocking can cause coronary vasoconstriction and systemic hypertension.

✓ **Fenoldopam:** Useful in patients with renal impairment or congestive heart failure.

Drugs for Hypertensive Urgency

✓ **Oral labetalol** can be used in hypertensive urgency.
✓ **Clonidine:** Central α-2 adrenergic agonist. Can be used in hypertension due to withdrawal syndromes. It can cause rebound hypertension, bradycardia, dry mouth.
✓ **Angiotensin-converting enzyme (ACE) inhibitors:** Can cause first-dose hypotension and renal failure in bilateral renal artery stenosis.

Specific Clinical Situations

✓ **Acute intracranial stroke:** Decrease BP only if SBP >220 mmHg. labetalol and nicardipine.
✓ **Hypertensive encephalopathy:** Labetalol and esmolol.
✓ **Acute coronary syndromes:** Nitroglycerine and labetalol.
✓ **Acute left ventricular dysfunction:** Nitroprusside (both systolic and diastolic dysfunction), nitroglycerine (ischaemic heart), labetalol (diastolic dysfunction), diuretics (systolic dysfunction).
✓ **Aortic dissection:** Rapid BP lowering is needed with SBP target ≤110 mmHg. Labetalol and opioids to control pain.
✓ **Phaeochromocytoma:** Phentolamine
✓ **Cocaine-associated hypertension:** Benzodiazepines, nitrates, and alpha blockers like phentolamine.

- Beta-blockers are avoided[Q] as they can cause unopposed alpha stimulation and can cause severe coronary vasoconstriction.
✓ **Alcohol withdrawal syndrome:** Clonidine and benzodiazepines.
✓ **Severe pre-eclampsia/eclampsia:** Labetalol, hydralazine, nicardipine, magnesium sulphate.
✓ **Perioperative hypertension:** SNP, NTG, labetalol, esmolol, analgesics.
✓ **Hyperperfusion syndrome[Q]:** Hypertension, focal seizures, and headache after carotid endarterectomy.
  - Due to re-establishment of blood flow. Labetalol and clonidine are used.

Prognosis

✓ Around 1% of patients with hypertension will develop a hypertensive crisis.

AORTIC ANEURYSM

Aetiology

✓ **Aortic aneurysm:** Segment of the aortic lumen whose *diameter exceeds 1.5 times the normal diameter for that segment.*
  - Normal diameter of aorta:
    - ❖ **Thorax:** 3 cm
    - ❖ **Abdomen** till iliac bifurcation: 2 cm
  - Up to 13% of patients with single aneurysm will have additional aneurysms.
  - **Abdominal aneurysms are more common** than the thoracic aneurysms.
  - Most encountered morphology is **fusiform:** Symmetrical dilatation of an aortic segment, involving the entire circumference of the vessel wall.

Clinical Features and Diagnosis

✓ **Thoracic aortic aneurysm (TAA)**
  - Around 40% of all aneurysms are asymptomatic at the time of diagnosis.
  - Abrupt increase in risk of rupture at a **diameter of 6 cm.**
  - Aortic root and ascending aorta (60%), descending aorta (40%).
  - **Causes:** Hypertension, bicuspid valve, Marfan's syndrome, Ehlers–Danlos syndrome, Takayasu arteritis, syphilis.

- *Aneurysms of descending thoracic aorta are mainly caused by atherosclerosis.*
- **Presentation:** Chest and back pain, superior vena cava syndrome, **dyspnoea** due to tracheal compression, **dysphagia** due to oesophageal compression, hoarseness of voice due to vocal cord paralysis.
- **Contrast CT angiography is the investigation of choice.**
✓ **Abdominal aorta aneurysm (AAA)**
  - **Risk factors[Q]:** Smoking, age >65 yr, male gender, hypertension, hyperlipidaemia.
    - ❖ **Infrarenal segment** of aorta is most heavily affected by atherosclerosis, and this is the segment **most commonly having abdominal aneurysms.**
    - ❖ **Risk of AAA in diabetes is half of that in non-diabetes.**
  - **Presentation:** *Most cases are asymptomatic and may present with hypogastric pain or lower back pain.*
    - ❖ Compression of the ureter or kidney can lead to hydronephrosis.
    - ❖ May present as a palpable, pulsatile mass in the midline.
  - **Contrast CT angiography is the investigation of choice.**
    - ❖ Ultrasound if patient is unsuitable for transfer.

Treatment

✓ **Thoracic aortic aneurysm**
  - Surgical repair for **diameter >5.5 cm** or for aneurysms expanding at the rate of **>0.5 cm per year.**
    - ❖ Rupture of a TAA is a surgical emergency. Open repair of the vessel using deep hypothermic circulatory arrest is done.
    - ❖ Retrograde endovascular stent placement may be useful for the repair of aneurysms of the descending aorta.
✓ **Abdominal aortic aneurysm**
  - Elective repair for males with **AAA >5.5 cm**, females with AAA >5 cm, or **rapid growth >1 cm/year.**
    - ❖ Rupture of an AAA is a surgical emergency. Open repair with replacement of the diseased segment with a Dacron graft is done most commonly.

- ❖ Open surgery and EVAR for ruptures AAA have equal mortality post-operative.
- ❖ Recommended to do EVAR for ruptures AAA under local anaesthesia if possible.
- ❖ *Target systolic blood pressure of 90* mmHg to maintain end-organ perfusion (110–120 mmHg in aortic dissection) and avoid crystalloids.

✓ **Complications post-ruptured abdominal aortic aneurysm repair are as follows**
- Colonic ischaemia (ligation of inferior mesenteric artery)
- Abdominal compartment syndrome
- Bowel paralysis
- Feeding intolerance (PN may be needed)
- Retro- and intraperitoneal bleeding
- Graft leak
- Intra-abdominal abscesses

✓ **Post-operative management for abdominal aortic aneurysm management.**
- **Cardiac output monitoring**
  - ❖ Measured after every 4 h and cardiac index target >2.5 L/min/m².
  - ❖ Use volume loading and adrenaline for this, and aim for PCWP between 5 and 15 mmHg.
  - ❖ K⁺ and Mg should be closely monitored to avoid arrhythmias.
  - ❖ Lactate monitoring^Q as possible sign of gut ischaemia.
- **Haemodynamic monitoring**
  - ❖ Haemoglobin target: >100 g/L.
  - ❖ CVP target: 4–12 mmHg.
  - ❖ MAP target: 85–105 mmHg.
  - ❖ Avoid hypertension with MAP >120 mmHg.
  - ❖ Drop in haemoglobin, acidosis, abdominal distension, big drain output, and respiratory distress from haemothorax can all be indicative of bleeding.
- **Lumbar drain insertion**
  - ❖ Reduces the risk of paraplegia post-operatively.
  - ❖ CSF drainage set at 10 mmHg.
  - ❖ Medical team informed if drainage exceeds >10 mL/h or 25 mL/4 h or 150 mL/24 h. As excessive drainage can lead to subdural haematoma.

- **Neurological monitoring**
  - ❖ Normal post-operative neurological monitoring and review of any new focal neurological deficit.
- **AKI prevention**
  - ❖ Monitor urine output with 2 mL/kg/h for first 4 h, and then 1 mL/kg/h.
- **GI management**
  - ❖ NGT in situ on arrival to unit and on free drainage.
  - ❖ Aspirate every 4 h till bowel sounds heard by the medical team.
  - ❖ NGT remains in place for 3–4 h.

Prognosis

✓ *Around 50% of patients with ruptured abdominal aneurysm don't reach the hospital, 50% of those who reach the hospital die before having surgery, and 50% of those who have surgery do not survive after the surgery.*

✓ *Approximately 1–2% mortality if fit for surgery electively.*

✓ *Glasgow aneurysm score^Q:* Used for assessing post-repair outcome of a ruptured aortic aneurysm.
- Variables used are: Cerebrovascular disease, renal disease, age, myocardial disease, and shock.

AORTIC DISSECTION

Aetiology

✓ **Aortic dissection:** Longitudinal cleavage of the muscular media, leading to the formation of a second false lumen.
- Cleavage typically progresses in the direction of blood flow from proximal to distal aorta.

✓ **Stanford classification^Q**
- **Type A:** Ascending aorta
- **Type B:** Descending aorta

✓ **The DeBakey classification^Q**
- **Type I:** Ascending aorta and the descending aorta both.
- **Type II:** Ascending aorta proximal to the brachiocephalic artery.
- **Type III:** Originates in the descending aorta distal to left subclavian artery.
  - ❖ **Type IIIa:** Limited above the diaphragm.

❖ **Type IIIb**: Extends below the diaphragm.

✓ **Incidence** is highest in the 6th and 7th decades of life among male patients with **hypertension.**
- Younger patients with connective tissue disorders like **Marfan or Ehlers–Danlos syndrome, vascular inflammatory disease (Takayasu), or trauma** may present with dissection as well due to medial wall degeneration.
- Also seen in bicuspid aortic valve[Q], **cocaine use,** coronary intervention, **bypass surgery,** and aortic valve surgery.
- Areas of the aorta with the highest stress, such as the right lateral wall of the ascending aorta and proximal segment of the descending aorta.

Clinical Features and Diagnosis

✓ **Chest pain** radiating to back. "Tearing or stabbing pain," diaphoresis, shortness of breath.
- **Complications** like aortic regurgitation, myocardial infarction, cardiac tamponade, haemoptysis, CVA, ischaemic neuropathy, mesenteric ischaemia, acute renal failure, lower limb ischaemia.

✓ **Chronicity of aortic dissection**
- **Hyperacute:** <24 h
- **Acute:** 1–14 d
- Subacute: 15–90 d
- Chronic: >90 d

✓ **Chest X-ray:** Widening of mediastinum, aortic knuckle enlargement, and displacement of aortic calcification. However, >20% of patients won't have mediastinal widening.
- **ECG:** ST-segment elevation in lead aVR in patients with type A dissection has prognostic value.
- **Transthoracic echocardiography (TTE):** Dilatation of aortic root, intimal flap in ascending aorta, aortic valve regurgitation, pericardial effusion.
  - ❖ Full length of aorta can't be evaluated.
- **ECG-gated CT angiogram** is the investigation of choice (sensitivity and specificity >95%).
  - ❖ "Tennis ball sign" may be seen due to visible dissection flap.

❖ Contrast is involved and can cause allergic reactions and contrast nephropathy.
- **Transoesophageal echocardiography (TOE)**[Q] can be used for evaluation of unstable patients and is superior to TTE for aortic dissection.

Treatment

✓ **Goals:** Decrease pain, blood pressure, and force of left ventricular contraction.

✓ *Targets: Hb >120 g/L, SpO$_2$ >95%, SBP 100–120 mmHg, HR 60–80 bpm.*

✓ **Initial management:** Wide-bore IV access and invasive BP monitoring with adequate analgesia.
- **Arterial access:** Left side for type A, right side for type B.
- Analgesia.
- Intravenous short-acting beta-blockers to decrease shear stress on the aortic wall.
  - ❖ Labetalol and esmolol are used commonly.
- Calcium channel blockers like diltiazem or verapamil in patients intolerant to beta-blockers.
- *Heart rate is controlled first, followed by vasodilation, to decrease blood pressure.*
- Vasodilators like sodium nitroprusside and glyceryl trinitrate can be used.

✓ **Type A dissection:** Open surgical repair with grafting of the ascending aorta ± arch. Aortic valve may or may not be replaced.
- Frozen elephant trunk technique is being increasingly used. Branched graft with stent in situ.
- Cardiopulmonary bypass with deep hypothermic circulatory arrest is used.

✓ **Type B dissection:** Treat uncomplicated disease medically.
- Treat complicated disease (refractory pain, malperfusion, rupture of the leak, rapid expansion of false lumen) with thoracic EVAR. Open surgery may also be an option.
- Prophylactic lumbar drain is put to prevent lower limb neurological deficit[Q].

✓ **Post-operative complications**
- Bleeding, spinal cord ischaemia[Q], stroke[Q], acute kidney injury.

✓ **Spinal cord perfusion optimization**[Q]
  - **CSF drain:** Ensure that the patient is flat, with a drain pressure of <5 mmHg and drain for 7 d.
  - **Oxygen delivery:** SpO_2 >95%, Hb >120 g/L, and a cardiac index >2.5 L/min/m².
  - **Patient status assessment:** MAP >90 mmHg, spinal cord perfusion pressure >80 mmHg.

Prognosis

✓ More than 20% of patients with acute aortic dissection die before reaching the hospital.
  - Aortic dissection mortality increases by 1–2% per hour after symptom onset.
  - A *30 d mortality for aortic dissection of any type is around 50%.*

ARRHYTHMIAS

Physiology

✓ **Potassium currents:** Involved in phase 3 (action potential) and phase 4 (diastolic depolarization).
  - **Na^+/K^+ pump**[Q]: Throws three sodium ions out for taking two potassium ions in. ATP-dependent and are blocked by digoxin.
  - Potassium has a large concentration gradient across the cell membrane and the greatest permeability at rest. It contributes the most to the resting membrane potential[Q].

✓ **Sodium currents:** Responsible for the depolarization phase of the action potential.
  - **Na^+/Ca^+ pump:** Throws three sodium ions out for taking one calcium ion in. Digoxin blocks the sodium–potassium pump, causing sodium to accumulate inside the cell. The sodium–calcium pump then pumps out that extra sodium to bring calcium in and cause increased inotropy.

✓ **Calcium currents:** L-type (slow inward current) and T-type (fast current).

✓ **Cardiac myocytes (RMP: −90 mV)**
  - Phase 0: Na^+ influx, upstroke, and initial rapid depolarization
  - Phase 1: K^+ efflux, early rapid repolarization
  - Phase 2: Ca^{2+} influx through slow L-type channels, K^+ efflux[Q], prolonged plateau phase
  - Phase 3: K^+ efflux, final rapid repolarization
  - Phase 4: 3 Na^+ out, 2 K^+ in, *resting membrane potential*

✓ **Pacemaker cells (RMP: −60 mV)**
  - Phase 0: Ca^{2+} influx through L-type channels and upstroke
  - Phase 3: K^+ efflux, repolarization
  - Phase 4: Pacemaker potential

✓ **Heart conduction system**
  - **Sinoatrial node (SA node):** At junction of right atrium and superior vena cava (SVC). Supplied by right coronary artery in 55% of cases and left circumflex artery in 45% of cases.
  - **Atrioventricular node (AVN):** Located within interatrial septum. Supplied by AV nodal artery (right coronary artery in 90% of cases)[Q].
  - **His bundle:** Formed by Purkinje fibres emerging from the distal AV node and divides into left and right bundle branch.

Morphology

✓ **ECGs:** Speed is 25 mm/s.
  - One small square (1 small box) = 0.04 s and one large square (5 small boxes) = 0.2 s
  - 10 mm (10 small boxes) = 1 mV

✓ **Rhythm:** Constant R–R interval or variable R–R interval.

✓ **Rate:** Divide 300 by the number of large squares between two QRS complex if regular or number of R waves over 10 s period multiplied by 6 if irregular.

✓ **Axis:** Normal axis 0–90°.

Lead	Normal Axis (0–90°)	Left Axis Deviation Physiological (0–30°)	Left Axis Deviation Pathological[Q] (−30 to −90°)	Right Axis Deviation[Q] (90–180°)	Extreme Axis (−90 to −180°)
Lead I	Positive	Positive	Positive	Negative	Negative
Lead II	Positive	Equiphasic	Positive	Positive	Negative
Lead III/aVF	Positive	Negative	Negative	Positive	Negative

✓ **P waves:** Checked in lead II. P wave shouldn't exceed 3 small squares. *If >3 small squares, it's right atrial enlargement.*
- *Bifid P wave*[Q] *is seen in left atrial enlargement.*

✓ **PR interval:** To look for any AV nodal block. Normal is 0.12–2 s.

✓ **QRS wave:** Broad (> 0.12 s) or narrow complex (< 0.12 s), depending upon supraventricular or ventricular origin.
- **Left ventricular hypertrophy (LVH)**
  - ❖ Voltage criteria **Sokolow–Lyon criteria**[Q]: If deepest S wave in V1 or V2 and amplitude of tallest R wave in V5 or V6 is ≥35 mm.
  - ❖ Non-voltage criteria: Increased R wave peak time >50 ms in leads V5/6 or ST-segment depression and T wave inversion in left-sided leads.
  - ❖ Voltage criteria must be used along with non-voltage criteria to be considered diagnostic of LVH.
  - ❖ Most common cause of LVH is hypertension.
- **Right ventricular hypertrophy (RVH**[Q]**):** QRS <120 ms, right axis deviation, dominant R wave in V1, dominant S wave in V5/6.

✓ J point: Point in ECG where the QRS complex joins the ST segment.

✓ **QT interval:** Increased in drug toxicities.

✓ **T wave:** Normal T wave is usually in the same direction as the QRS except in the right precordial leads. T wave is always upright in leads I, II, V3–6 and always inverted in lead aVR.

✓ **Abnormal ECG waves**
- **U waves**[Q]**:** 0.5 mm deflection after T wave.
  - ❖ Bradycardia (MC), hypokalaemia, severe hypothermia.
  - ❖ **Best seen in lead V2 and V3.**
- Tall T waves: Hyperkalaemia.
- **Osborne J waves**[Q]**:** Positive deflection seen in J point in precordial and true limb leads.
  - ❖ Characteristically seen in hypothermia.
  - ❖ **Other causes:** Hypercalcaemia, brain injury, subarachnoid haemorrhage, vasospastic angina, *type 1 Brugada syndrome*, normal variant, idiopathic ventricular fibrillation.
- **Delta waves:** Slurred upstroke at the beginning of the QRS complex.

- ❖ Seen in Wolff–Parkinson–White (WPW) syndrome.
- *P. pulmonale* (enlarged): COPD.
- *P. mitrale* (bifid): Mitral regurgitation.
- **Wellens pattern A:** Biphasic T wave in V2–3. ECG pattern plus chest pain signify critical stenosis of the left anterior descending artery.
- **Wellens pattern B:** Deeply inverted T wave in V2–3. ECG pattern plus chest pain signifies critical stenosis of the left anterior descending artery.

✓ **Short PR interval:** WPW syndrome
- **Long PR interval:** First-degree heart block, hyperkalaemia, beta-blockers, and digoxin.

✓ **Widened QRS:** Conduction deficits, hyperkalaemia, WPW syndrome, ventricular hypertrophy, drugs that inhibit sodium channels like TCAs, type 1a and 1c antiarrhythmics, antimalarial, and antiepileptics.

✓ **ST-segment changes**
- **Reverse tick ST depression** (down-sloping ST segments): Digoxin.
- **Saddle-shaped ST elevation** (concave ST elevation in all chest leads)[Q]: Pericarditis.
- **ST depression:** Conduction deficits, hypokalaemia.

✓ **Long QT syndrome**[Q] **(LQTS):** Blockade of rapid potassium outward current causes LQTS.
- **QT interval:** Time taken for ventricular depolarization and repolarization.
- Corrected QT interval (QTc): **Bazett's equation**[Q] ($QT/\sqrt{RR}$).
  - ❖ **Normal QTc for men:** <440 ms; for women: <460 ms.
- Causes of long QT syndrome
  - ❖ **Congenital:** Romano–Ward syndrome, Jervell and Lange–Nielsen syndrome.
  - ❖ **Acquired:** Myocardial ischaemia, subarachnoid haemorrhage, hypothermia.
    - **Hypokalaemia, hypocalcaemia, and hypomagnesaemia.**
  - ❖ **Drugs**
    - **Antiarrhythmics: Amiodarone**[Q], sotalol, quinidine, procainamide, disopyramide (Vaughan Williams class[Q] 1 and 3 drugs).
    - **Antibiotics:** Clarithromycin, **ciprofloxacin**, erythromycin, fluconazole, metronidazole, trimethoprim, and sulphamethoxazole.

- **Antipsychotics/antidepressants:** **Haloperidol**, amitriptyline, citalopram, chlorpromazine.
- **Others:** Methadone, **ondansetron**, domperidone, droperidol, dexmedetomidine, protease inhibitors, organophosphates, and grapefruit juices.
- **Presentation:** They can trigger afterdepolarizations, which can trigger torsades de pointes (TdP), palpitations, syncope, or sudden death.
- **Treatment:** Remove agent. Beta-blockers. ICD may be needed in high-risk patients not responding to beta-blockers.

✓ **Shortened QT interval^Q:** A QT <350 ms is abnormally short and can also cause ventricular arrhythmias.
- Hypercalcaemia, hyperkalaemia
- Acidosis and hyperthermia
- Digoxin

✓ **Brugada syndrome:** Sodium channel disorder causing sudden cardiac death in young patients.
- **Right bundle branch block** with coved ST-segment elevation >2 mm in >1 of V1–3, and negative T wave following the ST segment.
- Treated with **urgent implantable cardioverter**.

Tachyarrhythmias: *Heart rate >100/min.*

✓ **Supraventricular tachycardia (SVT):** Start at level above the bundle of His. They have usually narrow complex tachycardia, with QRS <120 ms.
- *However, SVT may have broad complex in the presence of pre-existing bundle branch block, rate-related aberrant conduction, or accessory pathway.*
- About 30% of patients with SVT or other arrhythmias have underlying sepsis; surgical complications can present with arrhythmias and are commonly seen in critically ill patients.

✓ **Ventricular arrhythmias:** Start at level below bundle of His. They have wide complex tachycardia with QRS >120 ms.

✓ **Mechanisms of tachyarrhythmias**
- **Abnormal automaticity:** New sites apart from SA node, AV node, and Purkinje cells with phase 4 depolarization characteristics. Hence, a new ectopic site with automaticity.
- **Abnormal conduction:** Seen in patients born with slow and fast AV nodal pathway.

A premature atrial contraction (PAC) is followed by a prolonged PR interval (conduction down the slow pathway), followed by a sudden-onset regular narrow complex tachycardia (retrograde conduction up through the fast pathway), and complete a circuit.

- **Triggered activity:** Heart contracts twice after being activated once. These are called afterdepolarizations. When afterdepolarization occur before a full repolarization of a preceding action potential, they are called early afterdepolarization (EAD). When afterdepolarization occurs after a full repolarization of a preceding action potential, it is called Delayed Afterdepolarization (DAD).

Regular Supraventricular Tachycardia of Atrial Origin

✓ **Sinus tachycardia**
- Sinus P wave morphology seen in leads II, III, and aVF.
- Gradual onset. P wave closer to the succeeding QRS complex (long R-P tachycardia).
- Seen in sepsis, pain, anxiety, fever, anaemia, thyrotoxicosis, beta-agonist activity.
- Exclude the diagnosis of paroxysmal atrial tachycardia or atrial flutter with 2:1 or 3:1 block.
- Beta-blockers may need to be given in patients with impaired diastolic filling.

✓ **Focal atrial tachycardia**
- Tachycardia origin other than sinus node. Increased automaticity at an ectopic atrial site.
- Sudden onset. P wave closer to the succeeding QRS complex (long R–P tachycardia).
- Heart rate generated is generally too fast and inappropriate, and treatment with beta-blockers and calcium channel blockers is needed.
- *Vagal manoeuvres and adenosine can decrease the ventricular response and allow for diagnosis of the atrial tachycardia from AVNRT. Adenosine won't terminate a focal atrial tachycardia.*
  - ❖ Flecainide and intravenous class III agents, such as ibutilide and amiodarone.
  - ❖ Overdrive pacing can terminate the tachycardia.

✓ **Atrial flutter (AFL):** Occurs due to re-entrant circuit involving the cavo-tricuspid isthmus in the right atrium.

- **Sawtooth**-like appearances are seen. Flutter rate is around **250–300**.
- Variable AV block is also common and can lead to irregular R–R intervals.
- Management is same as that of AF. Rule out under-overfilling, and pulmonary embolism is a common cause.
- Rate control can be challenging, and rhythm control may be used more often.
- AV nodal blocking agents like beta-blockers, calcium channel blockers are used to control ventricular rate.
- Overdrive atrial pacing may be used to cause cardioversion if an atrial wire is in place.
- Pharmacological rhythm control can lead to haemodynamic instability due to 1:1 ventricular conduction, and immediate electrical cardioversion may be needed.

Irregular Supraventricular Tachycardia of Atrial Origin

✓ **Multifocal atrial tachycardia:** Irregular narrow complex tachycardia with at least three distinct morphologies of P waves.

- Seen in **COPD**, and hypoxaemia should be corrected in these patients.
- Beta-blockers and calcium channel blockers are used for treatment.

✓ **Atrial fibrillation (AF):** Please see the section on atrial fibrillation.

✓ **Atrial flutter with variable block.**

Supraventricular Tachycardia of AV Node Origin

✓ **Atrioventricular nodal re-entrant tachycardia (AVNRT):** *Commonest cause of tachycardia in structural heart disease.* **Re-entry circuit is functional.**

- Often called as paroxysmal SVT and has ventricular rate between 150 and 250 rpm.
- Sudden onset. P wave closer to the preceding QRS complex (**short R–P tachycardia**).
- Seen in patients born with **dual AV nodal physiology (slow and fast AV nodal pathway).**
  - ❖ Normally, sinus rhythm transmits through both pathways.

- ❖ However, sometimes an atrial ectopic beat might travel through the slower pathway, while the faster pathway is refractory from the previous sinus beat.
- ❖ Once this ectopic impulse reaches the distal end of the fast pathway, it travels up the faster pathway in retrograde fashion and stimulates SA node.
- ❖ The SA node discharges again, and the cycle is repeated.
- Surface ECG shows a **premature atrial contraction (PAC), followed by a prolonged PR interval (conduction down the slow pathway), followed by a sudden-onset regular narrow complex tachycardia (retrograde conduction up through the fast pathway).** Retrograde P waves can be seen after each QRS complex.
- Vagal manoeuvres and adenosine are first-line treatment.
  - ❖ IV beta-blockers or calcium channel blockers (verapamil 2.5–5 mg IV) can be given for resistant cases.
  - ❖ Catheter ablation is the ultimate treatment.

✓ **Atrioventricular re-entrant tachycardia (AVRT): Re-entry circuit is anatomical.**

- Sudden onset. P wave closer to the previous QRS complex (**short R–P tachycardia**).
- Accessory pathways connecting atrium and myocardium are present.
- **Antidromic AVRT or antegrade conduction:** This pathway if it conducts from atrium to ventricle.
  - ❖ **In antidromic AVRT**, a PAC goes down the accessory pathway and comes up to the atrium through the AV node. As conduction is directly to ventricles, *a wide complex QRS is seen in them*.
- **Orthodromic AVRT or retrograde conduction:** If it conducts from ventricle to atrium.
  - ❖ **In orthodromic AVRT**, a PAC goes down the AV node and comes up to the atrium through the accessory pathway. ECG similar to AVNRT.
- **Treatment**
  - ❖ Stable orthodromic AVRT is treated with vagal manoeuvres, adenosine, and calcium channel blockers.
  - ❖ Stable antidromic AVRT is treated with amiodarone or procainamide.

- ❖ Unstable AVRT treated with urgent cardioversion.
- ❖ Catheter ablation is the ultimate treatment.
✓ **Wolff–Parkinson–White syndrome (WPW syndrome)/pre-excitation syndrome**[Q]: *Refers to the presence of a congenital accessory pathway and episodes of tachyarrhythmias*[Q]. Presence of pre-excitation and an associated SVT is characteristic. Accessory pathway (AP) is called **bundle of Kent.**
  - WPW syndrome has **two forms of tachyarrhythmias:** AVRT (80%) and AF/atrial flutter.
  - Pre-excitation is present only intermittently and is more pronounced during vagal manoeuvres or AV blockade by drug therapy.
  - **Two types of patterns seen in WPW syndrome**
    - ❖ **Type A WPW pattern**[Q]: Left-sided AP produces a positive delta wave in all precordial leads and a dominant R wave in V1. Can mimic a posterior MI.
    - ❖ **Type B WPW pattern**[Q]: Right-sided AP produces a negative delta wave in leads V1 and V2 with a dominant S wave in V1. Can mimic an inferior MI.
  - Surface ECG shows **short PR interval, a delta wave** (slow rise of initial portion of the QRS), **QRS >0.12 s, discordant ST segment and T wave** (opposite direction to the major component of the QRS complex).
  - **IV procainamide**[Q] and ibutilide[Q] are used for terminating it.
  - Calcium channel blockers block AV node and can precipitate VF[Q] and should be avoided. Beta-blockers block both accessory pathway and AV node and can be used for rate control.
✓ **Junctional tachycardia:** Heart rhythm originating from the AV node or bundle of His.
  - Heart rate >100/min, a narrow QRS complex, and a missing or inverted or retrograde P wave.
  - **Causes:** Primary (congenital) or secondary (post-operative, myocarditis, Lyme disease).
  - **Treatment:** Beta-blockers, amiodarone, cryoablation, overdrive atrial pacing.

Ventricular Fibrillation (VF)

✓ Disorganized rhythm that will always cause haemodynamic compromise.

✓ **ALS protocol for cardiac arrest with shockable rhythm** is used for VF, pulseless ventricular tachycardia, or torsade de pointes and involves cardiac defibrillation, chest compressions, epinephrine, and amiodarone.
✓ *VF is commonly caused by acute coronary ischaemia, and revascularization after resuscitation can improve prognosis.*
✓ After ROSC is achieved, lignocaine can be considered to reduce the risk of recurrence.

Polymorphic Ventricular Tachycardia (PMVT)

✓ Unstable rhythm with varying beat-to-beat QRS morphology and can degenerate into VF.
✓ *Caused by acute myocardial ischaemia, and hence, it should be excluded, and revascularization can improve prognosis here as well. Inotropic use in ITU and digoxin toxicity can also cause it.*
✓ *Catecholaminergic VT is an example of **delayed afterdepolarization (DAD).***
✓ Differential diagnosis: Pre-excited AF, AF with aberrancy, and artifacts.
✓ Non-sustained PMVT (<30 s or no haemodynamic instability) can cause sudden cardiac death in patients with history of myocardial infarction.
  - Primary preventive ICD is considered in post-infarct patients with LVEF <40% and a positive electrophysiology study.
  - Reassessment of ventricular function 40 d after acute MI or 90 d after revascularization is done in patients in need of ICP implantation.
✓ All patients with haemodynamic instability should be defibrillated.
  - Patients are generally given magnesium and lignocaine.
  - Class Ia and III agents should be avoided.
  - Beta-blockers are given in patient with VT due to catecholamine excess.

Torsades de Pointes (TdP)

✓ Its polymorphic VT with prolonged QT interval[Q].
  - It generally starts with a slow heart rate, followed by a premature ventricular complex which interrupts the T wave. It's a complication of the long QT syndrome, and causes

should be sought. It is an example of early afterdepolarization (EAD).

- **Sotalol** caused TdP in 2–4% of patients. Amiodarone increases the QT interval but rarely causes TdP.[Q] Hypokalaemia and hypomagnesaemia can also cause TdP.
- Procainamide can treat monomorphic ventricular tachycardia but can itself lead to torsades de pointes.
- Treated with defibrillation for pulseless TdP.
- **IV 2 g magnesium sulphate even when levels are normal,[Q] and pacing if baseline rhythm is bradycardia.**

Monomorphic Ventricular Tachycardias (PMVT)

- ✓ **VT:** Three or more consecutive ventricular beats at a rate of >100 bpm.
  - **Sustained VT** is VT that lasts >30 s or causes haemodynamic compromise.
- ✓ **QRS** morphology is the same for all the beats. *In ICU, wide complex tachycardia is treated as VT unless proven otherwise. If patient is haemodynamically compromised, cardiovert assuming VT.*
- ✓ **Non-sustained VT** should be treated as ventricular extrasystoles in a patient with normal LV function.
  - In a patient with LVEF <35% and NYHA heart failure class II to III, treat them by treating exacerbating factors like ischaemia and consideration of *implantable cardioverter defibrillator (ICD).*
- ✓ *Aetiology is mostly cardiac scarring from prior cardiomyopathy or infarction, and acute ischaemia is not a common cause for PMVT or TdP.*
  - Tricyclic antidepressants and other sodium channel blocking anti-arrhythmic drugs can also cause it.
  - Pulseless VT is defibrillated, whereas unstable patients with pulses are **cardioverted**.
  - In stable patients, use class I (procainamide or lidocaine)[Q] or class III (**amiodarone** or sotalol)[Q] antiarrhythmic drugs.
  - If in doubt of the origin of tachycardia, never give verapamil; always give amiodarone.
  - *Refractory ventricular tachycardia and fibrillation are treated with overdrive or underdrive pacing, coronary revascularization, intubation and mechanical ventilation, and cardiac assist device like IABP.*

- *Adenosine may be used in patients with high suspicion for SVT in haemodynamically stable patients with regular WCT.*
  - ❖ Adenosine is contraindicated in patients with AF with pre-excitation.
- ✓ Catheter ablation for VT in patients with RVOT VT, idiopathic left ventricular VT, and bundle branch re-entrant VT.
- ✓ **Differential diagnosis of a patient with broad complex QRS tachycardia[Q] (that dreaded question you don't want to be asked – sometimes you don't even know it exists):** SVT with pre-excitation, SVT with non-specific QRS morphology.
  - Wide complex tachycardia in a patient with age >35 yr and history of myocardial infarction, cardiac failure, and family history of sudden death is usually VT. **QRS >0.20 s.**
  - A heart rate of >170 bpm suggests SVT. Morphology of QRS complex on ECG is same to that seen prior to the onset of tachycardia. QRS between 0.14 and 0.16 s suggests SVT.
  - Irregular wide complex tachycardia (WCT) is commonly AF compared to regular tachycardia in VT.
  - **Axis:** *Northwest axis (−90 to −180°)* is suggestive of VT.
    - ❖ Dominant R wave in aVR and dominant S wave in I and II.
  - **Precordial concordance (lack of RS complex):** If QRS polarities are all negative or positive from V1 to V6 (precordial leads), it is likely to be VT.
  - **AV dissociation:** Highly suggestive of VT.
    - ❖ P and QRS complexes at different rates.
    - ❖ **Capture beats:** SA node transiently captures the ventricles and produces a normal QRS complex.
    - ❖ **Fusion beats:** When a sinus and a ventricular beat coincide to produce a hybrid complex.
  - **Brugada sign:** Distance from onset of R wave to nadir of S wave is >100 ms in leads V1–6.
  - Any pattern of atypical RBBB is considered VT.
    - ❖ RSR complex in **V1** with a taller left rabbit ear is suggestive of VT, whereas in RBBB, the right rabbit ear is taller.

❖ R/S ratio <1 (small R wave and deep S wave) in **V6** with left axis deviation is suggestive of VT.

❖ QS complex (completely negative complex with no R wave) in V6 is suggestive of VT.

● Any pattern of atypical LBBB is considered VT.

❖ **Josephson sign: Notched S wave in V1** is highly suggestive of VT.

❖ **Upstroke of R wave:** Slow in VT (>40 ms) and fast in SVT (<40 ms) in **V1** and **V2.**

❖ QS complex (completely negative complex with no R wave) in V6 is suggestive of VT.

Ventricular Tachycardia Storm

✓ ≥3 episodes of sustained VT/VF, requiring ICD therapy or external shocks within 24 h.

✓ Beta-blockers have been shown to improve mortality. Amiodarone should be started as well.

● Sedation and intubation may be needed if medical therapy fails.

● Thoracic epidural anaesthesia or stellate ganglion block (SGB) with bupivacaine has been used. Left-sided SGB has been used, and bilateral SGB might be needed.

✓ Electrophysiologist consultation is warranted.

Premature Ventricular Contraction (PVC)

✓ Ectopic ventricular contractions with wide QRS complex for <3 consecutive beats.

✓ Common in healthy population. PVCs >10,000 to 20,000 beats/24 h or >20% of all beats may cause PVC-induced cardiomyopathy.

✓ Beta-blockers, amiodarone, lignocaine can be given. SGB can be given in refractory cases. PVC ablation may be needed.

Accelerated Idiopathic Ventricular Rhythm

✓ Wide complex ventricular rhythm at a rate <100/min and is seen in first 12 h following reperfusion of acute myocardial infarction. It resolves without specific therapy.

● **Bradyarrhythmias:** Heart rate <60 beats per minute.

✓ Can be divided into failure of impulse generation by SA node and failure of impulse conduction system.

✓ **Failure of impulse generation by SA node:** Sinus arrhythmia, sinus bradycardia, sinus node dysfunction.

✓ **Failure of impulse conduction system:** Atrioventricular conduction block.

✓ **Common causes** are beta-blockers, calcium channel blockers, inferior wall MI, myocarditis, Lyme disease, systemic lupus erythematous.

Sinus Arrhythmia

✓ Change in beat-to-beat P–P interval, with unchanged morphology of the P waves.

● Physiological as normal response to change in vagal tone during respiration.

● Doesn't cause haemodynamic instability.

Sinus Bradycardia

✓ Seen normally in athletes or during sleep or pathologically due to increased intracranial pressure, hypothermia, and increased vagal tone.

Sinus Node Dysfunction

✓ Also known as **sick sinus syndrome**. It can manifest as a combination of bradycardia and atrial tachycardia (tachycardia–bradycardia syndrome). Can have concomitant AV nodal disease as well.

✓ Seen in old patients and due to drugs (beta-blockers, digoxin, calcium channel blockers), infiltrative disease (amyloidosis, sarcoidosis), trauma, myocardial ischaemia, inflammation (pericarditis), and infection (Chagas disease).

✓ Seen in 5–30% cases of acute myocardial ischaemia. No treatment required unless causing hypotension or continuing ischaemia.

Atrioventricular Block (AV Block)

✓ **First-degree AV block:** Prolongation of PR interval to >200 ms.

● Commonly seen with increased vagal tone or treatment with beta-blockers or non-dihydropyridine calcium channel blockers.

✓ **Second-degree AV block**

● **Type I second-degree AV block or Mobitz type 1 or Wenckebach-type block:**

Progressive prolongation of the PR interval, followed by a skipped beat.

❖ Occurs at the level of AV node. First-degree and Mobitz type 1 block rarely require intervention.

- **Type II second-degree AV block or Mobitz type 2:** Regular drop in beat after a fixed number of beats without PR prolongation. Ratio can be 2:1, 3:1, or 4:1.

❖ Occurs below the level of AV node, and wide QRS is seen.

❖ Atropine is ineffective in these cases[Q].

✓ **Third-degree AV block:** Complete block of propagation of AV impulse from atrium to ventricle. Complete dissociation of atrial beats (P waves) and ventricular beats (R waves) happen, and they are not related to each other.

- Some degree of complete AV block occurs in 12–25% of patients with acute myocardial infarction (inferoposterior MI).
- In anterior MI, generally the bundle branches are involved.
- Mobitz type 2 or third-degree AV block are often dangerous and temporary or permanent pacemaker is needed. Atropine routinely has got no effect in these patients.

✓ **Right bundle branch block (RBBB):** Right bundle branch block can be seen in normal people[Q]. Supplies right ventricle, and hence, problems of the right side can be diagnosed with it.

- ECG changes: **QRS >120 ms, rsR pattern in lead V1, deep notched S wave** in left-sided lead (**lead I,** aVL and **V4–6**). Secondary ST, T changes in V1–3.
- **Causes** are pulmonary embolism, pulmonary hypertension, COPD, Brugada syndrome, arrhythmogenic right ventricular cardiomyopathy.
- RBBB in a young adult may indicate atrial septal defect[Q].
- New RBBB should raise suspicion for acute cor pulmonale.

✓ **Left bundle branch block (LBBB):** Supplies left ventricle, and hence, problems of the left side can be diagnosed with it.

- ECG changes: QRS >120 ms, **deep S waves in V1 and V2, broad notched R wave** in lateral leads (I, aVL, v5–6), absence of septal Q waves in lateral leads.

- **Appropriate discordance:** Abnormal depolarization should be followed by abnormal repolarization. Hence, deep S waves are associated with ST elevation (<25% of preceding S wave), and tall, broad R waves are often associated with ST-segment depression.
- Causes are coronary artery disease, hypertension, valvular heart disease, myocarditis, post–aortic valve surgery.
- Development of LBBB in acute anterior MI signifies a poor prognosis. Backup temporary pacing should be considered in case of **bi-fascicular**[Q] and tri-fascicular block.
- **LBBB in a patient with myocardial infarction:** LBBB itself can show ST elevation on ECG and, hence, may be difficult to differentiate from MI. **Smith-modified Sgarbossa criteria**[Q] is used for diagnosis of MI in patients with LBBB.

❖ Concordant ST elevation: ≥1 mm in ≥1 lead.

❖ Concordant ST depression: ≥1 mm in ≥1 lead of V1–V3.

❖ Proportionally excessive discordant STE: >25% ST elevation of the depth of the preceding S wave.

✓ **Tri-fascicular block**[Q]: It refers to the presence of disease in **all three fascicles,** i.e. right bundle branch, left anterior fascicle block (LAFB), and left posterior fascicle block (LPFB).

- **Presentation:** Third-degree heart block + RBBB + LAFB (left axis deviation), or third-degree heart block + RBBB + LPFB (right axis deviation).

❖ **Bi-fascicular block: RBBB + LAHB/ LPHB.**

- **Causes:** Ischaemic heart disease, hypertension, hyperkalaemia, digoxin toxicity.
- These patients require pacemaker insertion.

Treatment

✓ **ALS guidelines for tachycardia**
- *If haemodynamically unstable*

❖ Synchronized DC shock, up to three attempts.

❖ Amiodarone 300 mg IV over 10–20 min; repeat synchronized DC shock.

- **If haemodynamically stable**
  - ❖ If QRS <0.12 s and regular, use vagal manoeuvres, adenosine 6 mg, 12 mg, 18 mg. If ineffective, give verapamil or beta-blocker.
  - ❖ If QRS <0.12 s and irregular, control rate by beta-blocker or diltiazem. If heart failure, consider digoxin or amiodarone. Anticoagulate if duration >48 h.
  - ❖ If QRS >0.12 s and regular, if VT, use amiodarone 300 mg IV over 10–60 min. If previous SVT with BBB, treat as regular narrow complex tachycardia.
  - ❖ If QRS >0.12 s and irregular, if AF with BBB, treat as irregular narrow complex tachycardia. If polymorphic VT, give magnesium 2 g over 10 min.
- ✓ **ALS guidelines for bradycardia:** *If haemodynamically unstable* (shock, syncope, myocardial ischaemia, heart failure) or *risk of asystole* (Mobitz type II block, *complete heart block*, recent asystole, or ventricular pauses >3 s).
  - Initial treatment is atropine, 6 doses of 0.5 mg IV each.
  - Adrenaline (2–10 mcg/min), isoprenaline infusion (5 mcg/min) or transcutaneous pacing.

- **Glucagon** in case of beta-blocker/calcium channel blocker poisoning.
- Dopamine or aminophylline are the alternative drugs.
- Ultimately, transvenous pacing needs to be done.
- ✓ **General principles of treating arrhythmias**
  - All antiarrhythmics are potentially proarrhythmic, and not all arrhythmias need to be treated. So correct abnormalities first if haemodynamics are stable.
    - ❖ Keep potassium in the upper range in patients with cardiac disease and cardiac surgery.
    - ❖ Magnesium levels in blood do not reflect tissue levels. Hence, replace generously.
  - Electricity is safer and quicker than drugs. So in a patient with compromised haemodynamics and fast rate, consider cardioversion. In patients with compromised haemodynamics and slow rate, consider pacing.
  - Treat all causes of treatable ischaemia as they are the major cause of dangerous VF and VT.
  - Check the position of intracardiac catheters, and withdraw a bit if in doubt.

Vaughan–Williams Classification of Anti-Arrhythmics[Q]

Class	Mechanism	Drugs	Action Potential
Ia	Sodium channel blockade	Quinidine, procainamide, disopyramide	• Prolongs action potential and refractory period
Ib		Lignocaine, phenytoin, mexiletine	• Shortens action potential and refractory period
Ic		Flecainide, propafenone	• No effect
II	Beta-blockers	Esmolol, propranolol, atenolol	• Slows rate at SA node and reduces AV conduction • Prolongs action potential and refractory period
III	K^+ channel blockers	Amiodarone, sotalol, bretylium	• Slows rate at SA node and reduces AV conduction • Prolongs action potential and refractory period
IV	Ca^{2+} channel blockers	Verapamil, diltiazem	• Slows rate at SA node and reduces AV conduction • Prolongs action potential and refractory period

✓ **Amiodarone:** Mainly potassium channel blocker[Q]. Na^+ and calcium channel blocker as well[Q].
  - Causes *corneal microdeposits, skin discolouration, thyroid dysfunction (hypo/hyperthyroid), pulmonary fibrosis*, and *liver dysfunction*.
  - **Type 1 amiodarone-induced thyrotoxicosis (AIT):** Excessive hormone synthesis due to excess iodine found in amiodarone. Thyroid antibodies and pre-existing thyroid disease are present. Treatment is to stop amiodarone along with use of anti-thyroid drugs and thyroidectomy.
  - **Type 2 amiodarone–induced thyrotoxicosis (AIT):** Excessive hormone release due to preformed hormones due to thyroiditis. Thyroid antibodies and pre-existing thyroid disease are absent. Treatment is to stop amiodarone, along with use of steroids.
  - Hepatic enzyme inhibitor leading to potentiation of drugs like warfarin and digoxin.
  - It is excreted in bile[Q] and needs no adjustment in renal failure.
  - It can't be removed by renal replacement therapy, as large volume of distribution and highly protein bound.
✓ **Digoxin[Q]:** Blocks Na^+/K^+ ATPase pump, which leads to increased intracellular calcium and, hence, inotropy.
  - Slows conduction at AV valve by increasing acetylcholine[Q] at muscarinic receptors.
  - Used to control rate in AF or atrial flutter.
✓ **Adenosine:** By activating A1 receptors and increasing potassium efflux, it slows electrical signals passing through the AV node.
  - Converts SVT into normal sinus rhythm if SVT is due to re-entry circuit involving AV node.
  - Helps in differentiating SVT from VT[Q].
  - Causes coronary dilation and, hence, coronary steal[Q].
  - Contraindicated[Q] in asthma, decompensated heart failure, and long QT syndrome.

ATRIAL FIBRILLATION

Epidemiology and Aetiology

✓ **Atrial fibrillation (AF):** Absence of P waves and irregular R–R intervals.

✓ **Paroxysmal:** If AF terminates spontaneously.
  - **Persistent:** If AF >7 d and terminated by electrical or pharmacological cardioversion.
  - **Permanent:** If sinus rhythm cannot be achieved.
✓ **Foci:** Around pulmonary veins.
✓ **Trigger:** Decompensated heart failure, sepsis, myocardial ischaemia, pulmonary embolism, thyrotoxicosis, cocaine use.
✓ New-onset AF in ICU differs in aetiology from AF in the community.
  - AF may occur in 5–15% septic patients. Underfilling/overfilling should be excluded.
  - Seen in post-surgical patients, and up to 40% patients will develop AF post-cardiac surgery.
  - AF can cause haemodynamic instability in patients with restrictive left ventricular filling like left ventricular hypertrophy due to loss of atrial kick.

Clinical Symptoms and Diagnosis

✓ Palpitations, chest pain, signs of heart failure.
  - Emboli[Q] to spinal arteries/brain can cause weakness in limbs and altered neurology.
✓ **Transthoracic echocardiography (TTE)[Q]:** Left atrial dilatation, valvular disease, low left ventricular ejection fraction.
  - Blood clot may be seen in heart chambers.
✓ **CHA_2DS_2_VASc score:** Assesses stroke risk in people with AF. Calculated in patients after >48 h of AF.
  - CHF, hypertension, age 65–74 yrs, diabetes, vascular disease, female sex score 1 point.
  - Age over 74 yr and previous stroke score 2 points.
  - Anticoagulation to be started in men[Q] with a score of ≥1 and women[Q] with a score of ≥2.
  - IV heparin and LMWH are used for anticoagulation initially.
    - ❖ All patients that underwent cardioversion should have anticoagulation for 4 wk irrespective of the CHA2DS2VASc score[Q].
  - Warfarin and novel oral anticoagulants like dabigatran, rivaroxaban, apixaban, and edoxaban are used for thromboprophylaxis.

✓ **HAS-BLED score:** Assesses the risk of bleeding in the people who are starting anticoagulation.
- Hypertension (SBP >160 mmHg), renal dysfunction, liver disease, previous stroke, previous major bleeding, unstable INR, age >65 yr, medication affecting coagulation (NSAIDs), significant alcohol/drug use.
- Score of 0, risk of bleeding in 1 yr is 1%; score 1, bleeding risk 3.5%; score 5, bleeding risk is 9%.
- For most people, the benefit of anticoagulation outweighs the bleeding risk.

Prevention and Treatment

✓ **Corrective measures:** Correct hypokalaemia, hypomagnesaemia, hypercapnia, hypoxia, fluid deficit, or fluid overload.
✓ **Rate vs rhythm control**
- In patients with cardiomyopathy or symptomatic heart failure, restoration and maintenance of sinus rhythm are useful[Q].
- *Otherwise, rate control is the preferred approach.*
- Older patients are more sensitive to the pro-arrhythmic effects of the drugs, with often permanent AF; hence, rate control is preferred in them as well.
- In young patients[Q], without having any haemodynamic stability, cardioversion to sinus rhythm is better.
- **If no haemodynamic compromise**, opt for rate control first.
  - ❖ **Beta-blockers** (bisoprolol, metoprolol, esmolol) or **calcium channel blockers** (verapamil or diltiazem) for rate control.
  - ❖ **Digoxin is ineffective for AF termination and is not recommended in postoperative patients.** However, it's the only agent that has no negative inotropic effect and may be helpful in patients with **decompensated heart failure**.
  - ❖ **Intravenous amiodarone** causes rate as well as rhythm conversion to sinus rhythm. **If EF <40%, amiodarone is drug of choice.**
  - ❖ In ICU patients, rate control is preferred because of high rates of recurrent AF.
  - ❖ If patient is stable and rhythm control is planned (patients with consistently rapid ventricular rates), if AF <48 h, do electrical cardioversion and give anticoagulation for 4 wk.

- ❖ If patients having AF for more than 48 h, perform a transoesophageal echocardiography, and if no left atrial appendage thrombus, perform cardioversion. If an atrial thrombus is detected, start anticoagulation and cardiovert after 3 wk[Q].
- **If haemodynamic instability:** Rhythm control is done using DC cardioversion (faster than pharmacological cardioversion) straight away irrespective of anticoagulation status[Q]. Rhythm control is also used for patients with consistently rapid ventricular rates.
  - ❖ If patient is haemodynamically unstable and pharmacological cardioversion is considered, then flecainide or propafenone is preferred as they work faster than amiodarone.
  - ❖ Flecainide is not suitable in structural heart disease.
✓ **Cardioversion:** Maximum energy is used. If sinus rhythm is temporarily present, use of anti-arrhythmic drugs will increase the likelihood of maintenance of sinus rhythm, and **amiodarone 300 mg over 30 min can help.**
✓ **Other Drugs**
- **Adenosine:** Rhythm will slow down to reveal no atrial activity and then revert back to tachycardia.
- **Vernakalant:** Atrial selective potassium channel blocker. At low heart rates, weak blocker of the activated sodium channel and the affinity for blockage increases as the heart rate increases. Reverse is also true, and quickly the binding is off. Contraindicated in advanced heart failure and SBP <100 mmHg.
- **Dronedarone:** Congener of amiodarone. Less thyroid and pulmonary effects. Contraindicated in heart failure. Oral preparation only.
✓ **Ablation[Q]:** Done around pulmonary veins and is known as pulmonary vein isolation.
- A left atrial thrombus on TTE is a contraindication for catheter ablation[Q].

PACEMAKERS

✓ **Indications of pacemaker[Q]:** American Heart Association (AHA)/American College of Cardiology (ACC) divides indications into three classes.
- **Class I** are conditions where a pacemaker is considered necessary and beneficial:

- ❖ **Sinus node dysfunction:** Documented symptomatic sinus bradycardia.
- ❖ **Acquired atrioventricular (AV) block:** Complete third-degree AV block with or without symptoms, symptomatic second-degree AV block (both Mobitz type I and II).
- ❖ **Chronic bi-fascicular/tri-fascicular block:** Intermittent third-degree AV block, type II second-degree AV block.
- ❖ **After acute phase of myocardial infarction:** Permanent ventricular pacing for persistent and symptomatic second- or third-degree AV block.
- ❖ **Hypersensitive carotid sinus syndrome:** Recurrent syncope caused by spontaneously occurring carotid sinus stimulation and carotid sinus pressure that induces ventricular asystole of more than 3 s.
- ❖ **Post-cardiac transplantation:** Persistent or symptomatic bradycardia not expected to resolve.
- ❖ **Hypertrophic cardiomyopathy:** Sinus node dysfunction and AV block.
- ❖ **Pacing to prevent tachycardia:** For sustained pause-dependent VT with or without QT prolongation.
- • **Class II** are conditions where pacemaker is indicated but there is conflicting evidence.
- • **Class III** are conditions in which permanent pacing is not recommended.
- ✓ **Overdrive/anti-tachycardia pacing**[Q]: Strategy is to terminate a tachyarrhythmia by pacing the heart at a rate faster than the intrinsic rate.
  - • Used in atrial flutter or ventricular tachycardia.
  - • Also used in bradycardia-induced torsade de pointes as they prevent bradycardia.
- ✓ **Indications for implantable cardioverter-defibrillator**
  - • **Class I indications** are
    - ❖ Cardiac arrest due to VF or VT, not due to a transient or reversible cause.
    - ❖ Spontaneous sustained VT.
    - ❖ Syncope of undetermined origin with clinically relevant, haemodynamically significant, sustained VT or VF-induced at electrophysiological study when drug therapy is ineffective.
    - ❖ Non-sustained VT with coronary disease, prior MI, LV dysfunction

and inducible VF, or sustained VT at electrophysiological study that is not suppressible by a class I antiarrhythmic drug.

- ✓ **Indications for cardiac resynchronization therapy (CRT)**
  - • **Class I indications**
    - ❖ Patients with LVEF <35%, sinus rhythm with LBBB, QRS ≥150 ms, and NYHA class II/III/IV symptoms while on optimal medical therapy.
  - • CRT with defibrillator may have possible benefit over CRT with pacemaker alone.
- ✓ **Types of cardiac pacing**[Q]: Lifesaving for brady-arrhythmia and some tachyarrhythmias.
  - • **Transcutaneous:** Used during refractory bradycardia in ALS protocol.
    - ❖ Consider sedation, and keep in mind that pacing thresholds increase during cardiac and thoracic surgery.
  - • **Transvenous/endocardial:** Used for atrial and/or ventricular pacing. Right IJV is used for approach as it is fastest and easiest.
    - ❖ Normally, ventricular single-chamber pacing is adequate. Right ventricle lead placement under fluoroscopy is done.
    - ❖ Avoid left subclavian as it might be needed for permanent approach later.
    - ❖ QRS complexes have an LBBB configuration.
    - ❖ Consider AV pacing if ventricular pacing is not successful.
  - • **Epicardial:** Pacing following cardiac surgery.
    - ❖ **Typical settings:** Atrial/ventricular output 10 mA, atrial/ventricular sensitivity 2 mV, rate 80/min, PR interval 150 ms.
    - ❖ Epicardial wires usually fail to sense and capture after a few days.
  - • **Resynchronization pacing:** Simultaneous right and left ventricular pacing has shown mortality benefit in chronic heart failure patients.
    - ❖ Benefits in acute heart failure are not confirmed.
  - • **Leadless pacemaker:** Pill-sized device implanted directly inside the heart. No leads involved.
    - ❖ It can pace only one ventricle and can't defibrillate.
  - • **Percussion:** Good old way during resuscitation.

Pacemaker Classification System: NASPE/BPEG Pacemaker Code (2002)[Q]

I	II	III	IV	V
Chambers Paced	**Chambers Sensed**	**Response to Sensing**	**Rate Modulation**	**Multisite Pacing**
O = none	O = none	O = none	O = none	O = none
A = atrium	A = atrium	I = inhibited	R = rate modulation	A = atrium
V = ventricle	V = ventricle	T = triggered		V = ventricle
D = dual (A + V)	D = dual (A + V)	D = I + T		D = dual (A + V)

✓ **Pacemaker terminology**
- **Sensitivity**[Q]: Minimum myocardial voltage required to be detected as a P wave or R wave in mV.
  - ❖ **Undersensing**[Q]: Pacemaker doesn't sense the native P or QRS wave and still paces asynchronously and can cause AF/VF.
  - ❖ **Oversensing**[Q]: Senses respiration or shivering, and hence, pacemaker fails to pace despite no native P or QRS wave.
- **Output:** Current (mA) produced by a pacemaker. Seen as a pacing spike on ECG.
  - ❖ **Output failure**[Q]: Failure to produce a pacing spike.
- **Capture:** Effective stimulation of cardiac depolarization by the pacemaker.
  - ❖ **Failure to capture**[Q]: Failure of pacing spike to produce QRS complexes.
- **Capture threshold**[Q]: Minimum amount of current (mA) needed to initiate depolarization of the paced chamber.

✓ **Some common pacing modes used clinically**
- **AAI**
  - ❖ Atrium paced and sensed.
  - ❖ If no electrical impulse sensed, then pacemaker will pace at the preset rate, and if electrical impulse sensed, then pacemaker will **inhibit itself**.
  - ❖ AV synchrony is maintained; however, unable to use in atrial fibrillation.
- **VVI**
  - ❖ Ventricle paced and sensed.
  - ❖ If no electrical impulse sensed, then pacemaker will pace at the preset rate, and if electrical impulse sensed, then pacemaker will **inhibit itself**.
  - ❖ Useful in atrial fibrillation[Q] and high-grade AV block; however, AV synchrony is lost, and risk of pacemaker syndrome is there.

- **DDD**
  - ❖ Both atrium and ventricle paced and sensed.
  - ❖ If both SA node and AV node are functioning, then pacemaker will just sense.
  - ❖ If either atrium or ventricle doesn't get the native cardiac impulse, the pacemaker will take over.
  - ❖ AV synchrony is maintained and useful in atrial fibrillation and high-grade AV block.
  - ❖ Pacemaker-mediated endless-loop tachycardia possible and pacemaker syndrome if incorrectly set up.
- **DDI**
  - ❖ Dual-chamber pacing without AV synchronization.
  - ❖ It lacks the "T" trigger option and can't trigger ventricular pacing after atrial event and, hence, better in AF as it results in AV dissociation if the atrial rate exceeds the set rate.
- **VOO**
  - ❖ Ventricle paced asynchronously without sensing.

✓ **Pacemaker checking:** Should be done daily and ideally during every shift.
- **Checking pacemaker threshold**
  - ❖ Set the pacemaker rate 10–20 beats above the native rate.
  - ❖ Start reducing the output until a QRS complex no longer follows each pacing spike.
  - ❖ The output at which capture is lost is called the **capture threshold**.
  - ❖ Typically, output is set at double this capture threshold.
- **Checking pacemaker sensitivity**
  - ❖ The patient needs to have a native rhythm.

- ❖ Put the pacemaker in an AAI, VVI, or DDD mode.
- ❖ Set the output as low as possible as you need to see the pacing spikes only.
- ❖ Set the pacemaker rate 10–20 beats below the native rate.
- ❖ Raise the sensitivity value until no cardiac activity is sensed (sense indicator on pacemaker stops flashing).
- ❖ Decrease the sensitivity value until all cardiac activity is sensed (sense indicator on pacemaker is flashing again). This sensitivity is called sensitivity threshold.
- ❖ Sensitivity is set at half of the sensitivity threshold.

✓ **Pearls of Wisdom**
- Intrinsic beats are always better and, hence, are preferred over a paced beat.

- Magnet^Q can turn the defibrillator function off in an ICD.
- AV node is prone to disruption after aortic valve surgery.
- Defibrillator pads should be placed as far from the pacing box as possible (at least 8–10 cm away)^Q.
  - ❖ The pacemaker must be checked as soon as possible post-defibrillation to check the pacemaker settings and functionality.
- **Electrolyte imbalances that can cause bradycardia:** Hyperkalaemia, hypermagnesaemia, hypercalcaemia.
- **Drugs that can cause bradycardia:**
  - ❖ **Sinus node affected:** Opioids, propofol, muscle relaxants
  - ❖ **AV block:** SSRIs, TCA

4

Pulmonary Problems

HIGH-FLOW NASAL OXYGEN (HFNO)

✓ **HFNO:** Nasal cannula to deliver warmed, humidified gases at flow rates of 40–60 L/min with fraction of inspired oxygen from 21 to 100%.
  - Nasal cannula connected to a specially designed **proprietary flow meter**.
  - Oxygen is routed through a heated humidifier that allows gas heating at 37°C and completely saturated with water.
  - *Normal breathing flow rates are 15 L/min, whereas flow rates during respiratory distress are up to 60–120 L/min. HFNO tries to match the peak inspiratory flow rates of dyspnoeic patients.*
  - PEEP generated exceeding 3–4 cm H_2O when flow rates are 60 L/min and mouth is closed.

✓ **Advantages of HFNO**[Q]
  - Generates a PEEP that stabilizes and recruits the alveoli. Requires mouth to be closed.
  - Reduces dead space and work of breathing.
  - Improves oxygenation and CO_2 clearance.
  - Improved degree of comfort, reduced dyspnoea, and decreased respiratory rate.
  - Humidified oxygen helps secretion clearance.

✓ **Low Chances of Success of HFNO**
  - Patients with tachypnoea, altered sensorium, hypercarbia, and inadequate oxygenation despite a high-flow rate have low chances of success of HFNO.
  - **ROX index:** Ratio of oxygen saturation (SpO_2/FiO_2)/respiratory rate.
    - ❖ It has been assessed as a predictor of HFNO treatment failure.

  - ❖ ROX <2.85 at 2 h, <3.47 at 6 h, and ROX <3.85 at 12 h are predictors of HFNO failure.

Uses of HFNO[Q]

✓ **Acute Hypoxaemic Respiratory Failure (AHRF)**
  - The American College of Physicians and ESICM recommend *the use of HFNO over NIV in patients with AHRF.*
    - ❖ NIV may cause lung damage through overdistension.
  - **FLORALI Trial (2015):** In patients with hypoxaemia without chronic respiratory failure or cardiogenic pulmonary oedema, no statistically significant difference in 28 d intubation rate was found between HFNO, NIV, and conventional oxygen therapy (COT).
    - ❖ Significant difference in 90 d mortality with HFNO compared to COT and NIV.
  - **FLORALI IM Trial (2022):** In **critically ill immunocompromised patients** with acute respiratory failure, no statistical difference in the mortality between HFNO and HFNO alternating with NIV.

✓ **Acute Heart Failure/Pulmonary Oedema**
  - Can be used in patients who are not tolerating NIV.

✓ **Covid-19 Patients**
  - **RECOVERY-RS Trial (2021):** In patients with AHRF and COVID-19, there was no difference in tracheal intubations or mortality within 30 d in HFNO-treated patients or COT.
    - ❖ Significantly less tracheal intubations or mortality within 30 d in CPAP-treated patients compared to patients on COT.

DOI: 10.1201/9781003476214-4

✓ **Preoxygenation**
- **FLORALI-2 Trial (2019):** In patients with acute hypoxaemic respiratory failure for intubation, **preoxygenation** with HFNO or NIV had no statistical difference in changing the risk of severe hypoxaemia.
- **ODEPHI Trial (2021):** In patients for gastrointestinal endoscopy, HFNO significantly decreased the rate of hypoxaemia compared to COT.

✓ **Prevention of Post-Extubation Respiratory Failure**
- Has been used to prevent respiratory failure after extubation to reduce the need for reintubation.

✓ **Post-Operative Respiratory Failure**
- **The BiPOP Trial (2015):** Among **cardiothoracic surgery** patients at risk for respiratory failure, the efficacy of HFNO is similar to that of NIV.

Additional Questions

✓ **Pulse Oximeter**[Q]: Two LEDs: 660 nm (red)[Q], 940 nm (infrared)[Q].
- **Beer's law**[Q]: Intensity of transmitted light decreases exponentially as concentration of substance increases.
  - ❖ **Lambert's law**[Q]: Intensity of transmitted light decreases exponentially as distance travelled by the substance increases.
- Each LED is switched on and off alternatively as the detecting photodiode is unable to differentiate between two wavelengths.
- **Isosbestic point**[Q]: Wavelength at which absorbances of oxyhaemoglobin and deoxyhaemoglobin are identical.
- **Meth**aemoglobin[Q]: 85% saturation fixed.
- **Carboxyhaemoglobin (CO poisoning)**[Q]: Falsely high readings.
- **Cyanide poisoning:** No effect on oxygen or haemoglobin saturation measurement.
- **Fetal haemoglobin or polycythaemia**[Q]: No effect.
- Motion artefacts (shivering), underperfusion (shock), electrical interference (diathermy), and nail polish can also lead to unreliable results[Q].

✓ **Venturi Mask**[Q]: Fixed performance device that works on Bernoulli effect. Fixed FiO_2 is delivered.

- Oxygen passes through a constricted nozzle and creates a subatmospheric environment which entrains air but in a fixed manner independent of the minute ventilation.
- If oxygen flow rate is increased beyond the recommended value of a venturi mask, $FiO2$[Q] will not increase.

✓ **Hudson Mask**[Q]: Variable performance device. Variable FiO_2 is delivered. FiO_2 dependent upon mask fit, oxygen flow rate, minute ventilation, and peak inspiratory flow rate.

NON-INVASIVE VENTILATION

✓ **Non-Invasive Ventilation:** Provision of mechanical ventilation without the need for an invasive artificial airway.
- **CPAP:** Continuous application of same positive pressure to the upper airway throughout the respiratory cycle.
- **BiPAP:** Provides ventilatory support by difference between inspiratory positive airway pressure (IPAP) and expiratory positive airway pressure (EPAP).
  - ❖ Hence, application of positive pressure to the upper airway, but different values during inspiration and expiration, respectively.

Indications

✓ **Recommended**
- **Exacerbation of COPD:** Reduced diaphragmatic work of breathing. Extrinsic PEEP counteracts intrinsic PEEP and pressure support assists the inspiratory muscle.
  - ❖ Reduces respiratory rate; improves dyspnoea and gas exchange.
  - ❖ Reduces intubation rates from 50 to 20%.
  - ❖ *Halves mortality* with NNT 10.
  - ❖ European Respiratory Society (ERS)/ American Thoracic Society (ATS) gives strong recommendation for the use of NIV as the first choice for ventilatory support in patients with hypercapnic respiratory failure (pH <7.35, $PaCO_2$ >6 kPa after 1 h of medical treatment[Q]).
- **Weaning for COPD patients:** NIV permits **earlier extubation** of COPD patients on invasive mechanical ventilation who have failed weaning.

- ❖ *Post-extubation NIV reduces mortality*, weaning failures, reintubation, and tracheostomy in COPD patients.
- **Cardiogenic pulmonary oedema:** *Helps reduce mortality.* CPAP (10–12.5 cm H_2O) reduces preload and afterload.
  - ❖ Increased FRC opens collapsed alveoli and improves compliance and oxygenation.
  - ❖ ERS/ATS strongly suggests NIV in patients with cardiogenic pulmonary oedema.
- **Acute hypoxaemic respiratory failure in immunosuppressed patients:** Initial enthusiasm about use of NIV in these patients has cooled down now due to newer studies suggesting that HFNO may be more efficacious in this population group.
  - ❖ ERS/ATS suggests early use of NIV in these patients.
- ✓ **Optional Use**
  - **Asthma exacerbations:** NIV use as early treatment allows more effective β-agonist bronchodilation.
  - **Cystic fibrosis:** Used when they develop chronic respiratory failure before an acute crisis starts.
    - ❖ During acute crisis, used to avoid intubation as a bridge to lung transplant.
  - **Acute hypoxaemic respiratory failure:** Not recommended in severe acute respiratory failure secondary to pneumonia/ARDS.
    - ❖ If it should be used, in mild cases at an early stage with prompt intubation for those that show lack of improvement.
  - **Flail chest:** ERS/ATS suggests the use of NIV in patients with chest trauma, especially those with flail chest.
  - **Extubation failure[Q]:** In patients with COPD and congestive heart failure intubated for acute respiratory failure, NIV has been shown to *decrease reintubation rates.*
    - ❖ However, HFNO is non-inferior to NIV and may be more beneficial as adverse effects are less.
  - **Post-operative respiratory failure:** When used prophylactically after major abdominal surgery or thoracoabdominal aneurysm repair, CPAP reduced the incidence of hypoxaemia, pneumonia, atelectasis, and intubations.

- **Neuromuscular problems as long as bulbar function is normal.**
- **Obesity hypoventilation syndrome.**
- ✓ **Predictors of NIV Failure**
  - GCS <12
  - RR >30/min, paradoxical breathing, excessive accessory muscle
  - PaO_2/FiO_2 <100
  - Hypercapnic respiratory failure with acidaemia, pH <7.10
  - Multiorgan failure
  - Lack of improvement in respiratory rate within 1–2 h
- ✓ **Absolute Contraindication of NIV[Q]**
  - Patient refusal
  - Undrained pneumothorax
  - Facial burns/trauma
  - Fixed upper airway obstruction
  - Up to 2 wk post-oesophagectomy
  - Active vomiting
- ✓ **Relative Contraindications of NIV**
  - pH <7.15
  - GCS <8
  - Confusion and agitation
  - Bowel obstruction
  - Poor compliance: Most common cause for failure of NIV
- ✓ **Complications**
  - Facial skin necrosis
  - Large mask leaks
  - Conjunctivitis
  - Gastric insufflation
  - Patient–ventilator asynchrony
  - Agitation, anxiety
- ✓ **Initiation of NIV[Q]:** Start with pressure support (PS) mode with IPAP as 8–10 cm H_2O and 4–5 cm H_2O for EPAP. Increase pressure gradually to get tidal volumes of 6–8 mL/kg.

INVASIVE MECHANICAL VENTILATION

- ✓ **Indications of Mechanical Ventilation:** Manage respiratory failure due to
  - Failure to maintain a patent airway (e.g. facial trauma, airway oedema, deep coma)
  - Failure to maintain adequate ventilation (e.g. respiratory muscle failure)
  - Failure to maintain adequate oxygenation (e.g. shunt, dead space ventilation)

✓ **Types of Ventilatory Modes**
- **Control modes:** Efforts of the patient are not considered. Triggering and cycling is by ventilator.
- **Assisted modes:** Sense patient's breathing efforts (e.g. pressure support mode).
- **Assist-control:** All modern ventilators with **control modes** are actually **assist-control**, in which if the patient triggers the ventilator, the breath will be assisted in the same way the control breath is delivered.

✓ **Mechanical Ventilation Breath**
- **Trigger^Q:** Signal initiating the breath.
  - ❖ **Time:** Trigger for controlled breaths.
  - ❖ **Pressure or flow:** Trigger for assisted breaths. Breath is triggered by drop in pressure or flow in the ventilator.
  - ❖ **Other triggers:** Neural sensing (diaphragmatic EMG signal) is used as neurally adjusted ventilator assistance (NAVA) in patients with severe airway obstruction and in children.
- **Target/Control:** Which factor is targeted and kept constant.
  - ❖ **Pressure:** Pressure controlled, pressure assisted, or pressure support.
  - ❖ **Volume:** Volume controlled and volume assisted.
- **Cycle:** How the inspiratory breath is terminated.
  - ❖ **Time:** In pressure-controlled and volume-controlled breaths.
  - ❖ **Flow:** In pressure support when flow falls below a specified fraction of the initial inspiratory flow.

✓ **Pressure-Controlled Ventilation^Q:** Time-triggered and time-cycled, pressure-targeted, variable flow.
- Flow decelerates throughout the cycle, and pressure is constant.
- Airway pressure trace doesn't allow assessment of airway resistance or plateau pressure.
- *Allows time for gas to equilibrate between fast- and slow-recruiting alveolar units.*
- No better than volume-controlled ventilation in ARDS.

✓ **Volume-Controlled Ventilation^Q:** Time-triggered and time-cycled, flow-targeted, variable pressure.
- *Pressure increases during inspiratory period, and flow is constant.*

- *Produces a square inspiratory flow pattern on ventilator^Q.*
- Constant flow allows measurement of mechanical properties of the respiratory system, like resistance, peak, and plateau pressure.

✓ **Synchronized Intermittent Mandatory Ventilation (SIMV):** A form of volume-assist controlled ventilation where the patient-triggered breath can be supported by parameters set by user.
- It will deliver a set tidal volume and respiratory rate to the patient, although if the patient takes a spontaneous breath within a set time window, the ventilator will synchronize the mandatory breath to the patient's.
- *Outside of this time window, any spontaneous patient breath can be either pressure-supported or unsupported, depending upon the parameters set by the user. It differs here as the patient's breath support in the other assist-control ventilator modes is the same as the controlled breaths.*
- Inspiratory flow is constant, and pressure decreases exponentially like a VCV.
- It doesn't consider volume of air in lungs at the start of the inspiration and, hence, can cause gas trapping in asthma.

✓ **Pressure-Support Mode:** Patient-triggered, pressure-targeted, flow-cycled mode with ventilator switching to expiration whenever it senses a reduction in the peak inspiratory flow.
- Constant pressure is provided during inspiration and is independent of patient's effort.
- Flow triggering (2–3 L/min) is more sensitive than pressure triggering (1–1.5 cm H_2O).
- Expiratory flow trigger: Flow % of inspiratory flow at which expiration starts.

✓ **Pressure-Regulated Volume Control (PRVC):** Lowest possible pressure to deliver preset tidal volume. Pressure-limited, time-cycled mode.
- Avoids high airway pressure.
- **Decelerating inspiratory flow pattern,** hence more oxygenation.
- It doesn't allow spontaneous breaths. *Pressure changes according to compliance and resistance of the patient.*

✓ **Airway Pressure Release Ventilation (APRV)^Q:** Time/effort-triggered, pressure-targeted, and time-cycled mode.

- In the absence of patient effort, it behaves like a pressure control ventilation with inverse ratio ventilation (high inspiratory time and low expiratory time).
- However, objective of APRV is to allow spontaneous ventilation. Patient is able to breathe spontaneously both on high and low pressure, thereby decreasing sedation use and neuromuscular blockers.
- Lowers **PEAK** airway pressures but increases **MEAN** airway pressure.
- This mode operates between higher and lower inflection points in PV loop.
- T-low (expiration) 0.5–1 s; T-high (inspiration) 6–8 s.
- **P-high** <20 cm H_2O; **P-low** (PEEP): 0–5 cm H_2O.
- Not ideal for asthma.
- **Ventilatory graphic:** Pressure time scalar shows a moderately high level of CPAP with spontaneous respiration. Pressure is released for short period of the time.

✓ **High-Frequency Oscillatory Ventilation (HFOV)**[Q]
- Tidal volumes of 1–3 mL/kg, smaller than dead space.
  - ❖ Produced by oscillations of pressure around the mean airway pressure[Q].
- Low peak pressure, higher mean airway pressure
- ↑ CO_2 clearance by decreasing frequency.
- Principles:
  - ❖ **Bulk convection:** Gas entrained when vacuum left in alveoli as oxygen absorbed into capillaries.
  - ❖ **Pendelluft:** Gas exchanged between lung units with different time constants.
  - ❖ **Taylor dispersion:** Gas exchanged between central gas column and peripheral airway.
  - ❖ **Coaxial flow:** Central rapid inspiratory column and outer slow expiratory column.
  - ❖ **Augmented molecular diffusion:** Oscillation moves molecules to enhance Brownian motion.
- **OSCAR (2014)** and **OSCILLATE (2013)** trials showed no mortality benefit in ARDS.
- Can be used in bronchopleural fistula and paediatric age group.

✓ **Proportional-Assist Ventilation (PAV): Closed-loop system**; it is a type of pressure support mode which adjusts inspiratory pressure according to the flow and volume generated by the patient.
- Assist provided by the ventilator is driven and terminated by the patient's effort.
- Ventilator stops pressure delivery when inspiratory flow decreases to zero.
- The ventilator automatically calculates the respiratory system resistance and elastance every 8 to 15 breaths by doing *short end-inspiratory occlusions*.
- PAV measures expiratory resistance assuming that both inspiratory and expiratory resistance are the same. In patients with obstructive disease, this can cause error.
- Reduces the work of breathing and improves synchrony. Outcomes have been shown to be better than PSV. *Patient should have some respiratory drive.*
- Setting up the ventilator: Ideal body weight, ETT size, maximum airway pressure, triggering, PEEP, and FiO_2 are set.

✓ **Neurally Adjusted Ventilator Assistance (NAVA): Closed-loop system**; electrically triggered, pressure-targeted, and electrically cycled.
- Utilizes electronic activity from the diaphragm using a specialized NG tube with built-in microelectrodes.
- Pressure delivery stops when diaphragmatic activity drops to a preset level which is normally a 70% decrease from the maximum value of electrical activity.
- If there is no electrical activity detected, ventilator switches to pressure support mode and breaths can either be pressure- or flow-generated.
- Setting up the ventilator: Electrical trigger is set at 0.5 μV.

✓ **Adaptive Support Ventilation (ASV): Closed-loop system**; uses artificial intelligence to select the appropriate tidal volume and frequency for mandatory breaths and appropriate tidal volume for spontaneous breaths.
- Calculates expiratory time constant to get an idea of TV for any patient. We put height, gender, percentage of mechanical ventilation, trigger, cycling, tube resistance compensation, PEEP, and FiO_2. No mortality benefits.

- **Ventilatory graphic** is seen with TV in Y-axis and respiratory rate in X-axis.

✓ **Respiratory System Mechanics**
  - **Peak inspiratory pressure (*Ppeak*):** Represents the sum of flow-related resistive pressure of airways (*Presist*) and elastic recoil pressure related to distension of alveoli, including PEEP. Presist normally = 4–10 $H_2O/L/s$.
    - ❖ Increased peak pressures: Treatment is bronchodilators, reduce secretion, change ETT to bigger tube depending upon the cause. Decelerating flows will also lower Presist.
    - ❖ Normally, peak pressures are 15 cm H_2O, with Pplat of 10 cm H_2O and Presist of 5 cm H_2O.
    - ❖ **Asthma[Q]:** High Ppeak, normal Pplat, with high Presist.
    - ❖ **Restrictive lung disease:** High Ppeak and high Pplat with low Presist.
  - **Plateau pressure (Pplat):** Pressure within the breathing circuit after an end-inspiratory pause gives plateau pressure by allowing equalization of pressure between alveoli and circuit. Pplat = Ppeak – Presist.
    - ❖ Pplat includes total PEEP, and auto-PEEP in this total PEEP can be determined by an end-expiratory occlusion manoeuvre.
    - ❖ Increase plateau pressures can be due to increased auto-PEEP, abdominal compartment syndrome, and aggressive volume resuscitation.
    - ❖ **Auto-PEEP[Q]:** Treatment is to reduce tidal volume, then add 80% of PEEPi (intrinsic PEEP) in patients.
  - **Driving pressure:** Pressure required to expand the alveoli against the elastic recoil forces of the lung and chest wall.
    - ❖ It is calculated as Pplat – PEEP.
    - ❖ Predictive of mortality in patients with ARDS, not so in other patients.
    - ❖ Driving pressure[Q] <15 cm H_2O is generally recommended to minimize ventilator-induced lung injury.
  - **Static compliance[Q]:** Change in volume of lung by the driving pressure.
    - ❖ **Static compliance** = TV/Pplat – PEEP. Normal value is 50–100 mL/cm H_2O.
    - ❖ Decreased lung compliance causes increase in the plateau pressure and decreases static compliance.

- ❖ **Bronchospasm affects dynamic compliance[Q]** more than static compliance as static compliance is pulmonary compliance during periods without gas flow, whereas dynamic compliance is measurement of lung compliance during gas flow.
- **Expiratory flows:** Expiration is ventilator mode independent, and same expiratory flows will be seen in both pressure- and flow-targeted modes.
  - ❖ Expiratory flows normally peak at 60% of the inspiratory flows and decline exponentially to zero before the next breath.
  - ❖ **Asthma:** Low peak expiratory rates, expiratory rates persisting until end-expiration. Square root–like shape in expiratory flow.
  - ❖ **Restrictive pulmonary process:** Expiratory flow is normal to be raised and often ends before the next breath begins.
- **Transpulmonary pressure:** Intra alveolar pressure – pleural pressure (oesophageal balloon pressure).
  - ❖ TPP is the principal force maintaining inflation.
  - ❖ When pleural pressure is non-significant, as in a patient who is being passingly ventilated and has a normal chest elastance, transpulmonary pressure is equal to alveolar pressure.
  - ❖ If we use oesophageal TPP to set PEEP, improvement in ventilation occurs.
- **Alveolar ventilation:** Minute ventilation – dead space ventilation.
  - ❖ Increasing tidal volume will increase CO_2 clearance more than increasing respiratory rate[Q].
  - ❖ Replacing HME filters which add 30–50 mL of dead space with humidifiers can increase alveolar ventilation.
- **Stress index:** Slope of the pressure time curve during volume control ventilation with constant flow.
  - ❖ Stress index = 1 means normal lungs.
  - ❖ Stress index >1 means overdistension with upward concavity of the curve towards the pressure axis.

❖ Stress index <1 means tidal recruitment with concavity away from the pressure axis.

✓ **Patient Ventilator Desynchrony**
  • **Triggering phase**
    ❖ **Ineffective trigger:** Patient's efforts can't trigger a breath. Auto-PEEP can cause ineffective trigger. Best detected by oesophageal pressure. Measures to correct it are eliminating auto-PEEP and decreasing sedation to increase effort by the patient. Flow triggering can also help.
    ❖ **Auto-triggering:** Ventilator delivers a breath without any patient effort. Hiccups, presence of water in circuit[Q], cardiac oscillations or circuit leaks like through the bronchopleural fistula can cause it. Characterized by absence of initial pressure drop below PEEP.
    ❖ **Double triggering:** Both breaths are by the patient. Two consecutive inspirations with an expiratory time interval of less than half of the mean inspiratory time. Seen in patients with short inspiratory timings, high respiratory drive, low tidal volume settings, and increased work of breathing. Can be seen in patients with coughing as well. Lowering PEEP, increasing inspiratory time, or changing patient to pressure support helps.
  • **Flow delivery phase**
    ❖ **Flow dyssynchrony:** Patient's inspiratory flow is insufficient to meet the patient's ventilatory demand. It is seen as a concave appearance on the pressure–time waveform in volume-controlled ventilation. Changing the mode to pressure targeting can help.
    ❖ **Excessive flow asynchrony:** Excessive flow in patients with low inspiratory efforts. Resolved by decreasing the tidal volume or pressure.
  • **Cycling phase**
    ❖ **Premature cycling:** Machine inspiratory time is less than neural (patient's) inspiratory time. This is often followed by double triggering. This represents that the patient's respiratory drive is high and the ventilatory demands

are not being met. Seen in ARDS and patients with restrictive lung disease.
    ❖ **Delayed cycling:** Machine inspiratory time is greater than neural inspiratory time. Seen in obstructed patients on pressure support mode and *is seen as sudden increase at the end of inspiration due to expiratory effort of the patient.*

✓ **Disease-Specific Ventilation**
  • **Normal gas exchange and mechanics:** Any mode, TV 6–8 mL/kg, PEEP 5 cm H_2O, inspiratory flow rate 50–60 L/min. Patient initiation of the breath is encouraged.
  • **ARDS:** PRVC mode, TV 6 mL/kg PBW, rate 26–35/min, inspiratory flow rate 50–60 L/min, high PEEP. Driving pressure <14 cm H_2O is recommended.
  • **Obstructive:** Controlled hypoventilation with permissive hypercapnia: TV 5–7 mL/kg, RR 10–14/min, I:E:1:4.
  • **Restrictive pattern:** Higher FiO_2 compared to high PEEP, and TV is preferred as high plateau pressure can cause haemodynamic instability.

✓ **Complications of IPPV**
  • Ventilator-induced lung injury: Acute lung injury due to mechanical ventilation.
    ❖ Barotrauma, volutrauma, atelectrauma, and biotrauma.
  • **Ventilator-induced diaphragmatic dysfunction:** Changes in diaphragm due to over- or under-assistance by the ventilator.
  • Hypotension, liver dysfunction (because of hypoperfusion), bronchopleural fistula, tracheal stenosis, dysphonia, dysphagia.

✓ **Spontaneous Respiration and Heart Mechanics**
  • During inspiration, intrathoracic pressure decreases and venous return to right ventricle increases.
  • This causes increased right ventricle output, which shifts septum to the left, decreasing left ventricle output during inspiration.
  • The reverse is seen with expiration.
  • These normal changes are exaggerated during cardiac tamponade, and a greater fall in BP during inspiration is known as pulsus paradoxus.

✓ **Invasive Ventilation and Heart Mechanics**
  • Increased intrathoracic pressure during inspiration.

- Decreased venous return.
- Decreased right ventricular output.
- Decreased left ventricular afterload.
- Decreased transmural pressure across the left ventricle.
- Increased LV output during inspiration.

✓ **Positive End-Expiratory Pressure**
- Improves oxygenation by increasing FRC, improving V/Q match, and decreasing shunt.
- Reduced work of breathing by shifting tidal volume towards the more compliant part of the pressure–volume curve.
- In preload-dependent patients, cardiac output decreases.
- In heart failure and fluid overloaded patients, left ventricular function improves.

Additional Questions

✓ **Requirements of a Portable Ventilator[Q] According to FICM Guidelines**
- Ability to vary FiO_2, PEEP, respiratory rate, tidal volume, and I:E ratio.
- Disconnection and high-pressure alarms.
- Ability to provide PCV, PS, and CPAP is desirable.

✓ **Functional Residual Capacity (FRC)[Q]:** It can be described as volume of air in lungs when the inward elastic recoil of the lungs is exactly the same as outward force of chest wall.
- **Factors causing increase in FRC**
  ❖ Males
  ❖ Height
  ❖ PEEP
  ❖ Asthma
  ❖ Emphysema
  ❖ *Standing*
- **Factors causing decrease in FRC**
  ❖ Age
  ❖ Supine position (20–25%) (**Most important respiratory change on lying down**)
  ❖ Pregnancy (20–30% at term)
  ❖ Obesity
  ❖ Anaesthesia

✓ **Closing Capacity[Q]:** Volume of lungs at which **smaller airway collapses** during expiration. In a **supine person aged 44 yr and a standing person aged 66 yr, closing capacity is equal to FRC.** Once the closing capacity is more than FRC, gas trapping happens.

- **Closing capacity = residual volume + closing volume**

✓ **Flow–Volume Loops[Q]**
- **Obstructive disease** (e.g. *COPD/asthma*). Peak expiratory flow rate (PEFR) is decreased, and residual volume is increased by gas trapping.
- **Restrictive disease** (e.g. *interstitial lung disease*). TLC is decreased. PEFR is reduced, but shape of expiratory curve is the same as normal curve.
- **Variable intrathoracic obstruction** (e.g. *bronchogenic cysts, intrathoracic tracheomalacia*). Inspiratory gas flow is normal as negative intrathoracic pressure helps keep airways open. Positive pressure produced during expiration closes airways and produces expiratory curve like obstructive disease. TLC and RV unaffected.
- **Variable extrathoracic obstruction** (e.g. *vocal cord paralysis, extrathoracic tracheomalacia*). Expiratory limb looks normal. Inspiratory limb shows marked reduced flow rates. TLC and RV unaffected.
- **Fixed large airway obstruction[Q]** (e.g. *tracheal stenosis, goitre*). Both limbs have reduced flow. TLC and RV unaffected.

✓ **Alveolar Gas Equation:** It tells the partial pressure gradient driving oxygen across the alveolar–capillary membrane.

- $P_AO_2 = FiO_2 (P_{ATM} - SVP) - P_ACO_2/RQ$
where:
P_AO_2 = alveolar partial pressure of oxygen.
FiO_2 = fraction of inspired oxygen.
P_{ATM} = atmospheric pressure.
SVP = saturated vapour pressure.
P_ACO_2 = alveolar partial pressure of carbon dioxide.
RQ = respiratory quotient.

WEANING

✓ **Weaning:** Process of liberating the patient from mechanical support and the endotracheal tube.
- Around 20–30% of patients are difficult to wean from mechanical ventilation.
- Patients who need reintubation have higher mortality rates of 30–50% compared to 5–10% for successful extubation[Q].
  ❖ Critical care units normally[Q] have reintubation rates of 10–15%.

- COPD patients, even if they fail weaning marginally, optimize them for few hours and extubate.
✓ **Weaning Failure:** Failure to pass spontaneous breathing trial or the need for reintubation and NIV support within 48 h following extubation.
  - **Simple weaning:** Extubating after one spontaneous breathing trial.
  - **Difficult weaning:** Extubating after 2 or 3 spontaneous breathing trial within 7 d from the first attempt.
  - **Prolonged weaning:** >3 attempts or >7 d from the first attempt.
✓ **Major Causes of Weaning Failure**
  - **Cardiac disease:** Coronary ischaemia, left ventricular diastolic dysfunction, anaemia, high-dose vasopressors.
  - **Respiratory problem:** Volume overload, inappropriate mechanical ventilation mode, residual infection, excessive secretions, diaphragmatic splinting[Q].
  - **Neurological dysfunction:** Critical illness neuromyopathy, altered mental status.
  - **Metabolic or endocrine diseases:** Acidaemia.
  - **Psychological factors:** Delirium, pain.
✓ **Predictors of Successful Weaning[Q]:** Identify patients likely to tolerate a spontaneous breathing trial.
  - Maximum inspiratory pressure of <-30 cm H_2O.
  - **Tidal volume** > 5 mL/kg.
  - **Forced vital capacity (FVC)** > 15 mL/kg.
  - Minute ventilation < 15 L/min.
  - **Rapid shallow breathing index (RSBI):** Respiratory rate/tidal volume < 105 (80% chances of successful extubation).
  - Spontaneous respiratory rate < 35/min.
  - PaO_2/FiO_2 >26.3 kPa.
✓ **Criteria for Successful SBT[Q]**
  - Respiratory rate < 35 breaths/minute
  - SBP > 80 and <180 or < 20% changes from the baseline
  - HR < 140/min or heart rate variability >20%
  - Sat > 90% or PaO_2 > 8 kPa on FiO_2 < 0.4
  - No signs of increased work of breathing
  - Good tolerance to spontaneous breathing trials
✓ **Spontaneous Breathing Trial Failure:** Failure if (reverse the criteria of successful SBT)
  - **Clinical criteria**
    - ❖ Diaphoresis

- ❖ Nasal flaring
- ❖ Cardiac arrhythmias
- ❖ RR > 35/min or apnoea
- ❖ Hypotension
- ❖ HR > 140/min
- **Gas exchange criteria**
  - ❖ ↑ $PaCo_2$ > 10 mmHg
  - ❖ Arterial pH < 7.32
  - ❖ Fall in SpO_2 > 5%
  - ❖ PaO_2 < 60 mmHg on FiO_2 > 0.4, PaO_2/FiO_2 < 20 kPa
✓ **Weaning Strategy**
  - Start weaning when FiO_2 40% and pulmonary compliance $\geq$ 50 mL/cm H_2O.
  - Tracheostomies often aid weaning, and ideal diameter is 8 mm.
  - Hypercapnia is not a very specific sign of weaning failure.
  - Weaning failure can occur because of respiratory drive, pain, weakness, and fatigue.
  - Handgrip strength testing can predict weaning failure.
  - Automated weaning strategies decrease extubating time compared to non-automated weaning, but no mortality benefit.
  - Tight glycaemic control helps weaning, but no mortality benefit.
  - Weak cough can also cause weaning failure.
✓ **Spontaneous Breathing Trial[Q]**
  - T-piece (physiological simulation), PSV mode, CPAP mode.
    - ❖ SIMV is not a suitable weaning mode as compared to others.
  - A 30 min duration normally.
    - ❖ Approximately 120 min for those that are high risk for reintubation, like elderly patients or those with heart failure or COPD.
✓ **Managing Weaning Failure**
  - **Protocol-based weaning:** Decreased duration of minute ventilation, reintubation rates, and ICU and hospital length of stroke.
  - Once-daily attempts at liberation from mechanical ventilation.
  - Increase muscle strength of respiratory muscles and early mobilization.
  - Optimize airway function, and use bronchodilation if needed.
  - **Cuff leak test** to check patients at high risk for post-extubation stridor. (Leak > 110 mL should be there after cuff deflation.)

- **Tracheostomy**
  - ❖ Studies have shown that tracheostomy can lower ICU and in-hospital mortality rates in carefully selected patients.
  - ❖ Reduces airway resistance and dead space in COPD patients.
- Optimize fluid balance by use of diuretics^Q in patients overloaded with fluid.
- Reduce afterload to heart by vasodilators and inotropes.
- Treat delirium, anxiety, and depression.
- Glucose control.
- HFNO is equivalent to NIV in rates of post-extubation respiratory failure.

✓ **Weaning from Tracheostomy:** Tracheostomy tubes should be changed every month.
  - Swedish nose
  - Cuff deflation time increased over days
  - Reducing the tracheostomy tube size
  - Fenestrated tube and speaking valve

✓ **Role of BNP and NT Pro:** NT Pro BNP stays longer in the blood and, hence, is easier to test and has better utility.
  - 14% change in BNP 2 h after SBT reflects cardiac cause of weaning failure.

✓ **Role of Diaphragm:** Critical care polyneuropathy of phrenic nerve is a frequent cause involving the phrenic nerve.

✓ **Maximal Inspiratory Pressure (MIP):** Maximum inspiratory pressure a person can generate during a forced inspiration, showing the strength of the inspiratory muscles.
  - **Normal:** Men, −75 cm H_2O; Women, −50 cm H_2O.
  - More negative values and absence of hypercapnia almost always exclude inspiratory muscle weakness, and values that are less negative do not prove muscle weakness, as this method depends upon cooperation and lung volume.
  - It has better negative predictive value.

Additional Questions

✓ **Absolute Humidity^Q:** Mass of water vapour per unit volume of gas. Measured in grams/cubic metre. Remains constant with increasing temperature.
  - **Relative humidity^Q:** Ratio of actual mass of water vapour in a volume of gas to the mass of water vapour required to saturate that

volume of gas. Decreases with increasing temperature.
- Fully saturated air at room temperature of 20°C contains 17 g/m^3.
- Fully saturated air at room temperature of 37°C contains 44 g/m^3.

✓ **Nebulizers^Q:** Heat and moisture exchanger (HME) (70%)^Q, cold water bath (30%), hot water bath (90%), cascade water bath (90%), ultrasonic nebulizer (>100%)^Q.
- Nebulizers produce very small droplet sizes and can lead to fluid overload by depositing water vapours in alveoli. They are thus used mostly for medication delivery.
- Active humidification^Q can cause water in circuit causing auto-triggering, obstruction, and infection, which can be prevented by using water traps, heated expiratory flow, and heating the downstream from the humidifier.
- HME^Q collects moisture from exhaled gases by condensation and returns it to dry inhaled gases for humidification. Typical pore size 0.2 μm.
  - ❖ ↑ Dead space and expiratory resistance^Q.

ACUTE RESPIRATORY DISTRESS SYNDROME

Epidemiology and Aetiology

✓ **Incidence:** 10% of patients admitted to ICU and 23% of intubated patients.

✓ **American European Consensus Conference (AECC) Criteria 1994:** They proposed the first definition of *acute respiratory distress syndrome* (ARDS).
- The four criteria for diagnosis were
  - ❖ Acute onset of hypoxaemia
  - ❖ PaO_2 to FiO_2 ratio ≤ 200 mmHg *irrespective of PEEP level*
  - ❖ Presence of bilateral infiltrates on chest radiograph
  - ❖ *Pulmonary artery wedge pressure ≤ 18 mmHg or no clinical signs of cardiogenic pulmonary oedema.*
- **Drawbacks of this definition:** Low specificity (51%) when compared to autopsy, PEEP not included in hypoxaemia criteria, no clear definition of the term *acute*, no clear definition for separating pulmonary oedema from consolidation in chest X-ray.

- AECC criteria has area under the curve (AUC) of 0.536 for prediction of mortality. Berlin criteria has AUC of 0.577.

✓ **Berlin Definition in 2012[Q]**
  - The four criteria for this diagnosis were:
    - ❖ **Timing:** Within 1 wk of a known clinical insult.
    - ❖ **Chest imaging (CXR/CT):** Bilateral opacities involving more than two quadrants – not fully explained by effusion/lobar/lung collapse/nodule.
    - ❖ **Origin of oedema:** Respiratory failure not fully explained by cardiac failure.
    - ❖ **Oxygenation:** $PaO_2/FiO_2 < 40$ kPa with PEEP/CPAP > 5 cm H_2O, corrected for altitude if > 1,000 m.
  - **Drawbacks of this definition:** ARDS severity assessed by a single blood gas measurement without prior standardization of ventilator settings.
    - ❖ Level of PEEP may have a major influence on oxygenation.

✓ **New Global Definition 2024:** Included non-intubated patients on HFNO, ultrasound lung as a modality, and pulse oximetry as a mode of measuring saturation as well.
  - Acute onset within 1 wk.
  - Bilateral opacities on Chest X-ray or CT scan or **B-lines/consolidations on USG[Q]**.
  - Respiratory failure not fully explained by cardiac failure.
  - PaO_2/FiO_2 ratio ≤ 300 or SpO_2/FiO_2 ≤ 315 (if SpO_2 ≤ 97%) with PEEP/CPAP > 5 cm H_2O in intubated patients or SpO_2/FiO_2[Q] ≤ 315 (if SPO_2 ≤ 97%) by HFNO on O_2 flow of 30 L/min in non-intubated patients[Q].

✓ **Causes of ARDS**
  - **Direct (pulmonary ARDS):** Pneumonia (most common cause), pulmonary contusion, fat embolism, smoke inhalation.
  - **Indirect (extra-pulmonary ARDS):** Sepsis, major trauma, pancreatitis, blood transfusion, bypass surgery. *Pulmonary ARDS is more common than extra-pulmonary ARDS.*

✓ **Pathophysiology of ARDS**
  - *Injury to the alveolar epithelium (direct injury) and endothelial capillaries (indirect injury), along with **neutrophil activation**, plays a critical role in the start of ARDS.*
  - **Ventilator-induced lung injury (VILI):** Use of mechanical ventilation itself can cause lung injury. Driving pressure ΔP = plateau pressure – PEEP is the major determinant of VILI.
    - ❖ **Barotrauma:** High pressures.
    - ❖ **Volutrauma:** High end-inspiratory volumes.
    - ❖ **Atelectrauma[Q]:** Repetitive opening and closing of alveoli. Prevented by PEEP.
    - ❖ **Biotrauma:** Biological response to mechanical stress. It increases *leucocytes, TNF, IL-6, and IL-8.*

Clinical Features and Diagnosis

✓ **Classification of ARDS**
  - **Mild ARDS:** PaO_2/FiO_2 26.7–40 kPa with PEEP ≤ 5 cm H_2O.
  - **Moderate ARDS:** PaO_2/FiO_2 13.4–26.6 kPa with PEEP ≤ 5 cm H_2O.
  - **Severe ARDS:** PaO_2/FiO_2 ≤ 13.3 kPa with PEEP ≤ 5 cm H_2O.

✓ **Histopathology:** *Diffuse alveolar damage is the hallmark feature and is defined by presence of hyaline membranes along with interstitial oedema, cell necrosis, and proliferation and fibrosis. Disease might resolve after proliferative stage or enter fibrotic stage. If present, all stages can be overlapping. Fibrotic stage can start as early as 24 h.*
  - **Exudative** (0–7 d): **Neutrophil sequestration, interstitial oedema**, exudates filled with fluid, protein, and cellular debris.
  - **Proliferative** (7–14 d): Organization of intra-alveolar exudates and **proliferation of type II alveolar cells,** fibroblasts, and myofibroblasts.
  - **Fibrotic phase** (>14 d): Collagen deposition in alveolar, vascular, and interstitial beds with development of microcysts.

✓ **Symptoms:** Median time of onset is between 1 and 2 d. Escalating oxygen requirements and need for respiratory support for decreased lung compliance.
  - **TRALI ARDS:** Within 6 h of blood transfusion.

✓ **Chest X-Ray:** Chest X-ray at onset may be normal, and it may take 2–3 d for bilateral ground-glass opacifications to appear.

✓ **Lung Ultrasound:** It can help to differentiate ARDS from cardiogenic pulmonary oedema. It is considered diagnostically more reliable than chest X-ray in patients with ARDS.

- Non-homogenous B-lines with interspersed lung regions, pleural line irregularity, and lung consolidation are suggestive of ARDS.
- Cardiogenic pulmonary oedema will have homogenous B-lines, left-sided pleural effusion, reduced left ventricular function, and a dilated IVC.

✓ **CT Scan:** Ground-glass opacities in the middle zone, consolidation in the dependent part of the lung, subpleural thickening. Pleural effusions rare. Small pneumothorax can also be identified.
  - Consolidation in the non-dependent regions may suggest a pre-existing or new ventilator-associated pneumonia.
  - Helps in prognosis as well. Early fibrosis on CT scan is associated with more mortality.
    - ❖ The extent of inhomogeneity is increased with the severity of ARDS and has direct correlation with increased mortality.

✓ **Bronchoalveolar Lavage:** To rule out other treatable causes (acute eosinophilic pneumonia, alveolar proteinosis, diffuse alveolar haemorrhage).

✓ **Covid ARDS:** Showed severe hypoxia despite preserved lung compliance. Vasocentric distribution of COVID-19 lesions with predominance of capillary congestion and microthrombosis.

Prevention and Treatment

✓ **Ventilator care bundles aim to reduce ventilator-associated pneumonia but do not reduce mortality in ARDS.**

✓ **Low tidal volume (ARDSnet Study 2000) has the biggest impact.** Prone ventilation (Proseva Trial) and early use of neuromuscular blockers within 48 h (Acurasys Trial) also showed mortality benefit in ARDS[Q].

✓ **Lung-protective ventilation:** Low tidal volume 6 mL/kg predicted body weight (PBW) with high PEEP. Plateau pressure < 30 cm.
  - **Males:** PBW (kg) = 50 + 0.91 [Height (cm) − 152.4]
  - **Females:** PBW (kg) = 45.5 + 0.91 [Height (cm) − 152.4]
  - In severe ARDS, high PEEP > 15 cm H_2O won't improve mortality. Higher PEEP in mild ARDS can be potentially harmful.
  - A flow rate of 60 L/min should be used on ventilator to meet patient's demand.

However, low tidal volumes and high flow rates (short insufflation time) can lead to ventilator patient asynchrony by causing **double-triggering**, where the patient continues breathing beyond the end of the ventilatory cycle and triggers a second ventilatory insufflation.

- **Permissive hypercapnia** is often needed to prevent VILI. pH >7.2 should be maintained. High respiratory rates up to 25 breaths per minute are used to avoid respiratory acidosis, but the effect of respiratory rate on mortality is unclear.
- **Evidence suggests that low tidal volumes can even help prevent progression to ARDS.**
- **Driving pressure ΔP** = plateau pressure − PEEP. Mounting evidence that ΔP <15 cm H_2O has mortality benefit.
- **High-flow nasal oxygenation (HFNO)**
  - ❖ **FLORALI Trial (2015)** showed that HFNO has mortality benefit in patient with acute lung injury and **may be safer than NIV with respect to long-term outcomes**.
- **Non-invasive ventilation**
  - ❖ **RECOVERY-RS Trial (2021)** showed that CPAP is better than conventional oxygen therapy in reducing the risk for intubation and had mortality benefit. They didn't find any difference between CPAP and HFNO.
  - ❖ The **LUNG-SAFE Study (2016)** showed that patients with PaO_2/FiO_2 < 150 mmHg treated with NIV had higher mortality than those treated with invasive ventilation.

✓ **Recruitment Manoeuvre:** No mortality benefit seen in Lung Open Ventilation Study (**LOVS Study 2008**). Causes barotrauma, hypotension.

✓ **Airway Pressure Release Ventilation (APRV):** Uses inverse ratio ventilation with spontaneous breathing.
  - Sustained high airway pressures and spontaneous breathing to increase recruitment with brief periods of pressure release to facilitate ventilation.
  - Spontaneous ventilation generates regionally variable transpulmonary pressures that favour recruitment.
  - Its role is still under investigation in management of patients with ARDS.

✓ **Neuromuscular Blockade**
- **ACURASYS Trial (2010):** Reduction in mortality benefit when NMBAs (cis-atracurium) used in moderate to severe ARDS.
- **ROSE Trial (2019):** No mortality benefit when cis-atracurium plus heavy sedation used in comparison to light sedation.
- NMBAs should be used early in the course of severe ARDS.
- A trial of NMBAs should be used before considering proning the patient as they increase chest compliance[Q].

✓ **Prone Position**[Q]**:** Improves ventilation of the previously dependent dorsal lung by reliving compression by heart.
- **PROSEVA Trial showed that early proning** (<48 h), normally for 16 h, which can be extended up to 24 h, helped in both moderate and severe ARDS patient, but not in milder patients. Reduced all cause 28 d and 90 d mortality in ARDS patients.

✓ **Conservative Fluid Management after Fluid Resuscitation:** No mortality benefit but increase in ventilator-free and ICU-free days.
- Diuretics should be considered if the patient has no sign of intravascular depletion.

✓ **Steroids:** Benefit more with low doses early in the course of disease during active proliferation stage.
- **Dexa-ARDS Trial (2020):** In patients with moderate to severe ARDS, early use of dexamethasone decreased duration of mechanical ventilation and mortality compared to usual care.
- **Meduri Trial (2007):** Low-dose, long-duration methylprednisolone improved lung function, duration of mechanical ventilation, ICU length of stay, and survival if used early in ARDS.
- **LaSRS Trial (2006): Late steroids rescue for ARDS.** Use of methylprednisolone in persistent ARDS (7–28 d after onset) did not improve 60 d mortality but did improve ventilator-free and ICU-free days.
- **Meduri Trial (1998):** Low-dose, long-duration methylprednisolone in unresolving ARDS improved ICU survival and lung function.

✓ **Pulmonary Vasodilators:** Used as rescue therapy in refractory hypoxaemia
- **Nitric oxide (NO)** improves oxygenation, but no survival benefit.
  - ❖ NO has been shown to increase the chances of renal dysfunction and then RRT.
  - ❖ Recommended dose is 20 ppm. Levels above 80 ppm can cause pulmonary oedema and methaemoglobinaemia.
- **Inhaled epoprostenol** also showed no mortality benefit but has fewer side effects as compared to iNO.

✓ **High-Frequency Oscillatory Ventilation (HFOV):** Constant mean airway pressure is increased by oscillating pressure variations at rates up to 900 cycles per minute.
- **OSCAR Trial (2014)** showed no mortality benefit, whereas **OSCILLATE Trial (2013)** showed increased mortality.
- Still used in paediatrics age group.

✓ **Extracorporeal Membrane Oscillation (ECMO):** VV ECMO is used for ARDS. Efficacy shown in neonates, but conflicting results in adults.
- Early initiation of ECMO is not recommended, and consideration can be given to transfer the patient to large centres with ECMO capability.
- Trials on the role of VV-ECMO have been explained in section on extracorporeal life support in Chapter 3.

Complications

✓ **Pneumothorax:** Due to mechanical ventilation is seen in 5–10% of patients. More common when plateau pressures >35 cm H_2O.

✓ **Ventilator-Associated Pneumonia:** Prolonged mechanical ventilation can cause it. Diagnosis can be difficult as patient will already have infiltrates on chest X-ray. Systematic quantitative tracheal cultures sent two to three times a week should be considered.

✓ **Acute Cor Pulmonale:** 20% incidence. Due to increased pulmonary vascular resistance and permissive hypercapnia, causing acidosis.

✓ **Haemodynamic Impairment:** Frequent in ARDS due to mechanical ventilation, causing decreased cardiac output, and mostly seen in patients with severe infections.

✓ **Persistent ARDS:** When ARDS is present after 5–7 d. CMV pneumonitis has been seen in some cases. BAL and CT scan should be done to identify all mimics.

Prognosis

✓ Mortality currently is 30%, with higher incidence amongst older people.

✓ Patients with ARDS due to trauma have better survival rates than other causes of ARDS.

- Mortality is same in ARDS due to pulmonary or extrapulmonary origin otherwise. Covid ARDS has the same mortality as classic ARDS.
✓ Majority of survivors will have a diminished diffusing capacity and exercise tolerance even after 6 months, while lung volumes and spirometry measurements will return to normal.
  - A 6 min walk distance remained markedly altered with persistent limitation even after years.

PRONING

✓ **Proning:** It is medical technique where a patient is placed in a facedown position.
✓ **Indications**
  - Moderate to severe ARDS with $PaO_2{:}FiO_2$ < 26.6 kPa (early < 48 h) and for at least 16 h.
  - High oxygen requirements (FiO_2 > 60–65%).
  - Surgical procedure (spinal and posterior fossa surgery).
✓ **PROSEVA Trial (2014): Early proning** (<48 h), normally for 16 h, can be extended up to 24 h; reduces[Q] all-cause 28 d and 90 d mortality in ARDS patients.
  - Helped in both moderate and severe ARDS patient, but not in milder patients.
✓ **Benefits of Proning**
  - Reduces[Q] plateau pressure and extravascular lung water.
  - Reduces IL-6 and inflammatory cells in bronchial lavage.
  - Prevents[Q] tidal hyperinflation.
  - Not beneficial in patients with fibrotic lung disease.
  - Better results in extrapulmonary ARDS compared to pulmonary ARDS.

Absolute Contraindications[Q]	Relative Contraindications[Q]
Spinal instability	Recent tracheostomy (<24 h)
Open chest post–cardiac surgery	High ICP/IOP
<24 h post–cardiac surgery	Facial fractures or multiple fractures
Central cannulation for VA ECMO and BiVAD	Pregnancy 2nd or 3rd trimester
	Morbid obesity
	Frequent seizures
	CVS instability despite resuscitation

✓ **Salient Features of Proning**
  - NG feed should be stopped and aspirated at least 1 h before proning.
    - ❖ Continuous feeding with low-volume, high-density feed (1.3–1.5 kcal/mL) preferred. Maximum rate of 65–85 mL/h is safe.
    - ❖ NGTs should be aspirated every 4–6 h, and maximum gastric residual volumes (GRVs) should be below 300 mL.
    - ❖ Low threshold for prokinetics, NJ feeding, and parenteral nutrition in the same order.
  - *RASS score of –5. Consider neuromuscular blocking agents.*
  - *Patient should be rolled towards the ventilator and ideally away from any CVC device.*
  - *Ensure chest drain below the patient and clamped for the minimal time.*
  - Minimum of five people, including one at airway and four others.
  - Patient should be nursed at **30° in the reverse Trendelenburg position.**
  - The position of hands and arms should be alternated every 2–4 h. Three people required.
  - While going from supine to prone, move the patient horizontally away from the ventilator.
✓ **Complications of Prone Positioning[Q]**
  - **Instability:** Airway displacement, haemodynamic instability, line/device displacement, and gastro-oesophageal reflux.
  - **Patient injury:** Pressure ulcers, ocular injury, nerve compression, and brachial plexus injury and stroke.
✓ **Conscious Proning in Patients Requiring >28% FiO_2:** Discontinue after 15 min if no improvement in patients.
  - Position changes every 1–2 h. Start with fully prone, then right lateral recumbent, the sitting up, and then left lateral position.
  - **Contraindicated** if respiratory distress, haemodynamic instability, altered mental status, and unstable spinal/thoracic/abdominal injury.
✓ **Prone Patient CPR**
  - Confirm cardiac arrest → shout for help → **start prone CPR (mid-thoracic level between scapulae)** → 100% FiO_2 via waters circuit → defibrillation pads (left midaxillary line + right scapula or biaxillary) →

effective CPR (end tidal CO_2/arterial pressure) → If yes, continue, and if no, turn the patient supine.

✓ **Prone Positioning on ECMO:** Not needed normally as ECMO can fully oxygenate and decarboxylate the patient.

- Indications for proning for patients on ECMO:
  - ❖ **Refractory hypoxia on ECMO** (e.g. patient's cardiac output is more than the ECMO flows, like sepsis or if ECMO pipes have restricted flow and, hence, ECMO flows are low.) These situations lead to some blood flow to lungs which can't be accommodated by ECMO flows.
  - ❖ **Failure to wean VV ECMO:** If the patient doesn't improve after being on ECMO for several days.
  - ❖ **Pulmonary toilet and drainage:** For specific conditions like pulmonary haemorrhage, postural drainage might be facilitated by the prone position.

✓ **Flexible Bronchoscopy in the Prone Position**

- Prone position can increase the mobilization of secretions from the distal to proximal airways. If ventilation is not improved on proning, additional bronchoscopy can help clear secretions.
- The internal diameter of ETT should be >1.5 mm than the bronchoscope.

ASTHMA

Epidemiology

✓ **Asthma:** Chronic inflammation of the airways characterized by *reversible bronchoconstriction and airflow limitation*[Q].

- Exaggerated airway smooth muscle cells contraction (main mechanism and reversible), airway oedema, **mucus hypersecretion**, and **airway remodelling** (seen in chronic patients and partially reversible) are seen.
- **Inefficient gas exchange:** Hypoxaemia initially with hypercapnia also adding up eventually due to muscle fatigue.
- **Dynamic hyperinflation:** Failure of respiratory system to return to functional residual capacity at the end of expiration.

- ❖ Increased airway resistance decreases airflow, and air is left behind in the alveoli.
- ❖ *The inspiratory threshold for breath initiation is increased as the respiratory muscles should first overcome intrinsic PEEP (PEEPi) before air can flow in.*

Clinical Features and Diagnosis

✓ **Two Types of Asthma Exacerbation:** *Up to 80% of asthma exacerbations are caused by viral infections, most commonly rhinovirus.*

- **Slow onset:** Symptoms progress over days and weeks. Airway obstruction with mucus is prominent, and there is eosinophilic predominance of inflammatory cells in the airway submucosa.
- **Rapid onset:** Symptoms progress over 2–6 h. Airway obstruction with mucus is not prominent, and there is neutrophilic predominance of inflammatory cells in the airway submucosa. Seen more commonly in patients with sensitivity to NSAIDs.

✓ **Risk Factors of Mortality:** *Previous history* of near-fatal asthma requiring mechanical ventilation, current user of or recently stopped using oral corticosteroids, *cigarette smoking*, patients with adverse *psychosocial factors*, *such as psychosis*, *depression*, and **food allergy** in a patient with asthma.

✓ **In Pregnancy:** Increases the risk of preeclampsia, gestational diabetes, placental abruption, and placenta previa. FHR should be monitored after 24 wk.

✓ **Dynamic Hyperinflation:** Can be diagnosed by slow filling of manual ventilator bag attached on ETT, capnography trace not reaching baseline, rise in plateau pressure in volume-controlled ventilation, or falling volumes in pressure-controlled ventilation.

- Expiratory flow not reaching zero in flow-time/volume graph[Q] and change of pressure waveform shape from linear to convex at the end of inspiration indicate a decrease in respiratory compliance.

✓ **Flowmeter:** Measures peak expiratory flow rate (PEFR), which is forced expiration from total lung capacity. Used for daily monitoring of asthma[Q].

- A pretreatment PEFR or FEV_1 <50% of baseline predicted value/patient's best-known value indicates a severe exacerbation of asthma.

- For patients with post–intensive treatment PEFR or FEV_1 <40% of predicted value, hospitalization is recommended.
- **Spirometry** can give values of tidal volume (TV) and functional vital capacity (FVC), but not functional residual capacity (FRC). FVC may be increased in asthma[Q]. Not used in acute exacerbation.
  - ❖ Spirometry showing reversible obstruction >12% after inhaled bronchodilators increases the likelihood of diagnosis of asthma.

✓ **Chest X-Ray and ECG:** Should be done to rule out other differential diagnosis and complications.

British Thoracic Society (BTS) Classification[Q] (One of the most important tables for revision in the last few days before exam)

Moderate asthma	• Increasing symptoms • PEFR > 50–75% predicted
Acute severe asthma	• PEFR > 33–50% predicted • Respiratory rates ≥ 25/min • Heart rate ≥ 110/min • Inability to complete sentences
Life-threatening asthma	**Clinical signs** • Altered consciousness • Poor respiratory effort • Cyanosis • Hypotension • Exhaustion • Silent chest • Tachyarrhythmia **Measurements** • PEFR < 33% predicted • SpO_2 < 92% • PaO_2 < 8 kPa • Normal $PaCO_2$ 4.6–6 kPa[Q]
Near-fatal asthma	• Raised $PaCO_2$[Q] • Requiring mechanical ventilation

Prevention and Treatment

✓ **Prevention in Community**
- Short-acting beta-2 agonist (salbutamol)
- Low-dose inhaled corticosteroid
- Long-acting beta-2 agonist (salmeterol)
- High-dose inhaled corticosteroid, or

add leukotriene receptor antagonist (montelukast)
- Oral steroids/monoclonal antibodies (omalizumab)

✓ **Initial Management in ICU**
- **Assessment of severity by clinical features/PEFR measurement.**
- **Oxygen** to maintain an SpO_2 of 94–98% (recommended by BTS), followed by nebulized beta-2 adrenergic agonists like **salbutamol**, oral **prednisolone**/IV hydrocortisone, and nebulized **ipratropium** bromide.

✓ **Inhaled Beta-2 Adrenergic Agonists:** Like salbutamol (2.5–5 mg nebulized or 200–400 mcg by puff).
- They reduce bronchoconstriction, and dose is repeated initially every 20–30 min.
- Nebulizers should be driven with oxygen at a flow rate of 6 L/min. However, their role is not superior to metered drug inhalers (MDIs), which can be used in absence of nebulizers.
- **They can cause type B lactic acidosis,[Q] and systemic beta-2 adrenergic agonists are not routinely recommended (dose is 3–20 µg/min)[Q].**

✓ **Anticholinergic Agents:** Like ipratropium bromide (0.25–0.5 mg nebulized or 80–160 mcg)
- They inhibit the vagal tone, leading to bronchodilation. Slower-acting than the beta-2 adrenergic agonists.
- They are used as adjuncts to beta-2 adrenergic agonists and never as sole therapy.

✓ **Corticosteroids:** Systemic steroids should be given within 1 h of presentation and taken at least 4–6 h to have beneficial effect.
- Oral steroids are as effective and can be used unless there is the possibility of impaired gastrointestinal absorption.
- Global Initiative for Asthma (GINA) Guidelines 2020 recommend 50 mg of prednisolone as single dose or 200 mg of hydrocortisone in divided doses in adults. A 5–7 d course is recommended.
- All patients should be prescribed inhaled corticosteroids on discharge. They are not recommended in acute setting.

✓ **Magnesium Sulphate:** *1.2–2 g IV over 20 min*[Q] can be used for *life-threatening asthma*. However, its use is *not recommended for routine use* in asthma exacerbations.

- Antagonizes calcium-mediated bronchoconstriction, decreases acetylcholine release at neuromuscular junction, and increases sensitivity of beta receptors to catecholamines.

✓ **Methylxanthines (Phosphodiesterase Inhibitors): IV aminophylline**[Q] 5 mg/kg loading over 20 min and then infusion of 0.5 mg/kg/h *only in near-fatal or life-threatening asthma.* It increases diaphragmatic contractility.
  - Drug monitoring is done to avoid toxicity. Can cause hypokalaemia[Q].

✓ **Heliox (21% He, 79% O_2)**[Q] may reduce work of breathing but doesn't relieve bronchoconstriction.
  - Reduces airway resistance in large airways due to reduced gas density.
  - *Heliox-powered delivery can be used to potentially avoid intubations for patients with severe, life-threatening exacerbations.*

✓ **Intravenous Ketamine**[Q], **Adrenaline Infusion, and General Anaesthesia with Isoflurane:** Has been used in refractory bronchospasm.
  - **Extracorporeal life support** has been used to support patient's refractory to conventional therapy.

✓ **Antibiotics:** Recommended only if evidence of bacterial infection like fever, purulent sputum, or radiographical evidence of pneumonia.

✓ **Mucolytic Agents:** Like N-acetylcysteine and leukotriene antagonists are not recommended in acute setting.

✓ **Non-Invasive Ventilation (NIV):** Has a role in treatment of acute asthma, but more trials are needed, and hence, no recommendation has been made for the use of NIV during asthma exacerbations.
  - May be used for 1–2 h and may be considered in patients with low risk of a severe attack for those not responding to medical therapy.

✓ **Mechanical Ventilation**[Q]: Indications are **respiratory muscle fatigue**, respiratory rate >35 breaths/min, **life-threatening** PaO_2 **<5.3 kPa**, hypercapnia >8 kPa, **pH <7.25, NIV failure,** inability to talk and manage secretions, **impaired mental status.**
  - **High-risk mortality intubation** due to switch to positive pressure ventilation from a highly negative intrathoracic pressure, hypovolaemia[Q], and loss of high existing sympathetic tone due to anaesthesia.

- Short- and rapid-acting IV benzodiazepine can relax the patient pre-intubation and allow preoxygenation.
  - ❖ Opioids should not be used as they can cause nausea and vomiting and provoke histamine release, worsening bronchospasm.
- **Mechanical ventilator settings**[Q]: Controlled hypoventilation with permissive hypercapnia: TV 5–7 mL/kg, RR 10–14/min, I:E: 1:4 with PaO_2 >8 kPa as target.
- **Reduce dynamic hyperinflation**[Q] by decreasing tidal volume and respiratory rate and accepting acidaemia. pH >7.2 is acceptable. *The goal is to return pH to normal and not $PaCO_2$.*
  - ❖ Prolong expiratory time by increasing inspiratory flow (60–100 L/min) and eliminating any end-inspiratory pause.
  - ❖ Sometimes the ventilator needs to be temporarily disconnected[Q].
- Paralysis may be needed but should be for minimal time as patients are at risk of myopathy. Boluses are preferred over continuous infusion.
- *Post-intubation hypotension may be due to dynamic hyperinflation.*
- **External PEEP around 80% of internal PEEP in patients with expiratory flow limitation as it reduces dynamic hyperinflation.**
- Role of mechanical ventilation is to support patient's respiration while corticosteroid starts working. Discontinuation should be tried in 1–3 d after intensive pharmacological therapy.
- **Barotrauma** is a major cause of morbidity and mortality and should be avoided by keeping plateau pressures low.
- **Mucus plugging** commonly occurs during acute exacerbation of asthma, and therapeutic bronchoscopy should be used cautiously as it can itself cause bronchospasm.

✓ **Ventilatory Parameters**
- **Intrinsic PEEP:** Performed by the end-expiratory occlusion manoeuvre and is called auto-PEEP.
  - ❖ End-expiratory occlusion is the value obtained after 2–5 s of occlusion.

- **Total respiratory resistance (R)** = Ppeak – Pplat / Inspiratory flow. Normal resistance <10 cm H_2O/L/sec.
  - ❖ Plateau pressures are measured after end-inspiratory occlusion for 3 s.
- **Compliance (C)** = change in volume / change in pressure = ΔV / Pplat – (ePEEP + iPEEP). Normal compliance >50 mL/cm H_2O.
- **Expiratory flow limitation:** Seen as a spike of high expiratory flow as air expires from the large open airways, followed by a flat part with a very low flat rate.

✓ **Pregnancy**[Q]: Asthma can either improve, worsen, or remain the same. Early MDT involvement should be done.
  - In pregnancy, both beta-2 adrenergic agonists and systemic corticosteroids are considered safe for use and should not be withheld in acute setting.

CHRONIC OBSTRUCTIVE PULMONARY DISEASE (COPD)

Epidemiology

✓ **Global Initiative for Chronic Obstructive Lung Disease (GOLD) Definition 2023:** Chronic respiratory symptoms due to abnormalities of the airway and/or alveoli, leading to progressive, *minimally reversible*, and chronic airflow obstruction.

✓ **Pathophysiology:** Increased airway resistance of small conduction airways (<2 mm diameter), **reduced lung elastic recoil** or **increased lung compliance** due to parenchymal destruction, and increased pulmonary vascular resistance are seen.
  - Collapsed airways are due to loss of tethering by destroyed lung parenchyma.
  - Time constant (τ) = R × C, where R is resistance and C is compliance. τ increases in patients with COPD and is represented by FEV_1 (maximal volume that can be expired in 1 s).
  - **Air trapping/dynamic hyperinflation:** Airway collapse leading to stopping of the airflow and trapping of air distal to the point of flow limitation. Leads to ↑ functional residual capacity (FRC)[Q] and ↑ residual volume (RV)[Q].
  - **Inefficient gas exchange:** Hypoxaemia and hypercapnia.

✓ **Acute Exacerbation of Chronic Obstructive Pulmonary Disease (AECOPD):** Acute deterioration of patient's baseline respiratory symptoms (**cough, sputum, and dyspnoea**). Fever is not a feature.
  - The most common cause is infection, either bacterial or viral.

✓ **Risk Factors for COPD**
  - **Patient factors:** Smoking, alpha-1 antitrypsin deficiency.
  - **Environmental factors:** Air pollution, industrial dust exposure.

Clinical Features and Diagnosis

✓ **Two Syndromes That Overlap:** Chronic bronchitis and emphysema.
  - **Chronic bronchitis:** Sleep apnoea, right heart failure, loss of hypercapnic respiratory drive.
  - **Emphysema:** Hyperinflation and greatly increased work of breathing.

✓ **Risk Factors for *Pseudomonas* Infection:** Immunocompromised, malnutrition, hospitalization for >2 d in last 90 d.
  - Age is not a risk factor.

✓ **Dynamic Hyperinflation:** Slow filling of manual ventilator bag attached on ETT, capnography trace not reaching baseline, expiratory flow not reaching zero in flowtime/volume graph, rise in plateau pressure.

✓ **ABG:** An increased HCO_3^- or compensatory respiratory acidosis on ABG suggests COPD.

✓ **Severity of COPD:** Diagnosed by spirometry with **FEV_1/FVC ratio of <0.7**[Q] and FEV_1 of <80% predicted.

GOLD Spirometric Classification

Gold Stage	Severity	Spirometry
I	Mild	FEV_1/FVC ratio < 0.7 and FEV_1 ≥ 80%
II	Moderate	FEV_1 ≥ 50% but < 80%
III	Severe	FEV_1 ≥ 30% but < 50%
IV	Very severe	FEV_1 < 30%

✓ **Modified Medical Research Council (MMRC) Dyspnoea Scale**
  - MMRC 0: Dyspnoea on strenuous exercise.
  - MMRC 1: Dyspnoea on walking a slight incline.
  - MMRC 2: Dyspnoea on walking on level ground.
  - MMRC 3: Must stop for breathlessness after walking 100 yd or after a few minutes.
  - MMRC 4: Dyspnoea resulting in being housebound or during dressing and undressing.

✓ **COPD:** Forms only 10% of patients with type 2 respiratory failure.

Prevention and Treatment

✓ **Prevention:** Smoking cessation. *Pulmonary rehabilitation* techniques like exercise training, breathing techniques, nutritional counselling.
  - **Short-acting beta-2 bronchodilator** (salbutamol).
  - **Long-acting beta-2 bronchodilator** (salmeterol/formoterol) + **long-acting muscarinic antagonists** (tiotropium/umeclidinium).
  - Add inhaled corticosteroids in cases with asthmatic features or frequent exacerbations.
  - Oral corticosteroids used in exacerbations.

✓ **Oxygen Titrated to Target Saturation of 88–92%:** With beta-2 adrenergic agonists, ipratropium, and steroids within the first hour.
  - High volumes of oxygen can worsen hypercapnia by:
    ❖ Changes in V/Q mismatch: As increased oxygen abolishes hypoxic vasoconstriction and increases dead space ventilation.
    ❖ Decrease in central respiratory drive.
    ❖ **Haldane effect:** Increased oxygenation increases offloading of CO_2 in lungs, which can't be cleared with already-maximized ventilatory efforts.

✓ **Beta-2 Adrenergic Agonists:** Metered-dose inhalers are as good as nebulizers. Nebulizer should be driven by compressed air rather than oxygen.

✓ **Anticholinergics:** Ipratropium bromide should be used in conjunction with beta-2 adrenergic agonists.

✓ **Corticosteroids:** Systemic steroids in first hour of presentation. Systemic steroids take 4 h to show any effect. Oral steroids are preferred over IV corticosteroids in hospitalized patients due to COPD exacerbation.
  - GOLD guidelines recommend oral prednisone 40 mg per day for 5 d in these patients.
  - Blood eosinophilia is a **promising biomarker** to direct corticosteroid therapy.

✓ **Antibiotics:** Infections (*Haemophilus influenzae*, *Streptococcus pneumoniae*, *Moraxella catarrhalis*, and *Pseudomonas aeruginosa*) are the most common precipitating factor for an acute exacerbation of COPD.
  - **Antibiotics should be given for 5–7 d.**
  - GOLD guidelines recommend use of antibiotics in the following patients:
    ❖ Patients requiring non-invasive and invasive ventilation.
    ❖ Presenting with increase in all three symptoms, like dyspnoea, sputum volume, and purulence.
    ❖ Presenting with increase in two aforementioned symptoms with purulence in one of the two symptoms.

✓ **Methylxanthines:** Not recommended currently and only used in severe cases.
  - **Heliox (79% helium and 21% oxygen)** is not routinely recommended in acute setting of COPD.
  - Mucolytic agents like N-acetylcysteine are not recommended.

✓ **COPD Patients:** Often also have chronic heart disease, and fluid should be given carefully.

✓ **Non-Invasive Ventilation:** If even after 1 h of medical management, patient remains acidotic, with **pH 7.25–7.35 and** $PaCO_2 > 6$ **kPa**, they should be offered NIV[Q].
  - **NIV has shown mortality benefit and decreases the risk of endotracheal intubation by:**
    ❖ Decreasing work of breathing
    ❖ Improving gas exchange
    ❖ Counterbalancing intrinsic PEEP
  - **Low GCS is a relative contraindication but may help avoid intubation.**
  - Initial IPAP of 10 cm H_2O and EPAP of 4–5 cm H_2O. The IPAP can be gradually increased by 2 cm H_2O increments every 10 min to respiratory rate ≤25 breaths/minute

and tidal volume 6–8 mL/kg. Avoid airway pressure above 20 cm H_2O.

  ❖ Titrate PEEP by 1–2 cm H_2O, assessing ineffective triggering attempts.

- CO_2 removal is proportional to alveolar ventilation (minute ventilation – dead space ventilation).

✓ **Invasive Mechanical Ventilation and Referral to ITU**

- **Indications:** Unsustainable increased work of breathing, severe hypoxaemia, decreased consciousness, inability to clear secretions, haemodynamic instability, and intractable arrhythmias.

- **Assist control mode** is recommended initially as patient initiates the breath and is more comfortable. Flow triggering is more comfortable for the patient.

- **Ventilatory settings** include tidal volumes between 6 and 8 mL/kg, respiratory rate 10–12 breaths/minute, I:E 1:4, and increased inspiratory flows (70–100 L/min).

  ❖ However, low tidal volumes and high flow rates can lead to **double triggering** if the patient continues effort beyond ventilator insufflation time. This can be prevented by switching back to long inspiratory time, reduced flow rates, adding an inspiratory pause, and switching from constant flow to a decelerating flow.

- **Dynamic hyperinflation** causes difficulty in triggering a breath as the patient must generate enough force to overcome the elastic recoil due to auto-PEEP.

  ❖ Intrinsic PEEP in mechanically ventilated patients is measured by end-occlusion manoeuvres, and in spontaneously ventilated patients, oesophageal pressure monitoring is needed.

  ❖ Intrinsic PEEP can lead to non-triggered breaths and a sense of dyspnoea.

  ❖ External PEEP is kept at 80% of intrinsic PEEP in patients with COPD.

- **Weaning** a patient with COPD can be difficult due to development of dynamic hyperinflation due to tachypnoea.

✓ **Extracorporeal Life Support:** Extracorporeal CO_2 removal to avoid mechanical ventilation has been used as mechanical ventilation and is associated with up to 30% in hospital mortality.

- Used when permissive hypercapnia poses a significant risk.
- However, it hasn't shown any mortality benefit.

✓ **Nutrition:** COPD patients are characterized by loss of weight and loss of muscle mass due to chronic steroid therapy, and early nutritional support is preferred.

- Care should be taken to avoid excessive carbohydrate feeding as it can lead to increased CO_2 production.

- **Pulmonary rehabilitation:** Can be started even during acute episode. Resistance training is started in early period. Even frail patients benefit.

✓ **Long-Term Oxygen Therapy (LTOT)[Q]:** Suggested on discharge for patients with a saturation < 92% and **resting** PaO_2 **of < 7.3 kPa.** It shows **mortality benefit** if used for >15 h.

- **LTOT also for** PaO_2 < **8 kPa** if secondary polycythaemia, peripheral oedema, or pulmonary hypertension is present.

Prognosis

✓ A 1-yr mortality for patient requiring NIV or ITU is 50%.

✓ **Poor prognosis factors** are new arrhythmias, failure to improve during current admission, ongoing acidosis, and an FEV_1 < 30%.

✓ **BODE index for estimating prognosis of 4-yr survival. Not recommended by NICE Guidelines** (hence, no need to cram as well).

- Score 0–2: 80% survival
- Score 3–4: 67% survival
- Score 5–6: 57% survival
- Score 7–10: 18% survival

	BODE Index Score		
Prognostic Factor	+ 1 Point	+ 2 Points	+ 3 Points
BMI	≤21		
Obstruction, FEV1 after bronchodilator therapy	50–64%	36–49%	
Dyspnoea (MMRC scale)	2	3	4
Exercise capacity (6 min walk distance)	250–349 m	150–249 m	≤149 m

PLEURAL EFFUSION

Aetiology

✓ **Pleural Effusion:** Non-physiological presence of fluid in pleural cavity. A pleural cavity can hold as much as 4–5 L of fluid.

✓ **Type: Pleural effusion** can be divided into exudative or transudative.
- Almost 20% of cases will remain undiagnosed for the causative factor.

✓ **Exudative:** Exudative effusion means that there is a disease process that is affecting the pleural cavity directly causing the pleura and its vasculature to be damaged (e.g. malignancy, pneumonia, TB, pulmonary embolism^Q, autoimmune diseases, asbestosis, and pancreatitis).
- **Empyema** is a serious form of complicated parapneumonic effusion and is characterized by pus in the pleural space.
- **Pulmonary embolism:** Unilateral effusion mostly that occupies less than one-third of the haemothorax.
  - ❖ Exudates mostly due to capillary leak caused by inflammatory mediators release due to pulmonary vasculature obstruction.
  - ❖ About 20% of patients may have transudates due to atelectasis.
- **Pancreatitis:** Unilateral mostly on the left side (60%). Elevated pleural fluid amylase higher than that of serum.
- **Coronary artery bypass surgery (CABG):** Small left-side pleural effusion with left-lobe atelectasis and elevation of the left hemidiaphragm on chest X-ray.
- **Abdominal surgery:** Seen in half of the patients who undergo abdominal surgery, especially upper abdominal surgery, due to atelectasis or diaphragmatic irritation.
- **Chylothorax^Q:** Lymphoma, post-pneumonectomy, CABG, penetrating injury of the neck.

✓ **Transudative:** Transudative effusion means that the pleura itself is healthy, and a disease process is affecting the hydrostatic and oncotic factors that either increase the formation of pleural fluid or decrease its absorption.
- *Atelectasis*, congestive heart failure (most common cause overall)^Q, post–myocardial infarction, hepatic hydrothorax, hypo-albuminaemia, peritoneal dialysis, nephrotic syndrome.
- **Atelectasis** causes increase in space between lung and chest wall, which causes increased fluid accumulation due to secretion from parietal pleural space.
- **Congestive heart failure:** Bilateral effusions, right > left, cardiomegaly.
- **Hepatic hydrothorax** results from movement of ascitic fluid through congenital or acquired diaphragmatic defects.
- **Hypoalbuminaemia (<18 g/L)** can present with bilateral pleural effusion, but rarely without anasarca.

✓ **Drugs That Can Cause Pleural Effusion:** Methotrexate, phenytoin, amiodarone, beta-blockers, and nitrofurantoin.

Diagnosis

✓ **Signs and Symptoms:** Chest pain which is sharp and worse with breathing.
- Dyspnoea and desaturation are the other symptoms.

✓ **Chest X-ray:** Needs 500 mL of fluid to be detected as pleural effusion by absence of costophrenic angle meniscus in a supine film. Its roughly 175 (lateral film) to 525 mL (PA film)^Q for an erect chest X-ray.
- Supine films can obscure a pleural effusion. Pleural effusion looks like increased homogeneous density over the lower lung field.

✓ **Ultrasound Chest:** Quantifies size and visualizes septations and then drainage under guidance.
- It can detect as low as 3–5 mL of fluid in pleural effusion.
- *Complex-appearing pleural effusions are more likely to be exudative.*
- Superior to chest X-ray for pleural effusions and comparable to CT scan in diagnosis of pleural effusions^Q.
- *Ultrasound is superior to CT scan for visualizing septations within a pleural effusion.*

✓ **Non-Contrast CT Scan:** Gives a better idea about amount of fluid, if fluid is loculated, and can help delineate possible causes.

✓ **CT Scan (with Pleural Enhancement):** Should be done in patients with undiagnosed exudative effusions and complicated infective causes. It should be done before drainage.

✓ **Diagnostic Thoracentesis:** Done in all patients with suspected pleural effusion, except those with a small amount of pleural fluid or patients with uncomplicated congestive heart failure.

✓ **Light's Criteria[Q]:** An exudate if:
- Pleural fluid protein/serum protein ratio > 0.5
- Pleural fluid LDH/serum LDH > 0.6
- Pleural fluid LDH > Two-thirds of the upper limit of normal range for serum LDH

✓ **Pleural Fluid Analysis**
- **Microscopy:** Culture and Gram stain.
- **Cell count and differentials:** Lymphocytes suggest TB or malignancy.
- **Biochemistry:** LDH and protein.
- **Cytology:** Malignancy, commonly lung, breast, and lymphoma.
- **pH:** if suspected infection, <7.2: **Empyema[Q]**.
- **Acid-fast bacilli:** If suspected TB.
- **Adenosine deaminase (ADA):** ADA <40 IU/L excludes the diagnosis of pleural TB, and levels >70 IU/L suggest pleural TB.
- **Triglycerides and cholesterol:** If effusion is milky, suggestive of chylothorax. *Triglycerides levels >110 mg/dL are diagnostic.*
- **Amylase:** If pancreatitis or oesophageal pathology
- **Serum albumin – effusion albumin <1.2 g/dL indicates exudative pleural effusion[Q]**.

✓ **Bronchoscopy:** After drainage, if there is suspected lesion in bronchial tree, evidence of volume loss, or a history of haemoptysis.
- Should be done under PCV to compensate for leaks with sedation.

✓ **Therapeutic Thoracentesis:** Main indication is relief of dyspnoea and to facilitate liberation from the mechanical ventilator.
- In mechanically ventilated patients, if there is suspicion for pleural infection, straight away ultrasound-guided small tube thoracostomy can be done and then taken out later if analysis doesn't show infection.
- Limit volume drained to 1.5 L, as excess volume drained can cause re-expansion pulmonary oedema[Q].

✓ **Haemothorax:** Diagnosed when haematocrit of pleural fluid >50% of peripheral blood.

Treatment

✓ **If Transudative Cause, Treat the Underlying Cause[Q]**
- Treat congestive heart failure with diuretics, inotropes, and afterload reduction and effusions resolve over days to weeks.
- Treat hepatic hydrothorax with diuresis and sodium restriction.

✓ **If Exudative, Respiratory Opinion, and a Diagnostic Tap Done[Q]**
- Thoracenteses can be safely done as long as there is around 2 cm[Q] of fluid on ultrasound even in patients receiving mechanical ventilation.
- **Parapneumonic effusion:** Any effusion due to bacterial pneumonia, lung abscess, or bronchiectasis.
  - ❖ Simple parapneumonic effusions resolve in 7–14 d without sequelae with antibiotics alone.
  - ❖ Early antibiotics and prompt adequate drainage is the mainstay of treatment of empyema. Treatment duration is 4–6 wk.
  - ❖ **MIST-2 Trial (2011)** has shown that intrapleural fibrinolytic therapy (10 mg of tPA) and 5 mg of DNase twice a day for 3 d was associated with improved radiographic resolution, lower surgical referrals, and hospital length of stay.
  - ❖ **Non-resolved cases may require VAT drainage, decortication, and rarely, thoracotomy.**
- **Haemothorax** should be drained immediately with large-diameter chest tube[Q]. Continuous rapid bleeding may require thoracotomy.
- **Malignant effusion:** Drainage of effusion with thoracentesis is often not sufficient, and insertion of chest tube followed by **pleurodesis** can prevent it from recurring.
  - ❖ **Long-term indwelling catheters** have also been used in these patients to drain effusion at home.
- **Chylothorax** is treated with **chest tube**, bed rest, and **TPN[Q]** to minimize chyle formation.
- **Diuretics:** Not effective in taking out exudative effusion. Fluid removal from pleural effusion and peritoneal cavity is slow.

✓ **Intercostal Chest Drain[Q]**
- Tube connecting the ICD to the underwater seal bottle should be wide and with a volumetric capacity exceeding half of the patient's maximal inspiratory volume.
- The end of the tube, within the underwater seal bottle, should not be more than 5 cm below the surface of water[Q].

- The drain should be at least 45 cm below the patient to prevent fluid from refluxing back in the chest.
- Suction must be applied between 10–20 cm H₂O.
- A **three-bottle system**^{Q} is used sometimes. First bottle acts as fluid trap, second bottle provides underwater seal, whereas the third bottle can be used for suction.
- **Flutter valves**^{Q} used for earlier mobilization.
- **Re-expansion pulmonary oedema**^{Q} can happen with over-draining. So don't drain over 1–1.5 L at a time with suction −10 cm to 20 cm H₂O.

PNEUMOTHORAX

Aetiology

✓ **Pneumothorax: Presence of Air in the Pleural Space**
- **Pneumothorax** in critically ill patients is most commonly due to invasive procedures and barotrauma^Q.

Clinical Features and Diagnosis

✓ **Classification of Pneumothorax**
- **Spontaneous:** Primary or secondary
- **Iatrogenic:** CVC insertion, barotrauma, surgical procedure
- **Traumatic:** direct or indirect injury to pleura or lung

✓ **Spontaneous Pneumothorax:** Pneumothorax in the absence of trauma or iatrogenic causes. *A greater than 2 cm size of rim* between the lung margin and the chest wall at the level of hilum is the cutoff between large and small pneumothoraxes.
- **Primary:** No history of lung disease. Seen in young people.
- **Secondary:** In patients with pre-existing lung disease or patient over 50 with significant smoking history.

✓ **Iatrogenic Pneumothorax:** Inadvertent consequence of diagnostic and therapeutic procedures.
- **Central venous catheters:** Delayed pneumothoraxes have been noted; in case of doubt, reorder a chest X-ray in 12–24 h.
  - ❖ Patients on mechanical ventilation should get a tube thoracostomy.

- **Barotrauma:** Pneumothorax seen in 1–15% cases of mechanical ventilation.

✓ **Trauma Pneumothorax:** Discussed in chapter on thoracic trauma.

✓ **Tension Pneumothorax:** Life-threatening complication when air enters the pleural space but is unable to leave.
- **Clinical diagnosis:** Ultrasound may be more sensitive and quicker than chest X-ray for helping diagnosis^Q.
- Tachypnoea, tachycardia, hypotension, cyanosis, hyperresonance, decreased breath sounds.
- Treatment is 14 G cannula into the second intercostal space^Q in the midclavicular line, followed by definitive chest drain.
  - ❖ ATLS^Q suggests cannula in the fifth intercostal space just anterior to midclavicular line.

✓ **Chest X-ray:** Standard erect PA inspiratory films are good enough for diagnosis.
- In supine films^Q, pneumothorax gas migrates along the anterior surface of the lung, making the diagnosis difficult.
- **Deep sulcus sign**^{Q} on supine film is indicative of pneumothorax. Costophrenic angle is abnormally deepened when the pleural air collects laterally, producing the deep sulcus sign.
- Tension pneumothorax: Contralateral mediastinal shift and ipsilateral diaphragmatic depression.

✓ **Ultrasound:** Detection of "lung sliding" (respirophasic to-and-fro movement of lung–chest wall interface) can rapidly exclude the anterior pneumothorax.

✓ **CT Scan:** May be needed for definitive diagnosis.

Prevention and Treatment

✓ **Entonox:**^{Q} Not used for analgesia as nitrous oxide can diffuse into the cavity and exacerbate a pneumothorax.

✓ **Primary Spontaneous Pneumothorax (PSP)**
- PSP should be managed conservatively in asymptomatic patients with **high-flow oxygen**^{Q}.
- PSP should be **aspirated**^{Q} with a cannula in cases of dyspnoea, hypoxia, or large pneumothorax (>2 cm).
- Use small-bore intercostal drains (8–14 Fr) if aspiration fails.

✓ **Secondary Spontaneous Pneumothorax (SSP)**[Q]
- Admit to hospital and give supplemental oxygen even if SSP <1 cm. Refer to respiratory physician within 24 h of admission.
- If pneumothorax is small (<2 cm) and patient is asymptomatic, attempt aspiration[Q].
- **A small-bore (8 to 12 F) chest drain**[Q] if aspiration has been unsuccessful or large PSPs.
- Routine use of suction and large-bore drains isn't recommended. If used (in persistent air leak >48 h), use high-volume/low-pressure suction.
- Refer to thoracic surgeons if persistent air leak or failure of lung to re-expand after 48–72 h[Q].
  - ❖ Pleurectomy via open thoracotomy (1% recurrence) or VATS (5% recurrence)
  - ❖ Surgical chemical pleurodesis
  - ❖ Medical pleurodesis

✓ **Bilateral or Tension Pneumothorax:** Should always be treated with chest drains and hospital admission.
- Iatrogenic and traumatic pneumothoraxes will also require chest drain insertion most of the time.

✓ **ICD Management: Triangle of Safety**[Q] between lateral border of pectoralis major and the anterior border of latissimus dorsi, just above the line joining the nipple at level of the fifth intercostal space.
- Small-bore drains[Q] are equally effective as wide-bore drains with fewer complications and less painful.
- Wide-bore ICD if haemothorax.
- Trocars should never be used.
- Bubbling chest drains should never be clamped.
- Purse-string sutures can be painful and should be avoided.
- Chest drain removal should occur during expiration[Q].

✓ **Indications for Removal of Chest Drain**
- Pneumothorax has resolved.
- No air leak present in the chest tube.
- Lung remains expanded after chest tube has been placed on water seal for 24 h.

Prognosis

✓ Intercostal drain infections are same in both wide-bore and narrow-bore drains.

Additional Questions

✓ Gas-filled cavities expand at higher altitudes[Q].

✓ **Body compensatory changes on high altitude**[Q]
- **Hyperventilation:** Fall in PaO_2 below 8 kPa, stimulates the peripheral chemoreceptors.
- Sinus tachycardia: Sympathetic stimulation.
- Hypoxic pulmonary vasoconstriction (HPV): It optimizes V/Q matching.
- Leftward shift of the oxyhaemoglobin dissociation curve: 2,3 DPG production increases.
- Polycythaemia: Increased erythropoietin secretion.
- Hypercoagulability: Due to increase haematocrit.

✓ **Effect on anaesthetic equipment at high altitude**[Q]
- Variable bypass vaporizer: **Partial pressure of the volatile agent remains the same.**
  - ❖ SVP of the volatile agent remains the same.
  - ❖ Therefore, same settings as at sea level.
- Measured flow vaporizer (desflurane): Partial pressure is halved as measured flow.
  - ❖ Concentration on dial should be increased compared to at sea levels.
- Flowmeters: Gases have a lower density.
  - ❖ Under-read at high altitudes.
- Bourdon pressure gauge: Over-read at higher altitude.
- Venturi-type O_2 masks: Deliver higher percentage of O_2 than at sea level.
- Gas and vapour analyzers: Under-reads.

BRONCHOPLEURAL FISTULA

Aetiology

✓ **Bronchopleural Fistula (BPF):** Unnatural communication between the bronchial tree and pleural space. Can be a difficult-to-treat condition.

✓ **Presents as**
- Failure to reinflate the lung despite chest tube drainage or continuous air leak after evacuation of pneumothorax.
- Complication of a thoracic surgery (within first 2 weeks).
- Complication of mechanical ventilation, usually for those with ARDS.

- Complications of trauma, tuberculosis, necrotic lung complication, chemotherapy, and radiotherapy.

Diagnosis

✓ **Clinical Presentation**
  - Tension pneumothorax, recurrent pneumothorax, subacute empyema.
  - Leads to failure of lung to expand, loss of tidal volume, and loss of PEEP.
✓ If there is continuous air leak for longer than 24 h after the development of pneumothorax, then a BPF is suspected.

Treatment

✓ **Failure of BPF to Resolve after 72 h:** Suggests lower probability of spontaneous closure, and pleurodesis (medical or surgical) should be considered.
✓ **Supportive Management:** Nutrition, antibiotics, clearing the empyema, and treating any bronchospasm.
✓ **Conservative**
  - **Adequate-size test tube:** Air leaks in BPF are between 1 and 16 L per minute.
    - ❖ The smallest internal diameter of tube that allows flows of 15 L/minute at 10 cm H_2O suction is 6 mm. 32-Fr chest tube has an internal diameter of 9 mm.
    - ❖ So larger chest tubes should be used, as a tube, too, can lead to tension pneumothorax.
  - **Drainage systems:** Use lowest amount of suction possible, as excessive suction can keep the fistula open.
  - **Mechanical ventilation:** Extubate patients as soon as possible.
    - ❖ If we can't liberate patients from mechanical ventilation, use lowest possible tidal volume, fewest mechanical breaths per minute, lowest level of PEEP, and shortest inspiratory time.
    - ❖ **Lung isolation:** Double-lumen tubes[Q] to preserve ventilation in the good lung.
    - ❖ **High-frequency ventilation (HFV):** Use of HFV in moderate to severe ARDS may be associated with increased risk of death.
    - ❖ **Flexible bronchoscopy[Q]:** Direct application of sealant (fibrin, gelatine) and endobronchial stents; valve has been used.
✓ **ECMO**
✓ **Surgery:** Pleurectomy is recommended over pleurodesis as lower pneumothorax recurrence rate in cases with persistent pneumothorax[Q]. Can be done by VATS (video-assisted thoracoscopic surgery) or open thoracotomy.
  - Mobilization of intercostal or pectoralis muscles
  - Thoracoplasty
  - Bronchial stump stapling
  - Pleural abrasion and decortication

Prognosis

✓ Mortality is higher with BPF which develops later and with higher than 500 mL/breath leak.

BRONCHOSCOPY

Anatomy of the Bronchus

✓ **Trachea:** Posterior wall is cartilage-deficient and has a muscle stripe that continues into the main bronchi. *Right main bronchus at a 25° angle and left main bronchus at 45° angle[Q].*
✓ **Right main bronchus:** Vertically placed and gives off right upper lobe bronchus at 90° at 3 o'clock position within 1.5–2 cm of carina and then continues as bronchus intermedius.
  - **Right upper lobe bronchus:** During bronchoscopy, right upper lobe divides into three equal segments (apical, anterior, and posterior bronchus), like the *Mercedes-Benz logo[Q].*
  - **Right middle bronchus:** Seen at 12 o'clock position. Divides into medial and lateral branches.
  - **Right lower lobe bronchus:** Apical (6 o'clock position), anterior basal, posterior basal, medial basal, and lateral basal.
✓ **Left main bronchus:** Horizontally oriented and twice as long as right main bronchus. Left main bronchus divides into upper lobe and lower lobe bronchus.
  - **Left upper lobe bronchus:** Divides into a superior division and an inferior division (lingular bronchus) at 9 o'clock position. Superior division branches into apical, anterior, and posterior bronchus, while lingular branch divides into superior and inferior branches.

- **Left lower lobe bronchus:** Apical (6 o'clock position), anterior basal, posterior basal, medial basal, and lateral basal.

Diagnostic Indications

✓ **Haemoptysis**
- Unless bleeding is massive, a flexible bronchoscope, rather than a rigid bronchoscope, is the initial instrument of choice[Q].
- In case of massive bleeding, the rigid bronchoscope is used to provide a secure route for ventilation and larger conduit for suctioning.
- Flexible bronchoscopy (FB) can be performed through the rigid bronchoscope to assess and temporize the source of bleeding beyond the main bronchi in cases of massive bleeding.

✓ **Diffuse Parenchymal Disease**
- Transbronchial lung biopsy (TBLB) in cases of suspected sarcoidosis, lymphangitic carcinomatosis, or eosinophilic pneumonia.
- TBLB has low yield for idiopathic interstitial pneumonias, inorganic pneumoconiosis, and pulmonary vasculitides.

✓ **Ventilator-Associated Pneumonia**
- Sensitivity of 70% and specificity of 80% for diagnosis.
- European guidelines advocate quantitative sampling with thresholds of 10^4 colony forming units (CFU) per mL for bronchoalveolar lavage (BAL) fluid and 10^3 CFU per mL for protected specimen brush (PSB)[Q].
- North American VAP guidelines recommend semiquantitative endotracheal suctioning cultures in immunocompetent adults.

✓ **Pulmonary Infiltrates in Immunocompromised Patients**
- Diagnostic yield of >95% for *Pneumocystis jirovecii* in HIV patients[Q].
- However, diagnostic yield in solid organ transplants and stem cell transplants is low.

✓ **Acute Inhalational Injury**
- Clearance of pulmonary debris and casts along with identifying the anatomic level and severity of injury.

✓ **Blunt Trauma Chest**
- Diagnosis of tracheal or bronchial laceration or transection, aspirated material, mucus plugging, and distal haemorrhage.

✓ **Post-Resectional Surgery and Lung Transplant**
- Identification of bronchopleural fistula due to suture line dehiscence, causing bleeding ʿ and pneumothorax following surgery.

Therapeutic Indications

✓ **Atelectasis:** Up to 90% success rate in case of lobar atelectasis[Q].
✓ **Foreign Bodies:** Rigid bronchoscope in the paediatric population.
✓ **Haemoptysis:** Endobronchial tamponade using a Fogarty catheter through a rigid bronchoscope.
✓ **Percutaneous Tracheostomy.**
✓ **Central Obstructing Airway Lesion:** Stents can be placed through the rigid bronchoscope.

Complications

✓ Fever due to cytokine release, bleeding, pneumonia, cardiac arrhythmias, bronchospasm, pneumothorax.
✓ *Mycobacterium tuberculosis*[Q] can cause contamination of bronchoscope.

Contraindications

✓ When the patient cannot cooperate, when adequate oxygenation can't be maintained during the procedure, in haemodynamically unstable patients, in untreated symptomatic asthmatic patients.
✓ Platelet count >20,000/μL for FB with BAL is recommended by the British Thoracic Society.
✓ In patients with high ICP, procedure should be done with deep sedation and paralysis.
✓ The lumen of the endotracheal tube should be at least 2 mm larger than the outer diameter of the bronchoscope.
  - A light-emitting diode[Q] illuminates the distal camera of a single-use bronchoscope.

Bronchoalveolar lavage: Performed by advancing the bronchoscope until the tip wedges in a distal bronchus in the area of clinical interest. Right middle lobe is used in diffuse disease. Three aliquots of saline, typically 35–50 mL, are then instilled and withdrawn. A total of 100 mL instilled with at least 30% retrieved constitutes an adequate specimen.

✓ **Indications**
  - **Non-resolving pneumonia**
  - Presence of infiltrates in the immunocompromised patient

- Presence of diffuse lung infiltrates
- Suspected alveolar haemorrhage
✓ **Pressure:** −20 kPa for non-guided BAL and −6 to −12 kPa for guided BAL.
✓ **Common investigation results**
  - Alveolar macrophages (normal >80%): Higher values in smokers.
  - Hemosiderin-laden macrophages: >20% in alveolar haemorrhage.
  - Neutrophils (normal <3%): Alveolitis, ARDS, idiopathic pulmonary fibrosis, granulomatosis with polyangiitis.
  - Eosinophilia (normal <1–2%): Low to moderate (5–20%) in asthma, drug-induced (minocycline, nitrofurantoin, penicillin), interstitial pneumonias. Moderate to marked (>20%) in allergic bronchopulmonary aspergillosis (ABPA), acute and chronic eosinophilic pneumonia.
  - Langerhans cells: >5% suggests pulmonary Langerhans cell histiocytosis.
  - Periodic acid Schiff stain: Pulmonary alveolar proteinosis.
  - Silver methenamine: *Pneumocystis jirovecii*.

RESTRICTIVE LUNG DISEASE

Aetiology

✓ **Restrictive Lung Disease:** Heterogenous set of pulmonary disorders characterized by reduced distensibility of the lungs, leading to reduced total lung capacity.
  - **Extrapulmonary causes**
    ❖ **Pleural condition:** Effusion, pneumothorax, chronic empyema, asbestosis
    ❖ **Thoracic wall:** Kyphoscoliosis, obesity
    ❖ **Abdominal wall:** Ascites
    ❖ **Neuromuscular:** muscular dystrophy, amyotrophic lateral sclerosis, polio, phrenic neuropathies
  - **Pulmonary causes**
    ❖ Interstitial lung diseases
    ❖ Acute respiratory distress syndrome
    ❖ Pulmonary oedema
    ❖ Surgical causes: Lobectomy, pneumonectomy
✓ **Interstitial Lung Disease (ILD):** Heterogenous group of parenchymal lung diseases characterized by varying degrees of inflammation and fibrosis. They are also called *diffuse parenchymal lung diseases* (*DPLDs*).

✓ **Classification of DPLD/ILD (ATS/ERS 2024 Consensus Statement)**[Q]
  - **Idiopathic interstitial pneumonias (IIPs)**
    ❖ **Idiopathic pulmonary fibrosis (IPF):** IPF is the most common form of ILD and carries the worst prognosis.
    ❖ **Non-IPF IIPs:** Acute interstitial pneumonias (AIP), cryptogenic organizing pneumonia (COP), desquamative interstitial pneumonias (DIP), non-specific interstitial pneumonias (NSIP), respiratory bronchiolitis interstitial lung disease (RB-ILD), lymphocytic interstitial pneumonia (LIP).
  - **DPLD of known cause**
    ❖ Drugs
    ❖ Environmental (asbestosis, silicosis)
    ❖ Collagen vascular disease
  - **Granulomatous DPLD**
    ❖ Sarcoidosis
  - **Other forms of DPLD**
    ❖ Langerhans cell histiocytosis
    ❖ Lymphangioleiomyomatosis (LAM)
    ❖ Pulmonary alveolar proteinosis
✓ **Classification of ILD by Clinical Behaviour**
  - **Reversible, self-limited:** RB-ILD
  - **Reversible, risk of progression:** DIP, COP, NSIP
  - **Irreversible and progressive:** IPF, NSIP
✓ **Sarcoidosis:** Second most common ILD. Granulomas in lung, liver, heart, brain, and skin.
  - Bilateral hilar lymphadenopathy on chest X-ray.
  - Spontaneous remission is common (up to 80% of cases in stage I).
  - Treated using prednisolone. Lung transplant for end-stage lung disease.
✓ **Lymphangioleiomyomatosis (LAM):** Affects women of childbearing age and is characterized by abnormal muscle-like cells growing and forming cysts in lungs, liver, and kidneys.
  - Lung transplant is needed ultimately.

Clinical Features and Diagnosis

✓ **Extra-parenchymal causes,** like pneumothorax, pulmonary embolism, and pleural effusions, should be ruled out.
✓ History, examination, and chest radiograph can give an idea about IIP or DPLD of known causes.
✓ **Diagnostic tests for DPLD of known causes:** Full connective tissue disorder panel, including

antinuclear antibody, rheumatoid factor, anti-cyclic citrullinated peptide antibody.

✓ **Spirometry**[Q]: Decreased FVC and FEV_1, but high FEV_1/FVC ratio.
  - Carbon monoxide transfer is used to measure diffusion capacity (DL_{CO}). V/Q mismatch will affect this.

✓ **CT scan:** High-resolution CT (HRCT) scans show fibrosis in IPF as reticulations, interstitial thickening, traction bronchiectasis, and honeycombing.
  - Inflammation is shown as ground-glass opacities.

✓ **BAL/transbronchial biopsy (TBBx):** Done in case where diagnosis of IPF is not clear on CT scan or other non-IPF causes of IIPs are suspected.

✓ **Surgical lung biopsy:** Definitive diagnosis of IPF in cases not diagnosed by BAL/TBBx.

Treatment

✓ **Oxygenation and ventilation:** Non-invasive ventilation or high-flow nasal oxygen can be used, and no difference in mortality between these two methods has been seen.
  - Mechanical ventilation is associated with high mortality rates amongst ILD patients.

✓ **Immunosuppression:** Corticosteroids form the mainstay if therapy for acute exacerbation of ILD.

✓ **Antibiotics:** Empirical antibiotics are started as these patients are frequently on corticosteroids.

✓ **Management of concomitant pulmonary hypertension.**

✓ **Lung transplantation:** ECMO may be needed as bridge therapy.

Prognosis

✓ Idiopathic pulmonary fibrosis has an estimated 5-yr survival rate of approximately 20%.
  - 5-yr survival rate of other ILDs
    ❖ LIP: 60%
    ❖ NSIP: 80%
    ❖ Sarcoidosis: 90%
    ❖ COP: 100%

PULMONARY HYPERTENSION

Epidemiology

✓ **Pulmonary Hypertension:** Defined as a mean pulmonary artery pressure (mPAP)[Q] ≥ 20 mmHg, assessed by right heart catheterization (AHA 2023 Guidelines). Normal pressure is 11–20 mmHg.
  - **Mild:** mPAP 21–30 mmHg
  - **Moderate:** mPAP 31–40 mmHg
  - **Severe:** mPAP >40 mmHg

✓ **WHO Classification of Pulmonary Hypertension**[Q]
  - **Group 1** (precapillary arteries and arterioles): Pulmonary **arterial** hypertension (PAH) from *pulmonary vasculopathy* (e.g. idiopathic, connective tissue disorders, drug-related, like fenfluramine, methamphetamines).
  - **Group 2** (post-capillary veins and venules): Pulmonary **venous** hypertension due to **left heart disease** (e.g. LV systolic/diastolic dysfunction).
  - **Group 3** (alveoli and capillary beds): Pulmonary hypertension due to **lung disease** and hypoxia (e.g. COPD, interstitial lung disease, OSA).
  - **Group 4: Chronic thromboembolic** pulmonary hypertension (CTEPH) (e.g. venous thromboembolism).
  - **Group 5:** Pulmonary hypertension with **unknown origin** (e.g. *sarcoidosis,* thyroid disease, *CKD*, neurofibromatosis).

✓ **Physiology:** Pulmonary circulation accommodates the entire cardiac output while maintaining both low pressure and low vascular resistance.
  - Under normal conditions, a 3- to 4-fold increase in cardiac output should not significantly increase pulmonary pressures and RV workload.
  - Right ventricle has a thin wall and normally a significantly lower afterload compared to left ventricle and thus fails quickly with acute increases in afterload.

Clinical Features and Diagnosis

✓ *Mean pulmonary artery pressure >40 mmHg suggests that pulmonary hypertension is chronic in origin.*
  - **Acute pulmonary embolism** can cause pulmonary hypertension, and >50% obstruction of pulmonary vasculature must occur before pulmonary hypertension happens.
  - Pulmonary hypertension complicates up to 80% of cases of **ARDS** but is mostly mild to moderate in severity.

- **Eisenmenger's syndrome:** Reversal of a previous left-to-right shunt due to development of pulmonary hypertension.
✓ **History:** Shortness of breath on exertion, chest pain, orthopnoea, paroxysmal nocturnal dyspnoea, and signs of right heart failure, like ankle swelling.
✓ **Examination:** Prominent P2, RV heave, pansystolic murmur due to tricuspid regurgitation, prominent JVP, hepatomegaly, ascites.
✓ **ECG findings:** Right axis deviation, right atrial enlargement *(P-wave >2.5 mm)*, right bundle branch block, and right ventricular hypertrophy.
✓ **Chest X-ray:** Enlarged main and hilar pulmonary arterial shadows (>18 mm diameter in men, >16 mm diameter in women) with peripheral pulmonary vascular attenuation (pruning).
✓ **CTPA:** CTEPH if unexplained pulmonary hypertension.
- **HRCT:** Interstitial lung disease.
✓ **Transthoracic echo (TTE)** is the investigation of choice initially.
- Non-invasive estimates of pulmonary artery pressures, LV and RV function, and evaluation of vascular diseases.
- RV dilation, RV hypertrophy (RVH), right atrial enlargement, and dilated IVC.
- *Peak tricuspid regurgitation velocity (TRV) can be used to estimate pulmonary artery systolic pressure*[Q].
  - ❖ RVH is seen in chronic cor pulmonale and leads to increased systolic pressures (>35 mmHg) and tricuspid regurgitation jets (>60 mmHg), distinguishing it from acute core pulmonale.
- Echocardiographic estimates of PAP correlate well with invasively measured PAP for patients with left-sided heart disease, but not so for patients with underlying lung disease.
✓ **Right heart catheterization (pulmonary artery catheter)** is the gold standard for diagnosis of pulmonary hypertension and must be performed to confirm the diagnosis and determine the aetiology and treatment.
- **Pulmonary capillary wedge pressure (PCWP):** Indirect measure of left atrial pressure. Measured by inflating a balloon at the tip of the catheter in a pulmonary artery branch.
- $PVR^Q = mPAP - PCWP$. Measured in wood units.
  - ❖ Cardiac output

- Elevated PAP, **pulmonary capillary wedge pressure (PCWP) >15** mmHg, and pulmonary vascular resistance **(PVR) < 3 wood units (WU)** suggestive of **pulmonary venous hypertension (left heart disease).**
- Elevated PAP, PCWP <15 mmHg, PVR >3 WU suggestive of **PAH, PH to hypoxaemic lung disease, or CTEPH.**
- **Mixed venous oxygen saturation:** Low values <60% are suggestive of low cardiac output and right ventricular failure.
- **Vasodilator testing** can be done, and *vasodilator responsiveness* is defined as decrease in mean PAP by at least 10 mmHg and to a pressure less than 40 mmHg, with no change or an increase of cardiac output. It is predictive of response to calcium channel blockers in patients with idiopathic pulmonary hypertension.

Treatment (same principles as right ventricular failure)

✓ **Oxygen therapy:** Reverses hypoxic pulmonary vasoconstriction and can result in decrease in PVR and an increase in cardiac output.
- Avoid hypoxia, hypercapnia, acidaemia, and hypothermia[Q].
✓ **Mechanical ventilation:** High risk of cardiovascular collapse during induction.
- Although it increases PAP, mechanical ventilation is well tolerated in patients with mild to moderate pulmonary hypertension.
- Low tidal volume and low PEEP[Q] while avoiding permissive hypercapnia.
✓ **Fluid therapy:** Optimal fluid balance to prevent right heart failure.
✓ **Sinus rhythm:** Loss of AV synchrony can cause haemodynamic instability; hence, AF and AV blocks should be avoided.
✓ **Pulmonary vasodilators:** *Intravenous epoprostenol is the only medication with proven survival benefit for patients with idiopathic PAH.*
- iNO has not shown any mortality benefit in these patients.
  - ❖ iNO increases cGMP,[Q] and tachyphylaxis happens over time.
  - ❖ iNO in high doses[Q] can cause exacerbation of cardiogenic pulmonary oedema, methaemoglobinaemia, and renal impairment.

✓ **Vasopressors/Inotropes**
- **Dobutamine** decreases PVR in mild to moderate pulmonary hypertension.
- **Milrinone:** Decreased PVR and improves right ventricular contractility.
- **Norepinephrine:** Used carefully as it can increase mPAP and PVR. Used to counteract systemic hypotension due to pulmonary vasodilators.
- **Vasopressin:** Low-dose vasopressin causes more increase in SVR compared to PVR.

✓ **Mechanical support:** ECMO and right ventricular assist devices (RVAD) are being increasingly used for these patients.

✓ **Surgical management:** Balloon atrial septostomy can be done. Lung transplant may be required in eligible cases.

Prognosis

✓ P-wave amplitude 2.5 mV or more in lead II and RVH are associated with increased risk of death.

✓ Pulmonary hypertension requiring ICU care has a poor prognosis and high mortality up to 40%. High mortality in pregnancy (10–20% mortality).

HAEMOPTYSIS

Aetiology

✓ **Haemoptysis:** Blood derived from the lungs or bronchial tubes.
- **Massive haemoptysis:** More than 600 mL/24 h. Seen in 5–15% of patients presenting with haemoptysis.
- **Non-massive haemoptysis:** Quantity smaller than massive haemoptysis and greater than blood streaking.
- **Asphyxiating haemoptysis:** Bleeding rates >150 mL/h.

✓ **Etiological Classification**
- **Non-massive haemoptysis:** Bronchiectasis, pneumonia, lung carcinoma, tuberculosis.
- **Massive haemoptysis:**
  - ❖ **Infection:** Tuberculosis, necrotizing pneumonia due to *Staphylococcus*, *Klebsiella*.
  - ❖ **Malignancy:** Bronchial cancer, metastatic cancer.
  - ❖ **Vascular:** Arteriobronchial fistula, pulmonary artery rupture.
  - ❖ **Inflammatory:** Bronchiectasis, diffuse alveolar haemorrhage due to vasculitis.
  - ❖ **Trauma:** Blunt/penetrating injury, iatrogenic injury.
- **Idiopathic haemoptysis:** No cause known in 11–19% of patients. Seen mostly in men between age 30 and 50 yr.

✓ **Pathogenesis**
- **Bronchial arteries** are the chief source of blood of the airways in up to 90% of cases.
- **Endobronchial bleeding:** Bronchial artery, **parenchymal bleeding (alveolar haemorrhage)**, pulmonary artery.

Diagnosis

✓ **History**
- **Recurrent episodes:** Bronchiectasis, chronic bronchitis, cystic fibrosis.
- **Orthopnoea and paroxysmal nocturnal dyspnoea:** Passive congestion of lungs.

✓ **Examination**
- **Pulsating tracheostomy:** Tracheoarterial fistula (3 d to 6 wk later).
- **Crackles:** Passive congestion of lungs, diffuse alveolar haemorrhage.

✓ **Routine Evaluation**
- **Complete blood count:** Infection, haematological disorder, chronic blood loss.
- **Urinalysis:** Haematuria may suggest systemic disease like SLE, Goodpasture syndrome, ANCA-associated vasculitis.
- **Coagulation studies:** Excessive anticoagulation.
- **ECG:** Pulmonary embolism.
- **Chest X-ray:** Localized honeycombing (bronchiectasis), diffuse infiltrates (bleeding from thrombocytopaenia, lung contusion, passive congestion of lungs), cavitary lesion (aspergilloma).
- **Flexible bronchoscopy:** Localization of site best within 24 h of bleeding. BAL can help in diagnosis of diffuse alveolar haemorrhage.
  - ❖ Helpful in patients that are too unstable to go for a CT scan.
- **Nasopharyngoscopy:** To diagnose causes of pseudo-haemoptysis, like nasopharyngeal bleeds.

✓ **Special Evaluation**
- **High-resolution CT scan:** Bronchiectasis, tuberculosis, aspergilloma, tumours.

❖ Can't visualize mucosa and associated bronchitis, telangiectasis, benign papilloma, and Kaposi sarcoma.

- **Angiography:** To localize source of bleeding
- **Sputum:** Cytology (malignancy), *Tubercle bacilli*, fungi
- **Immunological screen:** ANA, ANCA, complement, rheumatoid factor, cryoglobulins, anti-GBM antibody

Treatment

✓ **Supportive Care:** Bed rest and mild sedation, as patient may be distressed.
- Coughing may be necessary to clear blood from the airways; hence, antitussive effects should not be used.
- *Reverse any coagulopathy.*
- *Nebulized adrenaline[Q], 1 mL of 1:1,000 mixed in 4 mL of NaCl 0.9%.*
- *Endotracheal intubation* and mechanical ventilation may be needed[Q].
- *Volume resuscitation if needed.*

✓ **Definitive Care**
- **Non-massive haemoptysis**
  ❖ **Bronchiectasis, chronic bronchitis, cystic fibrosis:** Antibiotics, increased mucociliary clearance by β-adrenergic agonists, smoking cessation.
  ❖ Topical adrenaline, topical tranexamic acid (TXA) using bronchoscopy[Q].
  ❖ Corticosteroids in immunologic lung diseases.
- **Massive haemoptysis[Q]**
  ❖ Protect the uninvolved lung from aspiration of blood with *bleeding side down*, and intubation with wide, single-lumen ETT to facilitate bronchoscopy.
  ❖ Double-lumen tube may be necessary later to separate lungs.
  ❖ Tamponading[Q] of the bleeding site by using endobronchial balloon or blocker.
  ❖ In case of trachea-arterial fistula[Q], over-inflate the cuff balloon.
  ❖ **Bronchial artery embolization (BAE):** Angiographic embolization of the vessel is being used after initial stabilization and localization of bleeding site. Complications are chest pain, dysphagia, and paraplegia[Q]. Repeat embolization

is an acceptable treatment approach for recurrent haemoptysis.
❖ **Endoluminal therapy:** Laser (Nd:YAG), argon plasma coagulation (APC), electrocautery via rigid bronchoscopy can be used to stop bleeding in central airway lesions.
❖ **Surgery:** Emergency surgery reserved for traumatic injury to the chest, iatrogenic pulmonary artery rupture, or pulmonary artery haemorrhage in the context of a resectable lung cancer. Elective surgery for patients with aspergillomas and TB.

Prognosis

✓ Mortality is due to asphyxiation and not exsanguination, and mortality for massive haemoptysis is between 9 and 38%.

DROWNING

Epidemiology

✓ **Drowning[Q]: Respiratory impairment** because of submersion or immersion in a liquid and that a liquid–air interface is present at the entrance to the victim's airway, preventing the victim from breathing air.
- **Immersion:** Airway above liquid surface. **Submersion:** Whole body underwater.

✓ **Fatal Drowning:** The person dies during the drowning process.
- **Non-fatal drowning:** Person survives after drowning.

✓ **Near Drowning:** Initial survival following immersion in liquid. Death after this is by either ARDS or effects of hypothermia. This term, along with *dry drowning, wet drowning*, and *secondary drowning*, isn't used anymore.
- **Dry drowning:** Intense laryngospasm as the water enters the upper airway. Hence, the laryngospasm itself causes hypoxaemia, and lungs are dry.

✓ **Classification of Drowning Victims at Scene**
- **Class 1:** No evidence of inhalation of water.
- **Class 2:** Evidence of inhalation of water and adequate ventilation.
- **Class 3:** Evidence of inhalation of water and inadequate ventilation.
- **Class 4:** Absent ventilation and circulation.

✓ **Risk Factors[Q]:** Men, children <14 yr, floods, African Americans, alcohol use, illegal drugs, inadequate supervision, inadequate swimming skills, epilepsy, lower socioeconomic status.

✓ **Pathophysiology of Drowning[Q]**
- **Anoxia:** Initial breath holding is followed by uncontrollable hyperventilation, aspiration, bronchospasm, and death.
- **Hypothermia:** Malignant arrhythmias, ventricular fibrillation below 28°C, and asystole less than 20°C.

✓ **Diving Reflex[Q]:** When a **human face submerges** in **cold water.**
- It is mediated by ophthalmic division of the trigeminal nerve and leads to **apnoea, bradycardia,** and **peripheral vasoconstriction.**
- Seen in children predominantly.

✓ **Cold Water Immersion Syndrome[Q]:** Respiratory and autonomic responses after sudden immersion of **whole body in cold water.**
- **Stage 1: Cold shock reflex** (<5 min): Sudden immersion in cold water (all UK fresh water with temperature <25°C) causes an involuntary gasp (torso reflex), followed by **increased respiratory drive and tachycardia,** causing increased cardiac output.
- **Stage 2: Swimming failure** (5–30 min): Muscular coordination loss due to cooling of limbs, hyperventilation-induced tetany, and shivering.
- **Stage 3: Hypothermia (>30 min):** Temperature <35°C leads to arrhythmias, ataxia, dysarthria,
- **Stage 4: Circumrescue circulatory collapse:** Arrhythmias due to cooling of heart and hypovolaemia due to cold diuresis.

Clinical Features and Diagnosis

✓ Loss of surfactant leading to **ARDS[Q],** pulmonary oedema (up to 12 h later), pneumonia.
- **Hypoxic brain injury** (20%)
- Arrhythmias
- Disseminated intravascular coagulation
- Acute tubular necrosis, haemoglobinuria, metabolic acidosis
- Cervical injury uncommon (<0.5%)

✓ **Saltwater or freshwater drowning:** No significant differences in electrolytes abnormalities.
- Both cause aspiration of vomited gastric contents and both cause pulmonary oedema.

Prevention and Treatment

✓ **Prevention:** Education, swimming, flotation devices.

✓ **Initial resuscitation**
- **Dynamic risk assessment:** Ensure personal safety and always minimize the danger to yourself.
- Remove the patient from water in the **horizontal position** (counters sudden circulatory collapse on release of water pressure), and **remove clothes to avoid hypothermia.**
- **Cervical spine immobilization** should be considered in all patients.
- Resuscitation should start with **five rescue breaths** as soon as possible before standard 30:2 compressions to ventilations.
- Hyperthermia should be always avoided in the acute recovery period.
- **Rewarming** should preferably be performed with ECMO, and non-ECMO warming should be started if patient can't be taken to an ECMO centre in 6 h.

✓ **Organ failure management:** Mechanical ventilation for ARDS, neuroprotective measures.
- **Steroids and antibiotics are not recommended.**
- Exogenous surfactant has been used, but not of much benefit.

Prognosis

✓ **Poor prognostic signs**
- **Scene:** Long period of submersion (>10 min), long resuscitation period (>25 min).
- **Emergency department:** Asystole as rhythm, GCS <5, and acidosis with pH <7.1 on admission.

BRONCHIECTASIS

Aetiology

✓ **Bronchiectasis:** Progressive respiratory disease characterized by **permanent** dilation of the bronchi and presents with a clinical spectrum of sputum, cough, and recurrent respiratory infections.

✓ **Causes**
- **Post-infection:** *Pseudomonas aeruginosa, Haemophilus influenzae, Moraxella catarrhalis, Staphylococcus aureus, Streptococcus pneumoniae*

- **Post–lung disease:** Asthma, COPD, allergic bronchopulmonary aspergillosis
- **Genetic lung disease:** Cystic fibrosis, primary ciliary dyskinesia (Kartagener's syndrome)
- **Autoimmune diseases:** Inflammatory bowel disease, rheumatoid arthritis, SLE, Marfan's syndrome
- **Immunodeficiency diseases:** Isolated IgA deficiency, DiGeorge syndrome, combined immunodeficiency
✓ **Pathophysiology:** All these four processes interact with one another to promote development of bronchiectasis.
  - *Infection*
  - Inflammation
  - *Mucociliary clearance dysfunction*
  - Structural lung damage

Clinical Features

✓ **Presentation in ICU:** Recurrent chest infections, haemoptysis, chronic respiratory failure, cor pulmonale.
✓ **Chest X-ray:** Ring shadows and tram-track opacities.
✓ **CT scan** is the investigation of choice and shows
  - Bronchi that appear larger than the accompanying artery (signet ring sign)[Q]
  - Irregular wall and lack of tapering
  - Bronchus visualized within 1 cm of the pleural surface
✓ **Scoring systems for judging severity**
  - Bronchiectasis severity index (BSI)
  - FACED (FEV_1, age, chronic colonization, extension to lobes affected, dyspnoea)
  - Bronchiectasis Radiologically Indexed CT Score (BRICS)

Treatment

✓ **Prevention:** Smoking cessation, annual influenza vaccination.
✓ *Identify and treat underlying cause.*
✓ **Airway clearance:** Physiotherapy, exercise, mucoactive drugs.
✓ **Infections:** Antibiotic treatment (macrolides) covering *Pseudomonas*, inhaled antibiotics (colistin, gentamicin).
✓ **Breathlessness:** Bronchodilators, rehabilitation.
✓ **Steroids:** No role of routine inhaled/oral steroids. Used only in patients with underlying asthma or COPD.
✓ **Lung transplant:** For patients with cystic fibrosis. For non-cystic fibrosis bronchiectasis (NCFB), age above 65 yr is a relative contraindication.

Prognosis

✓ *Pseudomonas* colonization has a high risk of developing complications.

Cystic Fibrosis

✓ **Aetiology:** Autosomal recessive disorder[Q] diagnosed by neonatal screening for the defective cystic fibrosis transmembrane conductance regulator (CFTR) gene using heel prick test.
  - **Incidence:** 1:2,500 in UK.
  - Affects chloride ion channels, leading to impaired clearance of secretions that causes.
    - ❖ **Lung:** Bronchiectasis.
    - ❖ **Pancreas:** Exocrine pancreatic insufficiency, diabetes mellitus.
    - ❖ **Liver:** Bile duct obstruction, cirrhosis.
    - ❖ **Kidney:** Renal stones, CKD.
    - ❖ **Bowel:** Meconium ileus in newborns, constipation, distal intestinal obstruction syndrome (DIOS[Q]).
    - ❖ **Reproductive system:** Infertility.
✓ **Management**
  - **Prevention**
    - ❖ **Nutrition:** Increase calorie intake and oral pancreatic enzyme
    - ❖ **Exercise:** Regular exercise to improve lung function
    - ❖ Chest physiotherapy
    - ❖ **Mucoactive agents** (dornase alfa, hypertonic saline, mannitol dry powder)
    - ❖ Antibiotics for prevention
    - ❖ Influenza vaccination every year
  - **Treatment**
    - ❖ **Antibiotics** for exacerbations
    - ❖ **CFTR modulators**
      - *Ivacaftor/tezacaftor/elexacaftor (IVA-TEZ-ELX)* plus ivacaftor (IVA) alone for people 12 yr and above.
      - *Tezacaftor/ivacaftor (TEZ-IVA)* plus IVA for people 6 yr and over.
      - *Lumacaftor-Ivacaftor (LUM-IVA)* for people 2 yr and over.

❖ Bronchodilators.

❖ **Non-invasive mechanical ventilation:** For patients with moderate or severe lung disease.

❖ Steroids to treat nasal polyps.

❖ **Lung transplant.**

• **Prognosis**

❖ Recent advancements in treatment have increased median age of survival to up to 66 yr.

POST-OPERATIVE PULMONARY COMPLICATIONS

✓ **Post-Operative Pulmonary Complications:** Umbrella term for adverse changes in the respiratory system immediately after surgery.

• **Common complications:** Respiratory infections, respiratory failure, pleural effusion, atelectasis, pneumothorax, bronchospasm, aspiration pneumonia, ARDS, tracheobronchitis.

• **Post-operative respiratory failure:** Post-operative PO_2 <8 kPa, PaO_2:FiO_2 <40 kPa, or saturation <90% on pulse oximetry, requiring oxygen therapy. European Perioperative Clinical Outcome (EPCO) 2015 definition.

✓ **Risk Factors for Post-Operative Pulmonary Complications**

• **Non-modifiable**

❖ Age >60 or 65 yr

❖ Male sex

❖ **Surgery:** Cardiothoracic surgery, upper abdominal surgery, major vascular surgery, neurosurgery, head and neck surgery

• **Modifiable**

❖ ASA > II

❖ **Comorbidity:** COPD, OSA, congestive heart failure, chronic liver disease, renal failure

❖ Smoking

❖ General anaesthesia

❖ Neuromuscular blocking drugs and reversal

❖ Nasogastric tube

❖ Preoperative anaemia <100 g/L

❖ Urea > 7.5 mmol/L

❖ Low serum albumin

✓ **Sleep Breathing Disorders:** Can precipitate respiratory failure in post-operative patients in undiagnosed cases.

• **Snoring:** Noisy breathing due to **partially blocked airway** during sleeping.

❖ Common and affects 45% adults occasionally and 25% regularly.

• **Obstructive sleep apnoea (OSA): Complete obstruction** of the upper airway during sleep, resulting in repetitive breathing pauses, leading to oxygen desaturation and arousal from sleep.

• **Obstructive sleep apnoea/hypopnea syndrome (OSAHS):** OSA plus daytime sleepiness leading to cognitive impairment or cardiovascular morbidity.

❖ **Obstructive apnoea:** Stoppage of airflow despite continued breathing efforts ≥10 s.

❖ **Hypopnea:** 30–50% reduction in thoraco-abdominal movement for ≥10 s.

❖ **Severity** of OSAHS by using **apnoea-hypopnea index (AHI): Mild:** 5–14 events per hour of sleep; **moderate:** 15–29 events per hour of sleep; **severe:** >30 events per hour of sleep

❖ $PaCO_2$ **is normal**[Q] **during daytime-awake patient.**

• **Obesity hypoventilation syndrome (OHS)/Pickwickian syndrome**[Q]

❖ Condition in overweight people in which they are unable to breathe rapidly or deeply enough, leading to low O_2 levels and high CO_2 levels.

❖ Combination of obesity (BMI ≥30 kg/m^2), daytime hypercapnia ($PaCO_2$ ≥6.5 kPa), and sleep-disordered breathing.

❖ NIV preferred over CPAP in patients with OHS.

• **Risk factors for OSAHS:** Obesity, male gender, alcohol intake, smoking, reduced nasal patency.

• **STOP-BANG questionnaire**[Q]**:** Used to predict risk of OSA. **Low risk:** 0–2; **intermediate risk:** 3–4; **high risk:** >5.

❖ Snoring loudly

❖ Tiredness during daytime

❖ Observation of stopping of breathing during sleep

❖ Pressure, high BP

❖ BMI >35 kg/m^2

❖ Age >50 yr
❖ Neck circumference >40 cm
❖ Gender: male
- **Diagnosis of OSAHS**: Overnight polysomnography used for diagnosis (Gold standard)^Q.
- **Management of OSAHS**: Lifestyle measures like weight loss, smoking cessation, alcohol reduction.
  ❖ Nocturnal CPAP
  ❖ Mandibular repositioning device

❖ Surgery (uvulopalatopharyngoplasty, maxillomandibular advancement, tonsillectomy, hypoglossal nerve stimulation).

✓ **Physiological Changes in Obesity**^{Q}
- **CVS:** Ischaemic heart disease, hypertension, cor pulmonale, venous thromboembolism.
- **Respiratory:** ↓ FRC^Q, ↓ chest wall compliance, ↑ asthma, ↑ OSA, ↑ pulmonary hypertension, chronic hypercarbia.
- **Metabolic:** ↑ DM, ↑ fatty liver, ↑ GERD, ↑ hiatal hernia.

5

Neurological Problems

ACUTE CEREBROVASCULAR STROKE

Aetiology

✓ **Stroke:** Stroke is a serious condition in which blood supply to a part of the brain is cut off.
  - **85% of strokes are ischaemic:** Malignant infarct if >2/3 of territory of MCA is involved.
  - **15% of strokes are haemorrhagic:** *Hypertension* is the cause in 50% of these cases (deep grey matter in thalamus).
    ❖ Other causes of haemorrhage are cerebral amyloid angiopathy, ruptured AVMs.
  - **Transient ischaemic attack (TIA):** Neurological dysfunction resulting from cerebral ischaemia rather than infarction seen on imaging.
    ❖ Symptoms are less than 24 h.
    ❖ High risk of stroke (10%) within next 30 d of presentation.
✓ **Bamford or Oxford Stroke Classification**^{Q} according to the stroke territory involved.
  - **Total and partial anterior circulation systems (TACS/PACS):** Middle and anterior cerebral arteries involved. TACS if all three and PACS if 2 out of 3 are involved.
    ❖ Unilateral weakness ± sensory deficit.
    ❖ Homonymous hemianopia.
    ❖ Higher cerebral dysfunction (aphasia and visuospatial disorders).
  - **Posterior circulation syndrome (POCS):** Affects posterior cerebral circulation (vertebral-basilar system). Patient has one of these.
  - Brainstem signs like cranial nerve palsies and contralateral motor/sensory deficit.
    ❖ Cerebellar symptoms (ataxia, dysarthria)
    ❖ Isolated homonymous hemianopia, cortical blindness

- **Lacuna syndrome (LACS):** A subcortical stroke because of small vessel disease. Patients have an **absence of higher cerebral dysfunction** and one of the following.
  ❖ Sensorimotor stroke
  ❖ Pure sensory stroke
  ❖ Pure motor stroke
  ❖ Ataxic hemiparesis

Clinical Features and Diagnosis of Ischaemic Stroke

✓ **FAST (Face, arm, speech, and time)** used in community to recognize stroke. Maximal deficit at onset.
✓ **Recognition of stroke in the emergency room (ROSIER)**^{Q} is a validated tool used for diagnosis in ED and helps distinguish between stroke (score >0) and stroke mimics (score <0).
✓ Quantification of **NIHSS**^{Q} **(National Institutes of Health Stroke Scale)** score in the ER for severity of stroke along with neurological examination. 11 items scored with a total score between 0 to 42 (severe stroke).
  - Door to physician ≤10 min, Door to stroke team ≤15 min
  - Door to CT scan initiation ≤25 min, Door to CT interpretation ≤45 min
  - Door to Thrombolysis ≤60 min, Door to Stroke unit admission ≤3 h
✓ Stroke is a **clinical diagnosis.** Non-contrast CT scan (NCCT) scan to rule out haemorrhage followed by **CT Angiography (CTA) to evaluate blocked vessel for endovascular treatment.**
  - Repeat cranial imaging should be performed 24 h after reperfusion therapy.
✓ **CT Scan findings: Loss of grey-white matter differentiation**, hypo-attenuation of deep

nuclei, *cortical hypo-density* with associated parenchymal swelling and **gyral effacement.**

- Opacity from higher to lower: Bone > blood > grey matter (thalamus, basal ganglia) > white matter > oedematous brain tissue > CSF > air.
- **Hyperdense MCA clot** may be seen on CT scan if due to embolism.

✓ **CT Perfusion:** Helps guide **the intravenous (IV) or endovascular therapy for equivocal cases** and *when thrombectomy is indicated after 6 h.*

- It provides information about at-risk tissue (penumbra) and necrotic core as well as collateral supply.

✓ **MRI** is more sensitive to detecting hyper-acute stroke.

- **Diffusion-weighted imaging (DWI)** can show alterations minutes after the insult (Ischaemia = white area on MRI).
- **Perfusion-weighted imaging (PWI)** quantifies ischaemic penumbra tissue.
- **MRI angiography (MRA)** can visualize large vessel occlusion or stenosis.
- **MRI with fat suppression** technique can confirm a suspected dissection.

✓ **Additional tests:** Blood glucose, *markers of cardiac ischaemia, coagulation studies.*

- **ECG** (AF), **EEG** (suspected seizure), **TTE** (rule out emboli), **LP** (if suspected SAH, meningitis or vasculitis).
- *Anti-cardiolipin antibodies,* hypercoagulable testing, serum protein electrophoresis, and fibrinogen in patients younger than 50 yr.

✓ **Neurological complications of ischaemic stroke**

- **Haemorrhagic transformation** is seen in 5–6% of patients.
- **Cerebral oedema:** Develops within 24–48 h after the onset of stroke. Cerebellar swelling can compress brainstem, impair CSF circulation and cause hydrocephalus.

✓ **Differential diagnosis:** Hypoglycaemia, intracranial space-occupying lesions, seizures (Todd's paresis), encephalopathies (hyperglycaemic, hypertensive, hyponatraemic, hepatic, uraemic), sepsis, drug toxicities (lithium, carbamazepine, and phenytoin), and migraine (hemiplegic migraine).

Ischaemic Stroke Involvement by Territory

✓ **Frontal lobe:** Hemiparesis with unilateral facial weakness, personality change, impaired judgement.

- **Temporal lobe:** Memory impairment
- **Parietal lobe:** *Hemi-spatial neglect,* hemi-sensory loss, impaired perception, and spatial weakness.
- **Occipital lobe:** Homonymous Hemianopia.
- **Cerebellum:** Abnormal gait, Ataxia, Vertigo, Nystagmus, nausea, and vomiting.
- **Brainstem:** Ptosis, Ocular palsy, loss of pupil reactivity to light, impaired gag reflex

✓ **MCA Territory:** Contralateral motor weakness and sensory deficit **(face and arm > leg)**, aphasia (language disturbances), apraxia, ipsilateral eye deviation, homonymous visual field defects, impaired spatial perception, or neglect.

- **ACA Territory:** Contralateral motor weakness and sensory deficit **(leg),** urinary incontinence, apraxia, anosmia, bilateral muteness
- **Posterior circulation infarcts (usually embolic):** Ipsilateral cranial nerve palsy along with contralateral motor/sensory deficit, vertigo, dysphagia, Horner syndrome, cerebellar dysfunction, cortical blindness.

✓ **Lateral medullary syndrome (Wallenberg's syndrome)**[Q]: Stroke involving the vertebral or the posterior inferior cerebellar artery.

- **Ipsilateral:** Horner's syndrome, ataxia, loss of pain and temperature on face.
- **Contralateral:** Loss of pain and temperature below the neck.

✓ **Carotid artery dissection:** Seen in *younger patients or after trauma.*

- Signs of headache, neck pain, Horner syndrome and cranial nerve palsies in addition to ischaemic stroke.

Prevention and Treatment of Ischaemic Stroke

✓ **Primary prevention**

- Smoking cessation
- Statins (for LDL >100 mg/dL)
- Hypertension control (<130/80 mmHg) using ACEI/ARBs
- HbA1c < 7%

✓ **Class I evidence of improved outcomes**

- Stroke care in specialist units (Cochrane systematic review)

- IV thrombolysis within 4.5 h[Q]
- Endovascular therapy within 6 h[Q]
- Platelets inhibitors like Aspirin (160–325 mg) within 48 h
- **Decompressive craniectomy** as soon as possible and ideally within 48 h

✓ **Definitive treatment:** Time of stroke onset is the last time they were seen without neurological deficits[Q].

- **Thrombolysis:** After ruling out thrombocytopaenia and intake of warfarin, heparin or DOACs. Alteplase 0.9 mg/kg with a maximum of 90 mg over 60 min and first 10% given as a bolus in 1 min.
  - ❖ **NINDS trial (1995)** showed that Alteplase given within 3 h of symptoms onset of stroke reduced the incidence of disability at 3 months.
  - ❖ **ECASS III trial (2008)** showed that Alteplase can be effective till 4.5 h.
  - ❖ **EXTEND trial (2019)** showed that Alteplase can be beneficial between 4.5 and 9 h in patients who had viable ischaemic penumbra on perfusion imaging.
  - ❖ **Absolute contraindications:** BP >185/110 mmHg, INR >1.7, Platelets <100,000, full-dose LMWH within last 24 h or DOAC within last 48 h, Ischaemic stroke within last 3 months, severe head trauma within last 3 months, intracranial or spinal surgery within last 3 months, active internal bleeding.
  - ❖ **Relative contraindications:** Pregnancy, major surgery, or trauma within last 14 d, Acute MI in last three months, lumbar puncture within last 7 d, previous GI bleed.
- **Endovascular treatment:** Patients with large artery occlusion in **anterior circulation** (Internal Carotid Artery, proximal part of MCA) benefit from intra-arterial interventions in addition to IV rt-PA.
  - ❖ Urgent transfer of candidates for endovascular treatment should be done even if the IV alteplase is running.
  - ❖ *Mechanical thrombectomy and stent retrievers are superior to endovascular thrombolysis[Q].*
  - ❖ No change in clinical outcomes with use of endovascular treatment of occluded

basilar artery but still attempted due to no significant safety issues and intravenous thrombolysis is rarely effective.

- ❖ *Mechanical thrombectomy can be done up to 24 h after patient selection with CT-Perfusion/MRI-Perfusion.*
- ❖ *DAWN trial (2018):* Thrombectomy in patients of acute stroke within 6–24 h from onset had superiority regarding functional independence and disability at 90 d.
- ❖ *DEFUSE-3 trial (2018): Thrombectomy using perfusion imaging as guidance plus medical therapy in comparison to medical therapy alone within 6–16 h of stroke onset resulted in lower rates of disability and improved 90 d functional outcomes on the mRS.*

- **Supratentorial decompressive craniectomy for malignant MCA infarction**
  - ❖ **Malignant MCA infarction:** Rapid neurological deterioration due to cerebral oedema following MCA stroke.
  - ❖ **NICE Criteria[Q]: Age 18–60 yr, NIHSS score >15, MRI Infarct volume >145 cm³ or CT signs of infarct >50% of the middle cerebral artery territory** in patients within 48 h of symptoms.
  - ❖ Sub-occipital craniectomy along with a ventricular catheter for *cerebellar infarction.*
  - ❖ Benefit appears when surgery is performed early (within 48 h) after stroke onset.
  - ❖ **DESTINY trial (2007):** In patients between **18–60 yr of age with MCA infarction,** DC decreased mortality with no significant difference in disability.
  - ❖ **DECIMAL trial (2007):** In patients between **18–55 yr of age with MCA infarction,** DC decreased mortality with significant increase in disability at 12 months.
  - ❖ **HAMLET trial (2009):** DC within 48 h, reduced mortality but no effect on the chance of a good functional outcome.
  - ❖ **DESTINY II (2011):** In patients >**60 yr old,** improved survival but more functional debilitation.

✓ **Supportive management:** *NIHSS score >17 is an indication for ITU admission.*
  - **Intubated patient:** Maintain PaO_2 >10.6 Kpa. Self-ventilating: Saturation >94% in ITU.
  - **BP Control[Q]:** <185/110 mmHg for 24 h before and after thrombolysis and <220/120 mmHg except in those with severe comorbidities (aortic dissection, encephalopathy) not undergoing thrombolysis (NICE guidelines).
    ❖ <15% drop in the BP in first 24 h in those not receiving thrombolysis.
    ❖ IV labetalol, nicardipine are used to control blood pressure.
  - Hypotension should be treated with fluids (0.9% Saline) followed by vasopressors like norepinephrine.
  - **Intracranial pressure (ICP): Routine ICP monitoring is not recommended.** Mannitol 1g/kg or 3% hypertonic saline can be used.
  - **Glucose control** between 8–10 mmol/L in ITU. Hyperglycaemia seen in 40% of patients with stroke at admission. *It is a marker of illness severity.*
  - **Pyrexia** is in up to 50% of patients and is an independent predictor of a poor outcome. **Treat temperatures above >37.5°C.** *IV Metamizole/Diclofenac infusion can be used.*
  - **Swallow assessment should be done** soon after admission as dysphagia is common.
  - **Statins[Q]** should be started after 48 h if they are not already on it.
  - **Proton pump inhibitors** only if patient has a history of aspirin dyspepsia or dual antiplatelet therapy.
  - **Seizures:** Routine prophylactic anticonvulsant is not recommended. Treat documented seizures. *EEG to exclude non-convulsive seizures.*
  - **Steroids:** No role in management of cerebral oedema associated with acute ischaemic stroke.
  - Optimal timing of the tracheostomy has been controversial.
✓ **Venous thromboembolism:** Anticoagulants shouldn't be started within 24 h of thrombolysis.
  - Aspirin (160–325 mg) within 48 h of stroke onset but not until 24 h after thrombolysis[Q].
  - Patients with aspirin-related dyspepsia should be offered a proton pump inhibitor (PPI) as well as aspirin.

- **Aspirin and Clopidogrel in mild to moderate cases of stroke for 3 wk followed by Clopidogrel monotherapy[Q].**
- *Intermittent pneumatic calf compression should be started immediately.*
- For patients with non-valvular AF and small infarcts, start anticoagulation therapy and keep INR between 2–3.
- For patients with large acute infarcts, begin anticoagulation within 4–14 d of stroke onset.

Intracerebral haemorrhage: Bleeding into brain parenchyma.

✓ **Causes:** Hypertension, malignancy, amyloidosis, haemorrhagic transformation of ischaemic stroke, drugs like cocaine, amphetamines.
✓ *Clinical signs: Fast progression of symptoms in minutes, early excessive vomiting, headache, seizure, and coma.*
  - More than 50% of patients are comatose at presentation.
✓ **Territory wise symptoms**
  - **Putamen (30–50%): Lenticulostriate arteries[Q].** *Hemiplegia and hemisensory disturbances, homonymous hemianopia, paralysis of conjugate gaze to the side opposite the lesion.*
    ❖ Subcortical aphasia if dominant hemisphere and hemineglect if non-dominant side.
  - **Thalamus (10%):** Unilateral sensorimotor findings. May enter ventricular system and cause hydrocephalus.
  - **Pontine (10%):** Highest mortality. Quadriplegia, small pupils.
  - **Cerebellar (10%):** Dentate nucleus is most involved. Limb ataxia, *ipsilateral gaze palsy, lower motor neuron facial paresis,* nystagmus, vomiting, vertigo.
✓ CT scan is the modality of choice of acute haemorrhage. *CT angiography in younger patients to rule out aneurysms and AV malformations.*
✓ Reverse anticoagulation and liaise with haematology.
✓ **Recommended systolic blood pressure[Q] is between 130–140 mmHg, and should be done as fast as possible (within 1 h) and maintain this target for at least 7 d.**
  - Beta-blockers and nicardipine are recommended.

- **INTERACT 2 trial (2013):** No difference in death or major disability at 90 d in target of SBP of 140 mmHg vs 180 mmHg for 7 d in patients with spontaneous ICH.
- **ATACH-II trial (2016):** No difference in death or major disability in target of SBP of <140 mmHg vs <180 mmHg for 24 h in patients with spontaneous ICH.
- *Chemical prophylaxis may be started 48–72 h after cessation of bleeding for non-high-risk patients after neurosurgical consultation.*
✓ *Surgery may be indicated for lobar ICH in which patient continues to deteriorate, for cerebellar ICH or if hydrocephalus is present.*
  - **STITICH I—ICH trial (2005):** In patients with spontaneous intracerebral haemorrhage, early surgical haematoma evacuation, had no mortality benefit at 6 months.
  - **STITCH II—ICH trial (2013):** In patients with superficial spontaneous intracerebral haemorrhage, early surgical haematoma evacuation, had no mortality benefit at 6 months.
✓ Risk factors for mortality are calculated using **ICH score** which has parameters like age>80 yr, low GCS at presentation, *ICH volume >30 mL,* infratentorial origin of bleed and intraventricular extension of blood.

Additional Questions

✓ **Subclavian steal syndrome[Q]:** Subclavian stenosis proximal to the origin of the vertebral artery can lead to vertebra-basilar insufficiency (posterior circulation symptoms).
✓ **Pseudobulbar palsy[Q]:** Upper motor neuron paralysis. Spastic paralysis.
  - **Bulbar palsy:** Lower motor neuron paralysis. Flaccid paralysis.
✓ **Cerebellar hemisphere lesions[Q]:** Ipsilateral dysmetria, dysdiadochokinesis, intention tremor and fast beat nystagmus toward the lesion.
  - **Cerebellar vermis lesions[Q]:** Truncal ataxia and ataxic gait.

SUBARACHNOID HAEMORRHAGE

Aetiology

✓ **Subarachnoid haemorrhage:** Bleeding into subarachnoid space.

✓ **Traumatic subarachnoid haemorrhage** is the most common cause[Q].
  - **Ruptured cerebral aneurysm[Q]** is the most common form (85%) of non-traumatic subarachnoid haemorrhage (SAH). AV malformations, CVST, moyamoya disease are other causes.
✓ Median age is 53 yr. Females form two-thirds of cases.
  - **Risk factors[Q]:** Smoking, hypertension, cocaine, and high alcohol intake, Ehlers–Danlos syndrome.
  - **Location:** 30–35% are at junction of anterior communicating and anterior cerebral artery.
    - ❖ 30–35% around origin of posterior communicating artery.
    - ❖ 20% around middle cerebral artery bifurcation.
    - ❖ 20–30% of patients have multiple aneurysms.
✓ Saccular aneurysms don't have normal muscular media and elastic lamina layers hence prone to rupture.

Clinical Features

✓ A sentinel (warning) bleed occurs in 20% of patients and is characterized by **"thunderclap"** headache.
  - Common symptoms are severe headache, neck pain, nausea and vomiting, diplopia, photophobia, and seizures.
  - 50% of patients lose consciousness at time of rupture and patient may show *abducens nerve palsies due to raised intracranial pressure.*

Hunt and Hess Grading Scale for Prognosis

Grade	Symptoms	Mortality (%)
I	Asymptomatic or **minimal** headache	11
II	**Moderate to severe** headache, nuchal rigidity, **cranial nerve palsy**	26
III	Drowsiness, confusion, **focal neurological deficits**	37
IV	Stupor, moderate to **severe hemiparesis**	71
V	Deep coma, **decerebrate rigidity**	100

World Federation of Neurological Surgeons Scale (WFNS)[Q]

Grade	Motor Deficit	GCS	Risk of Severe Disability, Death (%)
1	–	15	13
2	–	13–14	20
3	+	13–14	42
4	±	7–12	51
5	±	3–6	68

Modified Fisher Scale

Grade	IVH	SAH Characteristics on Admission CT Head Scan	Risk of Symptomatic Vasospasm (%)
1	–	Localized thin or diffused thin	24
2	+	Localized thin or diffused thin	33
3	–	Localized thick or diffused thick	33
4	+	Localized thick or diffused thick	40

✓ **Diagnosis: Non-Contrast CT Scan is 100%** sensitive in first 6 to 12 h and 90% sensitive at 24 h in detecting SAH.
  - If CT scan is non-diagnostic, **lumbar puncture** is indicated[Q]. Diagnostic finding is **xanthochromia,** yellowish appearance of CSF following centrifugation.
    ❖ **Absolute contraindications:** Refusal and local infection.
    ❖ **Relative contraindications:** Coagulopathy and raised ICP.
  - **CT Angiogram** is done to identify an aneurysm in the emergency setting (sensitivities and specificities >98%).
  - **MR Angiogram** can be done several days later when a head CT may be negative.
  - **Four-Vessel Cerebral Angiography** is gold standard to localize the lesion and assess vasospasm and can be repeated in 1–3 wk if negative.
    ❖ It is done as soon as possible as endovascular treatment can be provided simultaneously.

  ❖ More invasive than CT angiogram as catheter is inserted directly in the artery.
✓ **Neurological Complications**[Q]
  - **Rebleeding:** 6% of patients in the first 24 h and carries a high mortality rate (>50%). Unlikely once the aneurysm has been secured.
    ❖ A blood pressure of <160 mmHg is recommended before the aneurysm is secured.
  - **Seizures:** 5–10% of patients will develop them.
    ❖ *Middle cerebral artery aneurysm and thick SAH blood clot increase the risk of developing seizures and highest risk is on the first day.*
    ❖ *Non-convulsive seizures can be seen later in course and should be sought after in a case with new onset drowsiness.*
  - **Hydrocephalus**[Q]**:** 20–30% of patients. More commonly in patients with severe grades of SAH. Can happen within first 24 h after SAH and occurs within first 3 d.
    ❖ Impairment of vertical gaze and progressive lethargy.
    ❖ **Ventriculostomy or lumbar drainage**[Q] is done when the clinical neurological examination deteriorates.
  - **Cerebral vasospasm (cVSP) and delayed cerebral ischaemia (DCI):** Most common cause of early death in SAH patient. *DCI is clinical manifestation of cVSP.*
    ❖ Seen between days 4–12 post-bleed. **Maximum between day 7 and 10**[Q]. Vasospasm related to amount of blood in CSF.
    ❖ Traumatic subarachnoid blood is not associated with vasospasm.
    ❖ **cVSP is evident on transcranial Doppler (TCD) for 70% of patients and 60% on angiography but clinically evident symptoms (DCI) in only 35% of patients.**
    ❖ **Transcranial Doppler: Flow velocities** >120 cm/s or **Lindegaard ratio (LR)**[Q]**:** a ratio of flows >3 between the middle cerebral artery compared with the ipsilateral internal carotid artery indicates vasospasm.
    ❖ **Digital subtraction angiography (DSA)**[Q]**:** Best investigation of choice

for vasospasm. CT angiography is up to 95% specific and correlates well with DSA.

❖ **EEG** showing reduced **alpha variability** can also be used for diagnosis.

❖ **CT perfusion** assessing the adequacy of perfusion can also be ordered to predict the need for endovascular intervention.

✓ **Cardiac complications**[Q]: Myocardial Infarction, stress cardiomyopathy, and neurogenic pulmonary oedema.

- Arrhythmias in up to 30% of SAH cases. **Elevated troponin and BNP** are seen but pathological Q waves are not seen commonly.
- ECG changes[Q] are T wave inversion, prolonged QT interval, and ST segment depression/elevation.

✓ **Metabolic complications**[Q]

- **Hyponatraemia:** 30% of patients. 4–10 d after admission. Cerebral salt wasting (CSW) and SIADH are the causes.
  - ❖ SIADH is treated by giving hypertonic saline instead of fluid restriction.
  - ❖ CSW is treated with isotonic fluids and fludrocortisone.
- **Hypernatraemia:** Diabetes Insipidus.

✓ **Inherited conditions with aneurysms**[Q]: Polycystic kidney disease, Ehlers–Danlos syndrome.

Prevention and Treatment

✓ **Resuscitation by ABCDE approach and Neuroprotective measures:** Set of manoeuvres done to prevent secondary brain injury.

✓ **Early goals of treatment are to identify and treat aneurysm by either coiling or clipping.**

- Treating patients in high volume SAH treatment centres *(>35 SAH/year) has shown mortality benefit.*
- *Prior to securing the aneurysm, SBP <160 mmHg[Q] or MAP <110 has been recommended to prevent rebleeding.* **BP control should not reduce the MAP below 90** mmHg.
  - ❖ Treatment is IV labetalol, nicardipine.

✓ **Coiling** better than clipped aneurysms seen in **ISAT trial (2005)**[Q].

- ❖ Coiling[Q] might lead to high recurrence rates but better for MCA aneurysms, wide necked aneurysms.

❖ Surgical clipping for anatomical challenged cases.

✓ **Vasospasm:** Oral Nimodipine 60 mg every 4 h for 21 d has mortality benefit but incidence of vasospasm in not reduced as the mechanism of action now is thought to be different from reducing vasospasm.

- **TXA or Triple H** (Hypervolaemia, hypertension, and haemodilution) therapy has no benefit.
  - ❖ Euvolaemia without hypertension is recommended before onset of cVSP.
  - ❖ **Hypertension-hypervolaemia therapy (HH-T) is indicated once clinically significant vasospasm (DCI) occurs.**
  - ❖ Haemodilution only in patients with erythrocytosis.
- **Intra-arterial infusion of vasodilators** such as verapamil, nicardipine, and milrinone has been used in patients with DCI and a repaired aneurysm.
- **Ventriculostomy and lumbar drain** to drain blood from CSF are often used to decrease the burden of blood in the CSF. Angioplasty can also be used.

✓ **Prophylactic anticonvulsants**[Q] indicated prior to securing the aneurysm and should be stopped as soon as possible. Agents other than phenytoin should be used.

- Patients who had seizures or at high risk of seizures should be continued on anticonvulsant therapy.

✓ **Supportive management:** Head elevation to improve cerebral venous return, good pulmonary toilet to avoid pneumonia.

- Fever is a common symptom. No benefit of intraoperative hypothermia though.
- Avoid hyperglycaemia and maintain blood glucose levels between 6–10 mmol/L.
- **Dexamethasone may help improve meningitis symptoms but are not recommended in the management of acute SAH.**
- **Venous Thromboembolism (VTE):** Pneumatic compression boots on admission. Antiplatelet and anticoagulant drugs should be discontinued and restarted once the aneurysm is secured.

Prognosis

✓ **Risk factors for poor outcome:** Female sex, co-morbid conditions, WFNS grade IV/V, posterior circulation aneurysm.

✓ Mortality rate from a ruptures aneurysmal subarachnoid haemorrhage (aSAH) is between 30–50%.

CEREBRAL VENOUS SINUS THROMBOSIS

Epidemiology and Aetiology

✓ **Cerebral venous sinus thrombosis (CSVT):** Thrombus formation in the cerebral venous system.
  • Accounts for 1% of all strokes and typically affects young patients (20–50 yr old)[Q] with a 3-fold female preponderance.
✓ The **superior sagittal** and **transverse sinuses** are most frequently involved sinuses[Q]. **Multiple areas** (two-thirds of patients) might be involved simultaneously and this differentiates it from arterial occlusion.
✓ **Risk factors**[Q].
  • **Thrombophilic conditions** like pregnancy, oral contraceptive use, antiphospholipid syndrome, malignancy, dehydration, nephrotic syndrome, heparin-induced thrombocytopaenia.
  • **Mechanical** causes like traumatic brain injury, post-neurosurgical procedures.
  • **Head and neck infections** like mastoiditis, sinusitis, otitis media, meningitis, cerebral abscess.
✓ **Pathophysiology:** *Venous congestion* leads to **haemorrhagic infarct** due to back pressure, **cerebral oedema**, and **hydrocephalus** due to *reduced CSF flow.*

Clinical Features and Diagnosis

✓ **Signs and symptoms:** *Headache exacerbated by lying down (MC complaint)*[Q], nausea, vomiting, papilledema, **abducens nerve palsy**, seizures, **hemiparesis (up to 40% of patients)**, dysarthria, aphasia, visual impairment, and encephalopathy.
  • Fever may be seen in patients with infected thrombophlebitis.
  • **Communicating hydrocephalus:** Venous sinuses play a role in draining CSF and hence thrombosis leads to hydrocephalus.
✓ **Laboratory studies for CSVT:** Thrombocytopaenia, raised D-dimer (>4000 μg/L)[Q], coagulation panel (low fibrinogen), and blood cultures if signs of thrombosis.

✓ **EEG** if seizure is a concern and evaluation of intracranial pressure with ultrasound to evaluate papilledema.
✓ **MR Venography (MRV) or CT venography (CTV)** are needed for diagnosis.
  • Filling defects (**empty delta sign**)[Q] can be seen in a dural sinus in CTV.
✓ **Non-contrast CT scan** may show direct signs like the clot itself (hyper-density in vessel) or indirect signs like haemorrhage in parenchyma or oedema due to clot.
  • **Dense triangle sign**[Q]: Clot in superior sagittal sinus.
  • **Dense cord sign**[Q]: Clot in a cortical or deep vein.
✓ **Invasive catheter angiography** may be used when CT and MRI are equivocal.

Treatment

✓ Haematology referral.
✓ **Anticoagulation:** Heparin anticoagulation. *Intracranial haemorrhage isn't a contradiction to anticoagulation (it's true, its true).*
  • **LMWH** is generally preferred and **unfractionated heparin is used** for patients who are critically ill and likely to require a procedure.
    ❖ **Oral anticoagulant:** Transition to OACs for 3–12 months depending on underlying cause and indefinitely in the presence of thrombophilia or recurrent VTE.
  • **Pregnancy:** Full anticoagulation throughout pregnancy and future pregnancy is not contraindicated[Q].
✓ **Seizures:** Prophylaxis only for individuals at high risk of seizures (supratentorial lesions with involvement of cortex, focal oedema, or neurological deficits).
  • Even a single seizure should be aggressively treated.
✓ **Catheter-directed endovascular therapy** (intrasinus thrombolysis or endovascular thrombectomy) as rescue therapy for progressive disease.
✓ **Impending herniation:** Neuroprotective measures along with decompressive craniectomy may be needed.
  • **Communicating hydrocephalus:** External ventricular drain (EVD) or lumbar

puncture and acetazolamide to treat isolated intracranial hypertension.
- ✓ **Underlying problems:** Antibiotics for infections and steroids for vasculitis.

Prognosis

- ✓ Mortality is 5%. Risk of permanent disability is 15–20%.

Additional Questions

Vaccine-induced immune thrombocytopaenia and thrombosis (VITT)[Q]**:** Seen in patients post–Covid-19 vaccination.
- ✓ **Clinical features:** Presents 5–30 d (median 12 d) after vaccination with both venous and arterial thrombosis (cerebral and abdominal) seen.
  - Thrombocytopaenia, D-dimer, and **anti-platelet factor-4 (PF-4)**[Q] antibody positive.
- ✓ **Treatment:** IVIg, plasmapheresis, steroids, and Rituximab.

STATUS EPILEPTICUS

Definitions

- ✓ **Epilepsy:** Patients with two or more seizures.
- ✓ **Status epilepticus (SE): Intensive Care Society (ICS) definition:** Seizure activity for 5 min or more without return of consciousness or recurrent seizures (two or more) without a period of recovery in between.
  - **Tonic–clonic status epilepticus:** GTCS is the most common form of status epilepticus[Q].
  - **Focal status epilepticus with preserved awareness:** A clonic activity is usually localized to the face or an extremity.
  - **Non-convulsive status epilepticus (NCSE):** Prolonged confusional state of **30 min or longer,** involving a variable level of altered consciousness with seizure activity on EEG.
    - ❖ Includes absence SE and focal SE with impaired awareness.
    - ❖ Signs like eye twitching, deviation, blinking, face twitching, delirium, aphasia, mutism, catatonia.
  - **Anoxic myoclonic status epilepticus:** Caused by toxic or metabolic encephalopathies, most commonly severe hypoxic ischaemic encephalopathy resulting from cardiac arrest.
- ✓ **Refractory status epilepticus (RSE):** *SE that doesn't respond to initial pharmacological therapy of one benzodiazepine and one non-benzodiazepine*[Q].
- ✓ **Super-refractory status epilepticus (SRSE):** SE that continues despite an adequate continuous infusion of *IV anaesthetic agents* for *more than 24 h.* Seen in autoimmune encephalitis.
- ✓ **Non-epileptic attack disorder (NEAD):** Involuntary physical reaction to psychological stress that resembles epileptic seizures but lack the abnormal electrical activity. Treatment is mainly psychological therapy.

Aetiology

- ✓ Structural brain lesion
  - **Stroke:** Up to 20% of cases
  - **Brain trauma:** Early seizures after trauma are predictive of long-term epilepsy
  - **Brain tumour**
- ✓ **Drugs**
  - **Changes or decreases of antiseizure drugs:** Up to 35% cases
  - **Toxic** e.g. theophylline, carbapenems, lidocaine.
  - **Withdrawal state:** Alcohol, benzodiazepine, and barbiturates.
- ✓ **Metabolic:** Hypocalcaemia, hypomagnesaemia, hyponatraemia, hypoglycaemia, hyperglycaemia, uraemia.
- ✓ **Central nervous system infections**
- ✓ **Autoimmune encephalitis**
- ✓ **Sepsis**

Clinical Features

- ✓ **Cardiovascular** Hypertension, tachycardia, hyperglycaemia. All because of sympathetic stimulation.
  - **Respiratory:** Increased bronchial secretions, aspiration pneumonia, neurogenic pulmonary oedema, apnoea.
  - **Metabolic:** Hypoglycaemia, hyperkalaemia, hyperthermia, lactic acidosis.
- ✓ **CSF Changes:** Mild pleocytosis with cell count <80 cells/μL. Mild transient elevation of CSF protein.
  - Lowering of CSF glucose doesn't occur and reduced CSF glucose points towards an infection/inflammation.

✓ Permanent neurological damage can happen even after 20 min of status epilepticus.
  • Non-epileptic seizures don't lead to tongue biting, faecal or urinary incontinence.
  • Febrile seizures are common in children but rarely lead to epilepsy.

Diagnosis

✓ Most general tonic–clonic and focal seizure cases are diagnosed based on clinical status.
  • NCSE are diagnosed by EEG with continuous electrographic seizure activity seen for ≥10 continuous minutes.
✓ Continuous EEG is advised for patients with ongoing depressed consciousness or patients with RSE or SRSE.
✓ Laboratory tests that should be sent are
  • Ammonia levels, urinary organic acids, blood amino acids.
  • **Vasculitis screen:** Antinuclear antibody (ANA), anti-neutrophil cytoplasmic antibody (ANCA), complement.
  • **Autoimmune encephalitis screen:** N-Methyl-D-Aspartate receptor (NMDAR), LGI1 and CASPR2 antibodies (voltage-gated potassium channels), $GABA_AR$ antibodies, $GABA_BR$ antibodies, Glutamic acid decarboxylase (GAD) antibodies, anti-neuronal (paraneoplastic) antibodies, Thyroid peroxidase (TPO) antibodies.
✓ **CT thorax, abdomen, and pelvis (CT TAP)** with contrast to look for evidence of occult neoplasia and indirect evidence of paraneoplastic limbic encephalitis.
✓ Anti-convulsant drug levels if on anti-convulsant to assess the compliance.

Treatment

✓ **Treatment Plan[Q]**
  • **Step 1:** Maintain airway, give oxygen, check blood glucose. **If hypoglycaemia, give dextrose 50%, 50–100 mL and thiamine 100 mg IV[Q].**
  • **Step 2:** First 5 min of seizure: Lorazepam 0.1 mg/kg IV or IO (max 4 mg[Q]) or Midazolam 0.5 mg/kg buccal or IM (10 mg max[Q]).
  • **Step 3:** 15 min of seizure: Second dose of Lorazepam 0.1 mg/kg IV (max 4 mg).
  • **Step 4:** 15–30 min of seizure: Fosphenytoin

20 mg/kg or phenytoin 20 mg/kg (maximum dose of 2000 mg) over 20 min or levetiracetam 60 mg/kg IV (up to 4500 mg) or Valproate IV 40 mg/kg (up to 3000 mg). **Call ITU[Q].**
  • **Step 5:** Seizure persists over 45 min: General anaesthesia should be given using propofol or thiopentone. **ITU transfer, CT scan, and EEG.**
✓ **Lorazepam** is initial drug of choice. Pre-existing anti-epileptic medication should be administered as they might have been missed any recent reduction in the dose reversed.
  • Prehospitally, patient can have **10 mg of PR Diazepam[Q]**, *repeated after 15 min if still fitting.*
✓ **Fos-phenytoin** is more expensive than phenytoin, but better drug profile as can be given intramuscularly, rapidly as phenytoin can extravasate into adjacent tissue and cause tissue necrosis.
✓ Muscle relaxants do not terminate seizures. **Propofol, midazolam, and thiopentone are recommended for refractory status epilepticus (60 min).** Thiopentone has strongest anti-convulsant effect.
  • **Thiopentone:** Iso-electric waveform in large doses whereas smaller doses show burst-suppression. It shouldn't be stopped until 12–24 h after last clinical seizure.
  • **Propofol:** Doesn't cause iso-electric waveform.
  • **Midazolam** doesn't cause iso-electric or burst-suppression even at higher doses. Tachyphylaxis seen with midazolam after 36–48 h.
  • Inhalational anaesthetics may need to be brought in as well.
  • **Goal is to produce a burst suppression for a period of 24–48 h[Q].**
✓ **CT head scan should be done followed by lumbar puncture. Start EEG monitoring immediately after these investigations.**
✓ **Neurology review** should be taken. Immuno-modulatory treatment like methylprednisolone 1mg/day for 3 days, intravenous immunoglobin (IVIG) and plasma exchange.
  • Second-line therapies include: Rituximab, Cyclophosphamide, Tocilizumab, and Anakinra.
✓ **Deep brain stimuli:** Thalamic nuclei, hippocampus, subthalamic nucleus and cerebellum.
  • Most common side effect associated with DBS was implantation site pain.

✓ **Ketogenic diet:** Treatment for super-refractory status epilepticus. High-fat and low-protein/carbohydrate diet given via NG tube.

Prognosis

✓ Mortality for refractory status epilepticus: 35–60%, 80% with anoxic status epilepticus.
  • Mortality after first episode of generalized convulsive status epilepticus: 16–20%.
  • Hospital mortality rate after NCSE is 18–50%.
  • Elderly with unknown aetiology have worse prognosis than younger patients with known aetiology.
  • Duration of status epilepticus longer than 30 min increases mortality.
✓ 40% of patients after the first episode of status epilepticus will develop subsequent epilepsy.
  • 25–30% risk of recurrent status epilepticus.
✓ Previous condition of pre-existing epilepsy, duration of seizure, level of consciousness and comorbid condition are risk factors that have effect on patient mortality and morbidity.

DISORDERS OF CONSCIOUSNESS

✓ **Consciousness:** State of perception of environment and self that relies on intact arousal and awareness.
  • **Arousal (wakefulness):** Ability to open the eyes spontaneously or on stimulation.
  • **Awareness (content):** Ability to interact with the environment.
✓ **Continuum of consciousness**[Q]
  • **Coma:** State of unresponsiveness in which patient doesn't open the eyes and has no signs of awareness.
    ❖ **Neither arousal nor awareness.**
    ❖ Most severe form of disordered consciousness.
    ❖ Coma can progress to either **brain death which is irreversible cessation of all brain functions including brain stem** or one of the below states.
  • **Vegetative state (VS):** *Wakefulness without awareness.*
    ❖ **Continuing VS**[Q]**:** If it lasts more than 4 wk.
    ❖ **Chronic VS**[Q]**:** If persists for more than 1 yr after traumatic brain injury and

more than 3 months after other brain injuries.
• **Minimally consciousness state (MCS):** *Presence of wakefulness* with *inconsistent* but reproducible goal-directed behaviour and awareness like eye tracking, blinking to threat, grabbing the bedsheets.
  ❖ **MCS plus:** Higher-level responses like command following.
  ❖ **MCS minus:** Lower-level responses like visual pursuit.
  ❖ **Continuing MCS:** If it lasts more than 4 wk.
  ❖ **Chronic MCS plus:** If persists for more than 18 months after traumatic brain injury and more than 9 months after other brain injuries.
  ❖ **Chronic MCS minus:** If persists for more than 12 months after traumatic brain injury and more than 3 months after other brain injuries.
• **Emerged:** Reliable and consistent responses.
• **Confused state:** Confusion, agitation, disorientation.
• **Normal recovery**
✓ **Locked-in syndrome**[Q]**:** Total paralysis of limbs without loss of consciousness. Due to destruction of **base of pons** and patient can only do vertical eye movements and blinking.
  ❖ They can hear, see, and feel pain.
✓ **Altered states of consciousness:** Depends on *reticular activating system in midbrain and upper pons and projections to higher brain centres* like thalamus, hypothalamus, and cortex. Lower pons and medulla that control respiration and cardiovascular system are not involved.
• **Confusion:** Awake with eyes open but disoriented and **unable to reason.**
• **Delirium:** Awake with eyes open but **impaired cognition**, agitation, autonomic instability, delusions, and hallucinations. E.g. Delirium tremens.
• **Somnolence:** Sleepy but responds appropriately to **commands.**
  ❖ Most common cause of somnolence in the hospital is iatrogenic sleep deprivation.
• **Obtundation:** Sleepy but responds appropriately only to **noxious stimuli.**

- **Stupor:** Sleepy but responds as groaning or grimacing to noxious stimuli.
- **Coma:** Unresponsive to noxious stimuli although posturing (decortication and decerebration) and spinal cord reflexes (Babinski) may remain intact.
  - ❖ **Psychogenic coma:** Appear comatose but have clinical (active resistance) and laboratory (EEG) evidence of being awake. E.g. hysterical personality, dissociative state.
- ✓ **Aetiology:** Traumatic brain injury, brain haemorrhage, and cardiac arrest are the most frequent causes of coma.
  - Metabolic encephalopathies form 20% of the cases (hypoglycaemia/DKA, hypercapnia, hyper/hyponatraemia, uraemia, hepatic or septic).
- ✓ **Initial stabilization:** Coma is a medical emergency[Q].
  - Initial ABCDE management plus 100 mg thiamine, 50 g glucose and 0.4 mg naloxone can be given to rule out reversible causes[Q]. Avoid pyrexia.
    - ❖ **TTM2 trial (2021)** showed no mortality difference in out of hospital cardiac arrest patients who were treated with hypothermia ≤33°C against normothermia.
- ✓ **Bedside examination:** Coma can be divided into structural and non-structural causes.
  - **Non-structural:** Signs of meningeal irritation and absence of focal neurological deficits suggests non-structural disease.
  - **Structural:** Lateralizing signs suggest structural lesion (neoplasm, infarct, haemorrhage, abscess).
  - Glasgow Coma Scale **(GCS) assessment** should be done. **FOUR** (eye response, motor response, brainstem reflexes, and respiratory pattern) can be used in mechanically ventilated patients.
    - ❖ **Best motor response:** Motor response itself has prognostic value. Noxious stimuli recommended is squeezing of the trapezius, pressure to the supraorbital notch or performing a jaw thrust.
  - **Pupils:** *Miosis:* Opiates; *Pinpoint:* Pontine lesions; *Mydriasis:* Midbrain lesions, atropine; *Asymmetry (anisocoria):* Uncal herniation

(dilated on the same site); and Horner's syndrome (small on the affected site).
- **Ocular movements:** Deviation of eyes at rest to side of lesion of motor cortex and hence away from the hemiparetic limbs. *Deviation of eyes at rest away from the side of lesion in pons and hence towards the hemiparetic limbs.*
- **Breathing pattern–*Kussmaul breathing*:** Deep and rapid regular breathing in severe metabolic acidosis and diabetic ketoacidosis. ***Cheyne–Stokes breathing*:** progressively deeper and faster breathing followed by a gradual decrease till apnoea seen in bilateral hemispheric lesions. ***Apneustic breathing*:** 2 to 3 s pauses after full inspiration seen in lesions of inferior pons.
- **Direct ophthalmoscopy:** Papilledema in optic disc (flame-shaped haemorrhage): Intracranial mass. Vitreous haemorrhage: subarachnoid haemorrhage.
- **Brainstem testing:** Pupillary response, corneal reflex, cough reflex should be checked. Oculocephalic (doll's eyes) and oculovestibular (caloric) stimulation also check the integrity of the brain stem.
- **Behavioural assessment:** To distinguish coma from vegetative state and vegetative state from minimally conscious state. Coma Recovery Scale-Revised (CRS-R) is the most sensitive test for it.
- ✓ **Ancillary tests**
  - **Blood tests:** Blood glucose, complete blood count, electrolytes, liver function tests with **ammonia**, kidney function tests, arterial blood gas analysis, coagulation studies, urine sample for toxicology, *serum osmolality, thyroid studies, serum cortisol,* **anti-NMDA receptor antibodies,** and **voltage-gated potassium channel antibodies.**
  - **CSF analysis:** Done to rule out meningoencephalitis or if CT scan is not able to detect subarachnoid haemorrhage. Cytology for cancer and antibodies for limbic encephalitis should be sent along with routine CSF tests.
  - **CT scan:** Can identify bleed, hydrocephalus, cerebral oedema, and loss of grey-white differentiation. *Contrast can be used for neoplasms and abscesses.*
    - ❖ CT Angiography to rule out large vessel thrombus or dissection.

- **MRI:** Better resolution than CT scan and highly sensitive for early ischaemic stroke and temporal lesions in early phase of HSV encephalitis.
  - ❖ **MR venography** can detect *cerebral venous sinus thrombosis* without contrast agents.
  - ❖ **MRI** can help in diagnosis of **posterior reversible encephalopathy syndrome (PRES).** It creates better superior images of posterior fossa and brainstem.
  - ❖ **MR spectroscopy** can distinguish tumour from **abscesses** and can confirm hepatic encephalopathy.
  - ❖ In post-cardiac arrest patients, volume lesion on DWI is associated with poor outcome.
- **EEG:** Helps in diagnosing **non-convulsive status epilepticus** (because of sepsis and metabolic dysfunction) and documentation of brain death.
  - ❖ New techniques of EEG can help to separate patients who will remain in vegetative state from those who will regain consciousness.
- **Somatosensory evoked potentials (SSEPs):** Documentation of prognosis and are less affected by drugs and hypothermia like EEG.
- ✓ **Prognosis of coma:** Assessment done once the acute insult is treated.

Cause of Insult	Factors Showing Unfavourable Outcome
Traumatic brain injury	Long-lasting elevated ICP, **Marshall** score on CT
Ischaemic stroke	Volume of ischaemia by MRI or perfusion by CT
Haemorrhagic stroke	Volume of haemorrhage on CT scan
Subarachnoid haemorrhage	**Fisher** score on CT

Additional Questions

- ✓ **Visual field defects due to lesions in pathway of vision[Q].**
  - **Optic chiasma:** Bitemporal hemianopia
  - **Optic radiation:** Homonymous hemianopia
- **Optic nerve**
  - ❖ **Partial:** Scotoma
  - ❖ **Complete:** Single eye complete vision loss

GUILLAIN–BARRÉ SYNDROME

Epidemiology and Aetiology

- ✓ **Guillain–Barré syndrome (GBS):** Rare disorder where the body's immune system attacks the peripheral nerves leading to muscle weakness or sometimes paralysis. Potential medical emergency as it can develop quickly into respiratory failure. Exists in many forms.
  - **Acute inflammatory demyelinating polyradiculoneuropathy (AIDP):** Affects *nerve roots.* **Demyelination predominant** (damage to myelin sheath).
    - ❖ **Acute inflammatory demyelinating polyneuropathy:** Progression of symptoms till 4 wk.
    - ❖ **Subacute inflammatory demyelinating polyneuropathy:** Progression of symptoms till 8 wk.
    - ❖ **Chronic inflammatory demyelinating polyneuropathy (CIDP):** Progression of symptoms beyond 8 wk.
  - **Acute motor axonal neuropathy (AMAN):** Affects axons of motor nerves mainly. *Axonopathy predominant* (damage to axons beneath myelin sheath). Rapid deterioration but quicker recovery as well.
  - **Acute motor sensory axonal neuropathy (AMSAN):** Affects axons of motor and sensory nerves. *Axonopathy predominant* (damage to axons beneath myelin sheath). A long time to recovery.
  - **Miller–Fisher syndrome[Q]:** Ophthalmoplegia, areflexia, and bulbar palsy.
- ✓ **Causes**
  - Infection with *Mycoplasma pneumoniae* precedes about 5% of cases of Guillain–Barré syndrome.
  - *Campylobacter jejuni*, CMV, HSV, and EBV are other common organisms.
  - SLE, **immunization,** general surgery, and renal transplant have all be studied as preceding events.
  - **IgG and complement mediated demyelination of peripheral nerves.**

- More common in males and bimodal distribution with peaks in young adults <40 yr and after 60 yr.

Clinical Features and Diagnosis

✓ **Signs and Symptoms**
  - **Ascending flaccid paralysis**, *areflexia*, and **autonomic instability.**
  - Symmetrical weakness in proximal and distal muscle groups with attenuation or loss of deep tendon reflexes.
  - Mild to moderate bilateral facial weakness.
  - Sinus tachycardia is the most common cardiac arrhythmia.
  - **Dysautonomia** can lead to hypotension, brady-arrhythmias, bladder paralysis, increased/decreased paralysis, and paralytic ileus.
  - Intra-arterial blood pressure monitoring should be initiated for wide fluctuations in blood pressure.
  - **Up to one-third of patients with Guillain–Barré syndrome will need intubation and ventilation for respiratory support within 2 wk after onset.**
    - ❖ Desaturation and hypercapnia are late signs.
  - 8–16% of patients with GBS can have one or more episodes of worsening after initial improvement.

✓ **Lumbar puncture:** CSF has increased protein in about 80% of patients at the end of first week but without pleocytosis (albumin-cytological dissociation)[Q]. CSF glucose is normal.

✓ **Nerve conduction studies**[Q]: *H-reflex abnormality* and *abnormal F-wave* occurs early in course of disease (after 4 d of onset).
  - **AIDP:** *Slowing of motor nerve conduction velocities* and **partial conduction block.** Amplitude of evoked motor responses and sensory response is reduced. *Fibrillation potentials and positive sharp waves late in course of disease.*
  - **AMAN:** *Compound motor action potentials (CMAPs) are low or even absent* and sensory responses are normal. *Anti-GM1 antibodies are seen in 10–42% of patients.*
  - **AMSAN:** Low-amplitude motor and sensory potentials.
  - **Miller–Fisher syndrome:** Reduced or absent sensory nerve action potentials (SNAPs). *90% of patients will have GQ1b antibodies.*

✓ **MRI:** *Enhancement of spinal nerve roots of cauda equina in addition to enhancement of cranial nerves.*

✓ **Erasmus GBS respiratory insufficiency score (EGRIS) score in GBS:** Predicts the probability of respiratory failure in the first week. ICU admission for score >4.
  - **Uses three characteristics.**
    - ❖ *Time from onset of weakness until admission.*
    - ❖ *Presence of facial and/or bulbar weakness.*
    - ❖ *Severity of muscle weakness at hospital admission defined by the MRC sum score*

Treatment

✓ **Indications for elective intubation**
  - **Vital capacity (VC)** <12–15 mL/kg by spirometry or *A reduction of >30% of VC from baseline. Test every 6 h. Most sensitive indication*[Q] *of respiratory muscle dysfunction.*
  - **Maximum inspiratory pressure (MIP)** less negative than −30 cm H_2O and **maximum expiratory pressure (MEP)** less positive than + 40 cm H_2O.
  - Oropharyngeal paresis with aspiration.
  - **Inability to count to 15 in a single breath.**

✓ **Suxamethonium** should be avoided owing to the risk of hyperkalaemia.

✓ **Autonomic dysfunction:** Use short-acting medications to control haemodynamic variability.

✓ **Immunoglobin therapy:** *Preferred due to relative ease of administration and tolerated well in patients with haemodynamic instability.*
  - 2g/kg divided over 5 consecutive days.
  - IViG is better than plasma in children but no difference in adult age group.
  - IViG doesn't have great effect after 2 wk of therapy.

✓ **Plasmapheresis:** Milder variety of GBS will benefit more from plasma therapy than IViG.
  - 200–250 mL plasma/kg over 7–14 d in 3–5 treatments. Albumin is replacement solution.
  - Safe in pregnancy and children.
  - Plasmapheresis is effective till 4 wk of onset.
  - *Combination of plasmapheresis and immunoglobin therapy is not recommended.*
  - **Corticosteroids are ineffective and might delay recovery**[Q].

✓ **Nursing care:** Avoid pressure sores. Avoid compression neuropathies.

Differential Diagnosis

✓ **Amyotrophic lateral sclerosis:** *Generalized muscle weakness with presence of brisk deep tenson reflexes and preserved sensation.*

✓ **Botulism:** Acute **descending motor paralysis** affecting cranial, respiratory, and **autonomic nerves.**

✓ **Myasthenia gravis:** Proximal muscle weakness. Ocular weakness predominates. Reflexes are spared. Muscular fatigability.

✓ **ICU-acquired weakness (ICUAW):** Flaccid paralysis with decreased reflexes. *Nerve conduction velocities are normal in ICUAW compared to decreased velocities seen in GBS.*

✓ **Multiple sclerosis**[Q]**:** Pseudobulbar palsy and internuclear ophthalmoplegia. Oligoclonal bands in CSF indicating increased IgG production by plasma cells. Slightly elevated CSF protein and normal CSF glucose.

Prognosis

✓ Mortality is 5–15%. Time to recovery is 3–6 months.
✓ *Up to 20% will have persistent disability after a year.*
✓ *Patients with a rapid onset of symptoms and requirement of mechanical ventilation are more likely to do bad.*

MYASTHENIA GRAVIS

Myasthenia Gravis

Epidemiology and Aetiology

✓ *Autoimmune disorder of neuromuscular transmission.*
- IgG autoantibodies block the post-synaptic acetylcholine receptors[Q] (anti-AChR antibodies) and are diagnostic.
- 10% of patients have autoantibodies against muscle-specific receptor kinase (MuSK)[Q] and seen more commonly in females less than 40 yr of age.
  - ❖ They tend to have more severe disease and respiratory crisis is more common.

✓ *Bimodal distribution:* 20–30 yr of age in females. 60–70 yr of age in males.

Clinical Features and Diagnosis

✓ **Clinical features:** Fatigable weakness, with proximal involvement of muscles.
- Extraocular weakness (diplopia and ptosis)[Q] are present in 85% of cases.

- **Oculomotor** (diplopia), **bulbar** (facial paresis, dysarthria, and dysphagia), and **proximal muscles** are the most affected.
- **Sensory innervation and reflexes are preserved.**

✓ **Osserman's classification of myasthenia gravis**
1. Ocular myasthenia (only ocular muscles)
2. Generalized myasthenia gravis
   a) Mild
   b) Moderate
3. Severe generalized myasthenia gravis
4. Myasthenic crisis with respiratory failure

✓ **Tensilon (Edrophonium) test**[Q]**:** An increase in strength within 45 s of 2–10 mg edrophonium (parenteral cholinesterase inhibitor) is a positive result.
- Low sensitivity and specificity.
- Edrophonium will make a cholinergic crisis worse.

✓ **Ice pack test:** Ice pack placed over the ptotic eyelid for 2–5 min and improvement of ptosis by at least 2 mm is considered a positive test.

✓ **Serological test:** *85% of patients with myasthenia have detectable serum antibodies which bind to AChR and sensitivity drops with purely ocular myasthenia.*
- 30–70% of seronegative patients will have antibodies against muscle-specific tyrosine kinase (**MuSK**).
- **CT chest** recommended as thymoma[Q] is present in 20% cases with 80% of patients having thymic hyperplasia.
- **Other autoimmune diseases:** Hypothyroid, SLE.

✓ **Nerve conduction studies**[Q]**:** EMG shows decremental reduction (at least 10%) in compound action potential with repetitive stimulation.
- *Clinically, motor nerve conduction is reduced and decreases with further repetition in myasthenia gravis but increases in Lambert–Eaton syndrome.*

✓ **Cholinergic crisis**[Q]**:** Patients on high anticholinesterase drugs like pyridostigmine.
- Overstimulation of nicotinic and muscarinic receptors.
- **SLUDGE syndrome:** Salivation, lacrimation, urination, defecation, gastrointestinal cramps, emesis.

✓ **Lambert–Eaton myasthenic syndrome (LEMS)**[Q]: Antibodies against presynaptic calcium channels.
  - Usually starts with proximal muscle weakness[Q] in legs and arms and absence of deep tendon reflexes.
  - Often linked to lung cancer. Repetitive nerve stimulation[Q] leads to improvements in symptoms.

Prevention and Treatment

✓ **Drugs to avoid in patients with myasthenia gravis**[Q]
  - **Antibiotics:** Aminoglycosides, fluoroquinolones, macrolides, tetracyclines, polymyxins.
  - **Cardiovascular:** Calcium channel blockers, beta-blockers, statins, magnesium, procainamide.
  - **Others:** Neuromuscular blocking agents, botulinum toxin, penicillamine, quinine.
  - Increased dose of suxamethonium[Q] needed due to resistance.

✓ **Myasthenia crisis**[Q]: Threatened or actual respiratory compromise. Respiratory muscle insufficiency or inability to handle secretions and oral intake.
  - Caused by infections, electrolyte imbalances, cholinergic crisis, thyroid dysfunction, and medications (aminoglycoside, fluoroquinolones, statins, lithium).
  - **Indications for elective intubation** (same in GBS: 20/30 rule).
    - FVC <20 mL/kg[Q]
    - Maximum inspiratory pressure not as negative as −30 cm H_2O[Q]
    - >30% decline from baseline.
  - **Plasmapheresis**[Q]: **Better than IVIG.**
    - 50 mL/kg of plasma removed per session and replaced with saline or 5% albumin.
    - 3–7 Sessions at 24–48-h interval.
    - Avoided in patients with haemodynamic instability.
  - **Intravenous Immunoglobin:** Dose of IVIG is 0.4 gm/kg/day for 5 consecutive days.
    - Pretreatment with paracetamol given for flu-like symptoms. Hydration to prevent thrombosis.
    - Avoided in patients with renal failure.

✓ **Long-term immunosuppression:** *Steroids for patients not responding to low-dose cholinesterase inhibitors on outpatient basis. High-dose steroids used during myasthenia crisis.*
  - **Azathioprine:** Used in patients not responding to steroids.
  - Mycophenolate mofetil and cyclosporine have also been used.
  - Rituximab and Eculizumab.

✓ **Cholinesterase inhibitors:** IV Pyridostigmine not needed while patient is intubated (can cause arrhythmias, coronary vasospasm) and oral pyridostigmine is started when patient can start eating.

✓ **Thymectomy** should be considered early in course of disease (<5 yr) in patients of age group 18–65 yr.

Neuromuscular Disorders

✓ **Classification**
  - **Hereditary**
    - **Pre-junctional:** Charcot-Marie-Tooth, Friedrich's ataxia.
    - **Post-junctional:** Duchenne, Becker's, myotonic dystrophy, myotonia congenita, hypokalaemia periodic paralysis, mitochondrial disorders.
  - **Acquired**
    - **Pre-junctional:** GBS, Multiple sclerosis, motor neuron disease.
    - **Junctional:** Myasthenia gravis, Lambert–Eaton myasthenic syndrome.
    - **Post-junctional:** Critical care myopathy.

✓ **Presentation**
  - Respiratory failure, cardiomyopathies, scoliosis, contractures.
  - **Charcot-Marie-Tooth:** It is not life-threatening, and most people have same life expectancy as a person without it.
  - **Fredrich's ataxia:** *Autosomal recessive.*
    - Most common type of hereditary ataxia.
    - Avoid negative inotropy in these patients.
  - **Duchenne muscular dystrophy:** *X-linked recessive.*
    - Proximal wasting of muscles.
    - Most common childhood muscular dystrophy.
  - **Becker's muscular dystrophy:** *X-linked recessive.*
    - Proximal wasting of muscles but milder than Duchenne's due to only partial absence of dystrophin protein.
  - **Myotonic dystrophy: Autosomal dominant**
    - Dysfunctional sodium/chloride channel.

❖ **Myotonia:** Inability of muscle to relax.
❖ Male hypogonadism, insulin resistance, thyroid nodules and increase parathyroid levels[Q].
❖ Avoid cold or stress.
❖ Avoid noradrenaline and beta-agonists.
• **Myotonia congenita: Autosomal dominant**
❖ Dysfunctional chloride channel.
❖ **Myotonia:** Inability of muscle to relax.
❖ Avoid cold or stress.
❖ Avoid noradrenaline and beta-agonists.
• **Hypokalaemic periodic paralysis:** Sudden onset of generalized or focal flaccid paralysis associated with low levels of potassium.
• **Mitochondrial myopathies:** MELAS (mitochondrial encephalopathy, lactic acidosis, stroke like episodes).
• **Multiple sclerosis:** Autoimmune demyelination. Relapsing or progressive forms.
❖ **Vision problems** lead the constellation of symptoms.
• **Motor neuron disease (MND):** Acquired progressive neurological disease that destroys motor neurons.
❖ Most patients die within 1–5 yr of diagnosis.
❖ Amyotrophic lateral sclerosis is the most common form of MND.
✓ **Management**
• Avoid volatile agents, suxamethonium[Q] due to risk of malignant hyperthermia.
• Use low doses of non-depolarizing neuromuscular blockers.
• Autonomic dysfunction management.

ICU-ACQUIRED WEAKNESS

Epidemiology

✓ ICU-acquired weakness: Defined as clinically detectable weakness in critically ill patients where no other cause could be found.
• Seen in up to 80% of ICU patients.

Clinical Features and Diagnosis

✓ **Classification[Q] of ICU-acquired weakness**
• Critical illness polyneuropathy (**CIP**)
• Critical illness myopathy (**CIM**)
• Critical illness neuromyopathy (**CINM**)
✓ **Critical illness myopathy:** Those with CIM can be further divided[Q] into **cachectic** myopathy,

thick filament myopathy or **necrotizing** myopathy.
• Symmetrical flaccid paralysis and decreased but **PRESENT** reflexes in all four limbs. Sparing of facial muscles, cranial nerves, and autonomic nervous system. *Proximal > distal weakness*[Q].
• Marked weakness of diaphragm and failure to wean from ventilator.
• **Risk factors[Q]: Steroids, muscle relaxants,** aminoglycosides, ARDS, prolonged acidaemia, hyperglycaemia.
• CIM accounts for 42% of weakness among patients in the surgical and medical ICU setting.
✓ **Critical illness polyneuropathy (CIP):** Symmetrical, sensorimotor, axon loss polyneuropathy[Q].
• Facial muscles are usually not affected. *Distal > proximal weakness* but generalized flaccid paralysis. Decreased or **ABSENT** reflexes.
• *Sensory loss of pain, temperature, and vibration sense.*
• **Risk factors[Q]:** Approximately 45% of patients with severe sepsis and multiple organ failure will have EMG evidence of *axon-loss polyneuropathy.*
❖ Hyperglycaemia is a risk factor as well[Q].
• Complication of systemic inflammation response triggered by sepsis.
✓ **Assessment**
• **Medical Research Council Sum Score (MRC-SS)** <48/60 indicates significant weakness and <38/60 indicates severe weakness.
• **Hand-held dynamometry and 6-min walk test** are used for quantification of muscle strength.
• **Respiratory muscles are assessed by** measuring maximum inspiratory and expiratory pressure, transdiaphragmatic pressure and thickening of diaphragm on ultrasound.
✓ **Nerve conduction studies[Q]:** No need for nerve conduction studies to diagnose it. Diagnosis of exclusion.
• CIP: Functional neuronal membrane in-excitability.
• CIM: Functional muscle membrane in-excitability.

Investigation	CIP	CIM	CINM
Creatine kinase	• Normal or slightly elevated	• **Elevated**	• Normal or elevated
CSF	• Normal cell counts • *Slightly elevated protein levels (<0.8 g/L)*	• Normal	• Normal cell counts • Slightly elevated protein levels (<0.8 g/L)
Nerve conduction studies	• ↓ CMAP amplitude • ↓ *SNAP amplitude* • **Normal conduction velocity** • **Normal conduction latency**	• ↓ CMAP amplitude • *Normal SNAP amplitude* • **Normal conduction velocity** • **Normal conduction latency**	• ↓ CMAP amplitude • ↓ SNAP amplitude • Normal conduction velocity • Normal conduction latency
Electromyography	• Spontaneous fibrillation potentials and sharp waves • **Long duration, high-amplitude polyphasic motor unit potentials (MUPs)**	• Spontaneous fibrillation potentials and sharp waves • **Short duration, low-amplitude polyphasic motor unit potentials (MUPs) with early recruitment**	• Features of both CIP and CIM
Direct muscle stimulation	• Nerve: muscle ratio <0.5 • **Normal direct muscle CMAP amplitude**	• Nerve: muscle response ratio ≥0.5 • **Reduced direct muscle CMAP amplitude**	• Variable
Muscle biopsy	• **Features of denervation and reinnervation** • Small angulated muscle fibres • Target and targetoid fibres, group fibre atrophy, fibre type regrouping	• **Cachectic myopathy** with myofibrillar degeneration • Thick filament myopathy with a **selective loss of myosin filaments** • Necrotizing myopathy with *muscle fibre necrosis*	• Both features of CIP and CIM
Nerve biopsy	• *Normal or **motor and sensory axonal degeneration***	• Normal	• Normal or motor and sensory nerve axonal degeneration

Prevention and Treatment

✓ *Glycaemic control,* avoid neuromuscular blockers and steroids, **more sedation holds**, avoid early parenteral nutrition.
✓ Deep vein thrombosis prophylaxis, positioning of limbs, regular full skin evaluations.

Prognosis

✓ *Higher 1-year mortality.*
✓ *5-years:* Lower handgrip force, shorter 6 MWT, lower respiratory muscle strength.
✓ Compared to patients with CIM, *patients with CIP have slower recovery over months and less complete recovery.*
✓ Patients with CIP may be left with *painful dysesthesias due to small fibre neuropathy.*

NEUROLOGICAL MONITORING

✓ **Basic Principles**
  • **Cerebral blood flow** is maintained over a cerebral perfusion pressure range of 50 to 130 mmHg.
  • Cerebral blood flow below 20 mL/100 gram/min can lead to irreversible brain damage.
✓ **Glasgow Coma Scale**[Q]
  • Originally intended for head trauma but is used for all disorders of consciousness.
  • The motor category has the best discrimination of the severity of brain injury.
  • Included in scores like **APACHE II** and **Trauma injury severity score (TISS)**.
  • **Severity**[Q]: Mild: 13–15, Moderate: 9–12, Severe: <8.

Glasgow Coma Scale

Eye response	• Spontaneous opening	4
	• Open in response to voice	3
	• Open in response to pain	2
	• Not opening	1
Verbal response	• Oriented, coherent speech	5
	• Confused	4
	• Inappropriate words	3
	• Unintelligible sounds	2
	• No response	1
Motor response	• Obeys commands	6
	• Localizes to painful stimulus	5
	• Withdraws from painful stimulus	4
	• Abnormal flexion to pain (decorticate)	3
	• Abnormal extension to pain (decerebrate)	2
	• No response to pain	1

✓ **Clinically:** Raised ICP can cause pupillary dilation. Abducens nerve is affected first due to long course[Q].
✓ **ICP Monitoring**
  • **ICP waveforms:** P1 (arterial pulsation), P2 (intracranial compliance), and *P3 (Dicrotic notch)*[Q].
  • **ICP waveform disturbances**[Q]
    ❖ **Lundberg A waves:** Always pathological and represent early herniation. Amplitude of 50–100 mmHg lasting 5–20 min.
    ❖ **Lundberg B waves:** Amplitude of 50 mmHg with frequency of 0.5–2/minute and are seen in normal individuals (e.g. REM sleep) or due to *vascular tone instability.*
    ❖ **Lundberg C waves:** Amplitude up to 20 mmHg. Frequency of 4–8/minute. Are seen in normal individuals and are due to interaction between cardiac and respiratory cycles.

ICP Measurement: Reference Point Is Foramen of Monroe-External Auditory Meatus[Q]

Technique	Critical Threshold for Raised ICP	Characteristics	Issues
Optic nerve sheath diameter (ONSD)[Q]	>5–6 mm	• Non-invasive technique and measured **3 mm behind the eyeball** by ultrasound, CT, or MRI	• Difficult in trauma patients • Operator-dependent
Automated pupillometry	NPi <3	• Pupils indicative of structural brain injury • **Neurological pupil index (NPi)** – combines pupil size, latency constriction velocity, and dilation velocity	• Difficult in trauma patients
ICP parenchymal bolt	>22 mm[Q]Hg	• Placed mostly in right frontal lobe • Infection <1%	• **Can't be recalibrated**[Q] • Local measurement of frontal lobe[Q] • Subject to zero drift over time • Can't drain CSF[Q]
External ventricular drain (EVD)[Q]	>22 mmHg	• Diagnosis of ICP and therapeutic as intrathecal medication can be given • Can be recalibrated; gold standard[Q]	• High infection rate (10%)

Cerebral Blood Flow Measurement

Technique	Critical Threshold	Characteristics	Issues
Transcranial Doppler (TCD)	• **Lindegaard ratio**[Q] **>3** suggests vasospasm **Flow in MCA:** • Normal 55 cm/s • Mild >120 cm/s • Moderate >160 cm/s • Severe >200 cm/s	**Lindegaard ratio:** • Middle cerebral artery flow velocity measured through the *temporal window* • Internal carotid artery measured through *submandibular window* • >6 suggests severe vasospasm[Q] • Can detect emboli in cerebral circulation	• Poor predictive value for delayed cerebral ischaemia post-SAH

Cerebral Oxygenation

Technique	Critical Threshold for Cerebral Ischaemia	Characteristics	Issues
Brain tissue oxygen tension (Pbt$_{O2}$)	<10–25 mmHg	• Intraparenchymal probes that measure local oxygen tension, CO_2 tension, and pH • Inserted through multilumen ICP bolts • **Assesses regional oxygenation**	• Haematomas, infection • Requires calibration
Near-infrared spectroscopy (NIRS)	rSO$_2$ <55%	• Near-infrared light penetrates skull and reflected by brain tissue and picked up probe • Trends better than actual values • **Assesses regional oxygenation**	• Difficult in head trauma patients
Jugular venous oximetry (SjvO$_2$)[Q]	<50%	• Dilatation of internal jugular bulb below the base of the skull • Catheter inserted in the vein as a CVC but directed in a retrograde direction • **Assesses global saturation**[Q]	• Regular calibration required • **Invasive** • Erroneous continuous measurement as protein material builds up on it

Cerebral Metabolism

Technique	Critical Threshold	Characteristics	Issues
Cerebral microdialysis (CMD)	• **Glucose <2** suggests decreased perfusion • **Lactate/Pyruvate >20–25** suggests ischaemia • **Glutamate >15–20** suggests excitotoxicity • **Glycerol >100** suggests cell membrane degradation	Catheter containing a semipermeable membrane is placed into the white matter and perfused with a microdialysate.	Invasive, expensive

Electrophysiology

Technique	Critical Threshold	Characteristics	Issues
Electroencephalogram (EEG)	• **Percentage alpha variability <0.1** • **Alpha–delta ratio (ADR) >10% decrease**, suggesting vasospasm	Indicated for diagnosis of non-status epilepticus and prognostication post–cardiac arrest	Affected by electrical equipment around; scalp fixation of electrodes possibly problematic
Somatosensory evoked potentials (SSEPs)	• Absence of N20 cortical waves	• Absence of N20 cortical waves within 3 d post-arrest a sign of poor prognosis post–cardiac arrest • Not influenced by neuromuscular drugs	Influenced by sedative drugs

NEURORADIOLOGY

✓ **Cerebral Oedema**
- **Vasogenic oedema:** Accumulation of fluid outside the cell in extracellular tissue after the blood–brain barrier is destroyed. Seen in neoplasm, inflammation, trauma, or haemorrhage.
  ❖ Can be reversible and primarily affects the white matter.
- **Cytotoxic oedema:** Accumulation of fluid inside the cell and the blood–brain barrier remains intact. Seen in cerebral ischaemia. Steroids are not effective.
  ❖ Often less variable and primarily affects the grey matter.

✓ **Computed Tomography**
- Uses multiple focused X-ray beams, a detector array and computerized production of an image.
  ❖ Image is formed by the differences in attenuation caused by the tissues in the path of these rays.
  ❖ **Attenuation is measured in Hounsfield units (HU)** with *water having zero* as reference. Bone: +1000, grey matter: +37 to +42 white matter: +20 to +30, fat −50 and air −1000.
  ❖ **Whiteness:** Bone > blood > muscle > brain > cerebral oedema > CSF > air.
  ❖ CT contrast used for suspicion of tumour, abscess, or vascular abnormality.
  ❖ **Subarachnoid cisterns/basal cisterns:** Collections of CSF and protect the brain. **Sylvian:** Between temporal

and frontal bones. **Cisterna magna:** Between cerebellum and medulla.
  ❖ **Earliest sign of raised ICP is loss of grey-white differentiation[Q].**
- **Indications**
  ❖ Acute neurological deficits
  ❖ Acute head trauma
  ❖ Suspected acute intracranial haemorrhage.
  ❖ Increased intracranial pressure
  ❖ Suspected hydrocephalus
  ❖ Suspected intracranial infections
  ❖ Aneurysm evaluation (CT angiogram)
  ❖ Cerebral venous sinus thrombosis (CT venogram)
- **Trauma CT scan:** A GCS score of 12 or less on initial assessment in the emergency department.
  ❖ *Indications for CT scan in 1 h:* GCS ≤12 or less on initial assessment, *GCS <15 after 2 h of initial assessment*, suspected open or depressed skull fracture, *sign of basal skull fracture* (haemotympanum, "panda" eyes, cerebrospinal fluid leakage from the ear or nose), *more than 1 episode of vomiting*, post-traumatic seizure, focal neurological deficits.
  ❖ *Indications for CT scan within 8 h* for patients who had some loss of consciousness: *Age > 65 yr*, any current bleeding or clotting disorder, *more than 30 min of retrograde amnesia after the event*, dangerous mechanism of

injury (a pedestrian or cyclist struck by a motor vehicle, an occupant ejected from a motor vehicle or a fall from a height of more than 1 m or 5 stairs).

❖ *Extradural haematoma*: Lens/egg shaped and won't cross the midline. *Subdural haematoma*: Crescent-shaped and crosses the midline, *Subarachnoid haemorrhage*: Extends into sulci, ventricles and basal cisterns, *Diffuse axonal injury*: Small punctate haemorrhages at the grey/white matter junction.

TBI Category	Characteristics
Diffuse injury I	• No visible pathology
Diffuse injury II	• Basal cisterns visible • Midline shift 0–5 mm • No high or mixed density lesion >25 mm³
Diffuse injury III	• Basal cisterns compressed or absent • Midline shift 0–5 mm • No high or mixed density lesion >25 mm³
Diffuse injury IV	• Midline shift >5 mm • No high or mixed density lesion >25 mm³
Evacuated mass lesion V	• Any lesion surgically evacuated
Non-evacuated mass lesion VI	• High or mixed density lesion >25 mm³ not surgically evacuated

- **Marshall score:** Higher categories have less chances of survival.
- **Rotterdam CT classification** and **Helsinki CT scores** have been developed recently and improve prediction accuracy of Marshall CT classification.
- **Intracranial haemorrhage:** Modified Fisher scale is used for aneurysmal bleeding and is given in chapter for subarachnoid haemorrhage.
  - ❖ **Acute haemorrhage**: Hyper-dense image, **Sub-acute haemorrhage:** iso dense (2–3 wk), and **chronic haemorrhage:** Hypo-dense (>1 month).
- **Ischaemic stroke:** Middle cerebral artery stroke may show some visualization of

embolic material^Q within the lumen on the CT scan.

- ❖ **Acute ischaemia:** Loss of distinction between grey and white matter in first few hours, hypo-density becomes visible by 12 h and hypo-density area with volume loss after 3–4 wk.
- **Infection:** Contrast is used for suspected abscess.
  - ❖ **Encephalitis:** Swelling and low density in the medial temporal lobes, insula or cingulate gyri. Bilateral and asymmetrical.
  - ❖ **Abscess^Q:** Ring-enhancing lesion surrounded by low-density oedema. Most frequently located in frontal and temporal lobes.
- **Diffuse hypoxic injury:** Brain looks swollen bilaterally with effacement of cisterns, sulci, and ventricles. Cerebral oedema is the characteristic finding in hypoxic brain injury after cardiac arrest.
- **Mass effect:** Midline shift and herniation seen. Midline shift ≥5 mm calls for urgent neurosurgical review^Q.
  - ❖ **Subfalcine or cingulate herniation:** Frontal or parietal masses cause cingulate gyrus to move under the falx cerebri to the opposite side.
    - Coma with asymmetric motor posturing (contralateral > ipsilateral).
  - ❖ **Uncal or trans-tentorial herniation:** Downward displacement of medial part of the temporal lobe under the tentorium cerebelli.
    - Ipsilateral third nerve palsy. Contralateral hemiplegia.
  - ❖ **Trans-foraminal or tonsillar herniation:** Downward displacement of the cerebellar tonsils at the level of the foramen magnum.
    - Sudden progression to coma with bilateral motor posturing in someone with cerebellar signs.
  - ❖ **Central trans-tentorial:** Downward displacement of diencephalon (thalamus).
    - Coma with decerebrate posturing and loss of brainstem reflexes.
  - ❖ **Transcalvarial herniation:** Displacement of the brain through a skull fracture or defect.
    - Focal neurological deficits depending upon location.

✓ **CT Perfusion:** Allows quick quantitative and qualitative evaluation of cerebral blood flow.
  • Generates imaging maps of cerebral blood flow (CBF), cerebral blood volume (CBV) and mean transit time (MTT) separately and CBF = CBV/MTT.
  • Red colour on imaging maps means higher values and blue means lower values.
  • **Indications:** Acute ischaemic stroke and delayed cerebral ischaemia (DCI) in subarachnoid haemorrhage.
    ❖ **Acute ischaemic stroke:** Identifies patients who will benefit from endovascular thrombolysis, by differentiating between infarcted areas and areas of penumbra (salvageable tissue).
    ❖ **Delayed cerebral ischaemia (DCI):** Increases sensitivity and specificity for the diagnosis of DCI.
✓ **Magnetic resonance imaging (MRI)**
  • MRI uses magnetic waves to create high-quality images with good anatomic detail.
    ❖ It uses the concept of varying amount of hydrogen atoms within different tissues. Hydrogen atoms have their own magnetic field which are aligned to a strong constant magnetic field generated by the MRI machine.
    ❖ MRI machine then generates a radio-frequency pulse which changes the spin of hydrogen atoms and misaligns them from the magnetic field of MRI.
    ❖ With time, hydrogen atoms return to their original relaxed state while generating a radiofrequency pulse themselves and become aligned with the magnetic field once again.
    ❖ This return to the original state happens at different rates and this differential rate is detected and converted into an image.
    ❖ MRI scanners use liquid helium^Q for superconducting magnets.

MRI Sequence	Tissues Involved
T1 weighted	• Normal grey-white contrast (white matter is white, and grey matter is grey). • Fat has high signal (white), and water has low signal (black). • **Standard and evaluates normal anatomy,^Q like atrophy.** • Post-contrast images are T1-weighted with fat suppression.
T2 weighted	• **Water has high signal (white). CSF is white.** • High signal in CSF, vasogenic oedema, gliosis, acute and subacute bleed. • **Shows pathology as white.**
FLAIR^Q (fluid attenuated inversion recovery)	• **Image is like T2 with CSF nullified in images, and only pathology is white. Fluid is dark.** • Good for white matter lesions, peri-ventricular region, periphery of the hemispheres. • Detects **vasogenic oedema.** • *Makes white pathology more white.*
Susceptibility-weighted imaging (SWI)	• 3D high spatial resolution images derived from gradient echo (GRE) MRI sequences in comparison to spin echo sequences used by T1- and T2-weighted images. • **Traumatic micro-haemorrhages** seen in diffuse axonal injury. • Blood appears hyperintense (bright). • Calcium appears hypointense (dark).
Diffusion-weighted imaging (DWI)/ apparent diffusion coefficient (ADC)	• Studies the random movements of water molecules. • DWI utilizes motion of hydrogen molecules, and ADC filters out the T2 effect and produces inverse images. • **Differentiates vasogenic from cytotoxic oedema**/white matter shearing and diagnosis of acute ischaemia. • **Sensitive for stroke; pathology is white in DWI.** • **Abscess and tumours are also white on DWI.**

- **Indications:** Same as CT scan but with higher resolution enabling detection of lesions especially in the *deep white matter and posterior fossa.* Also used for diagnosing **encephalitis** and **anoxic injury for prognostication** in post-cardiac arrest patients. Can easily diagnose *posterior reversible leucoencephalopathy syndrome (PRES)*[Q].
  - ❖ **Acute ischaemic stroke:** MRI is more sensitive in the first few hours. DWI will have high signal and low signal on ADC. T2 will have a high signal lesion.

- ❖ **Diffuse axonal injury (DAI):** In traumatic brain injury patients, MRI is sensitive in detecting non-haemorrhagic DAI as well. DAI is seen as high signal on T2/FLAIR and low signal lesions on DWI/SWI.
- ❖ **Hypoxic ischaemic injury:** Cytotoxic oedema can be detected by MRI and is characterized by high signal on T2/FLAIR and DWI. Restricted diffusion on MRI and hence low signal on ADC.

Additional Questions

- ✓ Vertebral arteries unite to form basilar artery at the base of the pons[Q].

Renal Problems

ACUTE KIDNEY INJURY

Epidemiology and aetiology: Incidence of AKI varies according to the criteria used.

✓ **Acute kidney injury (AKI) is defined**[Q] by **KDIGO** as
  - Increase in serum creatinine by ≥ 26.5 *mmol/L within 48 h* or
  - Increase in *serum creatinine ≥ 1.5 times* baseline within the prior 7 d or
  - Urine volume <0.5 mL/kg/h for 6 h

✓ **Incidence:** AKI develops in 5% of hospital admissions. AKI itself accounts for 1% of hospital admissions.
  - AKI develops in 5–25% of ITU admissions. **10% of these patients with AKI will require RRT.**
  - AKI and MOF can lead to 50% mortality. If RRT is requires then mortality can be as high as 80%.
  - AKI is seen in 50% of sepsis cases admitted to intensive care and sepsis is seen in 50% of cases with severe AKI in the ICU.
  - **The leading cause of AKI**[Q] **both in hospital and in ICU is sepsis (renal hypoperfusion).**
  - AKI incidence in **cardiac surgery is ~18%,** major abdominal surgery ~13% and > 50% in **liver transplant** and **emergency aortic surgery.**
  - **10% of patients that required RRT in ITU move to have CKD.**

✓ **Causes of AKI**
  - **Prerenal azotaemia:** Hypovolaemia, hypotension, *autoregulation failure* (NSAIDs by preglomerular vasoconstriction, ACEIs by post-glomerular vasodilation).

❖ Reduced renal perfusion decreases the flow of filtrate through the renal tubules. Urea reabsorption is increased but not that of creatinine. Hence plasma urea creatinine ratio is increased.

- **Intrinsic renal disease**[Q]
  ❖ **Acute tubular necrosis:** Due to ischaemia/nephrotoxins, necrosis of tubular cells. Delayed recovery of renal function compared to prerenal azotaemia. *Epithelial cell or muddy brown granular casts in urine.*
  ❖ **Glomerular diseases:** Signs of nephritis syndrome like hypertension, oedema, proteinuria. **RBC casts in urine**[Q].
  ❖ **Vascular diseases:** Bilateral renal artery occlusion, occlusion of smaller vessels due to TTP/HUS, vasculitis due to microscopic polyarteritis, or granulomatosis with polyangiitis.
  ❖ **Interstitial nephritis:** Allergic reaction with eosinophilia[Q] mainly due to medications, infections like Leptospira, *Legionella*, EBV, *Pyuria and **white blood cells in urine**[Q]. Acute pyelonephritis presents with similar urinary findings but rarely causes AKI.*

- **Post-renal failure:** Nephrolithiasis, ureteric obstruction, bladder neck obstruction due to prostate hypertrophy. Renal imaging is helpful in diagnosis. Urinalysis is not very useful.
  ❖ Painless gross haematuria due to papillary necrosis and NSAID ingestion can cause ureteral obstruction.

✓ **Risk Factors**
  - **Non-modifiable:** Age >65 yr, hypertension, chronic kidney disease, diabetes mellitus,

heart failure, chronic liver disease, COPD, obesity, cognitive deficits, malignancy.

- **Modifiable:** Sepsis, hypovolaemia, hypervolaemia, cardiac surgery, emergency surgery, trauma, burns, anaemia, gadolinium contrast.

✓ **Nephrotoxins**[Q]: Aminoglycosides, vancomycin, amphotericin-B, aciclovir, ganciclovir,

myoglobin (17 KDa), haemoglobin, uric acid, and myeloma light chains.

✓ **Causes of increased urea or creatinine without decrease in GFR:** GI bleeding, corticosteroids, increased protein intake, hypercatabolic state.

RIFLE Criteria[Q] for AKI Done in 2004: Predictive for Hospital Mortality

	Creatinine Criteria	Urine Output Criteria
Risk	• Increased creatinine × 1.5 or GFR drop by 25%	• UO <0.5 mL/kg/h × 6 h
Injury	• Increased creatinine × 2 or GFR drop by 50%	• UO <0.5 mL/kg/h × 12 h
Failure	• Increased creatinine × 3 or creatinine ≥4 mg/dL • Acute rise of ≥0.5 mg/dL or GFR drop by 75%	• UO <0.3 mL/kg/h × 24 h • Anuria × 12 h
Loss	Persistent ARF = complete loss of renal function >4 wk	
End-stage kidney disease	Loss of kidney function >3 months	

Staging of AKI by KDIGO[Q] Done in 2012

AKI Stage	Serum Creatinine Criteria	Urine Output Criteria
Stage I	• ↑ in s. creatinine by ≥26.5 µmol/L within 48 h • ↑ in s. creatinine to 1.5 –1.9 times from baseline within prior 7 d	• Urine volume <0.5 mL/kg/h for 6–12 h
Stage II	• ↑ in s. creatinine to **2–2.9 times** from baseline	• Urine volume <0.5 mL/kg/h for ≥12 h
Stage III	• ↑ in s. creatinine to **≥3 times** from baseline • ↑ in s. creatinine to 354 µmol/L • **Treatment with RRT** or in patients less <18 yr, ↓ in estimated GFR to <35 mL/min per 1.73 m²	• Urine volume <0.3 mL/kg/h for ≥24 h • Anuria for ≥12 h

✓ **Shortcomings of Diagnostic Criteria**
- **Serum creatinine** is affected by muscle mass and meat intake.
  - ❖ May take 24–36 h to rise after a renal insult.
  - ❖ Affected by volume status and may be missed in patient who has just been resuscitated.
  - ❖ Rise in creatinine is detected when kidneys have lost >50% of their functional capacity. It doesn't reflect small changes in GFR.
  - ❖ Reflects functional change in kidney function which lags behind the structural change that occurs early.

- **Urinary output** is influenced by physiological stimuli like ADH release triggered by stress, pain, or hypovolaemia.

Clinical Features and Diagnosis

✓ **Signs and symptoms:** *Signs of uraemia develop at GFR of less than 10 mL/min.*

✓ **Investigations:** Urine microscopy, urine electrolytes, urine osmolality, urine creatinine and serum calcium.
- **Urine dipstick:** Glomerulonephritis (haematuria and proteinuria), acute pyelonephritis (pyuria, nitrites), interstitial nephritis (eosinophils).

- **Renal ultrasound:** Enlarged kidney–Renal vein thrombosis, infiltrative diseases. Shrunken kidney and reduced corticomedullary differentiation: CKD, obstruction of urinary collecting tract.
- **Glomerulonephritis/vasculitis:** ANCA, ANA, Anti-GBM, Anti-ds-DNA, C3/C4, immunoglobins, *cryoglobulins*, hepatitis serology, HIV serology, **Renal Biopsy.**
- **Interstitial nephritis:** Serum eosinophils, eosinophiluria.
- **TTP/HUS:** LDH, platelets, reticulocytes, haptoglobin, bilirubin.
- **Rhabdomyolysis:** CK, myoglobin.
- **Myeloma:** Serum/urine protein electrophoresis, **renal biopsy.**
- **Cardio-renal syndrome:** Troponin, CK-MB, NT-proBNP.
- **Abdominal compartment syndrome:** Intra-vesicular pressure.

Laboratory Test	Pre-Renal AKI^Q	Intrinsic AKI^Q	Post-Renal AKI^Q
Urine osmolality	>500	<350	<350
Urine/serum osmolality	>1.5	<1.3	<1.5
Urinary Na$^+$ (mEq/L)	<20	>40	>40
FE$_{Na}$ (%)	<1	>1	>1
Urine-specific gravity	>1.018	<1.012	Variable
Urine/serum creatinine	>40	<20	<20
Urine/serum urea	>8	<3	<3
Urinary RBC	None	2–4+	Variable
Urinary WBC	None	2–4+	1+
Urinary sediment	Hyaline casts	Granular and cellular casts	Crystals and Cellular debris

✓ **In stage 1 AKI**, a non-invasive diagnostic work up of kidney function should be done.
- *Drug dosage review should be done in stage 2 AKI. Need for RRT and ICU admission should also be considered in stage 2 AKI.*

✓ **Furosemide stress test:** 1 mg/kg Furosemide given IV (1.5 mg/kg if Furosemide given in last 7 d).

- In patients with AKI stage 1 and 2 if urine output <200 mL in 2 h, risk for progression to stage 3 AKI and need for RRT is high.
- Responders don't have intrinsic renal failure.
- Non-responders: Conservative fluid therapy.

✓ **Kidney Biomarkers:** Apart from BUN and creatinine.
- **Cystatin C^Q:** Produced by all nucleated cells and release in plasma and cleared by kidneys.
  - ❖ Acute kidney injury will prevent its clearance and levels will rise.
  - ❖ A more sensitive marker of reduced GFR than creatinine as its levels is not dependent on muscle mass.
  - ❖ High cost is a limiting factor for use.
- **Urinary kidney injury molecule (KIM-1):** Transmembrane glycoprotein that is *upregulated by tubular cells* after ischaemic or nephrotoxic renal injury.
  - ❖ Kidney injury molecule-1 (KIM-1) suggests structural injury and is released during proximal tubule injury.
- **Urine IL-18:** Proinflammatory cytokine released in response to ischaemia-reperfusion injury of tubular cells.
  - ❖ Elevated within 6 h after renal injury and peaks at 12–18 h.
- **Neutrophil gelatinase-associated lipocalin (NGAL)**
  - ❖ Iron-carrying protein of 25 kDa size.
  - ❖ Urinary NGAL is produced by thick ascending limb and the collecting ducts.
  - ❖ Plasma NGAL is linked to infection and inflammation and is not produced by kidneys.
  - ❖ Both urinary and plasma NGAL can help to detect acute tubular necrosis (ATN).
  - ❖ Urinary NGAL upregulated after ischaemic or nephrotoxic renal injury and can be detected in urine within 2 h whereas plasma NGAL can detect the acute kidney injury within 24 h of insult.
- **Urinary TIMP-2 and IGFBP-7:** Markers of renal tubular stress. Also known as renal troponins. *Point of care test is available in USA.*

✓ **Contrast-induced nephropathy (CIN)[Q]:** *Defined as >0.5 mg/dL or an increase of 25% from the baseline within 48–72 h of contrast exposure.* Majority do not require dialysis.

- 14% incidence in critically ill patients after the contrast enhanced scans. Associated with larger volumes of *iodinated contrast (2 mL/kg)*.
- **Risk factors[Q]:** Age >75 yr, CKD, DM with CKD, renal transplant, heart failure, hypovolaemia, contrast osmolality, total contrast dose, concomitant exposure to nephrotoxic agents, intra-aortic balloon pump.
- Use **low osmolality contrast (600–800 mOsm/kg)** compared to high-osmolar agents (>1400 mOsm/kg). *Avoid diuretics, ACE inhibitors, and NSAIDs.*
- The risk of contrast-induced AKI is smaller than previously thought hence fear of contrast nephropathy shouldn't be the reason to postpone an urgent test[Q].

✓ **AKI recovery:** Absence of AKI by both creatinine and urine output criteria within 7 d after AKI onset.

- **Rapid reversal:** Recover within 48 h of AKI onset.
- **Persistent AKI:** AKI >48 h.
- **Acute kidney disease (AKD):** AKI >7 d.
- If AKI doesn't recover in next 90 d, CKD diagnosis is made if GFR <60 mL/min/1.73 m^2 or end-stage renal disease (ESRD) if GFR <15 mL/min/1.73 m^2.

Prevention and Treatment

✓ **Prevention:** Discontinue nephrotoxins like contrast agents, NSAIDs, ACEIs/ARBs, and aminoglycosides, magnesium containing drugs. Avoid hyperglycaemia.

✓ **Fluids:** Albumin is costly and no beneficial effect, hence crystalloids form the mainstay of therapy. Both normal saline and balanced crystalloids can be used.

✓ **Contrast-induced AKI: KDIGO guidelines suggest oral N-acetylcysteine (can cause anaphylaxis) along with IV isotonic crystalloids for volume expansion in CI-AKI.**

- 1 mL/kg/h for 12 h before and 1 mL/kg/h for 12 h after the procedure is recommended by KDIGO.

✓ **KDIGO suggests not using oral or IV NAC to prevent AKI otherwise in critically ill patients with hypotension or in post-surgical AKI.**

- **No MORTALITY benefit of both hydration and acetylcysteine** in preventing AKI.

✓ **Diuretics:** No benefit of diuretics and hence should be used only to treat volume overload and non-oliguric AKI.

✓ **Blood pressure:** Lower MAP targets of 60–65 mmHg are safe. In chronic hypertensive patient, higher MAP may prevent the occurrence or progression of AKI.

✓ **Nutrition:** Restrict sodium intake to *<2 g/day,* dietary phosphate less 2 g/day. Energy intake 20–30 kcal/kg/day.

- **Non-catabolic AKI patient without dialysis:** 0.8–1 g/kg/day
- **AKI on RRT:** 1–1.5 g/kg/day
- **Hypercatabolic patients on CRRT:** 1.7 g/kg/day

✓ **Glucose control:** Avoid hyperglycaemia and glucose levels between (6–10 mmol/L).

✓ **Fenoldopam:** Acts on dopamine D1 receptors. Causes vasodilation. Decreases SVR but increases IOP. No mortality benefits. Not recommended for CI-AKI.

- **Low-dose dopamine:** Increased chances of arrhythmias and higher mortality.
- **Alkaline phosphatase:** An ischaemic preconditioning has no role in prevention of AKI.

✓ **Timing of Renal Replacement Therapy:** No difference in need for RRT at 60 or 90 d with early or late initiation of RRT.

- **AKIKI trial (2016):** In critically ill patients with AKI, early renal replacement (at the time of randomization) had no mortality benefit over delayed dialysis (dialysis started once the patient had an urgent need or oliguria beyond 72 h).
- **ELAIN trial (2016):** In surgical ICU patients with early AKI and without a need for dialysis, early CVVHDF (within 8 h of KDIGO stage 2) had long-term mortality benefit over delayed dialysis (within 12 h of KDIGO stage 2).
- **IDEAL-ICU trial (2018):** In patients with septic shock and AKI without an urgent need for dialysis, early RRT (within 12 h of AKI) had no mortality benefit over delayed RRT (after 48 h of AKI if renal function had not recovered).
- **AKIKI 2 trial (2021):** In critically ill patients with AKI without an urgent

need for dialysis, a more delayed strategy (waiting to provide RRT once indicated) increased mortality compared to delayed strategy (after 72 h of oligura or BUN between 112 and 140 mg/dL).

✓ **Renal referral** if patient has ongoing RRT, renal transplant, AKI of unknown aetiology or suspected glomerular or vasculitis disease.

✓ **Bicarbonate** if pH <7.1. Bicarbonate 4.25% may reduce the need of RRT in patients with AKI stage 2 or 3 **but no mortality benefit.**

✓ **Steroids:** Used in acute interstitial nephritis, glomerulonephritis.

Prognosis

✓ AKI was independently associated with in-hospital mortality, irrespective of which definition was used.

- Patients with dialysis dependent ATN have mortality up to 70% compared to prerenal AKI which has good prognosis.
- Half of the patients with AKI are non-oliguric and have better prognosis than oliguric patients.

✓ KDIGO was more predictive for in-hospital mortality than RIFLE.

- No difference between AKIN and KDIGO in the prediction of in-hospital mortality.

✓ Amongst Stage 2–3 AKI patients, approximately 40% will not fully recover their kidney function at hospital.

Additional Questions

✓ Molecular weight > 70 kDa: Not filtered by kidney. Hence no albumin[Q]. Particles less than MW < 30,000 da are freely filtered.

✓ Hyaline casts[Q] are composed of Tamm–Horsfall proteins and are seen in normal healthy individuals.

✓ Percutaneous catheter angiography[Q] is the gold standard for investigating renal artery stenosis.

- CT angiography and MR angiography are other investigations that can be used for diagnosis.

✓ **Cardiorenal Syndrome**

- **Type 1:** Acute cardiac dysfunction leading to renal dysfunction.
- **Type 2:** Chronic heart failure leading to kidney failure.

- **Type 3:** AKD leading to acute heart failure.
- **Type 4:** CKD leading to heart failure.
- **Type 5:** Systemic disease leading to heart and renal failure. Hepatorenal syndrome, sepsis, amyloidosis are causes.

CHRONIC KIDNEY DISEASE

Epidemiology and Aetiology

✓ **CKD:** Abnormalities of kidney structure or function present for a minimum of 3 months with implications for health.

✓ **Diagnostic criteria (KDIGO 2024)[Q]:** CKD is renal dysfunction *(eGFR <60 mL/min/1.73 m²)* for **more than 3 months** plus 1 marker of kidney injury.

- Albuminuria (ACR >30 mg/g)
- Persistent haematuria
- Electrolyte and other abnormalities due to tubular disorders
- Urine sediment abnormalities
- Abnormalities detected by histology.
- Structural abnormality detected by imaging.
- History of kidney transplant

✓ **Causes:** Only 1% of patients with CKD will reach ESRD.

- **Diabetes (20–40%) is the leading cause of CKD followed by Hypertension (5–25%).**
- IgA nephropathy (10–20%) is also a common cause. Patients with CKD are at higher risk of AKI.

Classification[Q] of CKD by GFR and Albumin Creatinine Ratio (ACR)[Q]: A1, G1 and G2 Do Not Qualify as CKD

Category	GFR (mL/min/1.73 m²
G1	≥90
G2	60–89
G3a	45–59
G3b	30–44
G4	15–29
G5	<15

Category	ACR(mg/g)	Terms
A1	<30	Normal to mildly increased
A2	30–300	Moderately increased
A3	>300	Severely increased

Clinical Features and Diagnosis

✓ **Signs and symptoms:** Fatigue and weakness, swelling in ankles, feet or hands, shortness of breath, decrease appetite and weight loss, itchy skin, sleep disturbances, muscle cramps, high blood pressure, and breath that smells like ammonia.

✓ **Diagnosis**
  • **Estimated GFR (eGFR)** is calculated using **MDRD (Modification of Diet in Renal Disease)**[Q] calculation. It uses age, sex, creatinine, and ethnicity (Afro-Caribbean or not).
    ❖ National Kidney Foundation[Q] recommends calculating GFR using **CKD-EPI creatinine equation** and it calculates eGFR using sex, age, and creatinine and race is excluded.
  • **The Cockcroft–Gault formula** uses age, sex, weight, and creatinine to calculate creatinine clearance.

✓ Low-erythropoietin levels[Q] lead to decreased red cell survival and production.

Treatment

✓ Free drug fraction is increased and hence doses of highly protein bound drugs should be decreased.

✓ KDIGO guidelines suggest an **ACE inhibitor or angiotensin II blocking agent** in all patients with progressive CKD.

✓ Isotonic fluids should be used and hypo or hypertonic fluids should be avoided.

✓ **Drugs that may require dose alterations**[Q]: LMWH, warfarin, antibiotics like piperacillin/tazobactam. Meropenem, beta-blockers, opioids, and local anaesthetics.

✓ **General measures**
  • Protein intake reduction to 0.8g/kg/day is controversial.
  • **Good glycaemic control.**
  • **Reduced salt** intake <2 g/day.
  • **Anaemia** management by iron[Q] or erythropoietin.
  • **Lipid lowering by statins.**

Additional Questions

✓ **Nephrotic syndrome**[Q]: Proteinuria >3 g in 24 h, oedema, and hypoalbuminaemia.
  • Urinary loss of immunoglobulins and complement, hypovolaemia, hyperlipidaemia, and hypercoagulability due to urinary loss of antithrombin III and plasminogen.
  • Hypocalcaemia due to urinary loss of vitamin D-binding proteins.

RENAL REPLACEMENT THERAPY

✓ **Renal replacement therapy:** Life-supporting treatment to replace the normal function of the kidney when they are not functioning properly.

✓ **Working Principle**
  • **Haemodialysis**
    ❖ *Diffusion*[Q]: Only solute removal: From high concentration to low.
    ❖ **Smaller** molecules < **500 Da**[Q] are removed more readily as they have more velocities.
    ❖ Blood flow is countercurrent to dialysate flow to maximize concentration gradients.
    ❖ Urea, creatinine, and potassium move from plasma to dialysate whereas bicarbonate moves from dialysate to plasma.
    ❖ Alcohol, salicylate, and lithium can also be removed.
  • **Haemofiltration**
    ❖ *Convection*[Q]: Solutes and fluids: Hydrostatic pressure forms the pressure gradient and solutes small enough to pass through the pores are swept along with water by solvent drag.
    ❖ Moderate-sized molecules (**500–5,000 Da)**[Q] are better cleared with convection (CVVH).
    ❖ This technique doesn't change the plasma concentration of small solutes like BUN, creatinine, electrolytes, and glucose since water (ultrafiltrate) is removed in proportion to the solute.
    ❖ Theophylline and iron.

✓ **Haemodialysis**
  • **Intermittent haemodialysis (IHD):** Standard for patients with end-stage renal disease (ESRD).
    ❖ **Uses both diffusion (solute clearance) and convection (fluid removal).**
    ❖ **Blood flow:** 250–400 mL/min. **Dialysate flow:** 500–800 mL/min.
    ❖ **Ultrafiltrate:** 0–4 L/day as some convective part is there.

❖ Performed for a **few hours**, three to four times a week.

❖ Rapid shifts of fluid and solute can cause haemodynamic instability and it is hence less suitable for critically ill patient.

❖ *Disequilibrium syndrome:* Rapid removal of solute and water can cause delirium, seizures and dyspnoea. Hence blood flow rates are slowly started at 200–250 mL/min before going till 400 mL/min over several sessions as body is acclimatized to the high urea.

- SLEDD: Slow low efficiency daily dialysis
  ❖ Daily dialysis but with slow removal of fluid.
  ❖ **Blood flow:** 100–200 mL/min. **Dialysate flow:** 100 mL/min.
  ❖ **Ultrafiltrate:** 0–4 L/**day as some convective part is there.**
  ❖ Used at **night for 6–12 h** to allow patient mobility during the day.
  ❖ Complicates daily drug dosing.
  ❖ No mortality benefit seen.

✓ **Peritoneal dialysis (PD):** Peritoneum serves as a semipermeable membrane separating blood in the mesenteric vessels from dialysate in the peritoneal cavity.

- Mainly diffusion with some convection. Hence, solute and fluid both are removed.
- Dialysate is infused into the peritoneal space through a surgically placed Tenckhoff catheter.
- Tolerated better as fluid shifts happen slowly.
- **Continuous ambulatory peritoneal dialysis (CAPD):** Manual dialysate exchanges done during the day.
- **Continuous cycled peritoneal dialysis (CCPD):** Automated exchanges using a PD machine during the night.
- **Indications of PD in AKI**
  ❖ AKI in children
  ❖ Difficult vascular access
- **Contraindications of PD**
  ❖ Lack of trained staff
  ❖ Uncorrected mechanical defects like hernia
  ❖ Abdominal adhesions that limit dialysate flow
  ❖ Wound infections

❖ Intra-abdominal sepsis
❖ Malnutrition
❖ Inflammatory or ischaemic colitis
❖ Newly placed foreign bodies
❖ AKI in pregnancy.

- **Complications of PD**
  ❖ Blocked catheter
  ❖ Over-hydration/dehydration
  ❖ Constipation[Q] can decrease the efficiency of PD as it decreases dialysate flow

✓ **Haemofiltration (continuous renal replacement therapy):** Slow solute and volume removal over an extended period of time. Convection, dialysis or combination of both used.

- **Continuous venovenous haemofiltration (CVVH):** Only convection is the technique.
  ❖ *Used continuously for 24 h.*
  ❖ Blood flow: 200–400 mL/min. No dialysate flow as purely convective.
  ❖ Ultrafiltrate rate of **2–4 L/h.**
  ❖ **Ultrafiltrate taken out is replenished by using replacement fluid which can be given either of after the filter.**
- **Continuous venovenous haemodialysis (CVVHD):** Primarily diffusion is the technique.
  ❖ *Used continuously for 24 h.*
  ❖ Blood flow: 100–200 mL/min. Dialysate: 17–34 mL/min.
  ❖ Ultrafiltrate rate of **2–5 L/day** as primarily diffusion technique.
  ❖ No replacement fluid is given.
- **Continuous venovenous haemodiafiltration (CVVHDF):** Convection and diffusion.
  ❖ *Used continuously for 24 h.*
  ❖ Blood flow: 100–200 mL/min. Dialysate: 17–34 mL/min.
  ❖ Ultrafiltrate rate of **1–2 L/h.**
  ❖ **Ultrafiltrate taken out is replenished by using replacement fluid which can be given either of after the filter.**
- **Slow continuous ultrafiltration (SCUF):** Uses ultrafiltration and is mainly used for fluid overload. No dialysate or replacement fluid used.
  ❖ Blood flow: 100 mL/min. Ultrafiltrates: 100 mL–300 mL/h

✓ **Dosing of RRT[Q]:** Effluent volume: Therapeutic target measured in mL/kg/h.

- **CVVH:** Effluent volume is ultrafiltrate in this modality. Hence, 50 L of effluent volume means that 50 L of plasma has been fully cleared of urea.
- **CVVHD:** Effluent volume is spent dialysate in this modality. Spent dialysate is fully saturated with urea. Hence 50 L of spent dialysate is 50 L of plasma fully cleared with urea.
- **CVVHDF:** Effluent volume is ultrafiltrate plus spent dialysate.

✓ **Indications for RRT[Q]**
- Serum potassium >6.5 mmol/L refractory to medical management
- Refractory acidosis (pH <7.1)
- Oliguria/anuria leading to fluid overload
- Uremic complications like encephalopathy, pericarditis. Urea >35 mmol/L or creatinine >400 mmol/L
- Toxins

✓ **Trials:** See the section on AKI for clinical trials.

✓ **Toxins[Q]**
- **Dialysable: Salicylates, Theophylline/ Aminophylline, Barbiturates**
  - ❖ **Alcohol** (Ethanol, Methanol), Ethylene Glycol, Propylene Glycol
  - ❖ **Beta-blockers** (Sotalol, Atenolol),
  - ❖ **Anticonvulsants** (Carbamazepine, phenytoin, Valproic acid)
  - ❖ **Antibiotics** (most penicillins, cephalosporins, carbapenems, aminoglycosides)
  - ❖ Chloral hydrate, **metformin[Q]**, paraquat, **lithium[Q]**, methotrexate, and mushroom toxins
- **Non-dialyzable:** TCAs[Q], digoxin

✓ **Drugs characteristics that result in increased clearance by RRT[Q]**
- Small volume of distribution (<1 L/kg)
- Low degree of protein binding
- High water solubility
- MW up to 40 kDa can be cleared by CRRT

✓ **Solute clearance depends upon[Q]**
- Solute molecular size and properties
- Membrane sieving coefficient.
- Haemofiltration flow rate
- Dialysis flow rate
- Vascular access device lumen

✓ **Anticoagulation**
- **Filtration fraction (FF)[Q]:** Ultrafiltrate rate/plasma flow rate. Hence FF >20% will promote clotting.

- IHD can generally be performed without anticoagulation because of **high blood flows.**
- CVVH has high-ultrafiltrate rate and low blood flow, hence high chances of thrombosis.
  - ❖ **Pre-dilutional haemofiltration** involves infusion of replacement fluid before the filter.
- **Citrate[Q]** is first-line anticoagulation recommended by KDIGO unless contraindicated[Q] by liver disease or severe lactic acidosis. Unfractioned heparin is the next option.
  - ❖ Citrate binds to calcium and ionized calcium concentration in the filter <0.35 mmol/L results in anticoagulation.
  - ❖ Aim for post-filter ionized calcium of 0.2–0.35 mmol/L and total/ionized calcium ratio <2.5.
  - ❖ **Citrate prolongs circuit lifespan but otherwise no mortality benefit.**
  - ❖ **Citrate overload:** Citrate anticoagulation can lead to metabolic alkalosis due to conversion to bicarbonate.
  - ❖ **Citrate toxicity[Q]:** Acidic citrate is not metabolized and causes high anion gap metabolic acidosis.
- **Unfractionated heparin** bolus of 1000–2000 units followed by continuous infusion of 10 U/kg/h to maintain an APTT of 1.5–2 times the control.
  - ❖ This does cause some systemic anticoagulation.
- **KDIGO recommends Argatroban in patients with HIT** unless patients have severe liver disease.
- Other options are LMWH[Q], **prostacyclin[Q]** (causes systemic hypotension and not recommended by KDIGO).

✓ **Dialysate composition**
- **Bicarbonate:** 35 to 45 mEq/L. It is buffer and higher doses are used in patients with acidosis.
- **Sodium:** 138–145 mEq/L. Sodium levels are used initially in the session of dialysis to prevent hypotension and then tapered down gradually to prevent hypernatraemia.
- Potassium: 1–4 mEq/L. 1 mEq/L used for patients with severe hyperkalaemia.
- Calcium: 1–3.5 mEq/L. Higher calcium in hypocalcaemia.

- Chloride: 100–110 mEq/L.
- Magnesium: 1.5 mEq/L.
- *Composition of dialysate used in CVVHD is identical to replacement fluid used during CVVH.*

✓ **Dosing**
  - **ATN trial (2008):** No mortality benefit of high effluent flows (35 mL/kg/h) or intermittent haemodialysis/low efficiency dialysis six times per week compared to low effluent flow rates (20 mL/kg/h) or intermittent haemodialysis/low efficiency dialysis three times per week.
  - **RENAL trial (2009):** No mortality benefit of high effluent flows (40 mL/kg/h) compared to low effluent flow rates (25 mL/kg/h).
  - 25–30 mL/kg/h is recommended to achieve 20–25 mL/kg/h[Q].

✓ **Prescription for RRT[Q]**
  - **RRT dose (effluent rate):** 25–30 mL/kg/h.
  - **Blood flow rate:** 200–300 mL/min.
  - **Fluid balance target:** Negative or neutral balance
  - **Anticoagulation prescription:** Citrate, heparin, argatroban.

✓ **Effectiveness of RRT[Q] can be increased by**
  - ↓ Interruptions
  - ↓ Pre-dilution
  - ↑ Blood flow
  - ↑ Effluent dose
  - Improved vascular access

✓ **Vascular access:** Non-dominant arm is a likely site for future AV fistula and hence should be avoided. Subclavian insertion of vascular catheter is associated with vascular stenosis.
  - **Right IJV:** 15 cm, **Left IJV:** 20 cm, **Femoral vein:** 25 cm.
  - Cuffed tunnelled catheters are placed when the expected duration of dialytic support exceeds 2 wk.

✓ **Choice of modality: No benefit of CRRT over IHD in ITU mortality.**

✓ **Discontinuation:** Urine output >400 mL/day without diuretics is the only criteria with some evidence.
  - Otherwise UO >2300 mL/day with diuretics.

Additional Questions

✓ **Peritoneal dialysis (PD) peritonitis[Q]:** Presence of two of the following
  - Signs/symptoms like fever, abdominal pain, nausea, and vomiting.
  - White cell count >100/mL of effluent with >50% neutrophils after a 2-hour dwell.
  - A positive culture of an organism from the effluent (most commonly coagulase-negative Staphylococcus [30%], non-*Pseudomonas* Gram-negative organisms, and *Staphylococcus aureus*).
    - ❖ Antibiotics should be intra-peritoneal.

7

Fluids and Electrolytes

FLUIDS

✓ **Phases of fluid therapy (ROSE)**[Q]
- **Rescue:** Large fluid boluses to correct hypovolaemia. (Positive fluid balance)
- **Optimization:** Smaller fluid boluses with focus on optimizing cardiac output. (Slightly positive fluid balance)
- **Stabilization:** Maintenance fluids to maintain a state of euvolaemia. (Neutral fluid balance)
- **Evacuation/de-escalation:** Remove excess fluid using diuresis or RRT. (Negative fluid balance)

Important Trials Regarding Fluids

Trials	Year	Outcome
		Albumin[Q]
SAFE	2004	• **Albumin 4%** vs 0.9% normal saline for fluid resuscitation. • Primary end point: No mortality difference at 28 d. • **Traumatic brain injury** (TBI) subgroup had more mortality rates in albumin group in post hoc analysis.
FEAST	2011	• Fluid boluses in African children having severe infection. • Aggressive fluid resuscitation with **albumin 5%** or 0.9% normal saline increased mortality compared to no fluid boluses. • Population had a high incidence of malaria and anaemia not managed in standard critical care facilities.
ALBIOS	2014	• In patients with severe sepsis or septic shock, daily albumin does not improve mortality or any other clinically relevant endpoints.
		Colloids
CHEST	2012	• Hydroxyethyl starch (HES) vs 0.9% normal saline for resuscitation. • No mortality difference at 90 d, but HES increased the risk of renal failure and need for blood transfusion.
6S	2012	• HES vs Ringer's lactate. • In patients with severe sepsis, HES was associated with 90 d mortality, need for RRT, and use of blood products compared to Ringer's lactate.
CRISTAL	2013	• Colloids vs crystalloid in hypovolaemia in ICU. • Primary end point: No mortality difference at 28 d.
		Crystalloids
SPLIT	2015	• Plasma-Lyte 148 vs 0.9% normal saline in ICU patients. • **Primary end point:** No mortality difference, AKI within 90 d and length of stay.

DOI: 10.1201/9781003476214-7

Trials	Year	Outcome
SMART	2018	• Balanced crystalloids vs 0.9% normal saline in critically ill patients. • **Primary end point:** Balanced crystalloids *reduce major adverse kidney events (death, new renal replacement therapy, and doubling of serum creatinine).*
SALT-ED	2018	• Balanced crystalloids vs 0.9% normal saline in non-critically ill patients in ED. • Balanced crystalloids *didn't reduce hospital-free days but may have some impact in reducing major adverse kidney events.*
BaSICS	2021	• Plasma-Lyte 148 vs 0.9% normal saline in critically ill patient. • No mortality difference and no difference in renal outcomes. • TBI patients had better outcomes with normal saline.
PLUS	2022	• Balanced multi-electrolyte solution (BMES) vs 0.9% normal saline for fluid resuscitation. • Primary end point: No mortality difference at 90 d. • No difference in AKI between the groups.

Fluid Solutions

Fluid	Osmolarities (mmOsm/L)	pH
0.9% saline	308 (Na^+ and Cl^-: 154; K: 0)[Q]	5.5
Hartmann's solution	275–295 (Na^+: 131; K^+: 5)[Q]	6.5
5% dextrose	280	4.3
10% dextrose	560	4.3
0.18% saline/4% glucose	255 (Na^+: 30; K^+: 0)[Q]	3.5–6.5
4.5% albumin	330	7 ± 0.3
20% albumin	135	7 ± 0.3
10% mannitol	550	4.5–7
8.4% $NaHCO_3$	2,000	7.8

✓ **Role of albumin in critical care**[Q]
- **Spontaneous bacterial peritonitis (SBP):** 1.5 mg/kg within first 6 h and then 1g/kg on day 3.
- **Large volume paracentesis (>5 L)**[Q]: 100 mL of 20% albumin per 3 L of ascites drained.
- **Type 1 hepatorenal syndrome:** 1 g/kg on day 1 and then 20–40 grams/day until terlipressin is ceased.
- **Molecular adsorbent recirculation syndrome (MARS):** 20% albumin is used as a molecular adsorbent.
- **Burns:** May be used to produce less overall oedema.

✓ **Colloids**[Q]: Can cause coagulopathy, acute kidney injury and anaphylaxis.

Additional Questions

✓ **Most common**[Q] **intracellular cation is potassium and anion is phosphate**
- **Most common extracellular cation is Sodium and anion is chloride.**

HYPONATRAEMIA

Definition

✓ **Hyponatraemia** occurs in 20% of hospital admissions.
- **Hyponatraemia: <135 mmol/L**
  - ❖ Mild: 130–135 mmol/L
  - ❖ Moderate: 125–129 mmol/L
  - ❖ Profound: <125 mmol/L
- **Acute**[Q]: <48 h, **Chronic:** >48 h.
- **Corrected Na^+** = Measured Na^+ + 2.4 [Glucose (mmol/L) − 5.5]

✓ **Physiology:** Hypothalamic osmoreceptors sense thirst and release antidiuretic hormone that increase water retention by increasing the permeability of collecting tubules to water.
- **Plasma osmolality:** 2 × Na^+ + Glucose (mg/dL)/18 + BUN (mg/dL)/2.8 = 280–295 mOsm/kg.
- Urea can cross all cell membranes freely and glucose contributes normally less

than 8 mOsm per kg and hence effectively plasma osmolality = 2 × Na⁺.

✓ **Hypertonic hyponatraemia (dilutional)**[Q]: Hyperglycaemia, glycine, mannitol.

✓ **Isotonic hyponatraemia (pseudohyponatraemia)**[Q]: Hyperlipidaemia, hyperproteinaemia (multiple myeloma).

✓ **Hypotonic hyponatraemia:** *Two major causes are hypovolaemia and SIADH.*
  - **Hypovolemic hypotonic**
    ❖ *Urine Na⁺ <10 mEq/L* (extra-renal salt loss) seen in diarrhoea, vomiting, burns, pancreatitis.
    ❖ *Urine Na⁺ >20 mEq/L* (renal salt loss) seen in **Addison's disease, cerebral salt wasting syndrome (CSWS).**
  - **Euvolemic hypotonic**
    ❖ *Polydipsia*[Q]
    ❖ Syndrome of inappropriate ADH (SIADH), hypothyroidism, glucocorticoid insufficiency
    ❖ **Acute tubular necrosis**
    ❖ Drugs (**Thiazides, PPIs,** anti-epileptic drugs, antibiotics, and **SSRIs**)
  - **Hypervolemic hypotonic**[Q]
    ❖ Cirrhosis
    ❖ Heart failure
    ❖ Nephrotic syndrome
    ❖ Chronic kidney disease
    ❖ Pregnancy

Clinical Features and Diagnosis

✓ **Symptoms:** Nausea, vomiting, anorexia, confusion, or headache.
  - *Severe acute hyponatraemia* can present with muscle cramps, hyporeflexia, and cerebral oedema-induced seizures and coma.

✓ **Diagnosis:** Paired osmolality (Plasma osmolality, Urine osmolality).
  - **Urine osmolality <100 mOsm/kg suggests polydipsia.**
  - **Urinary sodium concentration:** Helps to differentiate hypovolaemia from SIADH/CSWS.
  - Addison's disease is diagnosed using ACTH stimulation test.

✓ **Syndrome of inappropriate antidiuretic hormone secretion (SIADH):** SIADH is seen in malignancies like **small cell lung cancer,** CNS tumours, psychiatric disorders, CNS bleed, vasculitis, SSRIs, ecstasy, and infections.

- A short Synacthen test or early morning cortisol level can be performed in suspected cases.
- **Diagnostic Criteria**[Q]
  ❖ Hypo-osmolality: <280 mOsm/kg
  ❖ Urinary concentration: U_{osm} >100 mOsm/kg
  ❖ Euvolaemia/slight hypervolaemia
  ❖ Urinary sodium > 40 mOsm/L
  ❖ Exclude hypothyroidism, diuretics, steroid deficiency
- First-line treatment as **fluid restriction to 800 mL/day** is recommended.
- **Hypertonic saline** or **demeclocycline** can be used in refractory cases. Demeclocycline takes 2–3 d to take effect and can cause renal failure.
- **Urea** in dose of 15–30 g in 1 to 2 divided doses has been recommended for treatment as well.

✓ **Cerebral salt wasting syndrome (CSWS)**[Q]: Diuresis and natriuresis. Low plasma osmolality, high urinary concentration and urinary sodium >20 mOsm/L.
  - Characterized by *dehydration and haemodynamic instability.*
  - Fluid resuscitation by **isotonic sodium containing fluids.** Hypertonic saline may be needed in patients with concomitant SIADH.
  - **Fludrocortisone** has been used to stop natriuresis.

✓ **TURP syndrome**[Q]: Use of *hypotonic 1.5% glycine.*
  - Restlessness, headaches, and visual disturbances.
  - *The height of the bag should be kept around 60–70 cm above the patient and less than 100 cm and surgical time should be less than an hour.*
  - Hypertonic saline should be given in TURP syndrome if sodium is <120 mmol/L aiming for a maximal increase of 1 mmol/L/h.

Treatment

✓ **An acutely agitated patient/symptomatic patient should be treated urgently with hypertonic saline to increase the sodium concentration by 5 mmol/L**[Q].
  - Total plasma sodium should not exceed approximately 8–10 mEq/L during the initial 24 h and stop hypertonic saline once sodium levels reach >120 mEq/L.

- 100 mL of 3% NaCl and can be repeated 3 times[Q], 10 min apart in patients with ongoing seizures.
- 3% NaCl @ 0.5–2 mL/kg/h in patients with moderate neurological symptoms.
✓ **Routine management:** Restrict water intake to below the level of excretion in those with oedematous states like heart failure and liver cirrhosis along with use of loop diuretic.
  - **Patients with polydipsia are also treated with restricted water intake.**
  - *Isotonic saline can be given to those who are hypovolemic or adrenal insufficiency. Each litre of saline infused raises the sodium by 1–2 mEq/L.*
    - ❖ The formula given below can help calculate sodium deficit in patients with true volume depletion. Not very accurate in patients with SIADH.
    - ❖ **Sodium deficit for initial therapy** = TBW × (target Na⁺ – current Na⁺).
    - ❖ *Total body water (TBW) values are 0.5 and 0.6 times the lean body weight in women and men.*
  - Plasma sodium levels in patients with chronic hyponatraemia should be raised at 0.5 mEq/L/h.
  - **Tolvaptan/Conivaptan (ADH-V2 antagonists)** are approved for used in SIADH or hypervolemic hyponatraemia. Can cause *hepatotoxicity.*
✓ **Central pontine myelinosis**
  - Rapid correction of chronic hyponatraemia can lead to it.
  - Total rate of correction in first 24 h is more important than the maximum in any given hour[Q].
    - ❖ 5% dextrose is often used to correct a rapid rise in plasma sodium levels.
    - ❖ DDAVP in dose of 2 mcg IV repeated every 6–8 h has been used to impede rapid rise in plasma sodium.
  - Oligodendrocytes appear to be more prone to apoptosis.
  - **Clinical signs** include dysarthria, dysphagia, oculomotor abnormalities, flaccid quadriplegia develop over next to several days.
    - ❖ Locked-in syndrome with large pontine lesions. Extrapontine myelinosis (EPM) have features like catatonia.

- **MRI** is the imaging modality of choice.
- **Treatment:** Patients are usually alcoholics or malnourished. It is rare in diabetic or renal dialysis because of protective high levels of glucose or urea.

Prognosis

✓ Significant hyponatraemia <125 mmol/L is an independent risk factor for mortality.

HYPERNATRAEMIA

Aetiology

✓ **Hypernatraemia:** Serum Na⁺ >145 mmol/L. *Primary problem is relative deficiency of free water[Q].*
  - These patients are primarily those who can not express thirst normally as even diabetes insipidus patients who are having polyuria can have normal sodium levels by increasing water intake.
✓ **Causes: Insensible fluid losses**, gastrointestinal losses, **diabetes insipidus[Q]** (lithium, hypercalcaemia, or cerebral injury), hypothalamic injury, **poly-uric phase of AKI**, hypertonic saline/sodium overload or antibiotic solutions.

Clinical Features and Diagnosis

✓ **Symptoms** normally if Na⁺ >155 mmol/L. Pyrexia, muscle cramps, drowsiness, seizures, and coma.
  - Brain shrinkage can lead to vascular rupture leading to intracerebral haemorrhage.
✓ **Urine osmolality** can help in diagnosis as ADH (intact hypothalamus and kidney) will lead to increase urinary osmolality.
  - Polyuria is sudden in central DI and gradual in nephrogenic DI.
  - **Water restriction test[Q]** is done for evaluation of polyuria with measurement of urine volume and osmolality every hour and plasma sodium and osmolality every 2 h.
    - ❖ *Test is continued till urine osmolality reaches 600 mOsm/kg indicating both ADH release and effect are intact.*
    - ❖ If urinary osmolality increases insufficiently, exogenous ADH is given to test if the release is a problem or the effect.
    - ❖ If increase in urinary osmolality is sufficient.

- Urinary sodium <20 mEq/L indicates volume loss.
- Urinary sodium >100 mEq/L is seen in sodium overload state.

✓ **Polyuria with high plasma sodium is diabetes insipidus (DI)^Q and polyuria with low plasma sodium is polydipsia.**

Treatment

✓ **Rate of correction: Acute hypernatraemia is corrected at a rate of 1 mmol/L/h.**
  - **Chronic hypernatraemia (>48 h):** Corrected at a rate of 0.5 mmol/L/h and no more than 10 mmol/L/day.
✓ **Water deficit:** Calculated as water deficit = current body water (plasma Na$^+$/140–1) where current body water = 60% body mass. Water needed to return the plasma sodium concentration to 140 mEq/L.
  - *Free-water deficit corrected over 48–72 h in chronic hypernatraemia.*
  - *Fluid boluses should be given enterally if possible.*
  - *In a patient with fluid overload and renal failure, haemodialysis or haemofiltration should be used.*
  - Insensible losses (40 mL/h) should be replaced as well.
✓ **Treatment of diabetes insipidus**
  - **Central DI:** DDAVP starting at the dose of 5 mcg every day.
  - **Nephrogenic DI:** Thiazide^Q with low-sodium diet.
    - ❖ Amiloride and NSAIDs have also been used for treatment.
    - ❖ Most patients have partial resistance and exogenous ADH in supraphysiological doses also helps.
  - **Thiazides** are preferred over **loop diuretics** in managing hypernatraemia as they promote natriuresis^Q.

HYPERKALAEMIA

Epidemiology and Aetiology

✓ **Hyperkalaemia:** Potassium above >5.5 mmol/L. Symptomatic hyperkalaemia >6.5 mmol/L.
✓ **Causes**
  - **Increased intake:** Blood transfusions, parenteral nutrition.
    - ❖ **Drugs:** Sando-K

- **Disturbed homeostasis:** *Metabolic acidosis*, malignant hyperthermia, rhabdomyolysis, tumour lysis syndrome, hyperkalaemic periodic paralysis.
  - ❖ **Drugs: Suxamethonium^Q, digoxin overdose^Q, beta-blockers^Q.**
- *Decreased excretion:* Chronic kidney disease, hypoaldosteronism.
  - ❖ **Drugs:** ACE inhibitors, **spironolactone^Q**, amiloride, NSAIDs, **tacrolimus^Q**, cyclosporine^Q, **trimethoprim^Q**, heparin.
✓ **Pseudo-hyperkalaemia:** During venipuncture leading to haemolysis.

Clinical Features and Diagnosis

✓ Most significant effect on resting potential of neural tissue is by potassium^Q.
  - **Impaired neuromuscular transmission:** Muscle twitching, cramps.
✓ Earliest and most sensitive change is **peaked T-wave^Q**: K$^+$: 5.5–6.5 mmol/L.
  - P wave gets wider and flatter: K$^+$ >6.5 mmol/L.
  - QRS gets wider as well: K$^+$: 7–8 mmol/L.
  - VF, Asystole or PEA.
✓ **Hypermagnesemia will have similar ECG effects like hyperkalaemia.**

Prevention and Treatment

✓ **Stabilize myocardial cell membrane:** 10% Calcium gluconate or calcium chloride.
  - Effect starts in minutes and lasts for 30–60 min.
  - Hypercalcaemia can itself cause digoxin toxicity and should be taken carefully in these patients.
✓ **Insulin with dextrose:** Produces a 0.5–1.5 mEq/L fall in plasma potassium concentration.
  - Effect starts in 15 min and peaks at 60 min and lasts for several hours.
  - 10 units insulin in 50 mL 5% dextrose.
✓ **Nebulized Salbutamol:** Produces a 0.5–1 mEq/L fall in plasma potassium concentration.
  - Effects are additive to effects of Insulin.
✓ **Sodium Bicarbonate:** Effective in patients with severe metabolic acidosis, cardiac arrest.
  - Action begins in 30–60 min. Dose is 45 mEq or roughly 50 mL of a 8.4% sodium bicarbonate.
  - Should be used with caution in patients with renal failure or heart failure.

✓ **Loop diuretics:** Used in patients with volume overload with working kidneys.

✓ **Potassium-binding resins**[Q]**:** Lokelma (sodium zirconium silicate)– Used for chronic hyperkalaemia.

✓ **Renal replacement therapy:** Refractory or severe hyperkalaemia.

✓ **Fludrocortisone:** Has been used in patients on calcineurin inhibitors, heparin, and post-infectious glomerulonephritis.

HYPOKALAEMIA

Definition

✓ **Hypokalaemia:** Serum potassium <3.5 mmol/L.

✓ **Potassium:** Major intracellular cation.

- 50% of ingested potassium appears in urine during the first 4 h. Rest of potassium load is transported into the cells.
- 90% of filtered potassium is reabsorbed by the time it reaches distal tubule. Aldosterone regulates the reabsorption by causing reabsorption of Na^+ in lieu of excretion of K^+.
- Intracellular Potassium transport is due to Insulin and beta-adrenergic stimulation.

✓ **Causes**

- **Decreased potassium intake:** *Starvation.*
- **Increased entry in cells:** Metabolic alkalosis[Q], insulin, beta-adrenergic stimulation, hypokalaemic periodic paralysis, **hypothermia**.
- **Increased losses:** *GI losses*[Q] *(Diarrhoea and vomiting)*, urinary losses[Q] (**diuretics**, hypomagnesaemia, aminoglycosides, aldosterone producing adrenal adenoma).

✓ **Classification by severity**

- **Mild:** 3–3.4 mmol/L
- **Moderate:** 2.5–3 mmol/L
- **Severe:** <2.5 mmol/L

Clinical Features

✓ Muscle weakness, cramps, paraesthesias, constipation, ileus.

✓ **ECG**[Q]**:** Atrial fibrillation, **U waves (V2–V4)**[Q], **prolonged QT interval, ST depression, and T wave inversion**.

- Duration of the action potential and refractory period are increased.
- Ventricular arrhythmias can occur in patients post-myocardial infarction or patients taking digoxin.

Treatment

✓ **Potassium deficit:** Loss of 200 to 400 mEq lowers the potassium levels from 4 to 3 mEq/L and another 200–400 mEq will take levels from 3 to 2 mEq/L.

✓ **Mild to moderate hypokalaemia** is normally asymptomatic and can be treated with oral potassium supplements.

- Oral potassium supplements can cause gastric mucosa irritation or ulceration, but the chances of rebound hyperkalaemia are low.

✓ **Severe or symptomatic hyperkalaemia** is treated with IV potassium with boluses of 40 mmol every 3–4 h.

- Rate of replacement shouldn't exceed more than 20 mmol/h (increases potassium levels at the rate of 0.25 mmol/h) as it can cause rebound hyperkalaemia.
- Rate above 10 mmol/h through peripheral IV confusions can cause pain and phlebitis.
- Up to 40 mmol/h can be given via CVC can be given.
- Hypomagnesaemia should be treated as well.
- Chronic hypokalaemia should be treated with potassium sparing diuretics as well.

MAGNESIUM METABOLISM

✓ **Magnesium:** Fourth most abundant cation in the body. Second most intracellular cation.

- Needed in body for parathyroid hormone (PTH) secretion and calcium secretion and maintenance.
- Neuromuscular function.
- Co-factor for enzymes.
- Na-K-ATPase function.

✓ **Physiology:** Two-thirds of magnesium is found in bone and only 2% is found in the extracellular space.

- Magnesium absorption is through the small intestine and is reabsorbed in the kidney tubules.

✓ **Mechanism of action as a drug in body**[Q]

- 1. Physiological NMDA receptor antagonist
- 2. Natural Ca^{2+} antagonist
- 3. Inhibits presynaptic release of acetylcholine (Ach)
- 4. Inhibits catecholamine release

✓ **Pharmacodynamic actions**
- **CVS:** Vasodilation via endothelial nitric oxide plus inhibition of catecholamine release. Decreases cardiac conduction and myocardial contractile force.
- **Respiratory:** Bronchodilation.
- **CNS:** Depresses the brain and causes sedation. Deep tendon reflexes are lost.
- **Uterus:** Relaxes uterus, used as a tocolytic.

✓ **Clinical uses of magnesium**
- **Asthma:** Used in refractory asthma. 25 mg/kg or 2 gram IV over 20 min.
  - ❖ **3Mg trial (2013):** Among patients with acute exacerbation of asthma, neither IV nor nebulized magnesium sulphate has any mortality benefit.
- **Pre-eclampsia and eclampsia:** A loading dose of 4 gram over 15 min followed by an infusion at a rate of 1 g/h for 24 h.
  - ❖ **Magpie trial (2002):** Significantly fewer eclamptic convulsions among women with magnesium sulphate than those in placebo with lower maternal mortality.
- **Fetal neuroprotection:** Magnesium sulphate to be offered to women carrying viable fetuses, who are very likely to deliver a premature baby within the next 24 h.
  - ❖ A loading dose of 4 gram over 15 min followed by an infusion at a rate of 1 g/h for 24 h.
- **Subarachnoid haemorrhage:** Prevention of vasospasm.
  - ❖ **MASH-2 trial (2012):** Intravenous magnesium sulphate didn't demonstrate any significant improve clinical outcome in patients with aneurysmal subarachnoid haemorrhage.
- **Hypomagnesaemia**
- **Analgesia**
- **Arrhythmias:** Torsades de pointes and tachyarrhythmias induced by adrenaline, digitalis, and bupivacaine.
- **Laxative and antacid**

✓ **Hypermagnesemia**
- **Causes**
  - ❖ **Increased intake:** Magnesium containing antacids, iatrogenic during pre-eclampsia.
  - ❖ **Decreased excretion:** Renal failure.
- **Magnesium toxicity**
  - ❖ 0.7–1.0 mmol/L: Normal blood levels

  - ❖ 2–3.5 mmol/L: Nausea and vomiting, ECG changes
  - ❖ **4–5 mmol/L: Loss of tendon reflexes (best way of monitoring toxicity)**
  - ❖ 5–7.5 mmol/L: Respiratory paralysis
  - ❖ 10–12.5 mol/L: Cardiac arrest
- **ECG[Q]:** Prolonged PR, QRS and QT interval. Peaked T waves and flat P waves.
  - ❖ Complete AV block and asystole.
- **Treatment:** Almost like hyperkalaemia.
  - ❖ **Cardiac stabilization:** IV administration of calcium gluconate diluted in 100 mL 5% dextrose over 5–10 min.
  - ❖ Furosemide 20–40 mg IV to increase magnesium excretion along with fluid hydration.
  - ❖ Dialysis when kidney function is impaired.

✓ **Hypomagnesaemia:** Serum magnesium concentrations below the normal range. Threshold may depend upon clinical laboratories. Commonly <0.7 mmol/L.
- **Causes**
  - ❖ **Reduced intake:** Prolonged starvation.
  - ❖ **Decreased intestinal absorption:** Steatorrhoea, diarrhoea.
  - ❖ **Increased excretion:** Osmotic diuresis due to hyperglycaemia, alcohol excess, diuretics.
- **Symptoms**
  - ❖ **CNS signs** of excitability like myoclonus, stridor, seizures.
  - ❖ **CVS signs** like hypertension and anginal pain.
  - ❖ **GIT symptoms** like nausea, vomiting and loss of appetite.
- **ECG:** Prolonged PR and QRS interval.
- **Treatment**
  - ❖ **Oral or parenteral magnesium:** 8–12 gram of magnesium sulphate over the first 24 h followed by 4–6 gram/day for 3–4 d.

CALCIUM METABOLISM

✓ **Calcium:** Needed in body for coagulation cascade, membrane potential maintenance, neuromuscular junction, neurotransmitter release and co-factor for enzymes.

✓ **Metabolism:** 99% of total body calcium is in bones. 1% is located in extracellular fluids.

- 50% of calcium in the extracellular fluids is bound to albumin and hyperventilation increases binding of calcium to albumin.
  - ❖ **Corrected total calcium (mg/dL)[Q] =** Measured total calcium (mg/dL) + {0.8 × [4 − serum albumin (g/dL)]}.
- **Parathyroid hormone (PTH):** Polypeptide secreted by chief cells of the parathyroid. Magnesium is needed for PTH secretion and end-organ response.
  - ❖ Increases calcium release from bones by activating osteoclasts.
  - ❖ Increases distal tubular reabsorption of calcium.
  - ❖ Decreases reabsorption of phosphate from proximal tubular cells.
  - ❖ Increases activity of 1, 25 D hydroxylase hormone.
- **Vitamin D:** Steroid hormone. 25-hydroxylation in liver followed by 1-hydroxylation in kidney.
  - ❖ Increased intestinal absorption of calcium and phosphate.
  - ❖ Reduces calcium losses in urine.
- **Calcitonin[Q]:** Polypeptide secreted by parafollicular (C-cells) of the thyroid.
  - ❖ Secreted in response to elevations in serum calcium.
  - ❖ Exogenous calcitonin enhances excretion of calcium, phosphate, magnesium, and sodium and is a potent inhibitor of bone resorption.
- ✓ **Uses in ICU**
  - **Massive transfusion:** Citrate can chelate calcium and cause hypocalcaemia.
  - **Hyperkalaemia:** Stabilize myocardial membrane.
  - **Calcium channel blocker overdose**
- ✓ **Hypercalcaemia**
  - **Classification**
    - ❖ **Mild:** 2.6–3 mmol/L
    - ❖ **Moderate:** 3–3.5 mmol/L
    - ❖ **Severe:** >3.5 mmol/L
  - **Causes[Q]**
    - ❖ **PTH-dependent hypercalcaemia:** More common in outpatient setting: Primary hyperparathyroidism (adenomas), tertiary hyperparathyroidism (CKD)[Q], familial hypocalciuric hypercalcaemia (FHH), multiple endocrine neoplasia (MEN) syndromes, **lithium.**

- ❖ **PTH independent hypercalcaemia: More common in hospital patients.** Hypercalcaemia of malignancy (breast, lung, or myeloma), granulomatous diseases (sarcoidosis), immobilization, milk-alkali syndrome, thyrotoxicosis, vitamin D and A intoxication, **thiazides.**
- **Symptoms**
  - ❖ **Neuropsychiatric:** Lethargy, **psychosis,** confusion, depression, generalized weakness.
  - ❖ **Renal:** Polyuria, polydipsia, renal tubular acidosis, **renal stones.**
  - ❖ **Gastrointestinal:** Abdominal pain, **constipation,** and nausea.
  - ❖ **Cardiovascular: Shortened QT interval,** hypertension, vascular calcification.
- **Hypercalcaemic crisis (Ca^{2+} > 4 mmol/L)** is most commonly caused by primary hyperparathyroidism[Q].
  - ❖ Anuria and AKI at calcium levels >4 mmol/L.
- **Milk-alkali syndrome:** Ingestion of calcium carbonate ingestion, alkalosis with an elevated bicarbonate level.
- **Investigations:** Serum PTH measurement. If low PTH levels, sources of malignancy should be sought.
  - ❖ PTH-related peptide (PTHrP) is raised in malignancies.
  - ❖ 1,25 D levels are raised in lymphomas and granulomatous disease.
- **Treatment**
  - ❖ Avoid thiazides and lithium[Q] in these patients.
  - ❖ **Hydration and diuresis:** IV saline to increase renal calcium excretion to aim for urine output of >75 mL/h. Frusemide 40 mg IV once hydration has been achieved.
  - ❖ **Haemofiltration:** In renal or cardiac failure patients here, we can't give adequate hydration.
  - ❖ **Calcitonin:** Rapid onset within 2 h, maximal effect within 24–48 h and low toxicity. Tachyphylaxis develops to drug action (4–7 d).
  - ❖ **Bisphosphonates:** Pamidronate or zoledronic acid can be given intravenously but are slow to act.

❖ **Donesumab:** Monoclonal antibody against RANKL. approved for use in treatment of hypercalcaemia of malignancy.

❖ **Steroids** in patients with myeloma.

❖ **Cinacalcet:** Used for chronic treatment of severe hypercalcaemia of patients with primary hyperparathyroidism. No role in active hypercalcaemia.

✓ **Hypocalcaemia:** Calcium <2.1 mmol/L.
  • **Causes**
    ❖ **PTH-related:** Hypoparathyroidism post-surgery, pseudohypoparathyroidism (target tissue resistance).
    ❖ **Non-PTH-related:** Alkalosis, renal failure, multiple blood transfusions, tumour lysis syndrome, vitamin D deficiency, hypoalbuminaemia (spuriously low).
  • **Symptoms:** Peri-oral numbness, tetany, laryngospasm[Q], seizures.
    ❖ **Chvostek's sign:** Muscle spasm on tapping the facial nerve.
    ❖ **Trousseau sign:** Carpal spasm precipitated by inflation of s blood pressure cuff above the systolic pressure.
  • **ECG: Prolonged QT interval**[Q], AV conduction block.
  • **Treatment**
    ❖ Magnesium replacement[Q].
    ❖ **Calcium gluconate 10% (0.23 mmol/mL):** 10–20 mL diluted in 100 mL 5% dextrose over 10 min. Infusion may need to be started after this.
    ❖ **Calcium chloride 10% (0.68 mmol/mL):** 10 mL given over 10 min.
    ❖ **Oral calcium supplementation:** 500–1000 mg calcium three times a day.
    ❖ **Vitamin D supplementation:** 25000–10,000 IU daily.

PHOSPHATE METABOLISM

✓ **Phosphate:** Major intracellular anion.
  • Oxidative metabolic pathway
  • Component of nucleic acids and phospholipids
  • pH buffering
✓ **Physiology:** 85% of total body phosphorus is found in bone.
  • Regulated by parathyroid and 1,25-D hormone.

✓ **Hyperphosphataemia:** Levels >1.45 mmol/L.
  • **Causes**
    ❖ **Increased intake:** Laxatives, fosphenytoin.
    ❖ **Disturbed metabolism:** Haemolysis, rhabdomyolysis, tumour lysis syndrome, metabolic acidosis.
    ❖ **Reduced losses (Most common)**[Q]: Renal failure or hypoparathyroidism.
  • **Spurious causes:** Amphotericin B, heparin, hyperglobulinaemia, hyperlipidaemia, hyperbilirubinaemia.
  • **Symptoms:** Symptoms are mainly due to accompanying hypocalcaemia. Myocardial and vascular calcification.
  • **Treatment:** Limit phosphate intake.
    ❖ Phosphate binder-like sevelamer or calcium acetate.
    ❖ Insulin-dextrose as a temporary measure.
    ❖ Renal replacement therapy for rhabdomyolysis.

✓ **Hypophosphataemia:** Levels <0.81 mmol/L.
  • **Causes**
    ❖ **Decreased intake:** Starvation, aluminum, calcium, and magnesium salts.
    ❖ **Disturbed metabolism:** Insulin, beta-2 agonists, respiratory alkalosis.
    ❖ **Increased loss:** Acetazolamide, metolazone, tenofovir, steroids, diuretics.
  • **Symptoms**[Q]: Impaired oxygen delivery to tissues due to decreased RBC 2,3 diphosphoglycerate levels, respiratory muscle weakness, ileus, cardiomyopathy, seizures, haemolysis.
    ❖ Chronic deficiency can cause haemolytic anaemia along with leucocyte and platelet dysfunction[Q].
  • **Treatment**
    ❖ **Mild hypophosphataemia:** Phosphate Sandoz tablets up to 6 tablets a day.
    ❖ **Severe hypophosphataemia (<0.32 mmol/L):** Phosphate polyfusor.
    ❖ Parenteral therapy should be given cautiously in patients with renal failure as can cause metastatic calcification. 50% less doses in these patients.

METABOLIC ACIDOSIS

Physiology

✓ **Acidaemia:** Blood pH <7.35. Blood pH 7.35–7.45 is necessary to keep intracellular pH at 7.20.

✓ **Regulation of H⁺ secretion**
- **Renal:** 4500 mEq of bicarbonate ions are filtered by kidneys and then 85% of it is reabsorbed from proximal tubule every day. *Kidneys also excretes 50–100 mEq of H⁺ generated each day.*
  - ❖ **Na+/H+ antiporter:** Sodium reabsorption is active with a counter transport of H⁺ secretion into lumen of PCT. This is at apical membrane.
  - ❖ H+ secretion into lumen allows reabsorption of bicarbonate via the use of the enzyme carbonic anhydrase. Both combine in lumen to form carbonic acid and dissociate into CO_2 and H_2O which are reabsorbed.
  - ❖ Therefore, for every one molecule of H+ secreted, one molecule of bicarbonate and Na^+ is reabsorbed into the bloodstream.
  - ❖ **Other buffers:** Phosphate (HPO_4^-/ $H_2PO_4^-$): Some in PCT but most in DCT and ammonia (NH_3/NH_4^-): PCT and DCT.
- **Respiratory:** In acute metabolic acidosis, lungs regulate acidosis by excretion of CO_2.
✓ **ABG analysis[Q]:** pH, H^+, PaO_2 and $PaCO_2$ are measured directly and HCO_3^-, base excess and SaO_2 are measured indirectly.
✓ **Base excess**
- **Actual base excess or deficit[Q]:** Refers to the amount of acid or base required to restore 1 L of blood to normal pH at a $PaCO_2$ of 5.3 kPa at body temperature.
  - ❖ Gives quantitative aspects of the metabolic acidosis and is present in blood only.
- **Standard base excess[Q]:** Base excess corrected to a haemoglobin of 50 g/L. This shows more accurate reflection of the overall acid-base balance of the body.

Metabolic acidosis: Categorized by using presence of absence of increased anion gap.
✓ **Anion gap[Q]:** Mainly due to negative charge of serum proteins, sulphates, organic acids and is underestimated in hypoalbuminaemia.
- $Na^+ + K^+ - (Cl^- + HCO_3^-)$. **Normal** is 12 ± 4 mmol/L.
- K is normally excluded as changes large enough to cause a difference in anion gap are either uncommon or are incompatible with life.

- Hence **ANION GAP** = $Na^+ - (Cl^- + HCO_3^-)$ and is normally taken as 8 ± 4 mmol/L.
- **Albumin correction:** Increase the baseline anion gap by 2.5 mEq/L for every 10 g/L fall in the albumin concentration.
✓ **High anion gap metabolic acidosis (HAGMA)[Q]**
- Lactic acidosis
- **Ketoacidosis:** Acetoacetic acid and β-hydroxybutyric acid cause it and not acetone as it is not an acid.
  - ❖ Diabetes mellitus
  - ❖ Starvation
  - ❖ Ethanol
  - ❖ Genetic/Metabolic disorders of amino acids
- Rhabdomyolysis
- Other acids
  - ❖ **Salicylates[Q]:** Mixed respiratory alkalosis with high AG metabolic acidosis.
  - ❖ Methanol
  - ❖ Ethylene glycol
  - ❖ Propylene glycol (parenteral medications like lorazepam)
  - ❖ **5-oxoproline (pyroglutamic acid):** Seen in chronic paracetamol intake
  - ❖ Toluene: In glues
  - ❖ Paraldehyde and formaldehyde
  - ❖ Iron, Isoniazid
  - ❖ Valproic acid
  - ❖ Cyanide, carbon monoxide
✓ **Normal anion gap metabolic acidosis (NAGMA)[Q]:** Decrease in bicarbonate is accompanied by increase in chloride. An infusion of Sodium bicarbonate will help in treatment of such patients.
- **Renal causes**
  - ❖ Renal tubular acidosis I, II, and IV
  - ❖ Acute renal failure
  - ❖ Acetazolamide (loss of bicarbonate)
- **Non-renal causes**
  - ❖ 0.9% NaCl-rich fluids.
  - ❖ Total parenteral nutrition (amino acid solutions).
  - ❖ **Diarrhoea:** Loss of HCO_3^- from GIT.
  - ❖ **Small bowel fistula:** Loss of HCO_3^- from GIT.
  - ❖ **Ureteric diversion:** Ileal conduit–Loss of HCO_3^- from GIT.
✓ **Osmolal gap (OG):** Difference between plasma osmolality measured by the lab and calculated using the formula:

$2 \times Na^+ + Glucose/18 + BUN/2.8$ or $2 \times Na^+ + Glucose + Urea$, all in mmol

- Normally measured osmolality is greater than calculated osmolality by <10 mOsm/kg.
- **Increased OG**
  - ❖ Toxins like ethanol, **methanol, ethylene glycol, isopropyl alcohol**, salicylate.
  - ❖ Metabolic disorders like high **ketones, lactates**, and **kidney injury.**

✓ **Chronic kidney disease:** Overlap between normal and elevated anion gap.
- GFR below 20–30 mL/min, anions such as sulphate and phosphate are increased causing raised anion gap. Above this GFR, normal anion gap metabolic acidosis exists.
- In uncomplicated CKD, plasma bicarbonate is greater than 12 mEq/L. A lower bicarbonate should call for a second acid/base disorder.

✓ **Renal tubular acidosis (RTA)^Q:** Classified into three types (1, 2, and 4). Type 3 is infantile version of type 1.
- **Type 1 RTA/Distal RTA (DCT):** Failure to excrete chloride and H^+. Nephrocalcinosis.
- **Type 2 RTA/Proximal RTA (PCT):** Renal bicarbonate losses.
- **Type 4 RTA/Hyperkalaemic RTA (Hypoaldosteronism):** Failure to excrete H^+.

✓ **Pyroglutamic acidosis (5-oxoprolinaemia)^Q:** **Pyroglutamic acid** is produced from γ-glutamyl cysteine by enzyme γ-glutamyl cyclotransferase and metabolized by 5-oxoprolinase.
- Low glutathione levels increase the levels of γ-glutamyl cyclotransferase and hence leads to high levels of pyroglutamic acid seen in chronic paracetamol, alcoholism, and chronic liver failure.
- **Inhibition on enzyme 5-oxoprolinase:** By Flucloxacillin, Vigabatrin, and Netilmycin, also leads to high levels of pyroglutamic acid.

✓ **Symptoms of metabolic acidosis:** Kussmaul's respiration (increase in tidal volume), tachycardia, decreased cardiac contractility, drop in consciousness, vasodilation in coronaries, muscle, and uterus but vasoconstriction in systemic, renal, splanchnic vessels.
- It shifts oxyhaemoglobin dissociation curve (ODC) to the right.

✓ **Diagnosis:** Access anion gap. Respiratory compensation is calculated to access mixed acid-base disorder.

- **Respiratory compensation:** In uncomplicated metabolic acidosis, pCO_2 is expected to fall by 1.2 mmHg (0.16 kPa) for each 1 mEq/L fall in bicarbonate. *Lower pCO_2 means respiratory alkalosis and higher pCO_2 means respiratory acidosis.*

  - ❖ **Winter's formula:**

    Expected pCO_2 (mmHg) = $[(1.5 \times Bicarbonate) + 8] \pm 2$

- **Delta ratio:** In patients with a high anion gap metabolic acidosis, monitor the change in anion gap (ΔAG) to change in bicarbonate concentration ($\Delta HCO3^-$).

  ANION GAP = $Na^+ - (Cl^- + HCO_3^-)$

  - ❖ **Delta ratio** = $\Delta AG / \Delta HCO3^-$ = AG – 12/24 – Bicarbonate
  - ❖ Delta ratio: < 0.4 = Pure NAGMA
  - ❖ Delta ratio: 0.4–0.8 = Mixed NAGMA + HAGMA
  - ❖ Delta ratio: 0.8–2 = Pure HAGMA
  - ❖ Delta ratio: >2 = HAGMA + Metabolic alkalosis/respiratory acidosis

- **Urinary anion gap:** $Na^+ + K^+ - Cl^-$. Used to calculate the aetiology of a normal AG metabolic acidosis with hypokalaemia.
  - ❖ A positive UAG suggests low NH_4^- like in renal tubular acidosis whereas a negative UAG implies high NH_4^- like in diarrhoea.

✓ **Treatment:** Treat the underlying cause.
- **Haemofiltration:** Patients with AKI.
- **Bicarbonate:** Patients with CKD take oral bicarbonate supplements regularly as a meta-analysis showed that it reduces the rate of developing ESRD.
  - ❖ Acidaemia of RTA type 1 can be corrected with bicarbonate or its precursor like citrate. Potassium citrate is preferred as it corrects potassium and citrate is converted to bicarbonate.
  - ❖ In acute metabolic acidosis, aim is to raise the arterial blood pH to >7.20.
  - ❖ No mortality benefit of giving bicarbonate in treating severe metabolic acidosis due to DKA.

✓ **ABG analysis by Stewart approach**[Q]
- **Strong ion difference (SID)**
  - ❖ Strong cations are Na^+, K^+, Ca^{2+}, Mg^{2+} and strong anions are Cl^- and SO_4^{3-}

    Strong ion difference (SID) = $(Na^+ + K^+ + Ca^{2+} + Mg^{2+}) - (Cl^- +$ other strong anions) = 40–44 mmol/L **or** SID $Na^+ - Cl^-$ 34 mM

  - ❖ The number of positive and negative ions in a solution must be equal.
  - ❖ Volume depletion causes increase in SID > 0 meaning alkalosis. Increase in SID < 0 means acidosis.
  - ❖ Normal saline has a strong ion difference of 0.
- **SID = $Na^+ - Cl^- = 34$ mM.**
  - ❖ **Step 1: [Na] – [Cl] disorder influence on BE:** $Na^+ - Cl^- > 34$ = High SID alkalosis, $Na^+ - Cl^- < 34$ = Low SID alkalosis. Deviation from 34 = BE attributable to SID changes. For example: $Na^+ - Cl^- = 24$ mM means BE – 10 mM if no other disorder and $Na^+ - Cl^- = 44$ mM means BE + 10 mM if no other disorder.
  - ❖ **Step 2: Albumin disorder influence on BE:** For each 10 g/L of albumin below 40 g/L, BE increases in positive direction by 3 mm (e.g. albumin = 20 g/L leads to BE + 6 mM if no other disorder).
  - ❖ **Step 3: Identify unmeasured anion:** If the ABG BE is different from BE calculated from Step 1 and Step 2, unexplained BE = Strong ion anion like lactates or unmeasured anions like ketones or poisons.
  - ❖ **Example:** BE from Step 1 = + 20 mM and BE from Step 2 = + 5 mM, then predicted BE = + 25 mM. If on the ABG strip BE is shown as – 5 mM and lactate as 10 mM, then unmeasured = 25–5–10 = 10 mM (can be ketones or any other ion).
  - ❖ **Step 4 is to use Boston rules to predict mixed acid base disorder by predicting pCO_2.**
✓ **Boston rules for mixed acid base disorder**[Q]: (10 mmHg = 1.33 kPa). For purpose of calculation normal pH = 7.4, pCO_2 = 40 mmHg (5.3 kPa) and Bicarbonate of 24 mmol/L.
- **Metabolic acidosis:** pCO_2 = *Bicarb/5 + 1 kPa [± 0.3]* **or** 1.5 × (Bicarb) + 8 mmHg [± 0.3].
  - ❖ If pCO_2 is higher than this, then an added respiratory acidosis.

- **Metabolic alkalosis:** pCO_2 will increase 6 mmHg for each 10 mEq/L increase in bicarbonate.
- **Respiratory acidosis**[Q]
  - ❖ Acute: Bicarbonate will increase 1 mEq/L per 10 mmHg increase in pCO_2.
  - ❖ Chronic: Bicarbonate will increase 4 mEq/L per 10 mmHg increase in pCO_2.
- **Respiratory alkalosis**
  - ❖ Acute: Bicarbonate will decrease 2 mEq/L per 10 mmHg decrease in pCO_2.
  - ❖ Chronic: Bicarbonate will decrease 4 mEq/L per 10 mmHg decrease in pCO_2.
✓ **Pearls of ABG analysis**
- Check acidaemia or alkalaemia.
- If acidaemia and respiratory, look for acute or chronic **compensation** or acute on chronic if in between values.
- If acidaemia and metabolic, calculate anion gap and correct it for albumin. Calculate osmolar gap.
  - ❖ Check Winter's formula for any secondary mixed based disorder/**compensation.**
  - ❖ Calculate delta ratio.
- If alkalaemia and respiratory, look for acute or chronic **compensation.**
- If alkalaemia and metabolic, check for urinary chloride.
  - ❖ Check for **compensation.**
- If normal pH, apply Stewart's approach to look for unmeasured anions.

METABOLIC ALKALOSIS

Aetiology

✓ **Alkalaemia:** Arterial pH >7.45.
✓ Factors that generate alkalosis may be different from those that maintain it.
- Excess bicarbonate generated can cause metabolic alkalosis but can be corrected by kidney.
- But **hypovolaemia** or **hypokalaemia** prevent renal correction of alkalosis and maintain alkalosis.
- Hypovolaemia cause alkalosis due to reabsorption of more bicarbonate from PCT and most hypovolemic disease states are associated with chloride depletion and hence are chloride responsive.

- However, giving chloride may be ineffective in patients with hyperaldosteronism who are already volume replete but have hypokalaemia due to absorption of sodium and losing potassium and hydrogen in urine.
- Citrate administration (precursor of bicarbonate) and milk-alkali syndrome can also cause metabolic alkalosis.

✓ **Causes**[Q]: Chloride-responsive alkalosis (urine chloride <20 mmol/L) and Chloride-resistant alkalosis (urine chloride >20 mmol/L).

- **Chloride-responsive alkalosis:** More common. **Diuretic use** and loss of gastric secretion due to **NG suction/vomiting**. Eating disorders with induced vomiting can also cause it.
  - ❖ **Diuretics**[Q]: Thiazide and loop diuretics.
  - ❖ **Vomiting:** Loss of H^+ and Cl^- leads to alkalosis as bicarbonate is reabsorbed for acid lost.
- **Chloride-resistant alkalosis:** Cushing's syndrome, Conn's syndrome (primary hyperaldosteronism), Bartter syndrome, and Gitelman syndrome (renal tubular chloride loss).

Clinical Features and Diagnosis

✓ Symptoms of **volume depletion** like weakness, muscle cramps or symptoms of **hypokalaemia** like polyuria or polydipsia.

✓ **Respiratory compensation:** pCO_2 rises approximately 0.7 mmHg (.1 kPa) for every 1 mEq/L elevation in plasma HCO_3^-.
- pCO_2 greater or less than predicted suggests the presence of respiratory acidosis or alkalosis.

✓ **Delta ratio: Delta ratio** = ΔAG / ΔHCO_3^- = AG – 12/24 – Bicarbonate.
- Monitor the change in anion gap (ΔAG) to change in bicarbonate concentration (ΔHCO_3^-).
- ΔAG more than double the ΔHCO_3^- signifies co-existing metabolic acidosis and metabolic alkalosis.

Treatment

✓ Rapid correction of metabolic alkalosis is usually not needed. Any exogenous source of alkali like bicarbonate, acetate, lactate, or citrate should be discontinued.

- Hypomagnesaemia or hypokalaemia should be corrected.

✓ **Chloride-responsive metabolic alkalosis:** KCl or NaCl should be given. Patients with vomiting may also benefit from drugs that reduce acid secretion.
- Isotonic solution of HCl may need to be given in patients with neurological signs of metabolic alkalosis.

✓ **Chloride-resistant metabolic alkalosis:** In a hypertensive patient, primary aldosteronism should be suspected and treatment can be spironolactone.
- Oedematous states like heart failure have low urine chloride secretion due to hypoperfusion but are non-responsive to chloride.
- Diuretics are already being used in these patients and they may benefit from acetazolamide administration.

Additional Questions

✓ **Gastric outlet obstruction**[Q]: Hypochloraemic, hypokalaemic, metabolic alkalosis. Initial increase in urine pH due to renal bicarbonate loss. Paradoxical aciduria occurs as sodium ion is preserved and hydrogen ions are thrown out in urine.

RESPIRATORY ACIDOSIS

Aetiology

✓ **Respiratory acidosis:** Acid-base disturbance initiated by a primary increase in CO_2 tensions of the body fluids.
- pH <7.35

✓ **Categorization of respiratory acidosis**
- **Acute respiratory acidosis:** Occurs when CO_2 accumulates quickly in the lungs.
- **Chronic respiratory acidosis:** Occurs when CO_2 accumulates gradually in the lungs.
- **Acute on chronic:** Acute retention of CO_2 in patients with chronic compensated respiratory disease (e.g. **pneumonia in a patient with COPD**).

✓ **Causes of acute respiratory acidosis**
- **Reduced alveolar capillary diffusion:** Asthma, pulmonary oedema, pulmonary embolism.
- **Decreased respiratory drive:** Drugs (opioids), cerebral oedema, brainstem injury.

- **Inadequate chest expansion:** Guillain–Barré syndrome.
- **Airway obstruction:** External (clothing), internal (oedema, foreign body).

✓ **Causes of chronic respiratory acidosis**
- **Reduced alveolar capillary diffusion:** COPD.
- **Decreased respiratory drive:** Obesity hypoventilation syndrome.
- **Inadequate chest expansion:** Scoliosis, muscular dystrophy.

Physiology

✓ Respiratory centre in the pons and medulla controls alveolar ventilation.
- Chemoreceptors for PCO_2, PO_2 and pH regulate ventilation.
- Central chemoreceptors in the medulla are sensitive to changes in pH level.
- **Disruption of the respiratory centre** can lead to disruption of ventilation leading to CO_2 retention.
- **V/Q mismatch of dead space** in respiratory disorders can also lead to CO_2 retention.

Clinical Features

✓ In acute respiratory acidosis, no time for compensation and hence pH falls, CO_2 increases and bicarbonate falls.
- In chronic respiratory acidosis, kidneys start compensating and retain bicarbonate. pH starts to return to normal.

✓ **Signs and symptoms**
- **Acute respiratory acidosis:** Drowsiness, hypotension, and headache due to vasodilation, rapid shallow breathing.
- **Chronic respiratory acidosis:** High blood pressure, heart failure symptoms, polycythaemia[Q], loss of coordination, and memory loss.

✓ **Investigations**
- **ABG:** Elevated CO_2 is seen. Elevated bicarbonate and polycythaemia signify a chronic process.
  - ❖ Acute: Bicarbonate will increase 1 mEq/L per 10 mmHg increase in pCO_2.
  - ❖ Chronic: Bicarbonate will increase 4 mEq/L per 10 mmHg increase in pCO_2.
  - ❖ If compensation doesn't occur in the above pattern, a mixed respiratory metabolic disorder may be present.

- Chest X-ray, CT scan chest, and CT head based on history.

Treatment

✓ **Treat underlying causes**
- Naloxone may be needed in opioid poisoning.

✓ **Oxygen therapy:** Lowest flow possible to prevent hypoxaemia.

✓ **Drug therapy:** Bronchodilators and mucolytics in case of asthma and COPD.

✓ **Mechanical ventilation:** In those with respiratory muscle fatigue and falling saturation.

RESPIRATORY ALKALOSIS

Aetiology

✓ **Respiratory alkalosis:** Systemic acid-base disorder characterized by reduction in arterial partial pressure of carbon dioxide.
- pH >7.45.
- Most common acid-base abnormality observed in critically ill patients[Q].

✓ **Classification**
- **As a component of disease processes:** Hyperventilation to compensate for metabolic acidosis, anxiety, salicylate toxicity.
- **Accidentally induced:** Hyperventilation due to inappropriate ventilatory settings.
- **Deliberately induced:** Hyperventilation for raised ICP.

✓ **Physiology**
- Hyperventilation is the mechanism responsible for lowered CO_2 in all cases of respiratory alkalosis.
- Low CO_2 will be sensed by the central and peripheral chemoreceptors and the hyperventilation is inhibited by higher centres unless patient's ventilation is controlled.

✓ **Causes**
- **Central causes:** Head injury, anxiety, pain, fear, salicylate toxicity, pregnancy.
- **Pulmonary causes:** Pulmonary embolism, pneumonia, asthma, pulmonary oedema.

Clinical Features

✓ **Signs and symptoms**
- **Cardiovascular:** Tachycardia, arrhythmias, hypotension, shift of haemoglobin oxygen dissociation curve to the left.

- **Electrolyte imbalance**
  - ❖ Hypocalcaemia: Circumoral tingling, carpopedal spasm
  - ❖ Hypokalaemia: Cramps, twitches, weakness
- **CNS:** Light-headedness, hyperreflexia, tinnitus, seizures, confusion.

✓ **Investigations**
- **ABG:** It will show decreased arterial CO_2.
  - ❖ Acute: Bicarbonate will decrease 2 mEq/L per 10 mmHg decrease in pCO_2.
  - ❖ Chronic: Bicarbonate will decrease 4 mEq/L per 10 mmHg decrease in pCO_2.
- Chest X-ray, CT head and chest based on history.

Treatment

✓ Treat the underlying cause.

✓ **Supplemental oxygen:** Hypoxaemia is an important cause of respiratory stimulation and hence giving oxygen can decrease the drive.

✓ Drug and fluid therapy to restore normal fluid and electrolyte balance.
- Rebreathing into a paper bag.
- Give anti-anxiety medications or sedatives.

8

Gastrointestinal Problems

UPPER GASTROINTESTINAL BLEED

Epidemiology and Aetiology

✓ **Incidence:** 50–150/100,000 adults per year
  - 80% or more patients with acute GI bleeding will stop bleeding eventually.
✓ **Upper gastrointestinal bleed (UGIB):** Bleeding from any point proximal to the duodenojejunal flexure.
  - **Causes**
    - ❖ **Portal hypertension:** Oesophageal varices (MC in developing countries), vascular malformations.
    - ❖ **Ulcerative:** Gastric or duodenal ulceration (MC in Western countries), oesophagitis.
    - ❖ **Tumours:** Polyps, carcinoids, lymphoma.

Clinical Features

✓ **History:** Blood in vomiting, appearance of blood in NG aspirate, melaena.
  - Massive upper GI bleed can present with rectal bleed as well and in patients with bright red blood in the stool and haemodynamically instability, upper endoscopy may be the first endoscopic evaluation.
  - History of NSAIDs, anticoagulants.

Risk Stratification

✓ **Glasgow–Blatchford score**: Uses only medical and laboratory data to *assess if a patient will need to have medical intervention* such as blood transfusion or endoscopic intervention or **admission to hospital.** *A score of >6 or more suggests patient needs intervention.*
  - ❖ **Clinical data:** SBP, pulse ≥100/min, blood urea, haemoglobin.
  - ❖ **Medical data:** Melaena, syncope, hepatic disease, cardiac failure.
✓ **Rockall Scoring System:** Assesses the risk of death in UGIB. *A score >8 suggests high mortality (35%).*
  - ❖ Age, shock (pulse rate and SBP), co-morbidities, diagnosis, and **evidence of bleeding at endoscopy** are the parameters used.

Treatment[Q]

✓ **Resuscitation:** Early intubation in those with ongoing hematemesis and altered mental status.
  - Fluid resuscitation along with blood products with two wide bore cannulas.
  - Targets: Hb >70 g/L, INR <1.5, fibrinogen >1.5 g/L, platelets >50 × 10⁹/L.
  - *Higher haemoglobin targets for patients with active cardiac ischaemia or ongoing massive bleeding.*
  - Tranexamic acid is not recommended currently for UGIB.
  - Prothrombin complex concentrate (PCC) for warfarin. Idarucizumab[Q] for dabigatran.
  - *Haemodynamically unstable patients with UGIB should be offered endoscopy immediately after resuscitation within 2 h and within 24 h in haemodynamically stable patients.*
  - Prokinetics like erythromycin or metoclopramide to induce gastric emptying.

✓ **Proton pump inhibitors (PPIs):** NICE guidelines advise against use of PPIs before endoscopy[Q].
  - Used only after endoscopy confirms recent non-variceal bleeding.
  - PPI reduced re bleeding, surgical intervention, and need for repeated endoscopic treatment and **reduced mortality in those with active bleeding or stigmata of recent bleeding.**
  - *Pantoprazole 80 mg bolus followed by 8 mg/h for 3 d.*
✓ **Terlipressin[Q]:** Synthetic analogue of vasopressin. It causes selective splanchnic vasoconstriction and **reduces variceal bleeding[Q] as well as mortality rates.**
  - Should be started in suspected variceal bleeding and given for 3–5 d.
✓ **Prophylactic broad-spectrum antibiotics** covering Gram-negative bacteria should be used for variceal bleeding and has mortality benefit.
✓ **Endoscopy therapy for non-variceal bleeding[Q]: Adrenaline** (1:10,000 or 1:20,000) injected in 0.5–1.5 mL aliquots to the four quadrants. Adrenaline is not recommended as monotherapy.
  - **Mechanical devices** include **endoscopic clips.**
  - **Thermal therapy** includes electrocautery and argon plasma coagulator (APC).
  - In stable patients, repeat endoscopy in the event of rebleeding with a view to further endoscopic treatment or emergency surgery.
  - In unstable patients who rebleed, interventional radiology or surgery should be done.
✓ **Endoscopy therapy for variceal bleeding[Q]:** *Endoscopic variceal ligation (EVL)[Q]* preferred over sclerotherapy for **oesophageal varices** and has mortality benefit.
  - *Endoscopic injection of N-butyl-2-cyanoacrylate injection* is recommended treatment for **gastric varices.** Gastric varices bleed less often but bleed profusely and dictate early consideration of trans-jugular intrahepatic portosystemic shunt (TIPSS).

Rescue Therapy for Variceal Bleeding

✓ **Sengstaken–Blakemore tube[Q]:** Temporary measure to ongoing massive haemorrhage when endoscopy has failed until further endoscopy, TIPSS, or surgery.

- **3 ports[Q]:** Gastric and oesophageal balloons, gastric aspiration port. Gastric balloon volume is 450–500 mL.
- Controls bleeding in 90% of cases. Relapse in 50% cases.
- General anaesthesia isn't mandatory and can be inserted via mouth or nose.
- Gastric placement is confirmed. Oesophagogastric junction is at 40 cm from incisors. So, tube is pushed till 55 cm mark. If in doubt, gastric balloon is inflated with 50 mL of air or contrast and a chest X-ray taken.
- Injection of total 250 mL of air or saline into the gastric balloon. Gentle traction is applied with a 500 mL bag of fluid.
- *Gastric port is aspirated to measure ongoing bleed.*
- Oesophageal balloon is inflated with 35–40 mmHg if ongoing bleed.
- Oesophageal balloon[Q] should be deflated for 15 min every four hours to assess for cessation of bleeding, gastric balloons are generally left inflated for 12–24 h.
- Tube is usually removed within 36–48 h[Q].
✓ **Minnesota tube** has 4 ports[Q] with an additional oesophageal port as well. Gastric balloon volume is 250–300 mL.
  - **Linton–Nachlas tube[Q]** has 2 ports (gastric suction and balloon inflation). Only one single 500–600 gastric balloon.
✓ **TIPSS:** Used in **uncontrolled bleeding or refractory ascites[Q].** Stent placement to create a portocaval shunt.
  - Increases encephalopathy. Better results in mortality reduction if performed early in patients (*within 72 h*) in selected patients with Child–Pugh class B or C cirrhosis.
✓ **Prophylaxis:**
  - *Helicobacter pylori* **eradication therapy** for all those tests positive for the infection.
  - **Non-selective beta-blockers** like carvedilol[Q] > propranolol are the drug of choice in prophylaxis against variceal bleeding as they reduce hepatic venous pressure gradient.
  - *Endoscopic variceal ligation (EVL)* is also effective as prophylaxis against variceal bleeding.
  - **Aspirin** can be restarted once haemostasis is achieved in patients taking low-dose

aspirin for secondary prevention of vascular events.

- *Primary prophylaxis against stress ulceration on the ICU reduces rate of UGIB but without overall effect on mortality.*

Prognosis

✓ Mortality due to UGIB was 7% among new admissions and 30% in those who bled as inpatients.

Additional Questions

You think you know it all and then the question in the exam will be like the following:

Q. Which of the following drugs can be used to reverse dabigatran?
  1. Idaruczuimab
  2. Idarucziumab
  3. Idarucizumab
  4. Idaruzicumab
  5. Sorry, I give up

LOWER GASTROINTESTINAL BLEED

✓ **Epidemiology and aetiology:** Incidence: 20–30/100,000 adults per year.
  - **Lower gastrointestinal bleeding (LGIB)** traditionally defined as bleeding distal to ligament of Treitz.
    ❖ With introduction of term "small bowel bleeding," LGIB is defined as bleeding distal to ileo-caecal valve.
  - **Small bowel bleeding:** Bleeding distal to the ampulla of Vater and proximal to the ileocaecal valve.
  - **Causes**
    ❖ **Commonest cause** of massive lower GI bleed (LGIB) is **Diverticulitis**[Q] (older patients) followed by **Angiodysplasia** (young patients).
    ❖ **Small bowel:** 5–10% of patients with GI bleeding have small bowel bleeding (Meckel diverticulum, radiation proctopathy, and angiodysplasia).
    ❖ **Upper GI:** 15% of LGIB will have altered blood with upper GI as source[Q].
    ❖ **Anal canal: Haemorrhoids** account for 5–10% of episodes of LGIB and are the most common cause of bright red in the

stool or toilet tissue in the ambulatory patient.
  ❖ **Other causes: Colorectal cancer**, inflammatory bowel disease, **mesenteric ischaemia.**

Clinical Features and Diagnosis

✓ **Symptoms:** Bright red or dark red blood around formed stools mostly with melaena in some cases. Rule out bloody diarrhoea as it is mostly because of infections.
  - **Bleeding colonic diverticula** are the leading cause of lower GI bleeding and causes arterial bleeding with more than half of bleeding coming from the right colon.
  - **Angiodysplasias** are small (3–15 mm) dilated communications between veins and capillaries that can cause bleeding in stomach, small bowel, or colon. They cause subacute and recurrent bleeding.
  - Lower rate of haemodynamic compromise compared to upper GI bleeding.

✓ **Stratification of patients:** Done based on **shock index (HR/SBP).** A shock index ≥1 is defined as unstable patient.
  - Patients with shock index ≥1 undergo CT angiography (CTA) and those with positive lesions on CTA are treated with angio-therapy or endoscopically.
  - Patients with shock index <1, undergo risk stratification using **Oakland score**[Q]. Patients with score ≥9 are categorized as stable major bleed and are booked for a colonoscopy on next available list.

✓ **Computed Tomography Angiography:** Fast, non-invasive, and can detect bleeding at a rate of >0.5 mL/min. **Used in haemodynamically unstable patients with active lower GI bleeding to localize the source of bleeding.**
  - In haemodynamically unstable patients with negative initial CTA, an upper GI endoscopy should be done.

✓ **Sigmoidoscopy:** Done in minimal bleeding in patients suggestive of a distal source near anal area (red blood coating formed stools, pain with defecation, tenesmus, and passage of fresh clots).
  - However, a colonoscopy almost always follows it as sigmoidoscopy cannot rule out a more proximal source.

✓ **Early colonoscopy (within 24 h)** to identify the bleeding source but early intervention didn't increase detection of stigmata of recent haemorrhage or decrease the rebleeding rates.

✓ **Video capsule endoscopy** (VCE) is considered test of choice in evaluating patients with suspected small bowel bleeding after negative upper and lower endoscopy.
  - Drawbacks are that accurate localization of findings is not possible and no therapeutic intervention can be done.
  - Can be done safely in patients with cardiac implantable devices and in ICU.

✓ **Enteroscopy:** Longer endoscope for small bowel lesions. Can be used directly in patients with high suspicion of small bowel bleeding, altered anatomy or when VCE is contraindicated.

Prevention and Treatment

✓ **Resuscitation:** First with fluids and then with blood products. 80–85% of bleeding will stop without intervention.
  - However, a colonoscopy almost always follows it as sigmoidoscopy cannot rule out a more proximal source.

✓ **Colonoscopy** *is done in haemodynamically unstable patients and positive CTA.*
  - Epinephrine injection, thermal cautery or haemoclip application is done in patients with bleeding diverticula.

✓ **Angio-therapy:** *Interventional radiology procedure done in patients with haemodynamic instability and positive CTA in whom lesions are not reachable by colonoscopy.*
  - *Angiography is followed by embolization and vasopressin infusion.*

✓ **Upper endoscopy** is done in **haemodynamically unstable patients and negative CTA** as up to 15% of these unstable patients can have an upper GI source of bleeding.

✓ **Laparotomy** may be needed for refractory cases.

Prognosis

✓ 3.6% mortality in patients admitted with lower GI bleed whereas patients developing GI blood loss during hospital stay have a mortality of 23%.

✓ Surgery or uncontrolled GI haemorrhage carries a 33% mortality rate.

STRESS ULCER PROPHYLAXIS

Gastrointestinal Function (Just to Improve Concepts, Don't Start Cramming Everything)

Area	Exocrine	Endocrine	Digestion	Absorption
Mouth	Lysozyme, amylase, lipase, ribonuclease, secretory IgA, mucin glycoproteins		Carbohydrates	
Stomach	Pepsinogen, **HCl**, *Intrinsic factor* B, HCO_3^-, mucins	Ghrelin, gastrin, motilin	Proteins and lipids	Water, ethyl alcohol, Cu, I^-, F^-, Mo
Duodenum	HCO_3^-, mucins	Cholecystokinin, GIP, secretin, motilin	Carbohydrates, proteins, and lipids	Ca^{2+}, Mg^{2+}, PO_4^{3-}, Fe, Se, thiamine, riboflavin, niacin, biotin, folate, and vitamins A, D, E, K
Pancreas	Trypsinogen, chymotrypsinogen, amylase, protease, lipase, nuclease, Na^+, Cl^-, Ca^{2+}, H2O, HCO_3^-	Insulin, glucagon, somatostatin, amylin, pancreatic polypeptide		
Bile	Bile acids, cholesterol, phospholipids, Na^+, K^+, Cl^-, Ca^{2+}, H2O, HCO_3^-			

Area	Exocrine	Endocrine	Digestion	Absorption
Jejunum	HCO_3^-, mucins, amylase, peptidase	GIP, secretin, motilin	Carbohydrates, proteins, and lipids	Monosaccharides, amino acids, fatty acids, glycerol, small peptides, Ca^{2+}, Mg^{2+}, PO_4^{3-}, Fe, Zn, Cr, Mn, Mo, thiamine, riboflavin, niacin, pantothenate, biotin, folate, vitamins A, C, D, E, K
Ileum	Mucins, HCO_3^-	Peptide YY		Bile salts and acids, Mg^{2+}, folate, vitamin C, D, K, B_{12}
Colon	Mucins, K^+, HCO_3^-	Peptide YY, GLP1–2		Short-chain fatty acids, Na^+, K^+, Cl^-, vitamin K, and biotin

- ✓ **Immunological function of gut:** Intact mucosa, peristalsis, saliva, acid, mucin, and bile provide immunity.
  - • Gut-associated lymphoid tissue (GALT) secretes IgA.
- ✓ **Acute gastrointestinal injury (AGI) classification**
  - • **AGI grade I: Risk** of developing GI dysfunction.
    - ❖ Nausea and vomiting, absent bowel sounds after abdominal surgery.
  - • **AGI grade II: GI dysfunction**
    - ❖ Gastroparesis with high GRVs, diarrhoea, *IAP 12–15* mmHg, visible blood in gastric content or stool.
  - • **AGI grade III: GI failure**
    - ❖ High GRVs despite treatment, worsening of bowel dilatation, *IAP 15–20* mmHg.
  - • **AGI grade IV: GI failure with impact on other organs**
    - ❖ Bowel ischaemia with necrosis, GI bleeding leading to haemorrhagic shock, *Oglivie's syndrome*, abdominal compartment syndrome.

Stress Ulcer Mucosal Disease

Aetiology

- ✓ 90% of patients in ICU have evidence of erosive disease in mucosa after 3 d.
  - • Only a small proportion of patients will have clinically evident bleeding.

- ✓ **Pathophysiology**[Q]: Hypoperfusion → Hypoxia → Epithelial cell damage → Breakdown of mucous bicarbonate barrier → Acid causes further injury → Mucosal ulcers.
- ✓ In stress ulcer mucosal disease, gastric fundus is affected the most and ulcers are painless[Q].
  - • In peptic ulcer disease, it's the gastric antrum and duodenum that are affected the most and ulcers are painful.

Clinical Features and Diagnosis

- ✓ **Phenotypes of GI bleeding from stress ulcers**
  - • **Occult bleeding** (15–50% of ICU patients). Blood detected only by haemoccult testing.
  - • **Overt bleeding** (5% of ICU patients). Gross or altered blood is visually evident in gastric aspirate or stool.
  - • **Clinically significant bleeding** (1–4% of ICU patients). Haemodynamic instability or a drop in haemoglobin of **>2 g/dL.**
- ✓ **Most common risk factors**[Q] are respiratory failure requiring *ventilation for >48 h* followed by the presence of a **coagulopathy (INR >1.5 or platelet count <50,000/mm³).**
- ✓ **Other risk factors:** Head injuries (Cushing ulcers), major burns (>35% body surface area, *Curling ulcers*), high-dose steroids, NSAIDs, trauma, renal and **hepatic failure**[Q], sepsis and septic shock, post-organ transplant.

Prophylaxis[Q]: Prevents acid causing mucosal damage. Doesn't prevent hypoperfusion.

✓ **IV Proton pump inhibitors (PPIs):** First-line agents in at risk patients. Blocks the H^+/K^+-ATPase pump on the gastric parietal cells.
  - **PPIs are more effective than H2RBs in reducing upper GI bleeding.**
  - PPIs can cause interstitial nephritis[Q] and hyponatraemia.
  - **REVISE Trial (2024):** In critically sick patients on mechanical ventilation, IV pantoprazole resulted in a lower risk of clinically important upper GI bleeding than placebo, however, with no effect on mortality.
  - **SUP-ICU (2018):** In critically sick patients at risk of GI bleeding, pantoprazole resulted in a lower risk of clinically important upper GI bleeding than placebo, however, with no effect on mortality.
✓ **Histamine-2 receptor blockers (H2RBs):** First-line agents in at risk patients. Blocks the action of histamine on H-2 receptors on the basolateral membrane of parietal cells.
  - H2RBs can cause tachyphylaxis and have shorter half-life.
  - **PEPTIC trial (2020):** In critically sick patients on mechanical ventilation, use of a PPI decreased the risk of clinically important GI bleeding in comparison to an H2RB but not effect on mortality.
  - **Overall. No mortality benefit with either PPIs or H2RBs[Q].** *They both increase the risk of VAP and chances of clostridium difficile infection[Q].*
✓ **Sucralfate:** Aluminum salt of sulphated sucrose.
  - They line the eroded mucosa and provide an additional layer of protection.
  - It is not as effective as PPIs or H2RBs in preventing stress ulceration.
✓ **Enteral feeding[Q]** is a prophylaxis for stress ulceration as well and no need of stress ulcer prophylaxis in those with established feeding.
✓ **Vasopressors:** Judicious use of vasopressors.

Prognosis

✓ *Patients with GI bleeding have mortality as high as 60% in patients with clinically significant bleeding.*

ACUTE LIVER FAILURE

Epidemiology and Aetiology

✓ *Acute liver failure (ALF): Triad[Q] of jaundice, coagulopathy, encephalopathy* in patients with previously normal liver function and <12 wk of illness duration[Q].
  - Around 400 cases in UK every year.
✓ **O'Grady classification for ALF[Q]:** Time from jaundice to encephalopathy.
  - **Hyperacute diseas:** <7 d
  - **Acute disease:** 1–4 wk
  - **Subacute disease:** 4–12 wk
✓ Severe forms of Wilson's disease, Budd–Chiari syndrome, and autoimmune hepatitis when diagnosed within the previous 6 months are also accepted as acute liver failure.
  - Patients with acute severe alcoholic hepatitis are considered acute on chronic liver failure since they have a long history of drinking.
✓ **Viral hepatitis (A, B, E)** is the commonest cause of ALF in developing world.
  - **Paracetamol poisoning** is the commonest cause in UK and is responsible for 70% of the cases. **NAPQI, the product of paracetamol poisoning is hepatotoxic.**
  - **Acute fatty liver of pregnancy (AFLP):** Defective β-long chain fatty acids oxidation in fetus.
  - **Drugs causing liver toxicity:** Amiodarone, HAART, NSAIDs, Omeprazole, Rifampicin, Isoniazid, Pyrazinamide, SSRIs, and TPN.
  - **Toxins:** Alcohol, Carbon tetrachloride, Amanita phalloides.
✓ **Secondary ALF:** Liver failure due to extra-hepatic organ injury.
  - Hypotension, hypoxia, sepsis.
  - Cholestasis is found in 20% of critically ill patients.

Clinical Features and Diagnosis

✓ **History:** Onset of encephalopathy, complete drug history, anaesthesia history, travel history, family history.
✓ **Examination**
  - Kayser–Fleisher rings: **Wilson disease**
  - Vesicular skin lesions: **Herpes simplex virus**
  - Hypertension: **HELLP syndrome**
✓ **Investigations**
  - Complete blood count, liver function tests (ALT is more specific for liver), kidney function tests, coagulation profile, blood and

urine culture, lactate dehydrogenase (LDH), arterial ammonia, amylase, and lipase.

- IgM anti-HBcore/HBsAg, Hepatitis A IgM antibody, Hepatitis E IgM antibody, Hepatitis C antibody, HSV PCR, CMV PCR, VZV PCR.
- HIV rapid antibody test.
- **Autoimmune markers:** Antinuclear antibody (ANA), anti-smooth muscle antibody, anti-liver/kidney microsomal antibody type-1, immunoglobulins (IGG)
- Toxicology screen and drug panel.
- **Right upper quadrant USG with Doppler:** Liver parenchyma, biliary tree dilation, patency of hepatic artery, hepatic vein, and portal vein.

✓ **Differential diagnosis by laboratory values**
- Acute liver failure should be differentiated from acute hepatitis as *acute hepatitis doesn't have features of encephalopathy.*
- **Acetaminophen:** Aminotransferases >3500 IU/L, low bilirubin, high INR.

- **Hepatitis B:** Aminotransferases up to 2000 IU/L with ALT>AST.
- **Ischaemic hepatic injury:** >1000 IU/L, elevated serum LDH.
- **Acute fatty liver of pregnancy/HELLP syndrome:** Aminotransferase <1,000 IU/L.
- **Alcoholic hepatitis:** Transaminases are only mildly elevated (200–300 U/L) and AST is higher than ALT with ratio of 2:1

✓ **Hepatic encephalopathy** is the hallmark of ALF. It leads to **cerebral oedema**, higher in acute > subacute liver failure.
- Encephalopathy may precede jaundice in patients with toxins leading to liver failure.
- Risk of cerebral herniation is there.
- **Patients with symptoms of ALF and hepatic encephalopathy should be immediately transferred to a transplant centre.**
- Ammonia levels are measured and levels >100 mmol/L predicts severe encephalopathy with 70% accuracy.

Grades of Encephalopathy Using West Haven's Criteria[Q]

Severity	Level of Consciousness	Cognition/Behaviour	Neurological Examination
Grade 0	Normal	Normal	May be impaired
Grade 1	Mild confusion	Reduced attention	**Mild asterixis**/tremor
Grade 2	Lethargy	Disorientation, inappropriate behaviour	**Asterixis**, slurred speech
Grade 3	Somnolent but arousable	Bizarre behaviour	Rigidity, clonus, hyperreflexia
Grade 4	Comatose	Comatose	Abnormal posturing

✓ **Coagulopathy:** Spontaneous bleeding is rare although both bleeding and thrombosis risk are there.
- Prophylactic PPIs as patients are at risk of bleeding.
- Viscoelastic testing like thromboelastography and ROTEM should be used for guidance.
- INR is used for prognostication hence INR is not corrected unless actively bleeding[Q].
- IV Vitamin K should be given as oral absorption is unreliable.
- *INR >1.5 should prompt discussions with transplant specialists for transfer.*

✓ **Metabolic dysfunction:** Hypoglycaemia, lactic acidosis, hyponatraemia
- Half-normal saline with bicarbonate may be required while waiting RRT.
- Infusions of concentrated dextrose solutions may be required.

✓ **Sepsis:** Fungal infections are also common and occur late during illness.

- High bilirubin is a late sign in acute liver failure.

✓ **Acute kidney injury (AKI):** Renal replacement therapy is needed in up to 30% of ALF patients due to acute renal failure.
- *Citrate anticoagulation is risky and should be avoided.*
- NAC dose should be increased as NAC is dialyzable.

✓ **Acute respiratory distress syndrome (ARDS):** Seen in 40% of patients with ALF.

✓ **Modified King's College Criteria (KCC)[Q]:** Identifies patients with acute liver failure who need a liver transplant. It combines original KCC with lactate criteria.
- It is not validated in trauma-related acute liver failure.
- Projected 5-year survival should be >50% post-transplant. Disease mortality calculated using UK model for end stage liver disease (UKELD).

Acute Liver Failure Following Paracetamol Overdose	Acute Liver Failure Due to Non-Paracetamol Overdose

• Arterial pH <7.3 after adequate fluid resuscitation or
 • A lactate level of >3.5 mmol/L (**lactate criteria**) at admission (4 h) or a lactate level >3 mmol/L after adequate fluid resuscitation (12 h after admission)[Q] or
 • All of the following
  • PT >100 s (INR >6.5)
  • Creatinine >300 mmol/L
  • Grade III-IV encephalopathy
	• PT >100 s (INR >6.5) with any grade encephalopathy or
	 • All three criteria from the following:
	  • Age <10 or >40 yr
	  • PT >50 s
	  • Bilirubin >300 mmol/L
	 • Onset of encephalopathy >7 d after the development of jaundice
	 • Unfavourable disease aetiology: Non-A hepatitis, non-B hepatitis, halothane hepatitis, drug-induced liver failure

✓ **Contraindications for liver transplant in acute setting**
- Current substance abuse
- Overwhelming septic shock
- AIDS
- Uncontrolled intracranial hypertension

✓ **Idiosyncratic drug-induced liver injury (iDILI):** Presents from 4 d later to up to 90 d with a median of around 7–14 d.
- Presents as raised ALT, AST, ALP, bilirubin and GGT.
- **Hy's law**[Q]: Presence of hepatocellular injury (↑ ALT/AST >3 × ULN) and jaundice (↑ bilirubin >2 × ULN) means increased mortality.
- NAC has been used in these patients as well.

✓ **Viruses:** Hepatitis A, B, and E can cause acute liver failure.
- **Hepatitis B lab tests**[Q]
  - ❖ Vaccinated: Surface antibody positive.
  - ❖ Acute hepatitis B: Surface antigen positive, core IgM positive.
  - ❖ Previous hepatitis B: Surface antigen negative, Core IgG positive.
- Reactivation of hepatitis B following systemic chemotherapy is a possibility and **Lamivudine/Entecavir/Tenofovir** therapy may be used in these patients undergoing chemotherapy.
- Hepatitis E can cause death in 20% of pregnant patients.

✓ **Acute fatty liver of pregnancy (AFLP):** Defective β-long-chain fatty acids oxidation in fetus.
- ALT and ASTs between 800–1000, coagulopathy, renal dysfunction, and hypoglycaemia.
- Early delivery of foetus is recommended.

✓ **Autoimmune hepatitis:** Positive autoantibodies and elevated gamma-globulins.
- Early use of **steroids** can help. May ultimately require a liver transplant.

✓ **Wilson's disease:** Autosomal recessive disease.
- *Copper accumulation in the body.*
- ALF in patients with psychiatric features as copper deposits in brain, liver, and cornea.
- Serum ceruloplasmin may be falsely elevated as it is an acute-phase reactant.
- **Coombs negative haemolytic anaemia**, AST:ALT ratio of greater than 2, normal or subnormal ALP, coagulopathy that can't be corrected by vitamin K, elevated serum copper, and elevated 24-hour urine copper.
- 95% mortality and liver transplant are needed.

✓ **Budd–Chiari syndrome**[Q]: *Hepatic vein thrombosis*[Q]. High mortality if you leave untreated.
- Abdominal pain, **ascites,** and hepatomegaly
- *Loss of hepatic venous signal and reverse flow in the portal vein in ultrasound.*
  - ❖ *Gold standard for diagnosis is hepatic venography.*
- **Anticoagulation** should be the first step.
  - ❖ *Restoration of veins by **angioplasty/thrombolysis** and decongestion of liver by **TIPSS** is increasingly being used.*
  - ❖ Patients with encephalopathy and renal failure require liver transplant.

✓ **Alcoholic hepatitis:** Alcohol misuse: >14 units per week (NHS definition)[Q].
- Transaminases are only mildly elevated (200–300 U/L) and AST is higher than ALT with ratio of 2:1[Q]. Bilirubin and GGT are raised. Leucocytosis with neutrophilia is seen.

- Jaundice, tender hepatomegaly, and fever. Diagnosis is clinical.
- Goal of treatment is to prevent progression to encephalopathy and AKI.
- **Steroids**[Q] can be given for treatment and **STOPAH trial (2015)** has shown mortality benefit at 28 d although outcomes at 1 yr were similar compared to pentoxifylline.
  - ❖ *Maddrey discriminant function score* (serum total bilirubin and PT) is used to predict the need for steroids. Score ≥32[Q] suggests use of steroids for treatment.
- **MELD score of at least 20 can be used for corticosteroid treatment.**
- **Pentoxifylline** is a non-selective phosphodiesterase inhibitor which blocks TNF synthesis and has been shown to have no mortality benefit.
- *Liver transplant is contraindicated in this situation.*
- Also, evidence of drinking whilst being on transplant list will lead to permanent removal of patient from transplant list.
- Abstinence from alcohol for **3 to 6 months** may change a patient from **Child–Pugh C to Child–Pugh A.**

Treatment

- ✓ **Airway and breathing:** HFNO is recommended over NIV. **Intubate electively if grade 3 or 4 encephalopathy.**
  - Propofol is used as preferred agent as it reduces ICP.
- ✓ **Circulation:** Aggressive fluid therapy initially and sodium containing crystalloids should be used.
  - Norepinephrine should be used once intravascular volume has been restored.
  - CVC and renal vascular catheter are inserted irrespective of urine output.
- ✓ **Prophylactic antimicrobials** should be given as sepsis is a common cause of morbidity and mortality. Antifungal prophylaxis should be given as well.
  - No mortality benefit of prophylactic antibiotics though.
- ✓ **Nutrition:** Should be given to all patients and NG tube is not a contraindication in patients

with oesophageal varices unless band ligation has been performed in previous 24 h.
- Protein intake: 1–1.5 g protein/kg/day.
- Thiamine supplementation.
- ✓ **Hepatic encephalopathy (HE):** ICP monitoring using a bolt is done in some centres when grade 3 and 4 HE is seen to help guide management.
  - Other indications for ICP monitoring are *patients on vasopressors and in renal failure, arterial ammonia >150 mmol/L, pupillary abnormalities.*
  - A CT head should be done before putting in a bolt to rule out other causes of rapidly altered mental status. Coagulopathy should be corrected before its placement.
  - **Routine seizure prophylaxis is not recommended. Phenytoin is recommended when used.**
  - **Cerebral oedema prevention:** Head of the bed to 30°, control of fever, serum sodium between 145–155 mmol/L.
    - ❖ Mannitol or continuous infusion Hypertonic saline for cerebral oedema. No mortality benefit of ICP monitoring.
  - *Lactulose, neomycin or rifaximin have no proven benefit for ALF*[Q].
  - **L-ornithine-L-Aspartate (LOLA)** increases the extrahepatic metabolism of ammonia to glutamine and has been used in these patients.
- ✓ **Liver transplant:** Definitive treatment of cerebral oedema and AKI. Offered to patients with predicted mortality of >90%.
  - One-year survival of 75–80% post-emergency liver transplant.
- ✓ **High-volume plasma exchange** is also being used as a modality now and has proven mortality benefit.
  - Given to patients who are ineligible for super urgent list and awaiting liver transplant but needs bridging.

Criteria for Transfer to Transplant Centre

Paracetamol Overdose–Induced ALF	Non-Acetaminophen-Induced ALF
pH <7.30 or bicarbonate <18 mmol/L	pH <7.30 or bicarbonate <18 mmol/L
Elevated lactate >4 mmol/L unresponsive to fluid resuscitation	Shrinking liver size

Oliguria and creatinine >200 mmol/L	*Oliguria and sodium <130 mmol/L*
INR greater than 3 on day 2 and greater than 4 thereafter	*INR greater than 1.8*
Altered level of consciousness	Encephalopathy or hypoglycaemia
Hypoglycaemia	Bilirubin >300 mmol/L

✓ **Specific treatment: N-acetylcysteine (NAC)** is given for all patients of ALF. It is given in patients with paracetamol poisoning, regardless of the paracetamol levels, timing of overdose, especially if there has been concern of a staggered overdose.
  • **12-h SNAP regimen:** 100 mg/kg over 2 h followed by 200 mg/kg over 10 h.
  • **21-h protocol:** 150 mg/kg over 1 h, 50 mg/kg over 4 h, 100 mg/kg over 16 h.
✓ *Penicillamine in case of Wilson disease.*

Prognosis

✓ 50% mortality without transplantation.
  • **Aetiology of ALF has prognostic significance for determining outcomes of patients listed for liver transplant.**
✓ **Probability of spontaneous recovery by degree of grades of encephalopathy.**
  • Grade I to II: 65–70%
  • Grade III: 40–50%
  • Grade IV: <20%
✓ **High lactates at initial presentation and not coming down after resuscitation is a high mortality indicator.**
  • Hypophosphataemia is a prognostic indicator in acetaminophen poisoning.
  • Prognosis is poorer in subacute presentation.
  • Patients with multiorgan failure have poorer prognosis compared to patients with just encephalopathy.

CHRONIC LIVER DISEASE

Epidemiology and Aetiology

✓ **Liver cirrhosis** is a pathological diagnosis and represents the end stage of **chronic liver disease** due to diffuse fibrosis and disruption of intrahepatic arterial and venous flow.
✓ **Acute decompensation of cirrhosis:** Signs and symptoms of both *portal hypertension* and *hepatic synthetic dysfunction* in patients with chronic liver disease.
  • Ascites
  • Hepatic encephalopathy
  • Variceal bleeding
✓ **Acute on chronic liver failure (ACLF)**
  • The European Association for the Study of the Liver-Chronic Liver Failure (EASL-CLIF) defines ACLF[Q] as *organ failure in a patient with acute decompensation of cirrhosis in a patient with or without prior episode of decompensation.*
  • **Organ failure** is defined using **Chronic-Liver Failure (CLIF)-SOFA score** that has six organ systems.
    ❖ **Circulation:** MAP ≥70 mmHg using vasopressors
    ❖ **Lungs:** PaO_2/FiO_2 ≤200 or use of mechanical ventilation
    ❖ **Brain:** Hepatic grade III or IV by West-Haven criteria
    ❖ **Liver:** Bilirubin ≥12 mg/dL
    ❖ **Kidney:** Creatinine ≥2 mg/dL
    ❖ **Coagulation:** INR ≥2.5
  • **Grading of ACLF**
    ❖ **ACLF grade 1**
      • Patients with single kidney failure
      • Patients with single liver, coagulation disorder, circulatory lung failure + serum creatinine between 1.5–1.9 mg/dL
      • Grade 1–2 hepatic encephalopathy + serum creatinine between 1.5–1.9 mg/dL
    ❖ **ACLF grade 2:** Patients with 2 organ failures
    ❖ **ACLF grade 3:** Patients with 3 organ failures
    ❖ **CLIF-ACLF 28 d mortality: Grade 1:** 20%, **Grade 2:** 30%, **Grade 3:** 80%.
  • *Systemic inflammation precipitated by infection, alcohol or gastrointestinal bleeding is the hallmark of ACLF.*
  • In contrast to acutely decompensated cirrhosis (28 d mortality of 5%), ACLF has a high short-term mortality (28 d mortality of 20%) like acute liver failure.
  • Clinical decision of futility in ACLF is not recommended without a trial of organ support.
  • Liver transplant is ultimately warranted in suitable cases.

✓ **Alcohol liver disease**
- Three histologic types: Steatosis, alcoholic hepatitis, and cirrhosis.
- 15% of heavy drinkers will develop cirrhosis.
- Single biggest risk factor is amount of alcohol ingested.
- Alcohol-related deaths are more common in males.

Clinical Features

✓ **Compensated Cirrhosis:** Patient with cirrhosis may remain asymptomatic for many years.
- Progression from compensated to decompensated cirrhosis at rate of 5 to 7% per year.

✓ **Decompensated Cirrhosis**: Ascites, variceal bleeding, encephalopathy, or jaundice are markers of decompensated cirrhosis. Median survival of 2 yr.
- Complications of one of these features (SBP, hepatorenal syndrome, hepatopulmonary syndrome) have worse prognosis. Median survival of 6 months.
- Sepsis, dehydration, electrolyte abnormality, sedative drugs, **portal vein thrombosis**, or GI bleed should be looked for in these patients presenting with decompensation.

✓ **Encephalopathy:** Liver cannot remove ammonia which enters blood and causes neurotoxicity and oedema.
- Early changes are often subtle like mood changes and insomnia.
- **West Haven criteria** is used for classification and is given in chapter on acute liver failure.
- **Precipitating factors:** Infection (SBP), GI bleeding, or drugs.
- Serum ammonia is a biomarker but no correlation with severity of hepatic encephalopathy.
- **Treatment**
  - ❖ **Cathartics:** Oral lactulose or lactulose retention enemas.
  - ❖ **Oral antibiotics**[Q]: Neomycin 500 mg PO QID or rifaximin 550 mg BD. Poorly absorbed from GIT.
  - ❖ **L-ornithine L-aspartate (LOLA)**[Q]: Removes ammonia from the blood by converting it to glutamine. No mortality benefit is seen.

✓ **Ascites:** Accumulation of fluid within peritoneal layer of the abdomen.

- Cirrhosis is reason for 75% of cases of ascites with mortality of up to 44% in 5 yr.
- It is most common manifestation of decompensated cirrhosis.
- **Simple:** Non-infected and not associated with hepatorenal syndrome. **Refractory:** Ascites that can't be mobilized or early recurrence that cannot be satisfactorily prevented by medical therapy.
- **Paracentesis:** Done in all patients with new onset ascites and in those in which the clinical condition changes like confusion, renal dysfunction, or GI bleeding.
  - ❖ *Done at 2 to 4 cm medial and cephalad to the anterior superior iliac spine either side of the abdomen.*
  - ❖ DIC is absolute contraindication. USG guided aspiration can be used in difficult cases.
  - ❖ Classified now by serum ascites albumin gradient (SAAG)[Q]: Serum albumin – ascitic albumin. **SAAG >11 g/L is suggestive of portal hypertension**. Diagnostic accuracy of 97%.
    - **High SAAG**[Q]**:** Cirrhosis, heart failure, Budd–Chiari syndrome, constrictive pericarditis.
    - **Low SAAG**[Q]**:** Cancer, TB infection, pancreatitis, serositis, nephrotic syndrome.
  - ❖ Albumin, cell count with differential and cultures are sent for investigation after paracentesis.
  - ❖ High amylase levels in ascitic fluid are seen in cases of pancreatic duct damage.
  - ❖ Routine correction of coagulopathy is not recommended before paracentesis. If platelet counts $<20 \times 10^9$, platelet transfusion may be helpful.
  - ❖ Main question is whether to drain ascitic fluid or not and to leave a catheter or not.
  - ❖ *Albumin needs to be given (1 bottle of 20% albumin for every 2/3 L of ascites removed).*
- **Hepatic hydrothorax** occurs in 13% of patients with ascites and is seen on right side mostly due to defects in the diaphragm.
  - ❖ Managed by thoracentesis, diuretics, and trans-jugular intrahepatic shunt (TIPS), and tube thoracostomy should be avoided.

✓ **Spontaneous bacterial peritonitis (SBP):** 10 to 30% of all bacterial infections in patients with cirrhosis and present in approximately 10% of all cirrhotic hospital patients.

- *SBP[Q] is diagnosed by neutrophil count >250/mL or growth of organisms in a culture of ascitic fluid.*
- **Risk factors[Q]:** Previous episode, GI bleed, high Child–Pugh score, ascitic protein <1 g/dL.

	Portal Hypertension	SBP	Tuberculosis
WBC count (cells/mm^3)	0–10	>500–1,000	50–300
Differentiation	Normal	>250–500 polymorphonuclear cells	50–300 lymphocytes
Microbes	None	Monomicrobial	TB-PCR
Glucose (mmol/L)	>3.6	>3.6	<3.6
Total protein (g/dL)	<1–1.5	<1	0.75–3
Serum-ascites albumin (g/dL)	>1.1	<1.1	<1.1
Ascites serum LDH	0.4	1	>1

- ***E. coli*[Q]** is commonest organism isolated. 60% of cases of SBP have no organism identified.
  - ❖ *No typical presentation and fever, confusion or diffuse abdominal pain may be present or absent.*
  - ❖ *Multiple organisms with high cell count can indicate presence of secondary bacterial peritonitis due to bowel perforation and intra-abdominal abscess.*
- **Treatment** should be started following a positive ascitic tap and shouldn't wait for microbiological culture results.
  - ❖ Broad-spectrum antibiotics like third and fourth-generation cephalosporins, carbapenems, and penicillin like piperacillin/tazobactam.
  - ❖ Discontinuation of diuretics and *administration of IV 20% albumin given at a dose of 1.5 g/kg (day 1) and 1 g/kg (day 3) reduces rate of renal dysfunction.*
- 1-yr mortality after a first episode of SBP is between 30 and 90%.
✓ **Portal hypertension:** State of relatively elevated pressure in the hepatic portal venous system and sinusoids.
  - Grading is by **hepatic venous pressure gradient (HVPG):** Mild: 5–10 mmHg, Clinically significant: >10 mmHg.
    - ❖ Salt restriction.
    - ❖ Diuresis by **spironolactone and furosemide**.

- ❖ Propranolol forms the medical management.
- **Variceal bleeding:** An annual incidence rate of 20% in cirrhosis and each has a 20% to 40% mortality rate.
  - ❖ Blood products, Terlipressin, prophylactic antibiotics are given.
  - ❖ Upper GI endoscopy and diagnostic paracentesis is done.
  - ❖ TIPS might be needed followed by liver transplant ultimately.
✓ **Hepatorenal syndrome (HRS):** Development of acute kidney injury (AKI) in those with chronic liver disease who have portal hypertension.
  - **Pathophysiology:** Generalized vasodilation in splanchnic circulation and renal vasoconstriction.
    - ❖ Liver transplant is the most effective treatment as it reverses these changes.
  - **HRS Type 1/HRS-AKI**
    - ❖ Acute and severe. Rapid decline (<2 wk) in renal function due to factors like bleeding or infections.
    - ❖ **Diagnostic Criteria[Q]**
      - Diagnosis of cirrhosis and ascites.
      - **Diagnosis of AKI:** Increase in serum creatinine ≥0.3 mg/dL within 48 h or 50% increase in serum creatinine from baseline, which is known/ occurred within the past 7 d AND/ OR urinary output ≤0.5 mL/kg for at least 6 h.

- No response after 2 consecutive days of diuretic withdrawal and plasma volume expansion with albumin 1 g/kg.
- Absence of shock.
- No current or recent use of nephrotoxic drugs.
- No macroscopic signs of parenchymal kidney injury defined as absence of proteinuria (>500 mg/d), microhaematuria (>50 RBCs/high-power field) and normal findings on renal USG.
  - ❖ **Treatment:** Terlipressin 0.5–2 mg QDS and *IV Albumin 1g/kg/day (up to 100g/day) for 24 h and then 20–40 g/day.*
  - ❖ Worse prognosis.
- **HRS Type 2/HRS-non-AKI**
  - ❖ Slow progressive decline in renal function with refractory ascites.
  - ❖ **Diagnostic criteria**^{Q}
    - **HRS–Acute kidney disease (AKD):** eGFR <60 mL/min per 1.73 m^2 for <3 months in absence of other structural causes or increase in serum creatinine <50% using last available outpatient serum creatinine within 3 months as baseline **plus diagnosis of cirrhosis and ascites.**
    - **HRS–Chronic kidney disease (CKD):** eGFR <60 mL/min per 1.73 m^2 for ≥3 months in absence of other structural causes **plus diagnosis of cirrhosis and ascites.**
  - ❖ **Treatment:** More prone to recurrence and less responsive to albumin and terlipressin.
  - ❖ Better prognosis than HRS type 1.
- ✓ **Hepatopulmonary syndrome (HPS)**^{Q}: Dilation of pulmonary precapillary and capillary vessels leading to hypoxaemia due to *ventilation-perfusion mismatch.*
  - Affects 10–30% of patients evaluated for liver transplantation and is frequently asymptomatic.
  - **Platypnoea** (dyspnoea worsening when moving from supine to upright position) and **orthodeoxia** (>5% or >4 mmHg decrease in partial pressure of PaO$_2$ after changing from supine to upright position) is seen in 20% of patients.
  - **HPS Diagnostic criteria**
    - ❖ **Underlying liver disease:** Portal hypertension with or without cirrhosis.
  - ❖ **Intrapulmonary vascular dilation:** Positive findings on *contrast echocardiography using IV injection of microbubbles*^{Q}.
  - ❖ **Oxygenation defect:** PaO$_2$ <80 mmHg or A—a gradient ≥15 mmHg (≥20 mmHg in patients >65 yr old) on room air.
  - **Disease severity:** Based on PaO$_2$ on room air.
    - ❖ **Mild:** ≥80 mmHg
    - ❖ **Moderate:** 60–79 mmHg
    - ❖ **Severe:** 50–59 mmHg
    - ❖ **Very Severe:** <50 mmHg
  - **Supportive treatment** with oxygen. *Mild to moderate HPS can be reversed by liver transplant.*
- ✓ **Porto-pulmonary hypertension (PoPH):** Presence of unexplained pulmonary arterial hypertension associated with portal hypertension with or without cirrhosis.
  - Vasoconstriction of pulmonary artery secondary to proliferation of the inner wall along with platelet aggregation.
  - Most patients are asymptomatic and have non-specific symptoms like dyspnoea and fatigue.
  - **Diagnosis:** Transthoracic echocardiography followed by **right heart catheterization (gold standard).**
  - *Treatment: Pulmonary vasodilators to be started with pulmonary pressures greater than 35 mmHg.*
    - ❖ *Liver transplant is done in selected patients as the post-transplant haemodynamic response is unpredictable.*

Prognosis

- ✓ **Child–Pugh score**^{Q} **is used to assess the prognosis of chronic liver disease**
  - Class A: 5–6 points, 100%, 1 yr survival
  - Class B: 7–9 points, 80%, 1 yr survival
  - Class C: >10 points, 45%, 1 yr survival

Parameter	1 point	2 points	3 points
Albumin (g/L)	>35	28–35	<28
Ascites	None	Mild	Moderate/severe
Bilirubin (mmol/L)	<34	34–50	>50
Coagulation (INR)	<1.7	1.7–2.3	>2.3
Encephalopathy	None	Grade 1–2	Grade 3–4

✓ **MELD score**[Q] quantifies end-stage liver disease for transplant planning. Was initially used to assess the outcome from TIPS.
- Scale based on the risk of the patient dying while awaiting transplantation. Based on bilirubin, INR, and creatinine.
- $3.78 \times \log_e(\text{bilirubin mg/dL}) + 9.57 \times \log_e(\text{Creatinine mg/dL}) + 11.20 \times \log_e(\text{INR}) + 6.43$

3-Month Mortality, %	MELD Score
1.9–3.7	<9
6–20	10–19
19.6–45.5	20–29
52.6–74.5	30–39
71–100	>40

BILIARY TRACT DISEASE

Physiology

✓ Amount of bile secreted at the level of canaliculus is approximately 500 mL.
- Conjugated bilirubin enters intestine where it is broken into urobilinogen in the terminal ileum. Some urobilinogen is reabsorbed in the portal vein but the majority of it is lost in the faeces as stercobilin (90%).

✓ **Prehepatic jaundice**[Q]
- Haemolysis (increased bilirubin production)
- Crigler–Najjar (impaired conjugation)
- Gilbert syndrome (impaired hepatic uptake of bilirubin)

✓ **Hepatic (unconjugated or conjugated)**
- Liver failure (unconjugated)
- Dubin Johnson syndrome (lesions of gene MRP2 involved in canalicular transport) (conjugated)
- Rotor syndrome (defective protein OATP1B1 and OATP1B3 involved in hepatic storage of bilirubin) (conjugated)
- Drugs: OCPs, Anabolic steroids, Haloperidol

✓ **Post-hepatic (Conjugated)**
- Gall stones
- Pancreatic carcinoma
- Primary biliary cirrhosis (PBC)
- Primary sclerosing cholangitis (PSC)

✓ **Conjugated hyperbilirubinaemia:** >50% conjugated bilirubin.
- **Unconjugated hyperbilirubinaemia:** <20% conjugated bilirubin.

Test	Prehepatic[Q]	Hepatic[Q]	Extrahepatic
Bilirubin (3–17 mmol/L)	↑ (unconjugated)	↑↑ (conjugated)	↑↑↑ (conjugated)
AST (<35 IU)	→	↑↑↑	↑
ALP (<250 IU)	→	↑	↑↑↑
Albumin (40–50 g/L)	→	↓	↓/→
Reticulocytes (<1%)	↑/→	→	→

Diagnostic Modalities

✓ **Obstructive jaundice**[Q]: Pale stools with dark urine because of conjugated bilirubin.

✓ **Laboratory tests**
- **Bilirubin:** Increased in obstructive jaundice, **sepsis**, haemolysis.
- *ALP: Non-specific for biliary disease but accompanying elevation of GGT helps to confirm its hepatobiliary origin.*

✓ **Abdominal X-ray:** Most common finding is **generalized ileus**.
- **Air in biliary tree:** Biliary-enteric fistula, prior sphincterotomy and infection with gas-producing organisms.
- Only 20% of gall stones are radiopaque.

✓ **Abdominal ultrasound:** Initial diagnostic test of choice in ITU.
- High sensitivity (95%) for detecting gall bladder stones but low sensitivity (25–60%) for common bile duct stones.
- Can detect **biliary ductal dilatation** and **acute cholecystitis** (thickening of gall bladder wall >3 mm, **gall bladder distension** **>5 cm** and pericholecystic fluid).

✓ **Radionuclide scanning:** Technetium-99m-labeled hepatic iminodiacetic acid (HIDA) scans can be used to cystic duct patency, and hence confidently **excluding the diagnosis of acute cholecystitis.**

- Structural abnormalities of bile tree like **bile duct leak.**
✓ **CT scan:** Low sensitivity for common bile duct stones like ultrasound.
  - Can detect biliary dilatation or local complications like liver abscess, pancreatic pseudocyst, **biloma, and free fluid in abdomen**.
  - Can detect acute cholecystitis with features like thickening of gall bladder wall >3 mm, gall bladder distension >5 cm, intramural gas, pericholecystic infiltration of fat and pericholecystic fluid.
✓ **Magnetic resonance cholangiopancreatography (MRCP)**
  - High sensitivity (90%) and specificity (95%) for common bile duct stones, strictures, and tumours.
  - Limited value for detecting stones <6 mm and impacted stones at the ampulla.
✓ **Endoscopic retrograde cholangiopancreatography (ERCP):** Used for therapeutic purposes.
  - Major ampulla in second part of duodenum is cannulated and biliary tree opacified with contrast injected through a catheter.
  - Biliary tree stones, strictures, and leaks can be seen. Stones can be removed, and strictures can be dilated during the same procedure.
  - Coagulopathy needs to be corrected. Complications are pancreatitis^Q (3.5%), cholangitis^Q (3%), and perforation^Q (0.6%).
✓ **Endoscopic ultrasonography**
  - More sensitive (95%) and specific (98%) than abdominal ultrasound for CBD stones.
  - *Can detect small <5 mm stones in bile ducts.*
✓ **Percutaneous transhepatic cholangiography**
  - Rapid, non-operative, percutaneous transhepatic biliary drainage.
  - Emergency procedure for biliary drainage when patient can't undergo ERCP or failed ERCP.

Biliary Tract Pathology

✓ **Biliary tract obstruction^Q:** Most common causes are stones, benign stricture, and malignancy.
  - **Classification of causes**
    ❖ **Intrinsic:** Stones, benign stricture, sclerosing cholangitis, cholangiocarcinoma.

    ❖ **Extrinsic:** Pancreatic carcinoma, pancreatitis, choledochal cyst, hepatic cysts.
    ❖ **Iatrogenic:** Post-operative stricture.
  - Obstruction without cholangitis is seen more commonly in malignancy.
    ❖ ERCP or PTC for stones, strictures, or palliation of malignancy. Surgery for those who have operable malignancy.
✓ **Primary biliary cirrhosis^Q**
  - Autoimmune disease with antimitochondrial antibody positive.
  - ↑ ALP and GGT and↑ AST/ALT.
  - **Liver biopsy:** Granulomas around bile ducts.
  - Liver transplant needed ultimately.
✓ **Acute cholangitis:** Life-threatening condition. Occurs due to partial or complete obstruction of biliary tract. Gram-negative or anaerobe bacteraemia seen.
  - **Charcot's triad^Q:** Fever, jaundice, and abdominal pain.
  - **Reynold's pentad^Q:** Fever, jaundice, abdominal pain, hypotension, and altered mental status.
  - Broad spectrum antibiotics with adequate biliary excretion like piperacillin/tazobactam, third-generation cephalosporins and a carbapenem.
  - Early/Urgent biliary drainage is a MUST in addition to medical therapy.
  - ERCP/PTC/Surgery can be used depending upon patient's condition and local expertise.
  - Mortality rate ranges from 10–50%.
✓ **Bile leak:** Extravasated bile may collect locally to form a biloma or may flow freely in peritoneum.
  - **Classification of causes**
    ❖ Post-surgical causes like cholecystectomy, hepatic resection, liver transplant, liver biopsy.
    ❖ Trauma: Liver laceration.
  - Biliary peritonitis may present with fever, ascites, and abdominal pain. Hepato-biliary scanning (HIDA) can be used for diagnosis followed by ERCP for stenting with or without sphincterotomy.
✓ **Acute cholecystitis:** Acalculous cholecystitis can cause significant morbidity and mortality.

- **Acute acalculous cholecystitis**[Q] is characterized by severe gall bladder inflammation without stone and cystic duct obstruction.
  - ❖ Due to dysfunction of gall bladder emptying.
  - ❖ Fever, leucocytosis, abdominal pain in the right upper quadrant.
- Broad spectrum antibiotics in septic patients. **Percutaneous cholecystostomy** for unstable patients with acute calculous or acalculous cholecystitis and failing medical therapy. Percutaneous cholecystostomy can be done at bedside without general anaesthesia.
- ERCP and EUS guided gall bladder drainage can be used in patients in whom percutaneous cholecystostomy is not possible.
- Cholecystectomy as soon as general condition improves.

ACUTE PANCREATITIS

Epidemiology and aetiology: 40–70 people/100,000 population

✓ **Inflammatory process** of the pancreas due to auto-digestive injury by activated pancreatic enzymes.
  - **Gall stones (40%)** and **alcohol (35%)** are two most common causes[Q].
  - **Alcohol-induced pancreatitis** happens in patients consuming >5 drinks/day for >5 yr. It is the commonest cause of chronic pancreatitis.
✓ **Drugs (3rd common cause): Valproic acid,** thiazides, furosemide, **azathioprine,** antiretrovirals, methyldopa, tetracycline, sulphonamides, metronidazole, nitrofurantoin, isoniazid, cisplatin, salicylate, piroxicam, statins.
✓ **Other causes:** Hypertriglyceridemia (>500 mg/dL), **hypercalcaemia** (TPN), pancreatic cancer, post-ERCP (3–5% incidence), cardiac surgery, **steroids,** hypothermia.
✓ **Infections:** *Mycoplasma pneumoniae, Salmonella, Campylobacter,* tuberculosis, *Legionella, CMV,* EBV, VZV, measles, *Mumps,* rubella, *Aspergillus,* toxoplasma, *Cryptosporidium.*
✓ **Scorpion and insect bites.**

Clinical Features and Diagnosis

✓ Abdominal pain radiating to back, nausea/vomiting, abdominal distension, hypoalbuminaemia, hyperglycaemia, hypocalcaemia, elevated WBCs, thrombocytopaenia.
  - One-third of patients with SAP will develop ARDS.
  - **Cullen's sign** (peri-umbilical ecchymosis) and **Grey–Turner's sign** (Flank ecchymosis)[Q] suggest retroperitoneal haemorrhage.
✓ *Severe acute pancreatitis (SAP) forms 15–20 % of cases of pancreatitis.*
✓ **Diagnostic criteria:** A diagnosis[Q] of acute pancreatitis is made with 2 out of the following 3 features.
  - Severe, acute, epigastric pain
  - Serum lipase or amylase at least 3 times the upper limit of normal
  - Features typical of pancreatitis on CT, USG, or MRI
✓ **Atlanta classification for severity**[Q]
  - **Mild:** No local or systemic complications, no organ failure
  - **Moderate:** Local or systemic complications, organ failure <48 h
  - **Severe:** Persistent organ failure >48 h
✓ **Organ failure is defined as score of 2 or more on the modified Marshall score.**
  - Score is based on PaO_2/FiO_2, SBP, pH, and serum creatinine.
✓ *Lipase levels three times the upper limit clinches the diagnosis.*
✓ **Amylase** is non-specific (raised in bowel ischaemia, salivary gland trauma). Shorter half-life than lipase and amylase levels come down in 3 to 5 d.
  - Rise in serum amylase along with clinical assessment is a poor indicator of severity in the first 48 h. No correlation between severity and levels of amylase.
  - Post-ERCP, an elevated lipase and amylase are common and in absence of abdominal pain, a diagnosis of pancreatitis should be avoided.
✓ **Ultrasound** should be done in all cases on admission and then all severe acute pancreatitis cases should have it done at 72–96 h.
  - Indicates the presence or absence of gallstones[Q] or dilation of the common bile duct.
✓ **Contrast-enhanced CT scan:** Investigation of choice when diagnosis is unclear initially

and when severe pancreatitis is suggested and should be done early in course for it.

- CT scan performed later can help in differentiating interstitial oedematous pancreatitis from necrotizing pancreatitis. Ideally at 72–96 h.
- Findings of normal pancreas should suggest an aetiology other than pancreatitis in these patients.
- Failure to improve after more than 7–14 d of illness suggests a complication and warrants a CT scan.
- Severe features include extensive fat stranding, peri-pancreatic fluid collections, and pancreatic necrosis.

✓ **MRI:** Main role is in diagnosing the cause of pancreatitis. More accurate than CT scan in defining the extent of pancreatitis associated necrosis.

✓ **Balthazar CT severity index**[Q] grades pancreatitis radiologically.

- **Score:** 0–3: mild, 4–6: moderate, 7–10: severe.

Pancreatic Inflammation	Points	Pancreatic Necrosis	Points
Normal pancreas	0	Absent	0
Focal or diffuse swelling of pancreas	1	<30%	2
Peri-pancreatic inflammation	2	30–50%	4
Single, ill-defined fluid collection	3	>50%	6
Two or multiple ill-defined fluid collections or presence of gas in/around pancreas	4		

✓ Scoring systems such as **Ranson**[Q]**, Glasgow, or APACHE II** may help in identifying patients for critical care admission.

- Ranson score >3 indicates severe pancreatitis and 15% mortality.

✓ **Glasgow Score:** Each positive finding scores 1. Score ≥3 predicts severe acute pancreatitis.

- **P:** Pa0$_2$ <8 kPa
- **A:** Age >55 yr
- **N:** WBCs >15 × 10^9/L

- **C:** Calcium <2 mmol/L
- **R:** Urea >16 mmol/L
- **E:** LDH >600 IU/L
- **A:** Albumin <32 g/L
- **S:** Glucose >10 mmol/L

✓ **BISAP Score (Bedside Index of Severity in Acute Pancreatitis):** Uses parameters in first 24 h to predict the risk of death bedside. **Score:** 0–2 <2% mortality, 3–5 >15% mortality.

- Blood urea nitrogen >8.9 mmol/L: 1 point
- Impaired mental status: 1 point
- >2 **SIRS** criteria present—1 point
- Age >60 yr: 1 point
- Pleural effusion on radiography: 1 point

Treatment

✓ **Aggressive fluid resuscitation (3 mL/kg/h)** of Ringer lactate is recommended in the first 12–24 h.

- Beyond 24 h however, it may lead to abdominal compartment syndrome.

✓ **Pain** is severe and difficult to control. Thoracis epidural analgesia offers advantages of sparring systemic opioids.

- Pethidine relaxes sphincter of Oddi and is a favoured analgesic in this context.

✓ **Supportive management** like invasive mechanical ventilation and RRT might be needed.

✓ **Early enteral feeding**[Q] has mortality benefit.

- Always start with NG feeding and if patient doesn't tolerate start NJ feeding.
- Medium-chain triglycerides enteral feeding solutions have been shown to improve feeding tolerance.
- TPN only if patient fails enteral feeding.

✓ **Antibiotics** (carbapenems and antifungal)[Q] only if signs of **infection in necrotic tissue** (gas in pancreas on CT) or **cholangitis** (jaundice) or **febrile neutropenia**. No prophylactic antibiotics[Q].

✓ **Surgery** for necrotic tissue should be delayed for at least 2–3 wk if possible and conservative management is preferred over early surgical intervention.

✓ **Early ERCP (<24 h)**[Q] is indicated only for gallstones with accompanying acute cholangitis or patients with persistent biliary obstruction (serum conjugated bilirubin >85 mmol/L.

- Pancreatic duct stents ± **rectal indomethacin may help prevent post-ERCP pancreatitis**[Q].

- Cholecystectomy should be done after about 6 wk for these patients once the initial episode of pancreatitis has subsided.
- ✓ **Probiotics** can cause increase incidence of gut ischaemia.
- ✓ Insulin[Q] can be used to decrease triglyceride levels by activating lipoprotein lipase which metabolizes chylomicrons in patients with elevated triglyceride levels.

Complications[Q]

- ✓ **Acute peri-pancreatic fluid collection:** Homogenous fluid collections without a wall, early in course of pancreatitis.
  - Attempts to drain are discouraged as they resolve spontaneously.
- ✓ **Acute necrotic collection:** Collection of necrotic tissue without a wall, early in course of pancreatitis. Infection of acute necrotic collection (translocation from gut) peaks at 3 wk.
  - PCT or CRP are anyway elevated due to inflammation and may not be helpful.
  - Clinical signs/deterioration because of sepsis and CT scan may be helpful. **Presence of gas bubbles within the necrotic tissue area are regarded pathognomonic and are found in 50% of cases.**
  - *Attempts to drain non-infected necrotic tissues are discouraged as they resolve spontaneously.* Even for infected necrotic tissue, conservative approach using antibiotics initially is being increasingly practiced.
  - **PANTER Trial (2010)[Q]:** "Step-up approach." Infective necrosis should be drained percutaneously first with the help of CT scan and if needed should undergo minimally invasive surgical necrosectomy.
  - **TENSION Trial (2018)[Q]:** "Endoscopic step-up approach" is non-inferior to surgical step-up approach. EUS-guided transgastric drainage of infected collections and if needed endoscopic transgastric necrosectomy.
- ✓ **Pancreatic pseudocyst (10–20% cases):** Homogenous fluid collection surrounded by a non-epithelized wall of fibrous tissue. Enclosed digestive enzymes due to leak from pancreatic ducts. Not seen before 4–6 wk.
  - Does not require invasive treatment unless they cause symptoms like biliary obstruction, gastric outlet obstruction or persistent symptoms like anorexia, weight loss and abdominal pains.
  - *Infected pseudocysts will require intervention.* EUS-guided cystoduodenostomy or cystogastrostomy can be done. Pancreatic duct stenting can be done if there is communication between the duct and cyst.
- ✓ **Walled-off necrosis:** Collection of necrotic tissue within a wall, seen after 4 wk or later.
  - *Sterile walled-off necrosis also does not require invasive treatment unless they cause symptoms like above.*
  - Surgical necrosectomy of walled off necrosis is done.
- ✓ **Pancreatic fistulas:** Pancreaticocutaneous fistulas or pancreaticoenteric fistulas are seen.
  - Minor leaks are treated by drainage and somatostatin or octreotide and major rupture by resection or stenting.
- ✓ **Perforation:** At the level of splenic flexure between left and transverse colon.
  - Surgical options include colectomy or loop-ileostomy.
- ✓ **Haemorrhage:** Severe complication that carries high mortality. Erosion of vessel wall by enzymes and pseudoaneurysm formation (3–4 wk later) of the pancreatic arteries.
  - Splenic artery is the most common artery involved. Angiography followed by embolization is needed.
  - Surgical drainage is needed in massive haemorrhage.
- ✓ **Splanchnic vein thrombosis:** *Therapeutic anticoagulation needed and can lead to haemorrhage later. Splenic and portal veins are involved.*

Prognosis

- ✓ 50% of patients will have spontaneous and uneventful resolution. Mortality of severe acute pancreatitis is 30%.
  - Deaths in first week of SAP are due to ARDS and SIRS response. Late peak of mortality is due to infections of necrotic debris.
- ✓ Severity of acute pancreatitis correlates with glucose, calcium, and transaminase levels but not with amylase levels and amount of necrotic tissue.
- ✓ **Chain of lakes** and **string of pearls** appearance in chronic pancreatitis.
- ✓ Diabetes mellitus and exocrine deficiency are long-term complications[Q].

DIARRHOEA

Aetiology: Incidence: 40–50% of patients in ITU will have diarrhoea during any illness.

✓ **Diarrhoea:** Defined as an increase of stool frequency >3 or more stools, stool weight >200 g/day and type 5–7 stools on Bristol stool chart.
  - **Acute:** Sudden onset and less than 2 wk.
  - **Chronic:** Passage of unformed stools for one month or more.

✓ **Causes**
  - **Iatrogenic: Antibiotics** (beta-lactams, clindamycin, azithromycin, quinolones), *Clostridium difficile* infection (CDI), **enteral feeding**, proton pump inhibitors.
  - **Diarrhoea as a primary manifestation of disease:** Diabetes (autonomic neuropathy), hyperthyroidism, adrenal insufficiency (secretory diarrhoea), graft-vs-host disease (GVHD)[Q], vasculitis.
  - **Diarrhoea secondary to underlying disease**: Infections in immunosuppressed patients, intestinal ischaemia[Q], GI bleeding, faecal impaction leading to overflow diarrhoea[Q].

✓ **Classification**
  - **Osmotic:** Increase in interstitial osmotic pressure.
    ❖ Moderate stool volume. Moderately watery. Flatulence.
    ❖ Improves after fasting.
    ❖ Seen in short bowel syndrome and post-laxatives like lactulose, magnesium salts.
  - **Secretory:** Enhancement of intestinal secretion by enterotoxins.
    ❖ Large volume and watery. Dehydration and electrolyte imbalance seen.
    ❖ No improvement after fasting.
    ❖ Enterotoxins from *Vibrio cholerae*.
  - **Inflammatory:** Intestinal mucosal damage due to inflammation.
    ❖ Systemic symptoms seen, and stool will have RBCs and WBCs.
    ❖ Infective diarrhoea due to *Shigella*.
  - **Motor:** Intestinal dysmotility.
    ❖ Seen while recovering from ileus.

Clinical Features

✓ **Antibiotic agents** cause a non-inflammatory diarrhoea characterized by nausea, cramping, and bloating and fluid and electrolyte losses are minimal.

- Passage of high frequency, small volume stools with urgency and tenesmus suggest distal, left-sided involvement of colon.
- Less frequent, large-volume stools are mostly due to proximal involvement of small intestine or right colon.

✓ **Overflow diarrhoea:** Fluid faeces may seep past the impacted faecal mass, leading to a loose unformed stool which is produced in relatively small amounts.

✓ **Severe diarrhoea:** Hyperchloremic metabolic acidosis and prerenal azotaemia.

✓ **Rule out laxative use or enema in the previous 48 h, enteral feeding and has a history of constipation and overflow.**

✓ **Investigations**
  - Stool culture for type 5, 6, and 7 stool.
  - *C. diff* toxin PCR
  - Faecal leucocytes (infection or inflammation)
  - Faecal fat (malabsorption)
  - Faecal calprotectin
  - Lactoferrin (dysentery and inflammatory bowel disease)

✓ **Stool osmolar gap** = 290 − [(stool {Na$^+$} + stool {K$^+$}) × 2]. Gap greater than 125 mOsm/L suggests osmotic diarrhoea.

✓ **Colonoscopy:** *C. difficile* colitis have distinct, adherent, raised plaques (pseudomembranes) and mucosa may be entirely normal looking.
  - CMV and HSV colitis can present as discrete ulcerations and widespread mucosal oedema on endoscopy.
  - *Mycobacterium avium* cellulare (MAC), *Cryptosporidium, Giardia,* and GVHD are diagnosed histologically.

Management

✓ **Resuscitation:** Correct fluid and electrolyte imbalance. **Suspected infectious cases of diarrhoea should be kept in an isolated room[Q].**

✓ **Antibiotics:** Patients with CDI are treated with **antibiotics.** All patients with complicated CDI should get a CT scan of abdomen and pelvis.

✓ **Nutrition:** Enteral nutrition should not be withdrawn, continue whenever possible in the absence of ileus. and the total amount can be reduced.
  - Avoid hyperosmolar formulas and put fibre in the formula.

- Lactose-free feeds should be used as diarrhoea can lead to loss of GI disaccharidase activity.
✓ Fistulas can be managed by bowel rest or surgery.
✓ Faecal impactions can be removed by manual disimpaction followed by cleansing enemas of water-soluble contrast agents.
✓ **Specific Treatment**
  - **Pancreatic enzymes:** Pancreatic enzyme deficiency.
  - **Cholestyramine:** Bile salt malabsorption (short bowel syndrome).
✓ **Antimotility agents** in non-infectious causes and diarrhoeas because of enteral feeding.
  - **Antiperistalsis agents should be avoided in infectious diarrhoeas.**
  - **Loperamide:** 4 mg initially followed by 2 mg after each stool. Max: 16 mg/day.
    ❖ Consider in patients with early severe diarrhoea after ileostomy.
  - **Diphenoxylate with Atropine (Lomotil):** 10 mL four times a day initially, and then titrate down.
  - **Deodorized tincture of opium:** 0.6 mL four times a day.
✓ **Antiemetic agents** for accompanying nausea and vomiting.
  - **Ondansetron^Q:** 5-HT3 receptor antagonist. QT prolongation.
  - **Metoclopramide:** 5-HT3 receptors and D2 receptor antagonist.
  - **Cyclizine:** H1 receptors and muscarinic receptor antagonist.

CONSTIPATION

Aetiology: Incidence in ITU varies between 15–80% depending upon definition.

✓ **Constipation:** Fewer than 3 bowel movements per week, sensation of incomplete evacuation, hard stool and difficulty passing stool with the need to strain or digital assistance for rectal emptying [Definition by American Gastroenterological Association (AGA)].
  - In ICU, we use the term "**paralysis of lower GI tract**" which means 3 d without stool passage. *Large bowel obstruction known as acute colonic pseudo-obstruction (Ogilvie's syndrome) is a common condition.*

✓ **Causes**
  - **Drug induced:** Opioids, anticholinergics, aluminum-based antacids, calcium channel blockers, anti-epileptics.
    ❖ Morphine has more probability of causing constipation than transdermal fentanyl.
  - **Mechanical factors:** Immobilization slows down intestinal peristalsis.
  - **Physiologic factors:** Electrolyte imbalance, mechanical ventilation, hypothyroidism.
  - **Dietary changes:** Early (<24 h) enteral nutrition can lead to less constipation.

Clinical Features

✓ Evidence has shown that constipation can lead to failure of enteral feeding and weaning from mechanical ventilation.
  - Also, constipation can lead to delirium, acid reflux, aspiration, bacterial overgrowth, and overflow diarrhoea.

Treatment

✓ **General Management**
  - Avoid narcotics and sedatives. Good glycaemic control.
  - Increase dietary fibre by liaising with dietician and increase mobility.
  - Ensure adequate fluid intake of at least 2 L a day.
  - Consider treatment with laxatives.
  - If still no bowel movements after laxatives, consider abdominal X-ray, digital rectal examination, and digital removal of faeces.
✓ **Naloxegol:** Peripherally acting opioid receptor antagonist. Used when traditional laxatives fail.
  - Does not alter central analgesic effect.
  - Onset of actions is 2 h and dose is 12.5–25 mg PO once a day.
✓ **Alvimopan:** Peripherally acting opioid receptor antagonist.
  - Approved for treatment of post-operative ileus following small or large bowel resections.
  - 12 mg BD for a total of 15 doses.
✓ **Neostigmine:** Antiacetylcholinesterase: Acts on colon.
  - Given in Ogilvie's syndrome.
  - Can cause abdominal pain, hypersalivation, vomiting, and bradycardia.

Classification of Laxatives[Q]

✓ **Bulk-forming agents:** These agents **increase the bulk** of the stool as fibre absorbs water, hence stimulating the intestine.
  - **Ispaghula husk:** Works like fibre and draws water.
    - ❖ May be used as bulking agent in diarrhoea as well, hence least likely to cause diarrhoea[Q].
    - ❖ Ensure adequate fluid intake.
    - ❖ Avoid in faecal impaction and intestinal obstruction.
    - ❖ Onset: 24–48 h, Dose: 1 sachet PO BD after meals.
✓ **Osmotic laxatives:** They draw water into the colon, softening the stool and making it easier to pass.
  - **Macrogols (polyethylene glycol/Laxido)**
    - ❖ Ensure adequate fluid intake.
    - ❖ Avoid in intestinal obstruction and intestinal perforation.
    - ❖ Onset: 24–48 h, dose: 1–3 sachets PO per day in divided doses
  - **Sodium citrate micro-enema (Micralax)**
    - ❖ First-line treatment for rapid relief of faecal impaction and acute constipation
    - ❖ Onset: 5–30 mins. One per rectum when required.
    - ❖ On resolution start macrogol maintenance.
  - **Phosphate enema**
    - ❖ Second-line treatment for rapid relief of faecal impaction and acute constipation
    - ❖ Can cause hypocalcaemia and hyperphosphataemia in ill patients and renal impairment.
    - ❖ Onset: 5–15 min. One per rectum when required.
    - ❖ On resolution start macrogol maintenance.
  - **Lactulose**
    - ❖ Used in constipation and hepatic encephalopathy.
    - ❖ Onset: 48 h. Dose: 15–60 mL three times a day.
✓ **Stimulants:** Increase motility and cause cramping. They can cause diarrhoea.
  - **Senna**
    - ❖ Useful in acute constipation where adequate fluid intake is difficult.

  - ❖ Used for opioid-induced constipation as well.
  - ❖ Liquid is unpalatable.
  - ❖ Avoid in intestinal obstruction.
  - ❖ Onset: 8–12 h, Dose: 5–10 mL liquid PO BD.
  - **Bisacodyl (Dulcolax)**
    - ❖ Prepares the bowel before surgery or colonoscopy.
    - ❖ Can cause abdominal cramps.
    - ❖ Onset: Oral: 6–12 h. Suppository: <60 min.
  - **Sodium picosulphate**
    - ❖ Prepares the bowel before surgery or colonoscopy.
✓ **Softening agents:** Reduce the surface tension of the stool, allowing water and lipids to enter the stool and, hence **softening the stool.**
  - **Glycerol:** Acts as a stimulant as well.
    - ❖ Laxative can be stopped once stools are soft and easily passed.
    - ❖ Onset: 15–30 min. One per rectum when required.
  - **Docusate:** Acts as a stimulant as well.
    - ❖ Useful in acute constipation where adequate fluid intake is difficult.
    - ❖ Used for opioid-induced constipation as well.
    - ❖ Avoid in intestinal obstruction.
    - ❖ Onset: 24–48 h, Dose: 100–200 mg PO BD. Max: 500 mg/24 h.

FULMINANT COLITIS AND TOXIC MEGACOLON

Aetiology

✓ **Fulminant Colitis:** Ill-defined entity that usually denotes most severe form of **uncomplicated acute colitis.**
  - Normally occurs in the disease course of ulcerative colitis and infectious colitis but occur in patient with Crohn's disease, ischaemic colitis, or irradiation colitis.
  - Fulminant colitis→ Dilatation of colon (Toxic megacolon).
✓ **Toxic Megacolon:** Acute **dilatation** of colon and can be due to inflammatory bowel disease, pseudomembranous colitis, CMV colitis or amoebic colitis.
  - Toxic megacolon occurs early in the course of ulcerative colitis, normally within first 5 yr of disease.

- Medications like **diphenoxylate with atropine** (Lomotil), loperamide, opioids and barium enema also increase the chances of development of toxic megacolon.
✓ **Inflammatory Bowel Disease (IBD)** is of two types: Ulcerative colitis and Crohn disease.
  - **Ulcerative colitis (UC):** Diffuse, continuous inflammation of the superficial mucosa of the large intestine.
    - ❖ **Acute severe ulcerative colitis (ASCU):** Progression of mucosal inflammation to deeper muscular layers of colon. It represents fulminant colitis.
  - **Crohn disease (CD):** Inflammation can appear anywhere in the digestive tract, from the mouth to anus and intermittent healthy areas are seen between inflamed spots.

Clinical Features

✓ **True Love and Witt's Criteria** for diagnosis of **Acute Severe Ulcerative Colitis (ASCU)**
  - Presence of ≥6 bloody stools per day and one of the following
    - ❖ **HR** >90/min or **temperature** >37.8°C or **Hb** <105 g/L or **ESR** >30 mm/h
✓ **Assessment for Fulminant Colitis:** Stool cultures and *C. difficile* toxin, CMV qPCR, QuantiFERON-TB Gold, hepatitis panel.
  - Abdominal X-ray to rule out toxic megacolon.
  - Early flexible sigmoidoscopy should be performed within first 48 h to assess severity of disease and obtain biopsies[Q].
✓ **Presenting Features of Toxic Megacolon:** Increased diarrhoea and bleeding, fever >101.5°F, tachycardia (HR >120/min), severe abdominal pain and diminished bowel sounds.
  - Peritoneal signs signify transmural inflammation and steroids can mask it.
✓ **Diagnosis of Toxic Megacolon:** Loss of haustration with segmental or total colonic dilatation (≥6 cm), pneumatosis cystoides intestinalis on abdominal X-ray.
  - CT scan will show segmental thinning of the colonic wall and nodular pseudopolyposis.

Management

✓ Treatment of fulminant colitis is based on two premises: intense medical treatment and early surgery in non-responders.

✓ Discontinue oral intake during fulminant colitis. NG tube for patients with associated ileus.
  - Aggressive resuscitation of fluids and electrolytes imbalances ($\downarrow K^+$, $\downarrow Mg^{2+}$, $\downarrow Ca^{2+}$, $\downarrow PO_4^{3-}$).
  - Gram-negative and anaerobic coverage by antibiotics although no benefits have been established.
✓ **Dilemma for Physician:** Severe flare up of IBD requiring intensive corticosteroid therapy or infectious colitis for which steroids might be harmful.
  - **Treat infectious colitis if suspected. Consider upfront colectomy** in toxic megacolon, perforation, or previous refractory ulcerative colitis. **All other cases get IV corticosteroids.**
✓ Treat CMV with Ganciclovir specially with >5 or more CMV nuclear inclusions on colonic biopsy.
✓ Treat *C. difficile* colitis with oral vancomycin and IV metronidazole along with resuscitation.
✓ **IV Corticosteroids** (Hydrocortisone 100 mg 6 hourly or methylprednisolone 20–30 mg BD).
  - Predicting the patients likely to fail corticosteroids therapy is important and includes predictors like ACE (Albumin <30 g/L, CRP >50 mg/L and Endoscopy showing severe colitis) or faecal calprotectin >1672 μg/g on day 3 after colonoscopy as well as elevated procalcitonin levels >0.10 μg/L.
  - Failure of reduction in bowel movements or improvement in CRP are other signs of failed steroid therapy.
✓ **Rescue Therapy** post-steroid failure involving cyclosporine or infliximab has been used.
  - **IV Cyclosporine (Calcineurin inhibitor) therapy** (2mg/kg) can be used for patients who failed corticosteroid therapy. Responders are transitioned to oral cyclosporine and azathioprine later.
    - ❖ Side effects of cyclosporine: Hypertension, nephrotoxicity, tremors, seizures, opportunistic infections (cotrimoxazole for PCP prophylaxis), $\downarrow Mg^{2+}$ and $\downarrow Ca^{2+}$.
  - **Infliximab (TNF-α inhibitor):** Accelerated loading dose regimen (3 doses within 24 d) or higher induction doses (10 mg/kg) significantly reduces the risk of colectomy at 3 months.

- **Vedolizumab (α4β7 integrin antagonist):** Maintenance therapy after induction with a calcineurin inhibitor.
- **Combination of cyclosporine with vedolizumab** can be used in patients who have failed azathioprine therapy in the past or older patients with comorbidities.

✓ **Indications for Surgery:** Surgery for patients who fail intensive corticosteroids by day 3 or at least one rescue therapy by day 7 in **ASUC.**

- **Surgery is advocated in toxic megacolon**[Q] if no improvement in patients despite 12–24 h of medical therapy.
- **In patients with *C. difficile* colitis:** Surgery is indicated for patients in septic shock, renal or pulmonary organ dysfunction or failure to respond to medical therapy after 5 d.

✓ **Surgical Options:** In older patients, one stage procedure of total proctocolectomy with end ileostomy is performed.

- Limited abdominal colectomy with ileostomy leaving the rectosigmoid or rectum alone using a Hartmann procedure is preferred by most surgeons. This gives the option of a subsequent restorative ileoanal anastomosis.

Prognosis

✓ Early recognition of toxic megacolon can lower mortality to around 15%.

✓ Hypoalbuminaemia, persistently increased CRP, small bowel ileus and deep colonic ulcers are poor prognostic factors for successful medical therapy.

✓ Colonic perforation (greatest risk factor), age >40 yr and delayed surgical intervention are factors causing increased mortality in toxic megacolon.

9

Endocrine Problems

PITUITARY

✓ **Physiology**
- **Anterior pituitary (adenohypophysis) (Chromophil cells)**
  - ❖ Develops from Rathke's pouch–oral ectoderm in roof of developing mouth.
  - ❖ Adrenocorticotrophic hormone (**ACTH**), thyroid stimulating hormone (**TSH**), follicle stimulating hormone (**FSH**), luteinizing hormone (**LH**), **Prolactin** and growth hormone (**GH**).
- **Posterior pituitary (neurohypophysis)**
  - ❖ Develops from neural ectoderm from floor of hypothalamus.
  - ❖ **Neurons from the supraoptic and paraventricular nucleus of the hypothalamus synthesize the hormones and then travel down the nerve axon connecting posterior pituitary.**
  - ❖ Secretes **ADH**^{Q} (**nonapeptide**, supraoptic) and **Oxytocin**^{Q} (nonapeptide, paraventricular).

✓ **Hormones secreted by hypothalamus:** CRH, TRH, GHRH, GnRH, somatostatin, dopamine.

✓ **Pituitary apoplexy**^{Q}: Hypoperfusion of pituitary due to infarction.
- Usually due to bleeding into a pre-existing tumour.
- **Sheehan's syndrome:** Pituitary hypoperfusion in the puerperium mostly due to haemorrhage.
- Patients present with signs of meningism^Q like sudden-onset headache, visual disturbances, and signs of cardiovascular collapse (cortisol deficiency).
  - ❖ Cranial nerves III, IV and VI palsy due to cavernous sinus compression.
- **Treatment** involves glucocorticoids, hormone replacement and surgery for mass effect.

✓ **Pituitary adenomas**
- Microadenomas <1 cm and macroadenomas >1 cm
- **Presentation of adenomas**
  - ❖ **Mass effect:** Headache, visual field defects, cranial nerve palsies.
  - ❖ **ACTH:** Cushing's disease or adrenocortical insufficiency
  - ❖ **GH:** Acromegaly or short stature
  - ❖ **TSH:** Hyper/hypothyroidism
  - ❖ **Prolactin:** Irregular menstruation, galactorrhoea, sexual dysfunction
  - ❖ **FSH and LH:** Ovarian hyperstimulation syndrome or hypogonadotropic hypogonadism
  - ❖ **ADH:** SIADH or diabetes insipidus
- **Diagnosis**
  - ❖ **Blood tests:** Can show too much or too less of hormone.
  - ❖ **MRI scan** for diagnosing the tumour. **CT scan** can be used as well.
- **Management of a post-operative case of transsphenoidal pituitary surgery**
  - ❖ HDU/ITU admission.
  - ❖ Avoid nasal CPAP and prevent post-operative retching.
  - ❖ Glucocorticoids replacement.
  - ❖ Manage complications like diabetes insipidus, CSF rhinorrhoea, meningitis.

DOI: 10.1201/9781003476214-9

THYROID METABOLISM

Thyroid Anatomy

✓ Landmarks: Thyroid cartilage: C4–5, Cricoid cartilage: C6.

Thyroid Physiology

✓ Principal hormones: Thyroxine (T4), triiodo-thronine (T3), and calcitonin.
  - Thyroid gland takes in iodide ion by active transport and peroxidase converts this iodide ion to atomic Iodine. Atomic iodine is added to tyrosine forming mono- or diiodotyrosine. These iodinated tyrosine residues couple up to form T4 or T3.
  - **T3 and T4 remain attached to thyroglobulin and are stored as colloid.**
  - Up to 80% of the T4 is converted to T3 by peripheral organs such as liver, kidney, and spleen.
  - T3 is 10 times more active than T4.
  - Only 0.02% of T4 and 0.3% of T3 is biologically active.
  - Rest is bound to plasma proteins like Thyroid-binding globulin, Transthyretin, and albumin.
  - T3 is responsible for 80% of metabolic activity.
  - Half-life of T4 is 7 d and T3 is 1 d.

Myxoedema Coma

Epidemiology

✓ **Myxoedema coma:** Seen in advanced untreated hypothyroidism. Mortality as high as 30–50%.
✓ *More than 95% of patients with hypothyroidism have primary thyroid disease* (autoimmune or ablative procedure on the thyroid)[Q].
  - Cold stress, narcotics/hypnotics, trauma, surgery, and infection can precipitate myxoedema coma among hypothyroid patients.
✓ **Sick euthyroid syndrome[Q] (SES):** Critical illness itself causes alterations in thyroid hormone concentrations and is characterized by low TSH levels, low total T3 levels, high total T4 levels initially followed by low total T4 levels.
  - Reverse T3 (rT3) is often increased in SES.
  - However, free hormone levels are normal and hence most patients appear euthyroid despite low total levels.

- Hence routine screening of thyroid dysfunction in ICU isn't recommended due to prevalence of sick euthyroid syndrome[Q].

Clinical Features

✓ **Diagnosis is clinical: Mental obtundation (coma and slow deep tendon reflexes),** bradycardia, **hypotension,** myxoedema facies, **hypothermia,** hypoglycaemia, atonic GI tract, pleural and pericardial effusions.
  - Laboratory tests just to confirm hypothyroidism. *T4 is low but TSH is high compared to **sick euthyroid syndrome patients in which both T4 and TSH are low.***
  - However, in hypothyroidism secondary to pituitary/hypothalamic disorder, even TSH will be low in patients with myxoedema coma.
  - T3 has no role in diagnosis as it is depressed not only by illness but also by fasting[Q].
✓ Evaluate for space occupying lesion within pituitary region for all patients with myxoedema coma.

Treatment

✓ **Hydrocortisone[Q]** 300 mg IV in three divided doses during the first 24 h even in the absence of hypotension.
✓ **Thyroid hormone[Q]:** Intravenous Levothyroxine (L-T4) or Liothyronine (L-T3) hormone.
  - L-T4 for all patients except the most severe cases of myxoedema coma. Dose is 0.2–0.4 mg/day and then repeated every 24 h.
  - In cases with poor response to L-T4, a loading dose of 5–20 µg of L-T3 can be given intravenously according to American Thyroid Association recommendations. This is followed by 2.5–10 µg of L-T3 every 8 h.
  - When the patient is stable and fully conscious, L-T4 can be given orally instead of the intravenous route.
  - IV dose of L-T4 is 75% less than the oral dose normally. Half-life of oral L-T4 is 7 d.
✓ **Hypothermia:** Passive rewarming as active rewarming increases oxygen consumption and can cause circulatory collapse.
  - **Antibiotics:** Pneumonia and urosepsis are precipitants in up to 80% of patients and should be treated aggressively.
  - **Hypoglycaemia:** 50 mL of 50% glucose.

- **Hyponatraemia:** Restrict free water. Hypertonic saline is serum sodium concentration less than 110 mEq/L.

Thyroid Storm

Epidemiology and Aetiology

✓ **Thyrotoxicosis:** Patients with thyrotoxicosis need hospitalization uncommonly.
✓ **Thyroid Storm**[Q] is decompensated form of thyrotoxicosis due to some physiological insult. Common precipitant for thyroid storm is **infection.**
  - Other precipitants are trauma, surgery and DKA.
  - Seen in 1% patients with hyperthyroidism.
  - May be seen 10–14 d after administration of radioactive iodine (I-131) in patients with large goitres who have not been treated with propylthiouracil (PTU) to deplete stored thyroxine (T4) or triiodothyronine (T3).

Clinical Features

✓ **Diagnosis based on clinical symptoms**[Q]
  - Fever, tachycardia, Hypotension or Hypertension, tachyarrhythmias like Atrial Fibrillation (commonest) leading to congestive heart failure.
  - **Delirium,** agitation, and hot flushed skin due to vasodilation.
  - Myopathy, weight loss, loose stools are seen and hepatomegaly with jaundice is a poor prognostic sign.
  - Classic signs of thyrotoxic Graves' disease like **ophthalmopathy** are seen in most patients.
✓ **Serum T4 may be normal or higher.** T3 may be less elevated due to marked impairment of conversion due to illness.
✓ **Burch–Wartofsky Point Scale (BWPS):** Scoring system that assigns points on temperature, central nervous system manifestations, gastrointestinal symptoms, cardiovascular symptoms and precipitating factors.
  - ❖ Score ≥45 is highly suggestive of thyroid storm.
✓ **Thyrotoxic periodic paralysis:** Rare complication of thyrotoxicosis characterized by elevated T3, T4, and hypokalaemia.
  - ❖ Presents with severe muscle weakness that can last for several days.

✓ **Differential Diagnosis** is malignant hyperthermia, neuroleptic malignant syndrome, and acute mania with life-threatening catatonia.

Treatment[Q]

✓ **Treat underlying illness**[Q]**:** Antibiotics, **Digoxin (double the dose) for cardiac arrhythmias.** Insulin if precipitating factor is Diabetic ketoacidosis (DKA), IV fluids.
✓ **Supportive care:** Cooling blanket and antipyretics. *Salicylates should be avoided as they can displace thyroid hormones from serum-binding proteins.*
✓ **Block peripheral effects of thyroid hormone: Propranolol** blocks the cardiovascular effects of thyroid hormone. *Propranolol decrease peripheral T4 to T3 conversion as well.*
  - 1 mg IV/min for a total of 2–10 mg followed by 40–120 mg PO q4–6h.
  - *Metoprolol (selective β-1 blocking agent)* can be used in patients with asthma.
✓ **Inhibition of thyroid hormone synthesis: Propylthiouracil** (Reduces T3/T4 production and *reduces peripheral conversion of T4 to T3*) or **Carbimazole** (Reduces T3/T4 production).
  - They should be started one hour before the administration of iodine (prevents release of stored hormone) to prevent stimulation of the thyroid gland.
  - Propylthiouracil (PTU): 800 mg PO stat and 200 mg 8 hourly.
  - Intravenous Methimazole (MMI) is available in Europe but not UK.
✓ **Blocks release of thyroid hormone from thyroid gland**
  - Saturated solution of potassium iodide: 5 drops PO q8h.
  - Lugol's solution: 10 drops PO q8h.
  - Lithium has been used in patients allergic to iodine.
✓ **Corticosteroids** (potent inhibitors of peripheral conversion of T4 to T3) can be used in these patients.
  - Dexamethasone: 2 mg q6h.
✓ **Cholestyramine:** 4g PO q6h binds T4 and T3 in the gut and may be useful when used early in a patient after an overdose.
✓ **Dantrolene may be used in a dose of 1 mg/kg.**
✓ Aspirin should be avoided[Q] as it will displace T3/T4 from plasma proteins.
✓ Surgery planned once patients is euthyroid.

Prognosis

✓ Mortality as high as 30% seen in untreated patients.

Additional Questions

✓ Commonest cause of hyperthyroidism in pregnancy is Graves' disease[Q].
✓ Hypothyroidism causes increased prolactin[Q] levels.

GLUCOSE METABOLISM

Diabetic Ketoacidosis

Epidemiology and Aetiology

✓ **Life-threatening complication** due to severe lack of insulin.
✓ Majority of episodes of DKA occur in patients with a previous diagnosis of diabetes mellitus. Seen classically in type 1 DM.
✓ Commonest cause for DKA is infection like UTI.
   • Non-compliance, stressors like alcohol, pancreatitis, myocardial infarction are other causes.
   • In 40% of cases, a cause is never found.

Pathophysiology

✓ Insulin causes a shift of glucose in cells and promotes lipogenesis by converting excess glucose into triglycerides.
✓ Initially during fasting, glycogenolysis and gluconeogenesis happens to supply glucose to brain.
   • **After 12 to 18 h of fasting**, peripheral tissues start using free fatty acids and leaving glucose for the brain.
   • **After 72 h of starvation**, brain starts using ketone bodies for fuel. All this while insulin remains low[Q].
   • **During stress and surgery**, functional insulin resistance develops due to release of epinephrine, glucagon, and cortisol.
   • A state of insulin deficiency promotes hyperglycaemia and lipolysis leading to ketone body formation.
   • When rate of hepatic ketoacid generation exceeds peripheral utilization, diabetic ketoacidosis happens.

Clinical Features and Diagnosis

✓ **Diagnostic Triad of DKA[Q]**
   • Capillary glucose >11 mmol/L
   • Ketonaemia ≥3 mmol/L or ketonuria ++ or more
   • Bicarbonate <15 mmol/L or venous pH <7.3.
✓ **Symptoms:** Patients are lethargic with dry skins, lips, and tongue. *Kussmaul breathing with sweet fruity odour in the breath.*
   • Patients may present with abdominal pain and DKA should be excluded in patients presenting with DKA.
✓ **Factors predicting severe disease: Admission to ITU**
   • Young patient aged 18–25 yr, elderly, and pregnant female.
   • Heart or kidney failure
   • Ketones >6 mmol/L
   • Bicarbonate <5 mmol/L
   • pH <7.0
   • Potassium <3.5 mmol/L on admission
   • GCS <12
   • O2 saturation <92 % on air
   • SBP <90 mmHg
   • HR >100/min or 60/min
   • Anion gap >16
✓ **Ketone bodies:** 3-beta-hydroxybutyrate (BHB), acetone and acetoacetate.
   • The commonly used **nitroprusside test** doesn't measure BHB as it a hydroxyl acid and not a ketone.
   • BHB can be measured directly, and its concentration is a better indicator of the severity of ketoacidosis.
   • *During severe acidosis, ketones bodies measured by nitroprusside test can show an initial rise rather than fall due to conversion of BHB into acetoacetate.*
✓ **Hyponatraemia** due to sodium loss in urine due to osmotic diuresis. Water also moves from intracellular space to extracellular space due to high plasma osmolality contributing to hyponatraemia.
   • Chloride may be high in patients with chronic ketoacidosis states and may be associated with slower recovery.
   • **Leucocytosis** can be there even in the absence of infection.
   • **Amylase** may be raised even in the absence of pancreatitis.

✓ **Differential Diagnosis**
- **Alcoholic ketoacidosis** which is euglycaemic and BHB should be measured as acetoacetate is suppressed. *Serum osmolality is generally not raised.*
- **Starvation ketoacidosis**[Q]: Slow onset and patient is better compensated metabolically.
- **Euglycaemic ketoacidosis**[Q]: DKA with abnormalities of ketones and pH but normal glucose.
  - ❖ Seen in SGLT-2 inhibitors like **Dapagliflozin** or young patients or pregnant females with high GFR.
  - ❖ Treated as same with measures taken when glucose reaches <14 mmol/L.

Treatment[Q]

✓ Treatment to be started with fluids followed by insulin treatment.
- 1 L 0.9% NaCl over 1 h with up to two repeated 500 mL boluses if SBP remains <90 mmHg. This is followed by:
  - ❖ 1 L over next 2 h with potassium supplementation.
  - ❖ 1 L over next 2 h with potassium supplementation.
  - ❖ 1 L over next 4 h with potassium supplementation.
  - ❖ 1 L over next 4 h with potassium supplementation.
  - ❖ 1 L over next 6 h with potassium supplementation.
✓ *Potassium replacement with 40 mmol/L if levels between 3.5 and 5.5 to achieve plasma potassium levels between 4 mmol/L and 5 mmol/L.*
- Potassium shouldn't be started before second bag of fluids unless potassium <3.5 mmol/L.
- **Peripheral potassium shouldn't be infused at >20 mmol/h peripherally.**
✓ Fixed rate intravenous insulin @ 0.1 units/kg/h. Continue long-acting insulin at usual dose.
- Add 10% dextrose 125 mL/h if glucose falls below 14 mmol/L and reduce rate to 0.05 units/kg/h.
- Insulin should never be stopped completely even if the rate is reduced to 0.5 units/h.
✓ **Overall Timeline of Management**
- **0 to 60 min:** Start fluids and insulin infusion and send investigations.
  - ❖ Hourly capillary blood glucose and ketones.
  - ❖ Venous bicarbonate and potassium at 60 min, 2 h, and 2 h thereafter.
  - ❖ 4-hourly plasma electrolytes.
- **60 min to 6 hr:** Fluid replacement and additional measures like airway protection if needed, urinary catheterization and thromboprophylaxis.
- **6 to 12 hr:** Referral to diabetes team. **Cardiovascular status re-evaluation to be done at end of 12 h.**
- **12 to 24 hr:** *Ketonaemia and acidosis should have resolved.*
✓ **Typical deficits in DKA in adults**
- **Water: 100 mL/kg**
- **Sodium: 7–10 mmol/kg**
- **Chloride: 3–5 mmol/kg**
- **Potassium 3–5 mmol/kg**
✓ **Response to Treatment**[Q]
- Capillary ketones falling by 0.5 mmol/L/h.
- Venous bicarbonate rising by 3 mmol/L/h.
- Plasma glucose falling by at least 3 mmol/L/h.
✓ *Resolution of DKA if patient's pH is 7.3 and ketones are <0.6 mmol/L.*
- Once ketonaemia is cleared, and patient is not eating and drinking, start VRII. If patient is eating and drinking, start subcutaneous insulin.
- Do not discontinue IV insulin infusion until 30 min after subcutaneous short acting insulin has been given.
✓ **Bicarbonate replacement** during DKA should be used only when hypotensive shock is unresponsive to rapid fluid replacement, buffering capacity is completely exhausted, respiratory responses are maximal and acidaemia is worsening.
- **Excess chloride** can impair renal bicarbonate absorption and itself lead to hyperchloraemic metabolic acidosis[Q].
✓ **Hypotension:** Normally resolves with fluid replacement. Refractory hypotension should prompt for evaluation of heart disease, bleeding, or adrenal insufficiency.
✓ **Oliguria:** It should improve after administration of fluid and an **atonic bladder** is common in these set of patients and should be sought for if oliguria persists.
✓ Mortality is <5%. Cerebral oedema is the leading cause of death.

Hyperosmolar Hyperglycaemia State

Aetiology

✓ Seen in type 2 DM patients mostly. Patients are mostly elderly. Like DKA, a precipitating factor may be present.

Pathogenesis

✓ **Relative insulin deficiency** to inhibit ketone body formation but not enough to prevent hyperglycaemia.

✓ **Renal impairment** is often present in these cases and hence they have low GFR and are not able to excrete glucose.

✓ **Cerebral impairment** is common in these patients, and they don't have adequate fluid intake normally.

Clinical Features

✓ **Hyperglycaemia, hypovolaemia**, and **increased serum osmolality**Q
- Blood glucose >**30 mmol/L.**
- Large fluid deficits with up to 10–30 L deficit and hence at greater risk of cerebral oedema.
- Serum osmolality of >**320 mOsm/kg and** absence of ketonaemia (<3 mmol/L) and pH >7.3.

✓ **Hyper-ketonaemia or severe acidosis are not featuring usually. If a significant anion gap is present, another cause of acidosis should be considered.**
- **Mixed DKA/HHS can happen as well.**

✓ *Gradual onset of symptoms.* Up to one-third of patients may have seizures.

✓ *Indications for admission to critical care*
- Serum osmolality >350 mOsm/kg
- Sodium >160 mmol/L
- pH <7.1
- Potassium <3.5 mmol/L or >6 mmol/L.
- GCS <12
- Oxygen saturation <92% on air.
- SBP <90 mmHg
- HR <60/min, >100/min.
- Creatinine >200 mmol/L.
- Urine output <0.5 mL/kg/h
- Hypothermia
- Serious comorbidity

Treatment

✓ **0.9% Saline should be given** until the osmolality stops decreasing.
- Sodium concentration should decline <10 mmol/L in 24 h due to increased risk of central pontine myelinolysisQ.
- Gradual decline osmolality by 3–8 mOsm/kg/h.
- Fluid rehydration should be 50% replacement in first 12 h (6–8 L).
- Start replacement with 0.45% saline once osmolality stops decreasing.

✓ **Fixed Rate Intravenous Insulin (FRII)** at 0.05 unit/kg/h should only be started if fluids alone are not decreasing the blood glucose levelsQ.
- Indications of FRII are BHB >1 mmol/L or ketonuria ≥2+.
- **Glucose concentration should decline by 5 mol/L/h.**

✓ **Resolution:** Takes longer than DKA
- Serum osmolality <300 mOsm/kg.
- Urine output >0.5 mL/kg/h
- Blood glucose <15 mmol/L.
- Cognitive state back to premorbid state.

✓ **Prophylactic anticoagulants** should be given as large vessel thrombosis as an important cause of mortality.

Mortality

✓ 20% mortality and more compared to DKA.

Hypoglycaemia

Definitions

✓ **Hypoglycaemia:** Blood glucose levels <3.9 mmol/L according to **American Diabetes Association (ADA)**
- Blood glucose levels <**3.5 mmol/L according to NICE guidelines.**
- **Whipple's Triad** defines hypoglycaemia as
  1. Documentation of low blood glucose
  2. Symptoms of hypoglycaemia
  3. Resolution of symptoms after administration of glucose.

Aetiology

✓ **Hormonal Imbalance**
- **Insulin overdose:** Most common cause
- Insulinomas

- Hypoglycaemic agents: Sulfonylureas and meglitinides (Repaglinide and Nateglinide)

✓ **Drugs**
  - Ethanol-induced hypoglycaemia (Alcoholic ketoacidosis)
  - **Beta-blockers:** Non-selective ones like propranolol, pindolol and nadolol.
  - Quinine
  - Pentamidine
  - **Salicylates:** In children as part of aspirin associated Reyes syndrome

✓ **Inadequate Gluconeogenesis**
  - Liver damage (90% of gluconeogenesis)
  - Kidney damage (10% of gluconeogenesis)
  - Sepsis
  - **Inborn errors of metabolism:** Glycogen storage disease
  - Exercise-induced hypoglycaemia

Pathophysiology

✓ Brain is the organ most dependent on glucose. *During starvation brain uses ketone bodies but this capability develops over hours to days.* RBCs and renal medulla are other tissues that require glucose obligatory.

✓ **During starvation,** the principal source of glucose is hepatic glycogen (60–80 grams), but this supply is exhausted by an overnight fasting.
  - Only about 20% of normal liver synthetic function is needed to maintain normal glucose homeostasis.

✓ Prolonged starvation requires glucose from muscle glycogen (120 grams) but this is not directly available due to absence of enzyme glucose 6-phosphatase in muscle.
  - Muscle glycogen is converted to lactate via anaerobic glycolysis and this lactate is transported to liver through the Cori cycle for gluconeogenesis.
  - Muscle also convert Pyruvate to Alanine, and this is transported to the liver for gluconeogenesis.
  - Glycerol derived from fat also contributes to gluconeogenesis.

✓ **Impaired Counterregulatory Response to Insulin** (Glucagon, epinephrine, growth hormone, cortisol, and thyroxine) can lead to hypoglycaemia.

✓ Ethanol causes hypoglycaemia by suppressing hepatic gluconeogenesis.

Clinical Features

✓ **Sympathoadrenal Symptoms** and signs like palpitations, anxiety, tingling and hunger.
  - These symptoms may be absent in patients on beta-blockers and diabetic autonomic neuropathy.
  - Severe symptoms include confusion, seizures, and coma.
  - Acute pulmonary oedema, supraventricular and ventricular tachycardias are seen as well.

✓ **Fingerstick Glucose** can be misleading if the patient is hypo perfused or in shock and hence arterial blood glucose is recommended.
  - **Urine ketones testing is helpful as hypoglycaemia with ketonuria rules out excess Insulin as a cause.**
  - Patients with Insulinoma will have raised C-peptide which is released along with insulin by pancreas and C-peptide is absent in a patient with intentional insulin use.

✓ **Target blood sugar** in normal ICU is 6–10 mmol/L[Q]. Overzealous correction can lead to hypoglycaemia.
  - **NICE-SUGAR (2009) Trial:** In critically ill cohort, patients with intense glucose target of 4.5–6 mmol/L had higher 90-d mortality compared to patients with glucose target of 6–10 mmol/L.

Treatment

✓ **Blood Glucose** <4 mmol/L should be treated. Enteral carbohydrate (15–20 gram) is preferred in cooperative patient. Glucose tablets or gel can be given.
  - All comatose patients should receive intravenous glucose. 50 mL of 50% dextrose over 3–5 min if central line is present (can cause local tissue pain) or 50 mL aliquots of 10% dextrose can be given via peripheral line.
  - This should be followed by an infusion of 5% or 10% dextrose.

✓ **Ethanol-Induced Hypoglycaemia:** Intravenous Thiamine (100 mg) should be given to prevent Wernicke encephalopathy.

✓ **Other Drugs:** Glucagon, Glucocorticoids, Octreotide, Diazoxide.

Prognosis

✓ Hypoglycaemia is a marker of poor outcome in critically ill patients.

PHEOCHROMOCYTOMA

Epidemiology and Aetiology

✓ **Pheochromocytoma:** Catecholamine secreting tumour of adrenal medullary cells.
- 10–30% of the cases are malignant and 25–35% of cases are familial and linked to genetic conditions like Multiple endocrine neoplasia type 2a and 2b.

✓ **Pathophysiology:** Adrenal gland divided into two parts:
- **Adrenal cortex:** Outer part of gland. Produces corticosteroid hormones.
- **Adrenal medulla:** Inner part of the gland. Chromaffin cells.
  - ❖ 20% Noradrenaline and 80% Adrenaline.

✓ **Synthesis of Catecholamines**
- L-Phenylalanine → L-tyrosine → L-DOPA → Dopamine → Noradrenaline → Adrenaline.
- **Tyrosine hydroxylase** is the rate limiting step of converting L-tyrosine to L-DOPA.
- **Excretion of catecholamines:** Metabolized by enzymes monoamine oxidase (MAO) and catechol-O-methyl transferase (COMT).
  - ❖ **Dopamine** → homovanillic acid (HMA)
  - ❖ **Noradrenaline** → metanephrine + vanillylmandelic acid (VMA)
  - ❖ **Adrenaline** → normetanephrine + vanillylmandelic acid (VMA)

Clinical Features and Diagnosis

✓ **5H's:** Hypertension, headache, hyperglycaemia, hypermetabolism and hyperhidrosis.
- Anxiety, palpitations, tremors.

✓ **Complications:** Pulmonary oedema, Hypertensive crisis, Takotsubo cardiomyopathy, stroke, mesenteric ischaemia, AKI.

✓ **Diagnosis:** Mostly an incidental finding on imaging.
- Blood/urine metanephrines is the initial test.
- CT scan is the gold standard test for diagnosis.

Prevention

✓ Foods rich in tyramine like cheese, chocolate, and red wine should be avoided.

✓ TCAs, MAO inhibitors, and caffeine can trigger spells as well.

Treatment

✓ **Pheochromocytoma Crisis (Preoperative)**
- Adequate hydration as these patients are severely vasoconstricted and have fluid deficit inside.
- **Alpha blockade** (Phentolamine and phenoxybenzamine) before **beta-blockers**^{Q} otherwise unopposed alpha action can cause severe hypertension.
  - ❖ **Phenoxybenzamine**^{Q} blocks irreversibly and is longer acting and is preferred.
- Short-acting beta-blockers for arrhythmias.

✓ **Intraoperative**
- Surgery is planned once patient is more stable with fluid optimization and effective beta blockade.
- Avoid release of catecholamine during surgery. Manage hypotension once the tumour is resected.
- **Arterial line** to monitor severe haemodynamic shifts.

✓ **Post-Operative**
- **Hypertension:** Due to incomplete resection of tumour or metastasis
- **Hypotension:** Due to abrupt catecholamine deficiency, hypovolaemia from blood loss and residual α/β blockade.
- Corticosteroid replacement if bilateral adrenalectomy.

Prognosis

✓ The most likely complication after removal of phaeochromocytoma which is one of known causes of hypertension is persistent hypotension^Q.

✓ 5-year survival of 95% in benign, non-metastatic disease.

✓ 5-year survival of 40–60% survival in malignant disease

ADRENOCORTICAL DISORDERS

Adrenal Glands: Adrenal glands divided into two parts.

✓ **Adrenal cortex:** Outer part of gland. Produces corticosteroid hormones.
- **Zona glomerulosa:** Outermost. Mineralocorticoids (Aldosterone)
- **Zona fasciculata:** Middle part. Glucocorticoids (Cortisol)

- **Zona reticularis:** Innermost. Androgens (Dehydroepiandrosterone)
✓ **Adrenal medulla:** Inner part of the gland. Produces catecholamines.

Overactive Adrenal Glands

✓ **Hyperaldosteronism:** Adrenal glands produce too much aldosterone.
- **Primary:** Bilateral adrenal hyperplasia (70% of cases), adrenal adenoma (Conn's syndrome)
- **Secondary:** Due to overactivity of renin-angiotensin-aldosterone (RAAS) like ascites, left ventricular failure, cor-pulmonale.
- **Clinical features:** Hypertension, low potassium, and metabolic alkalosis.
✓ **Cushing's Syndrome:** Adrenal glands produce too much cortisol.
- **ACTH dependent:** Pituitary tumour (Cushing's disease), ectopic ACTH producing tumour, ectopic CRH producing tumour.
- **ACTH independent:** adrenal gland tumour, exogenous corticosteroid use.
- **Clinical features:** Hypertension, diabetes mellitus, low potassium, muscle wasting, bruising.
✓ **Conn's syndrome:** Adrenal adenoma. Low renin hypertension. Diagnosed by increased aldosterone: renin ratio.

Adrenal Insufficiency

Epidemiology and Aetiology[Q]

✓ Prevalence of 1–3% in general population.
- **Critical Illness-Related Corticosteroid Insufficiency (CIRCI):** Sepsis is the most common cause of adrenal insufficiency in intensive care patients.
✓ **Adrenal crisis:** Acute deterioration in health status associated with hypotension, with systolic blood pressure <100 mmHg or systolic blood pressure ≥20 mmHg lower than usual, with resolving of features 1 to 2 h after parenteral glucocorticoid prescription.
✓ **Primary adrenal failure:** Addison's disease, TB, HIV, HIT (adrenal vein thrombosis).
- Adrenal crisis is more common in patients with primary adrenal insufficiency

compared to patients with secondary adrenal insufficiency.
✓ **Secondary adrenal failure:** Patients taking exogenous steroids for asthma, rheumatoid arthritis, inflammatory bowel disease.
- Daily use of 5 mg or more of prednisolone for longer than 4 wk by **all routes** may lead to ACTH deficiency.
- **Etomidate** can suppress cortisol production for up to 48 h by inhibiting *11-β-hydroxylase*.
- **Opioids (>100 mg of morphine daily)** can also cause functional adrenal failure.

Pathophysiology

✓ Cortisol (20 mg daily) released in pulsatile manner every day with plasma cortisol levels in morning as 140–700 nmol/L compared to 80–350 nmol/L at midnight.
- Diurnal variation is lost in stress and illness.
✓ **90% of Cortisol** is protein bound (80% to cortisol-binding globulin, 10 % to albumin).
- **10% of free cortisol** crosses lipid membrane and stimulates catabolism to release energy during times of stress.
- **Cortisol** causes fluid retention due to action on mineralocorticoid receptor and cardiac contractility along with vascular tone is maintained due to permissive action of catecholamines.
✓ Severe illness and stress stimulate the hypothalamic–pituitary–adrenal (HPA) axis, causing release of corticotrophin releasing hormone (CRH) from hypothalamus. CRH releases adrenocorticotropic hormone (ACTH)/corticotrophin from pituitary. ACTH releases cortisol from adrenal gland.
- During illness free cortisol increases by up to 5 times its normal values. Currently however, laboratories measure only total cortisol.
- **Critical illness-related corticosteroid insufficiency (CIRCI):** *Inappropriately low increase in cortisol levels* during acute illness leading to relative adrenal insufficiency.

Clinical Features

✓ **Presentation[Q]:** Weakness, fatigue, anorexia, vomiting, abdominal pain, and constipation.

Hyponatraemia is seen in up to 80% of patients and should be evaluated for adrenal insufficiency.

- Hypoglycaemia, hyperkalaemia, fever.
- *Hypotension resistant to fluid administration.*
- Eosinophilia and anaemia

✓ **Diagnosis:** Baseline ACTH and cortisol test before giving hydrocortisone in a critically ill patient should be done.

- Cortisol levels <15–18 μg/dL should prompt start of glucocorticoids.
- **ACTH stimulation test (Synacthen test)**[Q]: Not used in patients with septic shock as confounded by critical illness.
  - ❖ **250 μg of Corticotropin** leading to increase in cortisol level above 18 μg/dL after 60 min is considered responsive. Cortisol levels <9 μg/dL are suggestive of adrenal insufficiency.
- **Primary adrenal insufficiency:** Test for *21-hydroxylase autoantibodies* as well.

Treatment

✓ **Hydrocortisone (cortisol)** 100 mg bolus followed by 200 mg every 24 h before prolonged hypotension.

- Dexamethasone 4 mg every 24 h may be used as well but it doesn't have mineralocorticoid activity and should be used with Fludrocortisone.

✓ IV 0.9% normal saline bolus should be given tailored to patient's comorbid status.

✓ After resolving of crisis, hydrocortisone should be tapered to the patient's maintenance dose over next 3 d.

✓ Hypoglycaemia correction.

Prognosis

✓ Mortality rates double in patients with primary adrenocortical insufficiency.

- Recovery of adrenal glands can take up to one year even after just one month of corticosteroid intake.

Haemato-Oncology Problems

ANAEMIA

Epidemiology and Aetiology

✓ **Anaemia:** Haemoglobin concentration <120 g/L in women, <130 g/L in men.
  - Up to 60% of patients are anaemic upon admission to an ICU.
  - Majority of the patients admitted for more than 7 d will receive a RBC transfusion.
✓ *Most common cause of anaemia in ITU is blood loss.* Erythropoietin secretion is also decreased.
  - Patient's volume status should be considered first as resuscitation itself can cause dilutional anaemia.
✓ **Types of anaemia based on the size of RBCs**
  - **Microcytic (MCV <80 fL):** Iron deficiency anaemia, thalassemia, anaemia of chronic disease, sideroblastic anaemia.
  - **Normocytic (MCV 80–100 fL):** Acute blood loss, anaemia of chronic disease, haemolytic anaemia with low or normal reticulocyte count.
  - **Macrocytic (MCV >100 fL):** Vitamin B_{12} & folate deficiency^Q (chronic alcoholism, phenytoin), haemolysis with reticulocytosis, hypothyroidism.

Clinical Features and Diagnosis

✓ **Clinical features:** Fatigue, shortness of breath, palpitations, and pale skin.
  - In critically sick patients, diagnosed on routine blood tests.
✓ **Reticulocyte count** is the measure of bone marrow's ability to produce new RBCs and is the initial test.

- Reticulocyte count is **elevated** during haemolytic anaemias^Q, gastrointestinal bleeding, supplementation with iron or vitamin B12.
- Reticulocyte count is **low** during primary bone marrow disorders, parvovirus infection^Q, nutritional deficiencies, and anaemia of chronic disease.
✓ **Blood smear findings: Next test after reticulocyte count**
  - **Nucleated RBCs:** Haemolytic anaemia, post-splenectomy.
  - **Schistocytes:** MAHA including HUS/TTP/HELLP syndrome/DIC.
  - **Target cells:** Thalassemia, liver disease
  - **Spherocytes:** Warm autoimmune haemolytic anaemia (WAIHA)
  - **Bite cells:** G6PD deficiency.
  - **Teardrop cells:** Myelofibrosis.
  - **Rouleaux formation:** Multiple myeloma, Waldenstrom's macroglobulinaemia.

Treatment

✓ Packed RBCs are given if haemoglobin <70 g/L in ICU.
✓ IV iron has been used in non-critically ill patients.
✓ Erythropoietin can stimulate red blood cells production but critically sick patients often exhibit resistance to them.

Haemolytic Anaemias

✓ **Laboratory features:** ↑ Total and unfractionated bilirubin, ↑ LDH, ↓ Haptoglobin. ↑ reticulocyte count and nucleated RBCs. Can be due to

DOI: 10.1201/9781003476214-10

immune-mediated haemolysis or **microangiopathy haemolytic anaemia.**

✓ **Immune-mediated haemolysis**

- **Warm autoimmune haemolytic anaemia (WAIHA):** Warm antibodies react optimally with red cells at core body temperature (37°C).
  - ❖ Most commonly antibodies (**IgG**) are against Rh blood group.
  - ❖ Can be **idiopathic** or **secondary** to autoimmune and lymphomas.
  - ❖ **Evans syndrome:** WAIHA + Thrombocytopaenia.
  - ❖ **Clinical features:** *Positive direct Coomb's test*, spherocytes are seen on blood smear.
  - ❖ **Treatment:** Steroids, Rituximab, and splenectomy.
- **Cold agglutinin disease:** Cold antibodies react optimally with red cells below core body temperature (maximal reactivity at 4°C).
  - ❖ Most commonly antibodies are **IgM.**
  - ❖ **Idiopathic** or **secondary** to lymphoproliferative disorders.
  - ❖ **Clinical features:** Chronic condition leading to haemolysis and episodic cyanosis and ischaemia of the ears, tip of the nose and digits.
  - ❖ **Coomb's test is positive for Complement C3 but negative for IgG.**
  - ❖ **Treatment:** Avoidance of cold temperatures, rituximab, sutimlimab (Inhibitor of complement C1), plasmapheresis.
- **Paroxysmal cold haemoglobinuria:** IgG antibody binds to RBCs at cold temperature (<32°C) but haemolysis happens on rewarming and hence the name.
  - ❖ Upon warming the IgG dissociates from the RBCs but the complement remains fixed causing haemolysis.
  - ❖ This antibody is called **Donath–Landsteiner antibody** and is directed against the **P red cell antigen and diagnosis is by detection of this antibody.**
  - ❖ There is no cold-induced digital ischaemia.
  - ❖ **Coomb's test is positive for Complement C3 but negative for IgG.**
  - ❖ Primarily a paediatric disorder often seen following a viral infection.

- **Drug-induced haemolytic anaemia:** Piperacillin is the most common drug to cause immune haemolytic anaemia. Other drugs involved are Cephalosporins like Cefotetan, Isoniazid, Quinine, alpha methyldopa, levodopa, Procainamide.
  - ❖ **Treatment** is removing the offending drug.

✓ **Microangiopathic Haemolytic Anaemia (MAHA):** Vascular damage leads to thrombosis of small arterioles and fragmentation of erythrocytes. Hence, anaemia and thrombocytopaenia. Schistocytes are seen.

- **Differential diagnosis of MAHA**
  - ❖ Haemolytic uraemic syndrome (HUS)/ Thrombotic thrombocytopaenic purpura (TTP)
  - ❖ Disseminated intravascular coagulation.
  - ❖ HELLP syndrome
  - ❖ Malignant hypertension
  - ❖ Severe vasculitis
  - ❖ Intravascular foreign bodies
  - ❖ Prosthetic heart valves.
- HUS/TTP and DIC have been explained in the section by the same name.

Haemoglobinopathies

✓ **Sickle Cell Anaemia**

- *Autosomal recessive.*
- Valine is substituted for glutamic acid in the sixth position of the beta chain of haemoglobin[Q].
- Symptoms if patients are homozygotes for the defect.
- Hypoxia causes an unstable form of haemoglobin (haemoglobin S). Sickling at oxygen concentration of 85%.
- **Sickledex test[Q]:** Qualitative test for screening HbS. It doesn't differentiate between disease and trait.
- **Acute chest syndrome[Q]:** Fever, hypoxaemia, chest pain and new pulmonary infiltrates.
  - ❖ Fat embolism and infection are the most common causes.
  - ❖ Empirical antibiotic coverage with a cephalosporin and macrolide should be given to cover atypical bacteria.
  - ❖ Maintain hydration and oxygenation.
- **Acute stroke[Q]:** Acute thrombotic stroke or acute retinal artery occlusion.

- **Pulmonary hypertension**[Q]: Pulmonary hypertension due to nitric oxide scavenging by free haemoglobin released during haemolysis.
- **Acute cholecystitis**[Q]: Gall stones composed of bilirubin stones of calcium can lead to acute cholecystitis.
- **Sepsis**[Q]: Infections due to asplenia by capsulated organisms.
- **Aplastic crisis**[Q]: Secondary to folic acid deficiency or infection with parvovirus B19.
- **Iron overload**[Q]: Lifetime transfusions can lead to iron overload.
- **Osteomyelitis**
- **Renal failure**
- **Hyposplenism**
- **Treatment:** Hydroxyurea[Q] increases the amount of fetal haemoglobin and reduces the severity of symptoms as well as need for transfusion.
  - ❖ **Acute red cell exchange**[Q] is needed in acute infarction leading to stroke and acute chest syndrome with final haemoglobin S less than 30% and a final haemoglobin no higher than 80 to 100 g/L.
  - ❖ **Auto-splenectomy** can happen and vaccination against encapsulated bacteria such as *Neisseria meningitidis*, *Haemophilus*, Strep pneumonia, *Klebsiella*, *Salmonella* and Group B *Streptococcus* is needed.
- ✓ **Thalassemia:** Patients have deficiency of α or β chains.
  - Patients with thalassemia can develop high output heart failure.
  - Treatment is regular blood transfusions, chelation therapy and potentially bone marrow transplant.
- ✓ **Glucose-6-phosphate dehydrogenase (G-6-PD) deficiency:** Affects men of African American or Mediterranean descent.
  - G-6-PD is necessary to maintain glutathione in its reduced state in the erythrocyte.
  - Patients without the enzyme have oxidative haemolysis.
  - **Drugs to be avoided**[Q]: Dapsone, methylene blue, Nalidixic acid, Nitrofurantoin, Primaquine, Sulfacetamide, Toluidine blue.
- ✓ **Paroxysmal nocturnal haemoglobinuria**
  - Abnormal stem cell clone gives rise to red cells, white cells and platelets that lack proteins that are normally attached to the cell surface by a glycosylphosphatidylinositol (GPI) anchor.

- These proteins CD55 and CD59 are normally responsible for inactivating complement on the surface of red cells.
- PNH cells are susceptible to complement mediated lysis.
- **Presentation:** Pancytopaenia, arterial or venous thrombosis.
- **Eculizumab** has been approved for treatment.
- ✓ **Hereditary Spherocytosis:** Autosomal dominant disorder of red cell membrane skeletal proteins leading to a lack of anchoring of the red cell lipid bilayer to its skeletal backbone.
  - Lifelong haemolysis and can be accelerated by infection.
  - Coombs test will be negative and helps to differentiate it from WAIHA.
  - Treatment is blood transfusions, folic acid supplementation and splenectomy in some cases.

Other Causes of Anaemia

- ✓ **Haemolysis by infectious agents:** Malaria, Babesiosis, *Clostridium perfringens*, *Clostridium welchii*.
- ✓ **Iron deficiency anaemia**[Q]: ↓ MCV, ↓ ferritin, ↓ iron, ↓ transferrin saturation and ↑ total iron-binding capacity.
- ✓ **Megaloblastic anaemia:** Vitamin B12 and folic acid should be measured. Elevation of **homocysteine** and **methylmalonic acid (MMA)** is seen. Oval macrocytes and hyper-segmented neutrophils are seen on peripheral smear.
  - Methotrexate can also cause macrocytosis.
  - B12 is replaced before folate as folate replacement alone can lead to subacute degeneration of the cord[Q].
- ✓ **Anaemia of chronic disease/inflammation:** Blood loss, phlebotomy, decreased red cell production, decreased production of EPO, renal dysfunction.

THROMBOCYTOPAENIA

- ✓ **Thrombocytopaenia:** Platelet count below the 2.5th percentile of the normal platelet count distribution.
  - Platelets below 50×10^9/L seen in up to 15% of patients.
  - **Common causes**[Q]
    - ❖ **Decreased production:** Sepsis, recent cardiac surgery, alcohol excess, bone marrow failure.

- ❖ **Increased consumption:** HIT, VITT, ITP, TTP, DIC, HELLP syndrome, hypersplenism, intravascular devices with abnormal blood flow (IABP).
- ❖ **Dilutional:** Massive transfusion, fluid resuscitation
- ❖ **Distributive:** Hypersplenism, hypothermia.
- ❖ **Drugs:** Heparin, Abciximab, linezolid, vancomycin, cephalosporins, carbapenems, TMP-SMX
- **Clinical features:** Spontaneous epistaxis, easy bruising, hemarthrosis.
- **Initial assessment:** Patient bleeding or thrombotic.
  - ❖ **Bleeding** can be structural (gastric ulcer) or generalized.
  - ❖ **Thrombotic** in TTP and HIT.
- ✓ **Diagnostic approach:** Perform a peripheral blood smear.
  - **Platelet clumping:** Artefactual thrombocytopaenia
  - **Giant platelets ± white cell inclusion bodies:** Hereditary thrombocytopaenia
  - **True thrombocytopaenia:** Acquired causes.
    - ❖ **Isolated thrombocytopaenia:** ITP, HIV, HCV, HIT, DIC. Investigations based on clinical assessment.
    - ❖ **Blasts, nucleated RBCs:** Primary bone marrow disorder. BM aspiration and biopsy
    - ❖ **Micro-spherocytes, RBC clumping:** *Evans syndrome.* Reticulocytes, LDH, Bilirubin.
    - ❖ **Lymphocytosis, atypical lymphocytes, neutrophilia:** Consider infection. Order CRP, septic screen, virology (**hantavirus,** Ehrlichiosis, Lassa fever, **Ebola,** dengue)
    - ❖ **Schistocytes:** TTP/HUS/DIC. Order LDH, haptoglobin, bilirubin, PT, APTT, D-dimers, and fibrinogen.
- ✓ **Differential Diagnosis**
  - DIC, HLH, HIT and TTP present with modest thrombocytopaenia (50–100 × 10⁹/L).
    - ❖ **ITP** and **drug-induced thrombocytopaenia** will have severely low platelets (20 × 10⁹/L).
    - ❖ Patients with TTP will have really high LDH.
  - **Thrombotic microangiopathy with Coombs negative test:** Shiga toxin

associated HUS, invasive pneumococcal infection, Calcineurin inhibitors, *Ticlopidine* and quinine.

- ❖ *Thrombotic microangiopathy* can complicate both autologous and allogenic stem cell transplants.
- **Immune thrombocytopaenia (ITP)** presents with a rash in a systemically well patients.
  - ❖ Autoimmune disease in children.
  - ❖ Treatment is intravenous immunoglobulin and high-dose steroids.
- **Pregnant patient:** TTP, HELLP and fatty liver of pregnancy.
- **Drug-induced thrombocytopaenia:** Seen 1–3 wk after starting a new medication. Patients with vancomycin-induced thrombocytopaenia are resistant to platelet transfusions.
- **Post-transfusion purpura:** Severe thrombocytopaenia (<10 × 10⁹/L), one to two weeks after receiving blood products. *Patients lack the platelet antigen PLA1.*
- ✓ **Management:** Treat the underlying cause. Failure to detect a significant rise in the platelets count 30–60 min after platelet transfusion signifies peripheral destruction.
  - Platelet transfusion for non-bleeding patient at levels below 10 × 10⁹/L.
  - **Prophylactic platelet transfusion** should be avoided in patients with
    - ❖ TTP/HUS
    - ❖ Catastrophic antiphospholipid syndrome
    - ❖ HIT

Heparin-Induced Thrombocytopaenia

- ✓ **Heparin-Induced Thrombocytopaenia:** Prothrombotic state post-administration of heparin.
- ✓ **Type I Heparin-Induced Thrombocytopaenia (HIT): (Less common)** – Onset in 1–4 dᵠ.
  - Mild thrombocytopaenia without immune involvement and resolves without stopping heparin.
  - Direct action of heparin on platelet activity and involves heparin binding to PF4 and mild platelet aggregation.
- ✓ **Type II HIT:** Immune-related thrombocytopaenia. 1–5% incidence in UFH and <1% in LMWH.
  - **IgG** antibody against PF4ᵠ (stored in platelets α-granules) and heparin complex on

the platelet surface. However, presence of anti-PF4 antibodies is not diagnostic as not all antibodies are pathogenic.

- **Surgical** (cardiac and orthopaedic) and **female patients** are at a higher risk.
  - ❖ **Between day 4 and 10 is the maximum incidence rate**[Q].
- **HIT with thrombosis (HITT):** *Significant venous and arterial thrombosis in 30–70% patients even with thrombocytopaenia. It has the highest mortality associated with it.*
  - ❖ Pulmonary embolism, acute coronary syndrome and stroke.
  - ❖ Platelet count rarely falls below 20×10^9/L.

- ❖ **Typical onset HIT:** Platelet count falls at day 5–10 after Heparin.
- ❖ **Rapid-onset HIT:** Platelet count falls within 24 h after Heparin in patient exposed to heparin in previous 30–100 d.
- ❖ **Acute HIT:** Fever, chills, chest pain, hypertension within 30 min of heparin administration.
- ❖ **Delayed-onset HIT:** Platelet count falls after 10–14 d of heparin withdrawal.
- **Four T score for HIT**[Q]: *Those with pre-test scores <4 are unlikely to test positive for* HIT antibodies. 4–5 score makes HIT likely, *6–8 makes HIT highly likely.*

	0 Points	1 Point	2 Points
Platelet count decrease	<30%	30–50%	>50%
Time to thrombocytopaenia	≤3 d	≥10 d	5–10 d
Sequelae	None	Suspected thrombosis	New thrombosis
Alternative explanation	Definite	Possible	None

- **Laboratory diagnosis**
  - ❖ **Immunoassays:** ELISA: Detects the presence of HIT antibodies. Initial test which is very sensitive but not specific and a negative test hence rules out HIT.
  - ❖ **Functional assays:** Detect platelet activation by HIT antibodies in the presence of heparin. Sensitive and specific. **A positive immunoassay test** should be confirmed by a functional assay as antigen test is false positive in 10–50% of cardiac surgery, dialysis, or ICU patients.
- **Management**[Q]: Stop heparin if suspected and involve haematologist.
  - ❖ **Argatroban**, lepirudin, bivalirudin (direct thrombin inhibitor), Fondaparinux and **Danaparoid** (factor Xa and factor IIa inhibitor).
  - ❖ *Danaparoid is suitable in pregnancy and Bivalirudin in cardiac intervention.*
  - ❖ At least Lower extremity should be scanned for thrombosis. Anticoagulation for 3 months if thrombotic complications and 30 d without thrombotic complications.
  - ❖ *IVIG 1 g/kg has been used in patients with persistent thrombocytopaenia or thrombosis.*

- ❖ *Avoid platelet transfusion unless significant bleeding.*
- ❖ Warfarin should be avoided immediately as can lead to further thrombosis and necrosis.
- ❖ All future administration of heparin is avoided. *Heparin may be given for short periods for CABG after HIT ideally after >100 d.*

BLOOD TRANSFUSION

- ✓ **Blood Donation Ineligibility**
  - Have received blood products after 1 January 1980
  - Hepatitis B or C carrier
  - HIV positive
  - Cancer
  - Organ transplant recipient
  - Injected non-prescribed drugs like body-building drugs
- ✓ **Donated Blood Screening**[Q]
  - ABO and rhesus status
  - Red cell antibodies
  - Hepatitis B, C
  - Syphilis
  - HIV/HTLV
  - Malaria antibodies, *Trypanosoma cruzi*

antibodies, West Nile virus RNA if positive travel history

- CMV antibody (for transplant recipients)

✓ **Donated blood deterioration over time**

- Depletion[Q] of 2,3 DPG, ATP, Factor V and VIII.
- Accumulation of CO_2, H^+, K^+
- Activated clotting factors.
- Microaggregates of platelets, white cells, and fibrin.
- Increase in red cell fragility.

✓ **Methods to reduce antigenicity of stored blood**

- **Leucodepletion:** Introduced in 1999. WBCs are taken out.
  - ❖ Reduced risk of prions and CMV infection
  - ❖ Reduced risk of immune and non-immune transfusion reactions like TRALI
- **Solvent/Detergent-treated FFP:** Reduces the risk of transmission of HIV, Hepatitis B and Hepatitis C.
- **Irradiation:** Reduced T cell proliferation and subsequent graft versus host disease.
- **Triple saline wash:** Removes plasma proteins and antibodies.

✓ **Red Blood Cells:** One unit of packed RBC contains 300 mL of volume (200 mL RBCs + 50 mL plasma + 50 mL additive solution).

- Additive solution[Q] used in packed red blood cells commonly is SAGM that is saline, adenine, glucose, and mannitol.
- **Whole blood** has volume of 450–500 mL and has both plasma and platelets.
  - ❖ Except factors V and VIII (24 h only), most coagulation factors are stable during storage. Hence, whole blood is increasingly being transfused during trauma.
  - ❖ However, shelf life is only 5 d and higher incidence of haemolysis and graft versus host disease.
  - ❖ Additive is citrate phosphate dextrose (CPD).
- Packed RBCs are stored at 2–6°C[Q], for up to 35 d. Red cells cannot be returned to stock if outside for more than 30 min and should be transfused within 4 h of leaving controlled storage conditions.
- For RBCs transfusion, ABO incompatible units can be life-threatening. AB positive

are universal recipients. Group O RhD-negative is the universal blood group for emergency transfusion[Q].

Donor Blood Group[Q]	Antibodies in Donor Plasma[Q]	Compatible Plasma Recipient Patient's Blood Groups
A	Anti-B	A, O
B	Anti-A	B, O
AB	None	A, B, AB, and O
O	Anti-A and Anti-B	O

- **Transfusion Requirements in Critical Care (TRICC) Trial 1999[Q]:** Compared the transfusion trigger of <70 g/L as opposed to transfusion trigger of <100 g/L.
  - ❖ They found non-significant reduction in 30 d mortality in restrictive treatment group.
  - ❖ In patients with APACHE II score of <20 and patients younger than 55 yr, the mortality reduction in restrictive treatment group was statistically significant.
  - ❖ Significant increased rate of cardiac incidents in liberal arm group.
- **Carson et al. (2013):** Patients with **acute coronary syndrome** may benefit more from a liberal transfusion approach.
- **Transfusion Requirements in Septic Shock (TRISS) Trial (2014)[Q]:** Compared transfusion triggers of <70 g/L and <90 g/L in patients of septic shock and found no significant mortality difference in the 90 d mortality.
- **A higher transfusion trigger** may be beneficial in patients with stroke, TBI or subarachnoid haemorrhage (8–10 g/dL).
- **Lower threshold for transfusion** for those with chronic anaemia or **patients waiting for organ transplant.**
- Most common cause of anaemia in an old patient is bowel malignancy.
  - ❖ This will lead to iron deficiency anaemia.
  - ❖ In case of megaloblastic anaemia, replacement of Vitamin B_{12} should be done before folate to avoid development of neurological sequelae.

✓ **Platelets:** A bag of platelets has volume of 300 mL with 70% additive solution and 30% plasma. Additive is acid citrate dextrose (ACD).

- Should be stored at 20–26°C[Q] with constant agitation with shelf life of 5 d.

- They have risk of bacterial contamination and hence are cultured before being issued.
- One unit of apheresis platelets/pooled platelets[Q] increase the platelet count by 50,000/μL.
- Nearly one-third of the transfused platelets will be sequestered.
- Platelets transfusion is not needed above platelets count >50,000/μL for most invasive procedures.
- Platelets express HLA class 1 antigens, so in theory ABO compatibility isn't required.
  - ❖ However, due to possibility of contamination with RBCs and WBCs, **ABO Group-specific platelets are recommended** although out of the group can also be issued.
  - ❖ In emergency **AB group platelets** can be given. Serologic crossmatch is not required unless platelets concentrate have high RBC content.
- *HLA-matched platelets are used in patients with HLA antibodies.*
- *Platelet transfusion is relatively contraindicated in TTP.*
- Indications for use of platelets transfusion in adults.
  - ❖ Bleeding patients
  - ❖ <10,000 μL in normal patients
  - ❖ Lumbar puncture: 75000/μL
  - ❖ Neurologic or ophthalmologic surgeries: 100000/μL
✓ **Fresh frozen plasma:** Volume of 1 unit plasma: 200–300 mL.
  - Stored at −30°C[Q] and can be kept for up to 2 yr.
  - Shelf life at 4°C for 24 h.
  - FFP **doesn't need to be rhesus crossmatched but should be ABO compatible**[Q].
  - Plasma compatibility is the opposite to that of red cells and platelets with O being universal recipient and AB the universal donor[Q].
  - Dose is 10–15 mL/kg[Q] of FFP. Fibrinogen amount: 2–3 gram/L.
  - Plasma should not be used to correct isolated deficiencies of clotting factors when a concentrated replacement source is present (factor VIII for haemophilia).
✓ **Cryoprecipitate:** Prepared from plasma that has been snap frozen and then defrosted.
  - Stored at −25°C, for up to 2 yr.

- Contains factors **VIII, XIII, fibrinogen, vWF, and fibronectin.**
- Fibrinogen level <1.5 g/L in trauma patients and <2 g/L in pregnant female: **Give cryoprecipitate.**
- Treatment of massive transfusion involves mostly use of near-patient testing rather than laboratory tests.
- Dose is 1 single unit per 5–10 kg of body weight. Adult dose is hence around 10 units (2 pooled units as one pooled unit is made of 5 single units) and can increase fibrinogen levels by 3–4 g/L.
✓ **Human albumin solution**
- Prepared by cold fractionation followed by heating to 60 degrees for 10 h.
- Doesn't contain any clotting factors.
- Uses explained in chapter on fluids.
✓ **Prothrombin complex concentrate**
- Factors II, VII, IX, and X.
- Used for reversal of warfarin and bleeding patients.
✓ **Factor rVIIa**
- Off label use for major haemorrhage.
- Increased risk of thrombosis.

Transfusion reactions: Can be acute (<24 h) and delayed (>24 h).

✓ **Classification**
- **Mild:** Temperature <39°C or <2°C rise, with or without rash/pruritus.
- **Moderate:** Temperature >39°C or >2°C rise, with symptoms/signs other than rash/pruritus.
- **Severe:** Bleeding, respiratory compromise, circulatory collapse.
✓ **Febrile transfusion reactions (non-haemolytic reactions):** Recipient antibodies against donor WBC antigens. Complement activation leads to ↑IL-1, IL-6, TNF-α.
✓ **Haemolytic transfusion reactions:** Recipient antibodies against donor antigens.
- *Haemolysis → Fever, sense of impending doom, back pain, hypotension, red urine, DIC, renal failure, respiratory failure.*
- Drop in Hb and elevated bilirubin, decreased haptoglobin and increased LDH. Positive direct antiglobulin test (Direct Coombs test).
- Anti-ABO antibodies are IgM. Anti-rhesus D antibodies are IgG.

- **Acute**[Q]: ABO Incompatibility reaction. Anti-A or Anti-B antibodies are implicated and cause activation of complement[Q].
  - **Delayed (1–4 wk later)**[Q]: Non-ABO, RhD antigens.
- ✓ **Allergic reactions:** Allergic reaction to donor plasma proteins and can cause pruritus and urticaria.
- ✓ **Transfusion-related acute lung injury (TRALI)**[Q]: Donor antibodies against recipient WBC antigens.
  - ARDS (acute dyspnoea with hypoxia and bilateral chest infiltrates) with fever and hypotension within **6 h of transfusion.**
  - More common in blood products with more plasma (>60 mL) like FFP, platelets and cryoprecipitate.
  - Seen more commonly in blood donated by multiparous women[Q].
  - Seen in both RBC and immunoglobin transfusion.
  - Prevented by leucodepletion of blood[Q].
  - Intracardiac pressure is normal.
  - **Management** is supportive resuscitation with lung-protective ventilation (two-thirds of patients will require mechanical ventilation).
  - 10% mortality
- ✓ **Transfusion-Associated Circulatory Overload (TACO):** Respiratory distress due to pulmonary oedema like overload, hypertension, tachycardia, and positive fluid balance within 6 h of transfusion.
  - Treatment is diuresis.
- ✓ **Infections:** HIV, Hepatitis B, Hepatitis C, Malaria, Syphilis, variant CJD, CMV
- ✓ **Graft-versus-host disease:** Very rare. Donor T-lymphocytes attack host bone marrow cells
- ✓ **Transfusion-related immunomodulation:** Increased cancer recurrence
- ✓ **Dilutional coagulopathy due to massive transfusion**
- ✓ **Iron overload**
- ✓ **Post-transfusion purpura**
- ✓ **Hypothermia**
- ✓ **Citrate toxicity:** Metabolic alkalosis and tetany due to hypocalcaemia. Seen in massive transfusion
- ✓ **Management of a transfusion reaction**[Q]
  - Stop the blood transfusion immediately in all cases.

- Venous access should be maintained with physiological saline.
- ABC assessment done.
- Identification details of patients checked again with that of the blood bag.
- Blood bag should be visually checked for clumps or particulate matter or discolouration suggestive of bacterial contamination.
- Keep all blood products bags and labelling for return to laboratory for investigation.
- For patients with mild reactions, transfusion may be started with appropriate treatment and direct observation.
- For patients with moderate reactions, a medical review should be done, and transfusion may be started with appropriate treatment and direct observation.
- For severe reaction, call for help, start resuscitation and treat symptomatically.
- Anaphylaxis algorithm for suspected allergic reaction (wheeze, stridor).
- **Medicines and Healthcare Products Regulatory Agency (MHRA)** and **Serious Hazards of Transfusions (SHOT)** are sent a report.
- ✓ **Point of Care Coagulation Testing**
  - **Thromboelastography (TEG):** Uses a rotating cup containing a sample of blood activated by Kaolin. A wire hanging in the sample is attached to a strain gauge and as the blood clots, the wire is perturbed more and more by the movements of the cup.
    - ❖ Sample is heated at 37°C[Q] and hence hypothermia may affect the results.
  - **Rotational Thromboelastometry (ROTEM):** Cup is attached to the strain gauge and the wires act as a stirring device, sitting in the sample and moving the cup more and more as the clot forms.
  - Additional assays can be studied including
    - ❖ HEPTEM: Heparinase to eliminate the effect of heparin.
    - ❖ EXTEM: Using other activators such as tissue factors.
    - ❖ FIBTEM: Platelet deactivators to remove platelet function from the clot formation.

TEG[Q]	ROTEM[Q]	Description	Normal	Abnormality	Treatment
Reaction time (R value)[Q]	Clotting time (CT)	Time till initiation of fibrin clot formation	5–10 min	↑ R value ↓ factors	FFP, protamine
K value	Clot formation time (CFT)	Time to achieve 20 mm clot on assay	1–5 min	↑ K/CFT value ↓ fibrinogen	Cryoprecipitate, fibrinogen
α-angle[Q]	α-angle	Rate at which fibrin cross-linking occurs	50–75°	↓ α-angle ↓ fibrinogen	Cryoprecipitate, fibrinogen
Maximum amplitude (MA)	Maximum clot firmness (MCF)	Maximum strength of clot	50–75 mm	↓ MA/MCF ↓ platelet count	Platelets, DDAVP
LY-30	Clot lysis (CL)	Degradation of clot 30 min after MA/MCF	0–10%	↑ LY-30/CL ↑ clot breakdown	TXA

Additional Questions

✓ ABO compatibility is essential for RBCs and FFP transfusion. It is not essential but recommended for platelets transfusion. No compatibility matching for albumin or factor VIIa required.

HUS AND TTP

Epidemiology and Aetiology

✓ **Micro-Angiopathic Haemolytic Anaemia (MAHA):** Intravascular haemolysis due to red blood cells trying to pass through blood vessels obstructed due to clots (**thrombotic microangiopathy**).
  • Presents as TTP, HUS and DIC.
✓ **Thrombotic Thrombocytopaenic Purpura (TTP):** Incidence: 6–10 Cases/million.
✓ **Haemolytic uraemic syndrome (HUS)[Q]:**
  Typical form: Young patients with preceding diarrhoeal illness. **Atypical form:** Due to excess complement activation.

Clinical Features and Diagnosis

✓ **Thrombotic Thrombocytopaenic Purpura (TTP)**
  • Acquired due to antibodies against ADAMTS 13 (cleaves vWF)[Q]. Level <10%. Lower levels of ADAMTS13 causes accumulation of vWF and increased platelets clotting.
  • **Causes**
    ❖ **Autoimmune:** Triggered by SLE, cancer, HIV.
    ❖ **Genetic:** Inherited deficiency of ADAMTS13.
    ❖ **Drugs:** Quinine, statins, trimethoprim.

• **Triad** of **thrombocytopaenia, MAHA, and neurological involvement.**
• **Pentad** of fever, MAHA, thrombocytopaenia, AKI, and neurological involvement.
• Clinical features of TTP are like those of aHUS.
• TTP higher amongst females, Afro-Americans and obese patients
• TTP can present anytime during pregnancy compared to post-28 wk for HELLP syndrome.
• **Diagnosis of TTP:** *Based on clinical features while waiting for ADAMTS13 levels.*
  ❖ Most common symptoms are non-specific like abdominal pain, nausea, vomiting and weakness.
  ❖ **Low grade fever** and platelets rarely go less than 30×10^9/L. **TTP usually doesn't have significant coagulopathy (normal PT/INR).**
  ❖ **Haemolytic anaemia[Q]:** High unconjugated bilirubin, low haptoglobin, **high LDH**, high lactate, *Negative direct antiglobulin Coombs test.* **Schistocytes >1%.** *Normal complement levels.*
  ❖ Confusion, headache, seizures more common than focal neurological deficits. Coma is clinical manifestation in 10% of the patients.
  ❖ AKI is a late feature[Q].
✓ **Haemolytic Uraemic Syndrome (HUS)[Q]**
  • **Causes:** Enterohaemorrhagic *Escherichia coli* O157:H7 or *Shiga* toxin–producing *E. coli*.

- Classically seen in **children** and elderly.
- Triad of **thrombocytopaenia, MAHA, and renal failure**.
- **Diagnosis of HUS:** Non-immune haemolytic anaemia (schistocytes) and thrombocytopaenia.
  - ❖ Renal involvement more common. **Prodromal symptoms of bloody diarrhoea** (don't give antimotility drugs). 40% of patients will have seizures as well.
- **Atypical HUS (aHUS)** should be considered in patients with no history of preceding diarrhoea and normal ADAMTS13.

Treatment

- ✓ **Thrombotic Thrombocytopaenic Purpura (TTP)**
  - **Therapeutic plasma exchange** is the immediate treatment of choice.
    - ❖ Replacement with plasma (1–1.5 × plasma volume) is necessary in this plasma exchange.
    - ❖ Solvent/detergent treated FFP preferred[Q].
    - ❖ *LDH normalization is aimed.*
    - ❖ Mortality is 10–15% with and 90% without plasma exchange.
  - **Steroids** are indicated given the autoimmune nature of these cases.
  - **Rituximab** (can be used in acute severe stage), **caplacizumab**[Q] (anti-vWF Ig fragment), N-acetyl cysteine, Bortezomib, Recombinant ADAMTS13, Eculizumab.
  - **Platelet replacement is avoided unless bleeding.**
  - Aspirin may be considered once platelets improve.
  - **TTP in pregnancy (delivery of fetus).**
- ✓ **Haemolytic Uraemic Syndrome (HUS)**[Q]
  - No specific cure. Mostly supportive care.
  - Antibiotics are not indicated.
  - Eculizumab[Q] (risk of meningococcal meningitis) is used in aHUS.
  - Therapeutic plasma exchange not required.
  - Renal replacement therapy is indicated, and most patients recover some renal function.
  - Mortality is much lower.

VENOUS THROMBOEMBOLISM

- ✓ **Venous Thromboembolism (VTE):** Includes deep vein thrombosis and pulmonary embolism.
  - **PROTECT trial (2011)** showed that 7.7% of ICU patients developed VTE despite thromboprophylaxis.
  - **Virchow's triad**[Q]: Local injury to the vascular wall, circulatory stasis and increased coagulability.
- ✓ **Risk factors for first episode of VTE**
  - **Genetic risk factors**
    - ❖ Factor V Leiden (Most common inherited thrombophilia, slow rate of inactivation of factor Va)
    - ❖ Protein C and S deficiency
    - ❖ Antithrombin III deficiency
    - ❖ Hyperhomocysteinaemia
    - ❖ Dysfibrinogenaemia
    - ❖ Elevated factor VIII, IX, or XI
  - **Acquired risk factors**
    - ❖ Age ≥70 yr
    - ❖ Cancer (myeloproliferative neoplasms, pancreas, brain and stomach cancer, adenocarcinomas, chemotherapy/radiotherapy in last 6 months, metastasis)
    - ❖ Infections (sepsis, HIV, HCV, TB)
    - ❖ Surgery (Highest in first 6 wk, THR and TKR surgeries)
    - ❖ Trauma
    - ❖ Pregnancy (highest in third trimester and immediate post-partum period)
    - ❖ Immobilization (3 d or more)
    - ❖ Obesity (BMI ≥30)
    - ❖ Smoking
    - ❖ Antiphospholipid syndrome (APS)
    - ❖ Drugs (hormonal therapy, cisplatin, clozapine, quetiapine, olanzapine)
    - ❖ Central venous catheters (femoral and subclavian sites)
- ✓ **Clinical Features**
  - *Most DVTs begin in calves but presenting symptoms and signs are often not noted until more proximal veins are involved.*
    - ❖ Erythema, swelling, and pain.
  - 90% of DVT in pregnancy occur in the left leg and involve pelvic, iliofemoral and popliteal veins.
    - ❖ Increase in coagulation factors I, II, VII, VIII, IX, × and decrease in Protein S are the reasons for PE during pregnancy.

✓ **Diagnosis**
- Testing for inherited hypercoagulable conditions is expensive and is done in patients with strong suspicion.
  - ❖ Testing for HIT when clinically suspected and APS in patients with catastrophic APS is recommended in acute settings.
- **Wells score** is calculated to check the **pretest probability of DVT.** High probability ≥3[Q], Moderate probability 1 to 2 points and low probability is 0 to −2.

Wells Score for DVT Diagnosis	Score
Active cancer (within 6 months)	1
Recent immobilization of legs	1
Immobile for 3 d or major surgery within previous 12 wk	1
Localized calf tenderness	1
Swelling of whole leg	1
≥3 cm increase in calf size on the affected size	1
Pitting oedema on symptomatic leg	1
Presence of non-varicose collateral veins	1
Previous DVT	1
An alternative diagnosis at least as likely as DVT	−2

- ❖ **Proximal vein compression ultrasonography** is done straight away in patients with high probability scores.
- ❖ In cases with moderate probability, D-dimer is done, and a normal D-dimer essentially rules out DVT. An abnormal d-dimer in these cases warrants ultrasonography and **a negative ultrasound** calls for repeat ultrasound in 1 wk again.
- ❖ In cases with low probability, D-dimer is done, and a normal D-dimer essentially rules out DVT. An abnormal d-dimer in these cases warrants ultrasonography and **a negative ultrasound** rules out DVT.
- **Compression venous ultrasonography (Doppler not needed)** is the preferred test for diagnosis of symptomatic proximal DVT with sensitivity and specificity above 90%.
  - ❖ Can be done as a point of care test as well by trained intensivists.

- ❖ In patients with suspected high DVT probability, a proximal leg vein ultrasound scan should be performed within 4 h. If the ultrasound is negative, ultrasound scan can be repeated in a week.
- ❖ However, in a patient with high clinical suspicion but negative compression ultrasound further investigations like MRI and CT venography can also be done inpatient to rule it out.

✓ **Prevention and Treatment**
- **Mechanical thromboprophylaxis** (graduated compression stockings, intermittent compression devices and venous foot pumps) haven't shown any benefit in reducing the risk of death due to pulmonary embolism.
  - ❖ They prevent venous blood stasis and displace blood from superficial to the deep system.
- **Pharmacological VTE prophylaxis** reduces the risk of symptomatic DVT and PE by approximately 50%.
  - ❖ Unfractionated heparin (UFH), low-molecular-weight heparin (LMWH), Fondaparinux and direct oral anticoagulants (DOACs) like Dabigatran, Apixaban, Rivaroxaban have all been used.
  - ❖ LMWH and DOACs are acceptable choices for long-term management of VTE for patients with cancer.
  - ❖ Apixaban is preferred DOAC for patients with GI malignancies.
- **Contraindications to pharmacological thromboprophylaxis**[Q]
  - ❖ Platelets <50 × 10⁹/L or INR >1.5
  - ❖ Active bleeding
  - ❖ Recent central neuraxial blockade
  - ❖ New cerebrovascular accident within previous 2 wk
- **Treatment of VTE**
  - ❖ UFH and LMWH are used in critically ill patients.
  - ❖ LMWH in pregnant females as warfarin and DOACs are contraindicated.
  - ❖ Most critically ill VTE patients are shifted from systemic anticoagulants to warfarin or DOACs.
  - ❖ Bridging therapy with systemic anticoagulants is necessary for using warfarin

as warfarin produces a procoagulant state in first few days and can cause warfarin skin necrosis if not bridged. Continue systemic anticoagulation until INR of 2 has been achieved for at least 24 h.

❖ **In non-critically ill patients**, Apixaban and Rivaroxaban can be initiated for treatment of VTE without parenteral anticoagulant in whereas Dabigatran and Edoxaban should be preceded by at least 5 d of anticoagulant therapy.

❖ Fondaparinux is also an attractive agent for outpatient anticoagulation.

❖ IVC filter in cases at high risk of pulmonary embolism and contraindication to anticoagulation.

❖ **Duration of anticoagulation treatment:** Lifelong for unprovoked DVT and 3–6 months for post-surgery/trauma cases. Cancer cases should have it for at least 3–6 months or as long as the cancer is ongoing.

❖ **Thrombolysis** is done for symptomatic ilio-femoral DVT.

❖ **Catheter-directed thrombolysis (CDT)** is reserved for patients with extensive clot burden with concerns or acute limb ischaemia.

DISSEMINATED INTRAVASCULAR COAGULATION

Aetiology

✓ **Disseminated Intravascular Coagulation (DIC):** Uncontrolled, inappropriate, widespread activation of the thrombin system[Q].
  - Microvascular occlusion initially leading to organ dysfunction.
  - In severe cases, reduction in platelets and clotting factors can lead to haemorrhagic complications.

✓ **Causes**
  - **Sepsis:** Up to one-third of cases of **severe sepsis** have DIC. Gram-negative and Gram-positive sepsis have no difference in incidence.
  - Trauma, obstetric causes, burns, **tumours (acute promyelocytic leukaemia),** transplant rejections, severe pancreatitis are other common causes.

- **Drug-induced DIC:** Ceftriaxone, Carboplatin, Quinine.

Clinical Features and Diagnosis

✓ **Presentation[Q]:** Patient can be asymptomatic with only laboratory evidence of DIC.
  - Bleeding from different sites such as IV sites, surgical wounds.
  - **Thrombosis:** Unusual in acute DIC and mostly seen in cancer, trauma, and obstetric patients. Venous thrombosis is more common.
  - **Purpura fulminans:** Most severe form of DIC.
    ❖ Seen in meningococcaemia-induced DIC.

✓ **Organ dysfunction:** ARDS, renal failure, hepatic failure, neurological impairment, and skin sequelae.

✓ **Laboratory features[Q]:** Thrombocytopaenia, ↑ aPTT, ↑ PT, ↑ BT, ↑ D-dimers and ↓ Fibrinogen levels.
  - **Fibrinogen** is an acute phase reactant; levels may remain normal for some time initially[Q].
  - **Fibrin degradation products (FDPs)** are increased and have a high sensitivity (90–100%) but low specificity.
    ❖ **FDPs** are due to lysis of fibrinogen and non-cross-linked fibrin whereas **D-dimers** are due to lysis of already cross-linked fibrin.
  - **Schistocytes[Q]** (fragmented red blood cells) are seen on blood film.

✓ The **International Society on Thrombosis and Haemostasis (ISTH) DIC score[Q]** is used to diagnose patients with overt DIC (score ≥5)[Q].
  - Variables used are platelet count, prothrombin time, fibrinogen levels, and FDP/D-dimer results.

✓ **Differential Diagnosis**
  - DIC can be differentiated from thrombocytopaenic thrombotic purpura (TTP) by doing the ADAMTS13 test as levels remain >20–30% in DIC but are <10% in TTP.
  - Antiplatelet factor 4 antibodies to rule out heparin-induced thrombotic thrombocytopaenia (HITT).

Treatment[Q]

✓ *Treatment of the underlying cause of DIC is the cornerstone of its management.*

✓ **Prophylactic anticoagulation:** Low doses of UFH or LMWH should be used unless patient is bleeding.

✓ **Bleeding patients:** Give **FFP and Cryoprecipitate** to maintain Fibrinogen >1.5 g/L.

- Give platelets if levels are <50 × 10⁹/L in patients with bleeding and <20 × 10⁹/L in patients at risk of bleeding.

- Fibrinolytics are not recommended.

Prognosis

✓ The International Society for Thrombosis and Haemostasis (ITSH) DIC scoring system correlates with mortality.

IMMUNOLOGY

✓ **Immune Physiology**
- **Primary immunodeficiencies:** Genetic
  - Ataxia-telangiectasia (low IgG, IgM, IgA)
  - Combined variable immunodeficiency (low IgG, IgM, IgA)
  - Chediak–Higashi syndrome (abnormal neutrophil and cytotoxic T cells)
  - DiGeorge syndrome (T cell deficiency)
  - Bruton disease (X-linked agammaglobulinaemia)
  - Wiskott–Aldrich syndrome (neutropaenia)
- **Secondary immunodeficiencies:** Acquired and more common.
  - Infections
  - Medications
  - Malignancies

✓ **Pro-Inflammatory Cytokines**
- **IL-1:** Synthesized by mononuclear cells: Pyrogen, stimulates NO synthesis and lipid mediators, chemotactic factor for neutrophils and lymphocytes.
- **IL-6:** Synthesized by monocytes, macrophage, endothelial cells, and fibroblasts: Pyrogen, causes induction of immunoglobin synthesis, differentiation of B-lymphocytes, and activation of T cells.
- **IL-8:** Synthesized by monocytes, macrophage, endothelial cells, and fibroblasts: Chemotactic factor.

- **IL-12:** Synthesized by monocytes, macrophage, and B-lymphocytes: Activates cytotoxic T cells and natural killer cells.
- **TNF-α:** Synthesized by monocytes, macrophage, and B-lymphocytes: Fever, anorexia, weight loss. Apoptosis and stimulation of T cells and B-cells. Angiogenesis and multiplication of fibroblasts.

✓ **Anti-Inflammatory Cytokines**
- **IL-2:** Synthesized by Helper T cells: Stimulates proliferation of all types of T cells and activated B-cells.
- **IL-4:** Synthesized by Helper T cells, mast cells and basophils: Acts on the macrophage and blocks cytokine synthesis. Inhibits NO synthesis.
- **IL-10:** Synthesized by T cell, B-cell, monocytes, and macrophage: Inhibits the synthesis of cytokines, free radicals, and NO.

✓ **Causes of immunodeficiency**
- **Neutropenia:** Leukaemia, Chemotherapy with Doxorubicin and ARA-C, total body irradiation, aplastic anaemia: Infections by Gram-negative bacilli[Q], *Staphylococcus aureus*, *Aspergillus*, and Candida.
- **Cell mediated defects:** Hodgkin's lymphoma, Chemotherapy with Azathioprine, Bleomycin, corticosteroid use[Q] and protein energy malnutrition: Infections by *Pneumocystis jirovecii*, *Listeria monocytogenes*, Herpes virus, histoplasmosis, *Cryptococcus neoformans*.
- **Humoral defects:** Multiple myeloma, chronic lymphocytic leukaemia, chemotherapy with cyclophosphamide, methotrexate, and splenectomy: Infections by Capsulated organisms[Q] like *Streptococcus pneumoniae*, *Haemophilus influenzae*.
- **Complement defects:** Congenital deficiency, SLE and multiple myeloma, *Neisseria meningitidis*[Q].

✓ **Biological Agents** (whole list just for completion's sake, first few are the more important ones)
- **Rituximab:** Anti-CD-20 monoclonal antibody
  - Indications: Diffuse large B-cell lymphoma (DLBCL), low grade NHL, Chronic lymphocytic lymphoma (CLL), Rheumatoid arthritis, Wegener granulomatosis, microscopic polyangiitis

- ❖ Side effects: Febrile neutropenia, hypo-gammaglobulinaemia, Tumour lysis syndrome
- **Anakinra:** IL-1 antagonist
  - ❖ Indications: Rheumatoid arthritis, Juvenile idiopathic arthritis, Still's disease, Gout, Cryopyrin-associated periodic syndromes (CPS)
  - ❖ Side effects: Impaired neutrophil recruitment
- **Tocilizumab:** Anti IL-6 monoclonal antibody
  - ❖ Indications: Rheumatoid arthritis, Juvenile idiopathic arthritis, Giant cell arteritis
  - ❖ Side effects: Neutropenia
- **Adalimumab/Infliximab/Etanercept:** TNF-α antagonist
  - ❖ Indications: Rheumatoid arthritis, plaque psoriasis, psoriatic arthritis, ankylosing spondylitis, and inflammatory bowel disease (Adalimumab and Infliximab only)
  - ❖ Side effects: Neutropenia. Tuberculosis test^Q before starting Infliximab
- **Omalizumab:** Anti-IgE monoclonal antibody
  - ❖ Indications: Asthma, Chronic spontaneous urticaria
  - ❖ Side effects: Infection by parasites
- **Eculizumab:** Anti-complement C5 antibody
  - ❖ Indications: Paroxysmal nocturnal haemoglobinaemia (PNH), Atypical HUS
  - ❖ Side effects: Encapsulated organism infections
- **Alemtuzumab:** Anti-CD-52 monoclonal antibody
  - ❖ Indications: CLL, Multiple sclerosis, Graft vs host disease
  - ❖ Side effects: CD4+ depletion
- **Basiliximab:** Anti-IL-2 monoclonal antibodies
  - ❖ Indications: Immunosuppression for kidney transplant
  - ❖ Side effects: Autoimmune side effects
- **OKT3/Visilizumab:** Anti-CD3 monoclonal antibody
  - ❖ Indications: Immunosuppression for inflammatory bowel disease
  - ❖ Side effects: Autoimmune side effects

- **Bevacizumab:** Binds to VEGF-A
  - ❖ Indications: Non-small lung cell carcinoma, Colorectal carcinoma, Renal cell carcinoma, Breast cancer, Ovarian cancer, Fallopian tube cancer, cervical cancer
  - ❖ Side effects: Increased risk of infection
- **Sorafenib/Sunitinib:** Binds to Tyrosine kinase domain of VEGFR
  - ❖ Indications: Non-small lung cell carcinoma, Colorectal carcinoma, Renal cell carcinoma, Hepatic cell carcinoma, Gastric cancer, GIST, Pancreatic neuro-endocrine tumour, Thyroid cancer
- **Cetuximab:** Binds to EGFR/HER 1
  - ❖ Indications: Colorectal carcinoma, Head and neck squamous cell carcinoma
  - ❖ Side effects: Drug-induced neutropenia
- **Trastuzumab:** Binds to ErbB2/HER2
  - ❖ Indications: HER2-positive breast and gastric cancer
  - ❖ Side effects: Neutropenia
- **Natalizumab/Vedolizumab:** Binds to integrins
  - ❖ Indications: Multiple sclerosis, Crohn's disease
  - ❖ Side effects: Increased risk of infection
- **Imatinib:** Tyrosine kinase inhibitor
  - ❖ Indications: Ph+ CML and ALL, myelodysplastic syndrome, hyper-eosinophilic syndrome, GIST, systemic mastocytosis
  - ❖ Side effects: Neutropenia, reduced T cell activation and proliferation
- **Blinatumomab:** Bifunctional T cell engaging chimeric antibody binding CD-3 and CD-19
  - ❖ Indication: B-cell ALL
  - ❖ Side effects: Cytokine release syndrome and neurotoxicity
- **Pembrolizumab:** Immune checkpoint inhibitor and blocks PD-1 receptor.
  - ❖ Indications: Melanoma, head and neck cancer, lung cancer, bladder cancer, breast cancer, Hodgkin cancer
  - ❖ Side effects: Immune-mediated skin reactions like TEN and endocrinopathies like thyroid disorders, pituitary dysfunction
- **Sirolimus:** mTOR inhibitor
  - ❖ Indications: Solid organ transplants
  - ❖ Side effects: Impaired innate immunity, reduced neutrophil migration

HAEMATOLOGICAL MALIGNANCIES

✓ **Disease Burden:** 7–10% of patients with a haematological malignancy will require critical care input with respiratory failure as a leading cause (26%–91%).
  - 15% of patients with a haematological stem cell transplant will require ICU admission.
  - *Mechanical ventilation is associated with poor outcomes in patients with haematological emergencies.*
  - After matching for severity of illness, survival of patients with haematological malignancies and non-oncological patients is similar.

Classification of Haematological Malignancies

✓ **Haematological Malignancies:** Leukaemia (affecting blood-forming cells), Lymphoma (lymph nodes), multiple myeloma (affecting plasma cells in bone marrow), and others.
  - **Leukaemia**
    ❖ **Acute myeloid leukaemia**
    ❖ **Chronic myeloid leukaemia**
    ❖ **Acute lymphoblastic leukaemia**
    ❖ **Chronic lymphoblastic leukaemia**
  - **Lymphoma**
    ❖ Hodgkin's lymphoma
    ❖ Non-Hodgkin's lymphoma
  - **Multiple myeloma**
  - **Others**
    ❖ **Myelodysplastic syndromes** (MDS)/ **Myelodysplastic neoplasms:** Abnormal blood cells in the marrow

Individual Malignancies

✓ **Acute myeloid leukaemia (AML)**
  - Half of newly diagnosed patients are above 65 yr of age with 10% survival after 5 yr.
  - Accounts for up to 50% of haematological malignancy admissions to ITU.
  - **Hyperleucocytosis** (blasts >100,000/μL) can be an initial presentation and can cause respiratory failure, visual disturbances, renal failure, and intracranial haemorrhage. **Hydroxyurea ± leukapheresis** is used to reduce cell count.
  - **Induction chemotherapy:** 3 d of IV Idarubicin/Daunorubicin and 7 d of Cytarabine.

- **Post-remission therapy** includes chemotherapy ± allogenic haematopoietic stem cell transplant (HSCT).

✓ **Acute promyelocytic leukaemia**
  - Presents frequently with **acute disseminated intravascular coagulation (DIC)** with fatal haemorrhage.
  - Treatment with **all-trans-retinoic acid (ATRA)** and **arsenic trioxide (ATO)** targeting PML-RARα should be started early.
  - **Differentiation syndrome:** Seen in patients treated with ATRA and ATO. Presents with fever, peripheral oedema, pleuro-pericardial effusion, and acute renal failure. Treatment is Dexamethasone.

✓ **Acute lymphoblastic leukaemia (ALL)**
  - Patients with t(9;22)/BCR-ABL (**Philadelphia chromosome**) have poor prognosis.
  - **Induction chemotherapy:** Vincristine, Daunorubicin, corticosteroids, and L-asparaginase/cyclophosphamide.
  - **Post-remission therapy** is chemotherapy and HSCT.
  - **CNS Prophylaxis:** Intrathecal methotrexate ± cytarabine.
  - **Imatinib** targeting BCR-ABL has improved survival rates.

✓ **Chronic myeloid leukaemia (CML)**
  - Grows slowly and patients rarely need ITU.
  - Philadelphia chromosome is seen.
  - **Presentation:** Symptoms are because the CML cells crowd out the normal red blood cells, white blood cells and platelets.
  - **Treatment:** Most CML patients are treated with daily oral drug therapy.
    ❖ The use of Tyrosine kinase inhibitors has changed this disease from a life-threatening condition to a more manageable one.

✓ **Chronic lymphoblastic leukaemia (CLL)**
  - Variable course with some individuals having a slow growing tumour and some can have a quick progression.
  - It is the most common type of leukaemia in adults in the Western countries.
  - **Presentation:** Most patients are asymptomatic and those with symptoms, have them because the CLL cells crowd out the normal red blood cells, white blood cells and platelets.
    ❖ Most patients are old and is more common in male.

- **Treatment:** Involves wait and watch, chemotherapy, radiation therapy, splenectomy, and stem cell transplant.
  - ❖ Many people with CLL live good quality lives for years with medical care.
- ✓ **Aggressive non-Hodgkin lymphomas**
  - **Diffuse large B-cell lymphoma (DLBCL)** presents with enlarged lymph nodes.
    - ❖ **Chemotherapy:** Cyclophosphamide, doxorubicin, vincristine, and prednisone **(CHOP)** along with Rituximab.
  - **Burkitt lymphoma:** Fastest-growing human malignancy and presents with enlarged nodes and extranodal disease in abdomen and GI tract.
    - ❖ **Chemotherapy:** Cyclophosphamide, doxorubicin, vincristine, and anti-metabolite along with Rituximab with **intensive CNS prophylaxis.**
- ✓ **Hodgkin's lymphoma**
  - One of the most curable forms of cancer.
  - Reed–Sternberg cells^Q are lymphoid in origin and diagnostic of Hodgkin's lymphoma.
  - **Presents** most commonly with a painless swelling in a lymph node, usually in the neck, armpit, or groin.
    - ❖ Other symptoms include fever, night sweats, unintentional weight loss, persistent cough.
  - **Treatment:** Chemotherapy + Radiotherapy. Immunotherapy or a stem cell transplant can be used if other treatments don't work.
    - ❖ **ABVD regimen** can be sued Adriamycin (Doxorubicin), Bleomycin, Vinblastine, Dacarbazine (DTIC).
  - Risk of long-term problems like developing another type of cancer or infertility.
  - Good 5-year survival rate of 90%.
- ✓ **Multiple myeloma (myeloma)**
  - Cancerous plasma cells in the bone marrow that overcrowd normal cells.
  - Second most common haematological cancer after lymphoma.
  - Abnormal differentiation of B-cells into plasma cells and excessive production of immunoglobins known as **Para-proteins.**
  - Light chain of these immunoglobins are found in urine and known as **Bence-Jones proteins and can damage renal dysfunction^Q.**

- **Can present with dehydration, hypercalcaemia, hyper viscosity, or spinal cord compression.**
- Not curable but it can be treated to control the cancer and prolong life.
- Treatment is chemotherapy and steroids.
- ✓ **Myelodysplastic syndromes (MDS)/Myelodysplastic neoplasms**
  - Dysplasia in MDS emphasizes the abnormal growth aspect of cells.
    - ❖ In MDS, abnormal bone marrow stem cells produce increased numbers of immature blood cells.
    - ❖ Immature cells die prematurely and hence lower number of RBCs, WBCs, and platelets.
    - ❖ The cells that survive are mostly of poor quality.
  - **Causes:** *Primary:* No known cause, *Secondary:* Post-chemotherapy or post-radiation therapy.
    - ❖ Seen in people above 60 yr of age.
  - **Presentation: Anaemi**a, more frequent infections, and easy bleeding.
  - **Treatment:** Blood transfusions, chemotherapy and stem cell transplant depending upon type of disease.

Chemotherapeutic Agents

- ✓ **Chemotherapeutic agents:** Ultimate goal of chemotherapeutic agents is disruption of DNA and inhibition of proliferation of tumour cells.
  - **Corticosteroids:** Altered gene expression
    - ❖ Prednisone, Methyl prednisone
  - **Antimetabolites:** Act as false substrates and act as competitive inhibitors.
    - ❖ **Methotrexate** (pneumonitis, bone-marrow failure, hepatitis, nephrotoxicity, mucositis, seizure)
    - ❖ **Azathioprine** (hepatotoxicity)
    - ❖ Cytarabine (neurotoxicity, enterocolitis)
    - ❖ **5-Fluorouracil** (coronary/cerebral vasospasm)
    - ❖ 6-Mercaptopurine (biliary stasis, transaminitis)
  - **Alkylating agents:** Bind to DNA and cross link the strands.
    - ❖ **Cisplatin** (nephrotoxicity, hepatotoxicity)
    - ❖ **Busulfan** (endocardial fibrosis),
    - ❖ Chlorambucil

❖ **Cyclophosphamide** (SIADH, endocardial fibrosis, haemorrhagic cystitis)

❖ **Ifosfamide** (CNS toxicity, haemorrhagic cystitis)

- **Topoisomerase I and II inhibitors**
  ❖ **Daunorubicin/Doxorubicin** (cardiac toxicity)
  ❖ Idarubicin
  ❖ Mitomycin
  ❖ **Bleomycin** (Pulmonary fibrosis)
  ❖ Dactinomycin
  ❖ Etoposide
  ❖ Irinotecan

- **Mitotic inhibitors:** Mitotic spindle poisons.
  ❖ **Vincristine/Vinblastine** (neuropathy, hyponatraemia)
  ❖ Paclitaxel
  ❖ Docetaxel

Immunotherapy

✓ **Immunotherapy classification:** Utilizes body's own immune system to fight cancer. More details in chapter on immunology.

- **Monoclonal antibodies:** Bind to specific targets on cancers and make them better seen by our own immune system (e.g. trastuzumab).

- **Checkpoint inhibitors:** Drugs that block immune checkpoints and allow immune cells to respond more strongly to cancers (e.g. pembrolizumab).

- **Cancer vaccines:** Help to learn immune system cancer antigens (e.g. melanoma – T-VEC vaccine).

- **Cytokines:** Help to learn immune system cancer antigens. Used against myeloproliferative neoplasms (e.g. peginterferon alpha 2).

- **Chimeric antigen receptor-T therapy.**

✓ **Side effects of immunotherapy**
  - **Respiratory:** Pneumonitis
  - **Cardiovascular:** Myocarditis, arrhythmias
  - **Neurological:** PRES, encephalitis, meningitis
  - **GIT:** Hepatitis, diarrhoea
  - **Renal:** Nephritis, nephrotic syndrome
  - **Endocrine:** Hypo/hyperthyroid, diabetes mellitus

✓ **Chimeric antigen receptor therapy (CAR-T)**
  - **Principle:** *Curative* treatment that involves using patient's T cells and adding a gene for chimeric antigen receptor in vitro.
    ❖ Then these cells are infused in the patient's bloodstream again.
    ❖ These cells engage with **CD19 antigen** on tumour cells and kill them.
  - Used for B-cell ALLs, DLBCL, mantle cell lymphoma, follicular lymphoma, multiple myeloma, and high-grade B-cell lymphoma.
  - Pretreatment: Fludarabine and cyclophosphamide are used.

Haematopoietic Stem Cell Transplant (HSCT)

✓ **Haematopoietic Stem Cell Transplant (HSCT)**[Q]**:** Curative treatment for high risk leukaemias, lymphomas, myelodysplasia, multiple myeloma, aplastic anaemia and haemoglobinopathies.

- **Source of stem cells:** Bone marrow, Growth factor mobilized peripheral blood stem cells, umbilical cord blood.
  ❖ Children get marrow or cord blood whereas adults get peripheral blood cells.
  ❖ Marrow transplant recipients have higher chances of relapse but lower chances of graft vs host disease.

- **Allogenic:** Stem cells harvested from an HLA matched donor (graft vs host disease).
  ❖ Pre-transplant myeloablative conditioning is done using intensive chemotherapy or total body irradiation.
  ❖ **Post-engraftment immunosuppressive therapy** is required for allogenic HSCT to kill T cells in the graft to prevent graft-versus-host disease (GVHD).
  ❖ *Immune reconstitution is slow and B and T cell recovery takes 12–24 months and patient is at risk of infection.*
  ❖ **Prophylaxis** with antifungal agent is indicated during all periods of allogenic HSCT.
  ❖ **Prophylaxis** against HSV and CMV with acyclovir or valacyclovir is also recommended.

- **Autologous:** Own stem cells serve as donor (no graft-versus-host disease seen)
  ❖ High-dose preparative chemotherapy is used to kill tumour cells before transplant.

❖ Immune reconstitution is fast and **immunosuppressive therapy is not needed.**

❖ B and T cell recovery takes 6–12 months and patient is at risk of infection during this time.

✓ **Transplant-related complications:** Graft rejection, immunosuppressive regimen-related toxicity, infections and GVHD.

- **Graft rejection: Primary: Failure** to recover haematopoiesis immediately after the transplant. **Secondary:** Loss of established graft.
  - ❖ Recipient T cells are involved and re-transplantation may be needed in fulminant rejection.

- **Immunosuppressive regimen-related toxicity**
  - ❖ **Pancytopaenia:** Neutrophil recover first followed by platelets and then red blood cells. Irradiated blood products are used for them to eliminate lymphocytes to prevent GVHD.
  - ❖ **Liver sinusoidal obstruction syndrome:** Refractory thrombocytopaenia, tender hepatomegaly, jaundice seen in 10–60% of patients within 30 d post-HSCT. Treatment is mostly supportive, and mortality is high 20–50%.
  - ❖ Skin erythema, mucositis, diarrhoea, **idiopathic pneumonia syndrome,** diffuse alveolar haemorrhage, ARDS, AKI, thrombotic microangiopathy, hypertension, toxic encephalopathies, intracranial haemorrhage.

- **Infectious complications post-HSCT**
  - ❖ **Pre-engraftment (Transplant to neutrophil recovery, 20–30 d):** Neutropenic infections like Gram-negative bacilli, Gram-positive organisms, Candida. *Clostridium difficile* colitis is common.
  - ❖ **Post-engraftment (engraftment to day 100):** CMV, BK virus, PCP, Candida, and *Aspergillus*. **Risk of acute graft vs host disease.**
  - ❖ **Late phase (after day 100):** Encapsulated bacteria, VZV, *Aspergillus*, toxoplasma, PCP. **Risk of chronic graft vs host disease.**

- **Graft vs host disease (GvHD):** Transplanted cells (T cells) attack the recipient's body. *HLA disparity increases the risk.*

❖ **Acute GvHD:** Observed within first 10–100 d with peak in 30–50 d post-transplant. Triad of *Skin maculopapular rash, GI upset/diarrhoea, and liver dysfunction (hyperbilirubinaemia)*[Q].

- Tissue biopsy of skin, liver, or stomach is recommended for diagnosis and excluding opportunistic infections as cause.
- **Glucksberg–Seattle Criteria** is used to classify the severity of acute GvHD into grade I to IV with higher grades correlating to poorer outcomes.

❖ **Chronic GvHD:** Observed within first 90–600 d.

- *Above symptoms plus connective tissue and exocrine glands are involved.*
- Sclerotic skin, lichen planus like features, bronchiolitis obliterans, pancreatic insufficiency, cytopaenia are features.
- Biopsy is usually not necessary to confirm the diagnosis.

❖ **Prevention: ATG** has been used to decrease the incidence.

- **Tacrolimus** plus mycophenolate mofetil regimen is also being used.
- Ursodeoxycholic acid to improve liver function.

❖ **Treatment:** Glucocorticoids for GvHD. Ruxolitinib (Janus kinase inhibitor) for steroid refractory GvHD.

- **Antimicrobial prophylaxis for stem cell transplant patients.**
  - ❖ **Bacterial infections:** Indication is neutropenic patients for first 100 d. Fluoroquinolones.
  - ❖ **PCP prophylaxis:** All patients. TMP-SMX. Usually for 6 months and longer therapy only if they remain on immunosuppressive therapy.
  - ❖ **CMV prophylaxis:** Indication is CMV positive donor or recipient. Ganciclovir. At least first 100 d.
  - ❖ **HSV/VZV prophylaxis:** Indication is HSV/VZV seropositive patients. Acyclovir.
  - ❖ **Fungal prophylaxis:** Indication is prolonged neutropenia in HSCT patients. Fluconazole.

❖ **Hepatitis B:** Indication is HBsAg sero-positive patients. Lamivudine.

ONCOLOGICAL CRISIS

✓ **Tumour Lysis Syndrome (TLS):** Onco-logical emergency. 48–72 h post-treatment or spontaneously.

- **Causes:** Associated with haematological malignancies like acute leukaemias and high-grade non-Hodgkin lymphoma (Burkitt's lymphoma)[Q] along with solid tumours like hepatoblastoma.
- **Laboratory TLS: Cairo–Bishop Criteria:** Potassium >6 mEq/L, Phosphate >4.5 mg/dL, **Calcium <7 mg/dL**, Uric acid >8 mg/dL or >25% change in any variable.
  - ❖ Uric acid causes renal vasoconstriction and is poorly soluble in water.
- **Clinical TLS:** Laboratory TLS plus creatine >1.5 times the upper limit, cardiac arrhythmia, **hypocalcaemic seizure[Q]**, or sudden death.
- **Treatment[Q]:** Only oral anti-phosphorus agents (Sevelamer hydrochloride) available. Don't treat hypocalcaemia[Q] otherwise crystal nephropathy with uric acid can occur[Q]. *Only symptomatic hypocalcaemia should be treated.*
  - ❖ **Hyperhydration without bicarbonate guided by urine output (2 mL/kg/h),**
  - ❖ Alkalinization of urine minimizes precipitation of insoluble uric acid[Q] in tubules but should be avoided to prevent precipitation of calcium phosphate crystals.
  - ❖ **Rasburicase (most effective)[Q]:** Recombinant urate oxidase that converts uric acid into soluble allantoin. Used in established TLS. C/I in G-6 PD deficiency.
  - ❖ **Allopurinol[Q]:** Xanthine oxidase inhibitor. Used for prevention. Reduce dose in renal dysfunction.
  - ❖ **Hyperkalaemia** by insulin/dextrose, Hyperphosphataemia by phosphate binders.
  - ❖ Renal replacement therapy may be needed.
✓ **Cytokine Release Syndrome (CRS)[Q]:** Systemic hyperinflammatory response after chimeric

antigen receptor T cell (CAR-T) therapy (within 3–14 d), **Blinatumomab** or Pembrolizumab/ Nivolumab. Seen in 60–90% of cases.

- **IL-6** is the main mediator of CRS and patients present similarly to sepsis like fever, rash, malaise, hypoxia, hypotension and DIC.
- Cytopaenia, raised CRP, raised ferritin, deranged liver and kidney function tests are seen.
- Treatment is Supportive. **Tocilizumab** and **steroids** in severe CRS. Consider Granulocyte colony-stimulating factor (G-CSF) in neutropenia.
✓ **Immune Effector Cell-Associated Neurotoxicity Syndrome (ICANS):** *Seen post–CAR-T therapy.*
  - **IL-1 is the principal mediator** and patient presents with headache, tremors, speech impairment, delirium, and confusion.
  - Treatment: **Steroids** and **Anakinra.**
✓ **Superior Vena Cava (SVC) Syndrome:** Obstruction of return of blood through the SVC to the right atrium.
  - **Causes:** Lung cancer, non-Hodgkin lymphoma, thymic cancers, mediastinal lymph nodes.
  - Acute compression by tumour can lead to oedema of face and upper body along with dyspnoea and tachypnoea.
  - Chest X-ray and CECT scan thorax to confirm the clinical diagnosis.
  - **Treatment:** Chemotherapy and radiotherapy for responsive cancers. Endovascular stent placement in patients for palliation.
✓ **Epidural Cord Compression:** Due to metastasis or primary tumour involvement of the vertebral column (thoracic region in majority), paravertebral space or epidural space.
  - Metastatic cancers from **lung, breast, prostate**, haematopoietic, and genitourinary malignancies.
  - **Presentation:** Severe pain, **autonomic dysfunction**, *bladder, or bowel symptoms.*
  - Diagnosis is by MRI.
  - **Treatment:** Corticosteroids, radiation, and surgery.
✓ **Hypercalcaemia of Malignancy (HCM):** Most common emergency metabolic disorder associated with cancer.
  - **Causes:** *Multiple myeloma* and breast (osteolytic), **lung and urothelial cancer** (PTHrP).

- Increased parathyroid hormone (PTH) activity due to tumour production of parathyroid hormone-related protein (PTHrP).
- Malaise, fatigue, calciuria, osmotic diuresis, stones, renal failure, **psychosis,** and coma.
- **Treatment: Intravenous hydration** is the treatment of choice followed by loop diuretics.
  - ❖ Calcitonin and bisphosphates are used in severe cases.
  - ❖ Dialysis in cases with renal failure.
  - ❖ **Denosumab** targeting RANKL is approved for treatment of HCM.
- ✓ **Cardiac Tamponade:** Fluid accumulation within pericardial cavity affecting left ventricular function.
  - **Causes:** Lung and breast cancer, lymphoma and leukaemia.
  - Echocardiography is the most useful way to diagnose rapidly.
  - **Treatment:** Oxygen, IV fluids, vasopressor agents and **emergent pericardiocentesis** in severely hypotensive patients.
    - ❖ Radiation therapy specially in haematological malignancies is useful.
- ✓ **Hyperleucocytosis Syndrome:** Defined as TLC >100,000/μL. **Seen in AML > ALL,** low PaO$_2$ levels.
  - Due to obstruction of capillary bed in CNS, heart, and lungs.
  - **Pseudo hypoxaemia (leucocyte larceny)**[Q]: Spuriously low PaO$_2$ due to increased WBCs using oxygen.
  - Avoid Hb >8 till leucocytes fall below 50,000/μL due to risk of stroke.
  - **Treatment** is hydroxyurea and leukapheresis.

PLASMAPHERESIS

- ✓ **Plasmapheresis:** Process of **extracorporeal** removal of blood plasma from the patient.
  - **Plasma exchange:** Plasmapheresis + replacement of plasma with a substitute.
  - **Red blood cell exchange**[Q]: Red blood cells are removed and replaced with **donor RBCs.**
    - ❖ *Sickle cell disease*[Q], (acute stroke and stroke prophylaxis) category I, (acute chest syndrome and pregnancy) category II, and malaria.

- **Erythrocytapheresis:** Red blood cells are removed and replaced with **crystalloid or colloid solution when necessary.**
  - ❖ *Polycythaemia vera, hereditary haemochromatosis.*
- **Extracorporeal photopheresis (ECP):** Blood components like **white blood cells** are separated from the rest of the blood, combined with a **photoactive drug (psoralen)** and are then exposed to ultraviolet.
  - ❖ Acute and chronic GVHD, **Cutaneous** T cell **lymphoma (Sezary syndrome)**, heart transplant (cellular rejection), lung transplant (chronic lung allograft dysfunction, bronchiolitis obliterans)
- **Rheopheresis:** Process to decrease the viscosity of blood by separation of high molecular weight components like fibrinogen, vWF, LDL cholesterol and IgM.
  - ❖ Used in the treatment of diseases with impaired microcirculation like dry age macular degeneration.
- ✓ **Indications for therapeutic plasma exchange:** American Society for Apheresis (ASFA category)
  - **Category I (First-line treatment)**
    - ❖ **Neurological:** Guillain–Barré syndrome, Myasthenia gravis (acute exacerbation), NMDA antibody encephalitis, chronic inflammatory demyelinating polyneuropathy.
    - ❖ **Haematological:** Thrombotic thrombocytopaenic purpura (TTP), catastrophic antiphospholipid syndrome, thrombotic microangiopathy (complement related), hyperviscosity in hypergammaglobulinaemia.
    - ❖ **Renal:** Anti-glomerular basement membrane (GBM) disease, Focal segmental glomerulosclerosis in kidney transplant patients.
    - ❖ **Hepatic:** Acute liver failure, Wilson's disease (fulminant).
    - ❖ **Transplant:** Kidney transplant (antibody-mediated rejection and prophylactic desensitization) in ABO compatible patients and desensitization in living donor in ABO incompatible patients,

Liver transplant (desensitization in living donor) in ABO incompatible patients.

- **Category II (2nd-line treatment)**
  - ❖ **Neurological:** Acute disseminated encephalomyelitis (steroid refractory), multiple sclerosis (acute attack), voltage-gated potassium channel antibody-related diseases, paediatric autoimmune neuropsychiatric disorders (PANDAS) exacerbation, neuromyelitis optical spectrum disorder (acute attack).
  - ❖ **Haematological:** Autoimmune haemolytic disease (severe cold agglutinin disease), cryoglobulinaemia, acute and chronic graft vs host disease.
  - ❖ **Renal:** Myeloma cast nephropathy.
  - ❖ **Hepatic:** Mushroom poisoning, hepatitis B polyarteritis nodosa.
  - ❖ **Transplant:** Heart transplant (rejection prophylaxis and desensitization), Kidney transplant (antibody mediated rejection in ABO incompatible patients), haematopoietic stem cell transplant, major ABO incompatible.
  - ❖ **Miscellaneous:** Systemic lupus erythematosus (SLE), thyroid storm.
- **Category IV (retired categories where it is not used anymore)**
  - ❖ Amyloidosis (causes other than dialysis)
  - ❖ Amyotrophic lateral sclerosis
  - ❖ HELLP syndrome
  - ❖ Dermatomyositis and polymyositis
  - ❖ Inclusion body myositis
  - ❖ Multifocal motor neuropathy
  - ❖ POEMS syndrome
  - ❖ Rheumatoid arthritis
  - ❖ Idiopathic polyarteritis nodosa
  - ❖ Schizophrenia
- ✓ **Process of Plasmapheresis**
  - **Filtration: Used in ICU:** Blood passes through a filter (like RRT) and separated into different components.
    - ❖ **Centrifugation:** Used for donation: Blood is spun into separate components by density.

- Around 1–1.5 times the plasma volume is exchanged in 1 treatment, around 5 exchanges used for most patients.
  - ❖ 5% HAS used for replacement fluid.
  - ❖ Solvent/detergent treated FFP used in TTP[Q].
  - ❖ **Plasmapheresis** leads to removal of up to 60% of serum immunoglobins and complement.
- **Complications**
  - ❖ **Access related:** Haematoma, arterial puncture.
  - ❖ **Process related:** Dilutional coagulopathy, hypotension, anaphylaxis to replacement fluid, recirculation.
  - ❖ **Anticoagulation related:** Bleeding.

Immunoglobin Therapy (IVIG)

✓ **Immunoglobins:** Pooled blood products from over 1000 donors. Immunoglobulins are synthesized by B-cells with IgG being the most common and able to pass through the placenta to fetus.

- Immunoglobulin has two identical heavy and light chains held together by di-sulphide bridges. **Constant (Fc) region** for effector function and **variable (Fab)** for antigen recognition[Q].
- **Physiological role**
  - ❖ **Complement activation:** Tissue damage in myasthenia gravis and haemolytic anaemia.
  - ❖ **Antibody dependent cellular toxicity:** Activates natural killer (NK) cells.
  - ❖ **Neutralization:** Binds to toxins, bacteria and viruses and prevent them from binding to body cells.
  - ❖ **Opsonization:** Binds pathogen to Fab region and enhances phagocytosis.
  - ❖ **Mast cell activation:** IgE against parasite infections.
- **Mechanism of action**
  - ❖ Fab can neutralize autoantibodies, pro-inflammatory cytokines and complement components.
  - ❖ Fc part can supersaturate the receptors on host cells resulting in less receptors being available for autoantibodies.
  - ❖ Apoptosis of B-cells.

✓ **Production:** Cost is around 10,000 £ for a single 2 g/kg dose. Pooled plasma from many healthy donors and each unit is tested for HIV-1 and 2, hepatitis B and C.
- Exact composition of each batch will vary between products.
- Contains IgG, IgA, IgM, albumin, and buffer agents.
- Half-life is 2–3 wk.
- 50% of prescriptions in UK are for primary immunodeficiencies.
- Available as 50 mg/mL or 100 mg/mL preparation.
- Started @ 0.3 mg/kg/h while observing for any adverse reactions and slowly increasing it to 4.8 mg/kg/h.

✓ **Use in Intensive Care**
- **Guillain–Barré syndrome:** Recommended for those requiring mechanical ventilation. 2 g/kg given over 5 d.
  - ❖ Not given if >4 wk have elapsed since the time of diagnosis.
- **Myasthenia gravis:** Recommended in patients with a myasthenic crisis or before surgery to remove a thymoma. 2 gram/kg over two days.
- **Chronic inflammatory demyelinating polyneuropathy (CIDP):** Slowly progressive polyneuropathy which presents with weakness of proximal muscles, impaired sensation and areflexia.
  - ❖ Recommended for those patients presenting with rapidly progressive symptoms and weakness. Induction dose of 4 g/kg is given divided over two sessions.
- **Acute disseminated encephalomyelitis (ADEM):** Acute-onset autoimmune mediated demyelination of the CNS. Preceded by a viral illness. Encephalopathy, motor and sensory defects and cranial nerve abnormalities.
  - ❖ High-dose steroids (Methylprednisolone 1 g/day for 3–5 d) are first-line treatment.
  - ❖ IVIg in dose of 0.4 g/kg for 5 d for patients who are refractory to steroids.
- **Toxic shock syndrome:** Recommended in patients with suspected or confirmed life-threatening streptococcal toxic shock syndrome who fail to response to antibiotics.

- *Clostridium difficile:* Used in severe infections despite optimal medical management.
  - ❖ Recommended dose is 0.4 mg/kg which can be repeated once.
- **Haemophagocytic lymphohistiocytosis (HLH):** Second-line treatment after steroids and IL-1 antagonist Anakinra.
  - ❖ 2 g/kg given in 5 divided doses.
- **ANCA-associated vasculitis:** Steroids and plasma exchange are first-line therapy and IVIg used is second-line treatment.
- **Catastrophic antiphospholipid syndrome:** Steroids and plasma exchange are first-line therapy and IVIg used as second-line treatment.
- **Vaccine-induced immune thrombocytopaenia and thrombosis (VITT):** Potentially fatal complication post-Covid-19 vaccination.
  - ❖ 1g/kg dose given as early as possible.
- **Chimeric antigen receptor therapy (CAR-T):** New treatment for haematological cancers which itself can cause cytokine storm.
  - ❖ 0.4–0.6 g/kg per month to prevent subsequent episodes.
- **Necrotizing fasciitis, Steven–Johnson syndrome/toxic epidermal necrolysis**: No longer recommended in guidelines.

✓ **Side Effects**
- **Constitutional:** Fever, chills, hypotension, anaphylactoid reactions.
- **CNS:** Headache, paraesthesia^Q (due to citrate anticoagulation causing hypocalcaemia), aseptic meningitis, posterior reversible encephalopathy syndrome (PRES).
- **CVS:** Hypertension, chest pain, tachycardia.
- **Respiratory system:** Transfusion-related acute lung injury (TRALI)^Q.
- **Renal:** AKI presenting between day 5 to 10.
- **Venous thromboembolism**
  - ❖ **Prevent IVIG-related thrombosis:** Give adequate pre and post-infusion hydration.
  - ❖ Start slow and gradually increase dose rate.
  - ❖ Premedicate with anticoagulants in high-risk patients.

PORPHYRIA

Aetiology

Porphyria: Disorders of Haem Synthesis

Compound	Enzyme
Succinyl CoA and glycine	ALA synthetase
ALA	ALA dehydrogenase
Porphobilinogen	Hydroxymethylbilane synthase
Hydroxymethylbilane	Uroporphyrinogen synthetase
Uroporphyrinogen III	Uroporphyrinogen decarboxylase
Coproporphyrinogen	Coproporphyrinogen oxidase
Protoporphyrinogen IX	Protoporphyrinogen oxidase
Protoporphyrin IX	Ferrochelatase
Haem	

✓ **Acute Porphyrias**
- **Acute intermittent porphyria[Q]:** Hydroxy-methylbilane synthase/Porphobilinogen deaminase
- **Variegate porphyria:** Protoporphyrinogen oxidase
- **Hereditary coproporphyria:** Coproporphyrinogen oxidase
- **5-ALA dehydratase deficiency porphyria:** ALA dehydrogenase

✓ **Non-Acute Porphyrias**
- **Porphyria cutanea tarda:** Uroporphyrinogen decarboxylase
- **Erythropoietic protoporphyria:** Ferrochelatase
- **Congenital erythropoietic protoporphyria:** Uroporphyrinogen synthetase
- X-linked erythropoietic protoporphyria: ALA synthetase 1 and 2

Clinical Features and Diagnosis

✓ **Risk factors:** Hormonal variation, pregnancy, alcohol, infection, pain, surgery.

✓ **Clinical features:** Diffuse abdominal pain, hypertension, tachycardia, pain in legs and back, paraesthesia, weakness in distal muscles, seizures, psychiatric symptoms like depression, hallucinations.

✓ **Diagnosis:** High clinical suspicion.
- Urine sample for urinary porphobilinogen: Protect from light.
- Plasma and faecal porphyrins.

Treatment

✓ **Management**
- **Haem arginate[Q]:** For hyponatraemia, seizures, neuropathy, refractory pain, or vomiting.
    ❖ 3 mg/kg once daily for 4 d.
    ❖ Use CVC as can precipitate in veins.
- **Supportive care:** Intubation and ventilation, beta-blockers for cardiovascular instability, and avoid hyponatraemia.
    ❖ Analgesia for pain symptoms.
    ❖ Benzodiazepines for seizures.
    ❖ Antipsychotics for psychiatric symptoms.
- Follow-up with porphyria specialist.

✓ **Drugs to Be Avoided**
- Thiopentone (Induces ALA synthetase)[Q], Ketamine, Etomidate, Dexmedetomidine, Halothane.
- Amiodarone, diltiazem, verapamil, hydralazine.
- Phenytoin, Valproate, Nitrazepam.
- Clarithromycin, erythromycin, clindamycin, fluconazole, rifampicin, sulphonamides.
- Ergometrine, mifepristone.

11

Trauma and Burns

TRAUMA TRIAGE AND INITIAL MANAGEMENT

- ✓ Road traffic accidents are the leading cause of death for people between age 15–29 yr.
- ✓ **Major trauma:** Defined as an injury severity score (ISS) >15.
  - Life-threatening injuries that can be life changing as they may result in long-term disability.
- ✓ **Major trauma centre:** A hospital providing tertiary trauma care. It has 24/7 trauma team with all relevant specialties and consultant presence within 30 min, ability to perform resuscitative thoracotomy, massive haemorrhage protocol and rehabilitation services.
  - If a patient triggers on a prehospital trauma triage tool and major trauma centre (MTC) is within 45 min travel time^Q, they should be taken there directly.
  - If the patient is too unstable or MTC isn't accessible in 45 min^Q, stabilization should occur at the nearest Trauma unit before secondary transfer to the MTC.
- ✓ **National Major Trauma Registry (NMTR):** Clinical audit for trauma cares across the whole of UK. Previously known as **Trauma Audit and Research Network (TARN).**
  - Collects data on the acute care pathway of patients with major traumatic injury whose length of stay is more than 3 overnight stays or are admitted to critical care.
  - **Few standards/quality indicators include**
    - ❖ The trauma team leader should be available within 5 min of arrival of the patient.
    - ❖ Detailed radiological report.

documented within 1 h from the start of the scan.
- ❖ Patients with significant haemorrhage should be given TXA within 3 h of injury and receive a second dose according to CRASH-2 protocol.

Pre-Hospital Major Trauma Triage Considerations

- ✓ **National Expert Panel on Field Triage Recommendations in 2021**
- ✓ **Red Criteria:** High risk of injury with transport to the highest-level trauma centre available within the region.
  - **Abnormal physiology**
    - ❖ Unable to follow commands (motor <6)
    - ❖ SBP <90 mmHg in patients between age 18–64 yr and SBP <110 mmHg in patients >65 yr
    - ❖ RR <10/min or >29/min
    - ❖ Room air saturation <90%
  - **Anatomical indicators**
    - ❖ *Open or depressed skull fracture*
    - ❖ Suspected spinal injury and motor or sensory loss
    - ❖ Penetrating trauma to head, neck, torso, and extremities proximal to knee and elbow
    - ❖ Chest injuries with altered physiology
    - ❖ *Pelvic fractures*
    - ❖ *>2 proximal long bone factures*
    - ❖ Severe extremity injury (crush injuries, degloving, pulseless activity)
    - ❖ Amputation proximal to wrist or ankle
    - ❖ Active bleeding requiring a tourniquet or wound packing

DOI: 10.1201/9781003476214-11

✓ **Yellow Criteria:** Moderate risk for serious injury and patients sent to a trauma centre as available nearby.
- **Mechanism suggesting serious injury**
  ❖ High-risk auto crash
    - *Partial or complete ejection*
    - Significant intrusion of roof (>12 inches at occupant site and >18 inches at any site) or need for extraction
    - *Death in passenger compartment*
    - Child (0–9 yr) unrestrained or in unsecured child safety seat
    - Vehicle telemetry data consistent with severe injury
  ❖ *Fall from height >10 feet (all ages)*
  ❖ *Pedestrian/bicycle rider thrown, run over, or with significant impact*
  ❖ Rider separated from transport vehicle with significant impact
- **EMS judgement**
  ❖ *Low level falls in young children (age <5 yr) or older adults (age >65 yr) with significant head impact*
  ❖ Children (Paediatric trauma centre)
  ❖ Suspicion of child abuse
  ❖ Pregnant patients
  ❖ Burns
  ❖ Patients on anticoagulants

Injury Scores

✓ **Anatomical injury scores**
- **Abbreviated Injury Scale (AIS):** Classifies each injury on a scale of 1 (minor) to 6 (incompatible with life) with 0 for no injury.
  ❖ Each injury classified on severity, involved body surface area, imaging, clinical examination, GCS score, and autopsy data.
- **Injury Severity Scale (ISS)**[Q]
  ❖ Six regions are considered (head and neck, face, thorax, abdomen, pelvis, and limbs, external).
  ❖ Each injury in every region is assigned a score derived from AIS. The highest AIS score from each region is used.
  ❖ Only three regions with most severely injury scores are taken and squared and added to produce the ISS score.
  ❖ Values from 0 to 75 are there and an AIS score 6 takes score automatically to 75.

❖ *Severe injury is defined as ISS above 15.*
❖ **Major trauma centres:** Receive trauma victims with injury severity scores (ISS) >15. Increase in odds of survival of trauma patients is statistically significant.
❖ It correlates with mortality, morbidity and length of hospital stay.
- **New Injury Severity Scale (NISS):** Three injuries rather than regions with maximum score are taken and squared and added.
  ❖ Better than ISS in penetrating torso injury and traumatic brain injury (TBI).

✓ **Physiological Injury Scores:** Better then anatomical scores in acute setting like prehospital and emergency department.
- **Glasgow Coma Scale (GCS):** Has been used for patients with head injury.
- **Emergency Trauma Score (EMTRAS):** Takes four parameters and gives a score from 0 to 3 to them. Predicts mortality and can be used in other scores. EMTRAS >8 predicts high mortality.

Parameters	0	1	2	3
Age	<40 yr	40–60 yr	61–75 yr	>75 yr
GCS	13–15	10–12	6–9	3–5
Base excess	>−1	−1 to −5	−6 to −10	<−10
Prothrombin time	<80%	80–50%	49–20%	>20%

- **Revised Trauma Score (RTS):** Assigns score from 0 to 4 to these 3 parameters: Glasgow Coma Scale (**GCS**), systolic blood pressure (**SBP**), and respiratory rate (**RR**).
  ❖ Total score of 12 and can be used as a triage tool with score <11 triggering transfer to a trauma centre.
  ❖ Can be used as an outcome predicting model.
- **Trauma Score and Injury Severity Score (TRISS):** Mathematical model with score >75% indicating preventable mortality and potentially preventable mortality (50–75%). It takes these parameters in account.
  ❖ Severity of the lesions (ISS)
  ❖ Vital parameters (RTS)
  ❖ Age (0 if 55)
  ❖ Injury mechanism (blunt or penetrating)

Mechanism of Injury

✓ **Blunt injuries:** Most common mechanism. Severe head injuries are the most common cause of death in patients with blunt trauma.

✓ **Penetrating injuries:** 5% of severe injuries in Europe. Up to 50% of severe injuries in some cities in USA.

✓ **Blast injuries:** Seen in war zones. Produces damage at the interface of media of differing densities.

✓ **Thermal injuries:** Due to fires and electric shocks.

Initial Management

✓ **Primary assessment and interventions:** **Primary survey** is a set of clinical and ultra-sonographic examination to detect acute life-threatening injuries that require immediate resuscitation. All interventions are done alongside the problems identified.

- **Cervical spine stabilization:** Manual in line stabilization of cervical spine (MILS).
- **A/B (immediate airway/breathing problems):** RSI should be done where indicated within 45 min of initial call to emergency services.
  - ❖ **Obstructed airway:** Remove the obstruction and maintain patency using simple manoeuvres like jaw thrust, oropharyngeal airway, mask ventilation, endotracheal intubation, or surgical airway. Give 100% Oxygen.
  - ❖ **Tension pneumothorax:** Needle decompression in 5th intercostal space just anterior to mid axillary line (ATLS guidelines) followed by chest tube insertion. Finger thoracostomy may be needed if needle decompression fails.
  - ❖ **Open pneumothorax:** Treated with a chest tube inserted at a separate side and covering the wound with an occlusive dressing. ATLS recommends occlusive dressing sealed on three sides acting like a flutter valve.
  - ❖ **Massive haemothorax (1500 mL or more):** Fluid resuscitation and chest tube drain.
  - ❖ **Flail chest:** 2 or more ribs broken at 2 or more places. Manage the underlying injury with intubation and ventilation if necessary.
  - ❖ **Cardiac tamponade:** Pericardiocentesis or emergency clamshell thoracotomy in case of cardiac arrest.
- **C (Catastrophic haemorrhage):** Radial pulse if present indicate a systolic blood pressure of 70 mmHg and central pulse indicate a systolic blood pressure of approximately 40–50 mmHg.
  - ❖ Look at significant sites of blood loss: **Blood on the floor plus 4 more.** Chest, abdomen, pelvis and long bones.
  - ❖ **Direct compression of wound, proximal arterial compression,** tourniquet, splint the limb to stop bleeding. Use a pelvis binder in cases of shock even without signs of pelvic fracture to address catastrophic bleeding.
  - ❖ Bilateral finger thoracostomy before chest compression in case of traumatic cardiac arrest.
  - ❖ Two large-bore IV cannulas should be secured immediately.
  - ❖ **Permissive hypotension** with targeting a systolic pressure 80–90 mmHg and MAP of 60 mmHg until definitive surgical control.
  - ❖ **Haemostatic resuscitation:** Restrictive fluid management with early use of blood products in case of ongoing haemorrhage. Tranexamic acid bolus 1 g followed by 1 g over 8 h should be given.
  - ❖ O negative or O positive packed red cells in case of severe shock and uncontrolled haemorrhage.
- **D (Disability):** Evaluated using Glasgow Coma Scale and pupil size and reactivity.
  - ❖ Any patient with severe trauma should be considered as having cervical spine injury unless proven otherwise.
  - ❖ Mean arterial pressure targets are higher in traumatic brain injury (GCS ≤ 8) with pressure around 80 mmHg to prevent cerebral hypoperfusion.
- **E (Exposure):** Patient should be completely undressed to avoid missing any injury.
  - ❖ Antibiotic prophylaxis with amoxicillin-clavulanic acid for 48 h should be considered in first 48 h and gentamicin in case of soiled wounds.

- ❖ Tetanus vaccination should be ensured in large, soiled wounds.
- ❖ Avoid hypothermia.
- **Imaging:** Chest X-rays, pelvic X-rays, and Focused Assessment with Sonography for Trauma (FAST) are performed together with primary survey
  - ❖ **Chest X-ray:** Can identify pneumothorax, position of endotracheal tube and signs of diaphragmatic rupture (stomach pouch in the thorax).
  - ❖ **Pelvic X-ray:** Identify pelvic fractures as source of bleeding.
  - ❖ **FAST[Q]:** Structured approach for diagnosing internal haemorrhage in trauma patients.
    - **Right hypochondrium:** Effusion in peri-hepatic space and right haemothorax
    - **Left hypochondrium:** Effusion in peri splenic space and left haemothorax
    - **Suprapubic view:** Effusion in pouch of Douglas
    - **Subxiphoid view:** Pericardial effusion
    - **Pleural views right sided:** Pneumothorax
    - **Pleural views left sided:** Pneumothorax
- ✓ **Secondary Assessment:** Whole-body CT scan with IV contrast for complete injury assessment.
  - Whole body CT scan involves a CT head without the contrast and a contrast enhanced CT from skull base till mid-thigh.
  - The sickest but transportable patients benefit the most from a whole-body CT scan.
- ✓ **Damage Control Surgery (DCS):** Haemorrhage forms the main cause of death pre-hospitally and first few hours after arrival in emergency department and if initial resuscitation doesn't give a satisfactory response[Q], DCS should be considered.
  - Set of abbreviated surgical procedures that aim to control the bleeding rapidly.
  - It focuses on immediate physiological restoration rather than anatomical reconstruction.
  - Next phase after physiology restoration in theatre is resuscitation in ICU and then

re-exploration for anatomic reconstruction in theatre 24–48 h later.
- ✓ **Thromboprophylaxis:** LMWH should be given within 24 h unless contraindicated.
  - Use combined pharmacological and mechanical prophylaxis and continue until the patient is mobilized.
- ✓ **Nutrition:** Enteral nutrition should be started within 24 h if possible and built over next 5–7 d.
- ✓ **Antibiotics:** Prophylaxis after trauma is generally not recommended unless specific conditions like open head and neck injury, open thoracic injury, hollow viscus perforation, open extremities, fracture, and limb amputation.
  - Short prophylaxis of 48 h should be given in these cases.
- ✓ **Pain:** Multimodal pain management with opioids, anti-inflammatories like acetaminophen, muscle relaxants, neuropathic agents, and regional blocks with local anaesthetics.
- ✓ **Sedation:** Ketamine and dexmedetomidine provide both sedation and pain relief.
- ✓ **Secondary Survey[Q]:** Head to toe examination of other potential causes of severe illness.
  - **Tertiary survey:** Documentation of all injuries post-investigations. Usually done 48–72 h after initial admission.

MAJOR HAEMORRHAGE

Epidemiology and Aetiology: Medical emergency.
- ✓ **Definition of major haemorrhage**
  - Replacement of the circulating volume in 24 h
  - 4 units of blood in 1 h with continuous blood loss
  - Loss of 50% of circulating blood volume within 3 h.
  - Loss of 150 mL/minute.
- ✓ **Pathophysiology of blood loss**
  - Decrease in blood volume causes decrease in discharge rates of **baroreceptors located in the carotid sinus and aortic arch**.
  - Decrease cardiac output also activates chemoreceptors.
  - Stroke volume is restored to levels lesser than pre haemorrhage values whereas SVR is restored to higher values before the onset of blood loss.

Clinical Features and Diagnosis

Haemorrhagic Shock Classification

	Class I	Class II	Class III	Class IV
Estimated blood loss	<15%	15–30%	30–40%	>40%
Blood loss	<750 mL	750–1500 mL	1500–2000 mL	>2000 mL
Heart rate	<100	100–120	120–140	>140
Blood pressure	Normal	Normal	Reduced	Reduced
Pulse pressure	Normal	Reduced	Reduced	Reduced
Respiratory rate	Normal	20–30	30–40	>40
Urine output	Low Normal	Low	Very Low	None

✓ **Haemorrhagic shock** with significant blood loss will present with narrowed pulse pressure[Q].
  - It happens just before a significant drop in BP.
✓ **Trauma-induced coagulopathy:** Defined as 50% prolongation of aPTT/PT, an INR ≥1.5 or Fibrinogen <1.5 g/L. Seen in two phases.
  - **Acute traumatic coagulopathy (ATC)[Q]:** Develops within first 30 min of trauma even before the resuscitation is started. Due to endothelial damage and hypoperfusion (Base deficit >6 mmol/L)
  - **Dilutional coagulopathy:** Due to dilution of haemostatic factors and hypothermia.
✓ **Trauma "diamond of death":** Acidaemia, hypothermia, coagulopathy, and hypocalcaemia.
✓ **Massive transfusion in paediatrics:** >40 mL/kg of blood products[Q].
✓ **Complications of massive transfusion:** Hypothermia, coagulopathy, hypocalcaemia, hyperkalaemia, lactate acidosis, alkalosis due to citrate from packed red cells, multiorgan dysfunction.

Treatment

✓ **Initial approach:** Advanced trauma life support (ATLS) protocol with an ABCDE approach and **a massive haemorrhage situation should be declared.**
  - 2 large bore (16 G) venous access should be available.
✓ **Damage control resuscitation (DCR)[Q]:** Comprises of 3 components.
  - **Permissive hypotension:** Titrate support to central pulse. Restrict fluid resuscitation and allowing a lower-than-normal perfusion pressure.

❖ An initial target for SBP 80–100 mmHg with MAP of 60 mmHg until bleeding is controlled.
❖ In patients with a traumatic brain injury, a higher target is necessary for perfusion (MAP = 80 mmHg).
❖ Urine output >1 mL/kg/h.
● **Haemostatic resuscitation:** Use of blood products as first line of resuscitation fluid after severe injury.
  ❖ **Tranexamic acid:** 1 gram stat within 3 h of injury followed by 1 gram over 8 h. TXA reduces the risk of death in bleeding trauma patients (CRASH-2 trial).
  ❖ Give RBC: Plasma: Platelets in ratio of 1:1:1.
  ❖ **PROPPR trial (2015)[Q]:** In patients with severe trauma requiring massive transfusion, *no mortality difference in administration of red cells: platelets: FFP in ratio of 1:1:1 vs 2:1:1.*
  ❖ Maintain Hb levels between 70 and 90 g/L.
  ❖ **PT and APTT <1.5 times the normal control.** Give FFP: 15 mL/kg.
  ❖ **Fibrinogen >1.5 g/L[Q] (>2 g/L in pregnant female[Q]):** 1 L of plasma has 2–3-gram fibrinogen and an initial supplementation of 2–4-gram fibrinogen is indicated.
  ❖ **Platelet count above 50 × 10⁹/L.** Platelets above 100 × 10⁹/L in patients with ongoing bleeding or TBI.
  ❖ FFP and platelets should be given as soon as possible in massive haemorrhage as it is easier to prevent coagulopathy than to treat it once coagulopathy is established.

❖ **Factor VIIa**[Q] only as off-label use in trauma patients. Initiates direct thrombin generation on the platelets. No evidence of any mortality benefit. Decision for use only at consultant level.

❖ Ionized calcium within the normal range

❖ **DDAVP**[Q]: 0.3μg/kg: Increases factor VIII and vWF and hence improves platelet function.

❖ Blood should be given by standard **170-micron filter** to remove cellular microaggregates and clots.

❖ **Platelets should be given through a dedicated new set as the cellular debris from the previous RBC transfusion can lead to clotting.**

❖ **Cell salvage** is often used when blood loss is anticipated greater than 1000 mL.

❖ Avoid hypothermia and acidosis.

• **Damage control surgery**[Q]: Initial emergency surgery aimed at control of haemorrhage, decompression of compartments, and decontamination of wounds, while definitive anatomical repair is delayed until the patient becomes stable.

❖ Operative time should be kept below 90 min.

✓ **Interventional radiology:** For arterial embolization of pelvic haematomas and rectus sheath haematomas.

✓ **Pharmacological thromboprophylaxis:** Within 24 h after bleeding has been controlled.

✓ **Organizational management**

• Trust wide major haemorrhage protocol.

• Access to O negative emergency blood in key clinical areas.

• Emergency blood packs (4 units of RBCs and 4 units of FFPs)

• Team briefing after the episode.

TRAUMATIC BRAIN INJURY

Epidemiology

✓ 70–90% of traumatic brain injury (TBI) cases are mild.

• Bimodal incidence with peaks in teenagers (road traffic accidents) and the elderly (falls).

• Males are affected more.

✓ **Main aim in early stage of management of TBI is to prevent secondary brain injury.**

✓ 10 % of all patients with severe head injuries have **Extradural haematoma (EDH).**

• **Subdural haematomas (SDH)** are most frequent extra-axial (above brain) haematomas in patients with TBI.

• **Parenchymal lesions are the most frequent lesion in TBI.**

✓ **Blunt cerebrovascular injury:** Non-penetrating injury to major arteries supplying the brain. Signs of stroke seen. Denver criteria is used for diagnosis.

Clinical Features

✓ **History and Examination:** GCS (especially motor score) at the time of accident. Possible medical reason for the accident (seizure, cardiac arrest, stroke) and use of anticoagulants or antiplatelet therapy.

• Assume all patients with head injuries have fractures of spine and treat them accordingly until such fractures have been ruled out.

• **Basal skull fracture:** Peri-orbital haematomas, bruising behind the ear (Battle's sign), rhinorrhoea or otorrhoea.

• **GCS score:** Most commonly used score to communicate the severity of the injury. Supra-orbital pressure or Trapezius pinch is used in unconscious patients to avoid spinally mediated responses.

• **Cushing's triad**[Q]: Seen in tonsillar herniation. Hypertension, bradycardia, and irregular respiratory pattern.

✓ **Investigations:** All routine investigations plus creatinine kinase, troponin, and amylase/lipase.

• **ITACTIC Trial (2020)** found no overall benefit for using **TEG** in trauma patients with haemorrhagic shock but patients with TBI with an increased survival at 24 h.

✓ **CT Scan Indications within 1 hr**[Q]: Decline of GCS of 2 points, *GCS score of 12 or less on initial assessment*, GCS score of 14 or less at 2 h after the injury, suspected open or depressed skull fracture, *possible basal skull fracture*, post-traumatic seizure, *focal neurological deficits*, 2 or more episodes of vomiting.

• **Loss of consciousness with amnesia:** Do CT scan within 8 h *if age >64 yr* or *coagulopathy* or had a *dangerous mechanism of injury.*

- *A repeat CT scan is suggested in all patients with a severe or moderate injury within 6 h after the initial CT scan.*
  - ❖ *Low threshold for repeat CT scan for patients with traumatic subarachnoid haemorrhage, fractures, or a known history of antiplatelet or anticoagulant therapy.*
- **Trauma CT scan:** CT head, CT cervical spine, CT angiography of thorax, abdomen, and pelvis.
- CT scan is better for skull base and midface.
- **Marshall classification**[Q] of CT scan used to differentiate focal from diffuse lesions. It is a part of IMPACT score for prognostication.
  - ❖ Six grades (I–VI) with the worse having higher grade.
  - ❖ Parameters involved are basal cistern involvement, evacuation of lesions, density of mass lesions and shift in midline.
- ✓ **MRI is more sensitive than CT scan** especially for lesions in **posterior fossa, brainstem**, and superficial cortical areas.
  - MRI is good for improving the diagnostic specificity of multiple petechiae in brain.
  - MRI is sensitive for axonal injury and hence MRI is part of the prognostic picture.
- ✓ **Intracranial pressure (ICP) monitoring:** Raised ICP occurs in approximately 50% of all patients with mass lesion and 30% of all patients with severe diffuse injuries. Normal ICP in adults is <15 mmHg.
  - **Signs**[Q] are compression of ventricles and midline shift, sulci effacement, loss of grey/white matter differentiation and brain parenchymal herniation.
  - **Indications**[Q] are GCS <8 and CT evidence of TBI like potentially evolving contusions, Diffuse axonal injury type III or IV, anisocoria.
    - ❖ **In patients with GCS <8 and a normal CT scan, if one of the following risk factors are present (age >40 yr, motor score <4 or SBP <90 mmHg), ICP monitoring is indicated.**
    - ❖ GCS <12 who cannot be serially assessed neurologically.
  - **Exclusion criteria:** Patients with fixed bilateral pupils, untreatable lesions, advanced age and comorbidities.
  - Relative contraindication in coagulopathy and sepsis.

- Most commonly used sites are **intraventricular (therapeutic as well, high risk of infection but most accurate and hence preferred)** or intraparenchymal (ease of insertion but recalibration not possible).
  - ❖ Extradural and subarachnoid have been used as well.
- ICP monitoring in high volume centres has shown superior outcomes but no mortality benefit.
- Foramen of Monroe is the standard reference point but for simplicity the external auditory meatus can be used.
- Positive pressure ventilation raises[Q] the ICP due to decreased cerebral venous drainage.
- ✓ **Micro-dialysis catheter:** Passed through ICP bolt into parenchymal and tells about cerebral blood flow and metabolic indicators like lactate, pyruvate and glucose.
  - Lactate/Pyruvate ratio >40 suggests hypoxia. Gives changes in ratios even before ICP rise.
- ✓ **Brain tissue oxygen tension:** Low oxygenation is a predictor of poor outcome and treatment guided by brain tissue oximetry has been shown to improve outcomes.

Complications

- ✓ **Seizures:** Seen in patients with operated haematomas, penetrating injury, focal neurological signs, and intracranial sepsis.
  - 25% of TBI patients will have early seizures (<7 d) and up to 42% will have late seizures (>7 d).
  - Seizure in a comatose patient is a medical emergency and should be treated immediately.
- ✓ **Catecholamine storm:** Cardiac stunning, neurogenic pulmonary oedema, ST segment elevation, left ventricular apical ballooning on Echocardiography.
  - Troponin positivity may be seen.
- ✓ **Paroxysmal sympathetic hyperactivity (PSH):** Transient increase in sympathetic (HR, BP, RR, Temperature and sweating) and motor posturing due to loss of cortical inhibitory pathways.
  - Clonidine and beta-blockers have been used.
- ✓ **Traumatic axonal injury (TAI)** without an intracranial mass happens in almost

half of patients with severe head injury. MRI (T2-weighted or FLAIR sequences) is suggested.

- **Grade 1:** Junction of cortex and white matter
- **Grade 2:** Corpus callosum
- **Grade 3:** Thalamus and brainstem

✓ **Post-traumatic hydrocephalus:** Two-thirds of patients suffering from severe brain injury. 25% within two weeks of injury, 90% within 6 wk. Slowly progressive and suspected when there is a decline in the patient progress. CSF shunts needed.

✓ **Post-traumatic meningitis:** 5–15% incidence. *Organisms colonizing the nasopharynx such as Streptococcus pneumoniae, Haemophilus influenzae, Neisseria meningitidis and Staphylococci species.*
- Ventricular catheter associated ventriculitis is caused by *Pseudomonas aeruginosa*, *S. aureus* and *S. epidermidis*.

✓ **Subdural empyema:** Serial CT scanning needed in case with high degree of suspicion.

✓ **Sunken skin flap syndrome:** Post-large decompressive craniectomies. After weeks to months.
- Fluctuating headaches, focal signs, epileptic seizures, and disturbances of consciousness.

Prevention and Treatment (British Trauma Foundation, 4th Edition Recommendations)

✓ **Secondary brain injury prevention^Q:** *Main objective of TBI management.* Avoid hypoxia, hypercapnia, and hypotension to prevent secondary insult. *Patients with moderate to severe TBI are managed in the ICU.*
- **High-flow oxygen** by mask to all patients with TBI regardless of its severity. Avoid low levels of oxygen i.e. SpO_2 <90% or PaO_2 <60 mmHg. *Keep PaO_2 >10 kPa^Q.*
- **Early use of EtCO$_2$ monitor** and keep *pCO_2 between 4.5–5 kPa^Q* **(Tier 2 recommendation).**
  - ❖ **Therapeutic hyperventilation** is the fastest way to lower ICP. If hyperventilating, do it for less than 30 min and on 100% O_2.
  - ❖ **Rebound hypertension** is a risk for hyperventilation. It should not be utilized in the first 24 h after injury.

- **Optimize cerebral venous drainage**
  - ❖ 30-degree head up
  - ❖ Avoid tight endotracheal tube ties.
  - ❖ Avoid excessive PEEP
- **Blood pressure:** If hypotension happens, check for extra cranial injury first.
  - ❖ Permissive hypotension, a strategy for haemorrhagic trauma, should be used carefully for patients with TBI due to concerns for *cerebral perfusion pressure^Q (CPP). CPP of 60–70 mmHg should be the target* **(Tier 1 recommendation).**
  - ❖ Avoid hypotension^Q i.e. SBP <90 mmHg. *Aim for SBP >100 mmHg for patients 50 to 69 yr old or ≥110 mmHg or above for patients 15–49 or over 70 yr old.*
  - ❖ Balanced crystalloids are preferred. Avoid colloids in these patients.
  - ❖ No role of hypertonic saline as resuscitation fluid.

✓ **Tranexamic Acid (TXA):** 1 g of TXA followed by a 1 g infusion over 8 h.

✓ **Reversal of Anticoagulation:** Vitamin K 10 mg IV on day 1 followed by 5–10 mg on day 2 and 3.
- Reversal by PCC is faster and superior to plasma transfusion in patients on warfarin. FFP if patient needs volume due to extra-cranial injuries.
- Dabigatran can be reversed by Idarucizumab, PCC, haemodialysis, and haemofiltration.
- Rivaroxaban and Apixaban can be reversed by Andexanet alfa.
- Aspirin: Platelet transfusion for patient undergoing urgent neurosurgery.
- TEG or ROTEM guided therapy should be performed especially in first 72 h.

✓ **Surgery:** Open and depressed fractures need neurosurgical intervention, ideally within first 8 h.
- **Isolated extradural haematoma (EDH)** is due to bleeding of the middle meningeal artery^Q. Patients may be neurologically intact initially (Lucid interval).
  - ❖ *It needs urgent evacuation if mass effect or progressing and has good outcome.* An EDH greater than 30 cm^2 should be surgically evacuated regardless of the GCS score.

- ❖ Rapid deterioration with ipsilateral pupillary dilation and contralateral hemiparesis.
- ❖ Egg-shaped on CT scan, doesn't cross suture line[Q].
- **Subdural haematoma (SDH)**[Q] is due to shearing of bridging cortical veins.
  - ❖ It will exert mass effect and have worse prognosis. Most patients are unconscious immediately after the trauma. *Evacuation for size over 1 cm or a midline shift greater than 5 mm should be surgically evacuated regardless of the patient's GCS score.*
  - ❖ Crescent shaped on CT scan, can cross suture line.
- **Intraparenchymal contusions**: They are observed over hours and days and not evacuated routinely.
  - ❖ Lesions with a dense haemorrhagic core are called *intraparenchymal haematomas and need urgent evacuation.*
  - ❖ **Contused brain lobes are also treated surgically.**
✓ **Supportive treatment**
- **Hypothermia: No consensus currently on therapeutic targeted hypothermia in TBI patients** (Tier 3 recommendation).
  - ❖ **Eurotherm3235 Trial (2015):** In patients with ICP >20 mmHg after TBI, therapeutic hypothermia (32–35°C) plus standard care didn't result in better outcomes compared with standard care alone.
  - ❖ **POLAR trial (2018):** In patients with severe TBI, early hypothermia of 35°C didn't improve neurological outcome.
- *Steroids: No role of steroid in traumatic brain injury.*
  - ❖ *CRASH trial (2005): Increases the chance of death from all causes and hence not indicated.*
- **Euglycaemia:** 6–10 mmol/L.
- **Enteral nutrition** should be started shortly after admission while reaching full intake by day 3 in ICU.
- **Antibiotic prophylaxis:** For depressed skull fractures and penetrating brain injury.
- **Tracheostomy:** Optimal timing of tracheostomy in TBI still needs to be identified.
- *Seizure prophylaxis during the first 7 d after*

severe injury should be given. No mortality benefits. (Tier 1 recommendation).
- ❖ *Phenytoin is recommended for first 7 d. Levetiracetam can be used as well.*
- **Induced coma:** Prophylactic administration of barbiturates doesn't improve outcomes. Pentobarbital is used for this purpose.
  - ❖ Barbiturates can be used as a rescue measure when medical and surgery treatment has been unsuccessful.
- **Venous Thromboembolism:** Intermittent pneumatic compression systems within 24 h.
  - ❖ LMWH started 24 or 48 h after admission or completion of surgery after a neurosurgical consultation.
✓ **Intracranial Pressure (ICP)**[Q]: *It is to be treated if above 22* mmHg[Q].
- **Lundberg A waves:** 50–100 mmHg and 5–20 min long. Always pathological.
- **Lundberg B waves:** up to 50 mmHg and 0.5–2/min. Due to vascular hyperaemia.
- **Measures to control ICP**
  - ❖ Head up 30° position, check dressings don't compress the jugular veins (Tier zero recommendation).
  - ❖ Avoid increased intrathoracic pressure and intra-abdominal pressure.
  - ❖ Treat fever, shivering or pain (sedation and analgesia) (Tier 1 recommendation).
  - ❖ **CSF drainage via a ventricular catheter for ICP ranging 20–25** mmHg (Tier 1 recommendation).
- **Osmotherapy (Tier 1 recommendation).**
  - ❖ Mannitol 1 g/kg IV every 6 hrs[Q].
    - Initial action is by expanding plasma and causing reflex compensatory cerebral vasoconstriction followed by effect due to osmotic diuresis.
    - Mannitol contraindicated in renal failure.
    - Repeated doses can cross blood–brain barrier and cause brain oedema.
    - No difference between boluses or continuous infusion of mannitol.
  - ❖ Hypertonic saline 3% to 30%. 15 to 30 mL boluses of 23.4 % NaCl every 4–6 h.

- ❖ **No mortality benefit of hypertonic saline or mannitol in treating raised ICP. No single agent is superior.**
- **Hyperventilation** *and* **barbiturate coma can also be used as an emergency measure.** (Tier 3 recommendation).
- **Decompressive craniectomy:** in patients with severe head injury with refractory intracranial hypertension (Tier 3 recommendation).
  - ❖ **DECRA Trial (2011)**[Q]**:** In patients with severe diffuse traumatic brain injury and refractory intracranial hypertension, decompressive craniectomy causes *reduced ICP and ICU length of stay but worse neurological outcomes at 6 months.*
  - ❖ **RESCUE ICP Trial (2016)**[Q]**:** In patients with severe diffuse traumatic brain injury and refractory intracranial hypertension, decompressive craniectomy caused lower mortality and higher rates of vegetative state at 6 months.
- ✓ **Hypernatraemia (Na >150 mmol/L).** Central or neurogenic diabetes insipidus (DI) or osmotic diuresis.
  - DI: High urine output (>3 mL/kg/h), low urine SG (1001–1005), low urine osmolality (<150 mOsmol/kg), and urinary Na <50 mmol/L. Treatment is Desmopressin + parenteral free water.
- ✓ **Hyponatraemia (Na <135 mmol/L) in TBI patients.** Cerebral salt wasting syndrome (CWS) and SIADH.
  - **SIADH:** High urine sodium and low urine output.
    - ❖ **Treatment:** Fluid restriction, Loop diuretics
  - **CWS:** High urine sodium and high urine output.
    - ❖ **Treatment:** Fludrocortisone acetate (0.1–0.2 mg/day) and hypertonic intravenous sodium.

Prognosis

- ✓ **Factors suggesting poor prognosis by BTF**
  - **GCS (particularly motor score)** is of prognostic benefit[Q].
  - Age and bilaterally absent pupillary light reflex are also poor prognostic indicators.

- Even a single pre-hospital systolic blood pressure (SBP) <90 mmHg can lead to unfavourable outcome.
- ✓ **Increased D-dimer**[Q] **are associated with progressive haemorrhagic brain injury and a potential poorer outcome.**
- ✓ *Recovery is most rapid in the early weeks. 90% of recovery is in the first 6 months.*
- ✓ *Glasgow Outcome Scale–Extended (GOS-E) is used to access functional outcome scale following brain injury.*
  - *Scale from 1 to 8 with 1 being dead and 5–8 showing good recovery.*

SPINAL CORD INJURY

Epidemiology and Aetiology

- ✓ Vast majority of **spinal trauma injuries** occur in cervical region (55%). Around 10% of patients with cervical spine injury will have another non-contiguous vertebral fracture.
  - Up to 10–15% of major trauma patients will have a cervical injury.
  - Commonest region in thoracic and lumbar region for fractures is between T12 and L2.
  - **Spinal cord injury without radiographic abnormality (SCIWORA) is seen in 10–15% of patients.**
- ✓ **Classification of spinal cord injury**
  - **Traumatic:** Road traffic accidents, falls, sports injuries.
  - **Non-traumatic:** Degenerative disease (spondylosis), tumour (primary and metastatic), abscesses.
- ✓ **Neurological dermatomal anatomy**
  - **Upper extremity:** C5: Elbow flexion, C6: Wrist extension, C7: elbow extension, C8: Long finger flexion, T1: Finger abductors.
  - **Lower extremity:** L2: hip flexion, L3: Knee extension, L4: ankle dorsiflexion (towards face), L5: great toe extension, S1 ankle plantar flexion.

Clinical Features and Diagnosis

- ✓ **American Spinal Injury Association (ASIA) Impairment Scale [AIS]**[Q]**:** Neurological injury score based on motor, sensory, reflex, and rectal function. *Neurological level of injury is the lowest segment with intact sensation and antigravity (grade 3 or more) motor function.*

- **Grade A:** Complete neurologic injury with no motor or sensory sensation preserved in the sacral segments (S4–S5).
- **Grade B:** Preserved sensory function but not motor function below the neurological level and includes the sacral segments (S4–S5).
- **Grade C:** Preserved motor function below the neurological level and more than half of key muscles below the neurological level have a grade less than 3.
- **Grade D:** Preserved motor function below the neurological level with at least half of key muscles below the neurological level have a grade more than 3.
- **Grade E:** Normal neurological function.
✓ **Anterior cord syndrome[Q]:** Loss of pain and temperature sensation (Aδ and C fibres)[Q] and motor response below the level of injury. Due to disruption of anterior spinal artery.
  - Vibratory sense and proprioception are preserved.
  - Worst prognosis of incomplete spinal cord injuries.
✓ **Posterior cord syndrome:** Loss of proprioception with preserved motor, pain, and light touch.
  - Due to disruption of posterior spinal artery.
✓ **Central cord syndrome[Q]:** *Most common incomplete cord injury.* Most common form of cervical spinal cord injury as well.
  - More pronounced motor deficit in the upper extremities compared to the lower extremities.
  - *Mixed upper motor neuron (UMN) and lower motor neuron (LMN) signs in upper limbs and UMN signs in lower limbs.*
  - Loss of pain and temperature sensation in upper limb.
  - Sacral sparing seen. Overall, good but incomplete recovery.
✓ **Brown–Sequard syndrome[Q]:** Hemi-section of spinal cord.
  - Seen in stabbings.
  - Ipsilateral motor, vibratory and proprioception deficit below the level of the injury and contralateral loss of pain and temperature sensation.
  - Excellent overall prognosis.
✓ **Conus medullaris syndrome**
  - **Spinal cord injury** at level of **T12 to L2.**

- **Symmetric** lower extremity motor deficits and bowel and bladder dysfunction (spasticity)[Q].
- **Significant back pain,** symmetrical perineal or saddle loss of sensation.
- *Combination of upper (predominant) and lower motor neuron dysfunction.*
- Reflex or automatic bladder with overactivity, urgency, and incomplete emptying[Q].
- Surgical emergency and treatment within 48 h.
✓ **Cauda equina syndrome**
  - *Nerve root* compression in the *lumbosacral region.*
  - **Bilateral leg pain (asymmetric),** bowel and bladder dysfunction (flaccidity)[Q], saddle anaesthesia, and lower extremity motor and sensory deficit.
  - **Mostly a lower motor neuron dysfunction and absent reflexes.**
  - Overflow urinary incontinence due to loss of bladder motor function so that the bladder fills passively[Q].
  - Surgical emergency and treatment within 48 h.
✓ **Injury levels[Q]**
  - **Above C3:** Diaphragmatic paralysis. Early tracheostomy.
  - **C3–C5[Q]:** Impaired diaphragmatic function. Quadriplegic. 80% of patients will require ventilation within 48 h.
  - **T1–T11:** Intercostal muscles. Impaired sputum clearance.
  - **T6–L1:** Abdominal muscles: Impaired sputum clearance.
✓ Patients with high spinal injury develop gastroparesis[Q] due to unopposed vagal activity to stomach.
  - Abdominal breathing in a patient with spinal cord injury may suggest impending respiratory failure[Q].
✓ **Neurogenic shock[Q]:** Hypotension and bradycardia. Due to injury to upper thoracic sympathetic outflow *(above T6).*
  - Can last up to 1–3 wk.
  - Norepinephrine is preferred due to both alpha and beta properties.
✓ **Spinal shock[Q]:** Flaccid paralysis with **acute loss of reflexes** followed by spasticity below the level of lesion.
  - *Examined by checking the bulbocavernosus reflex.*

✓ **Autonomic dysreflexia**[Q]: *Seen in cord injuries at or above level of T6.*
  - Commonest triggers are distension of bladder or bowel.
    ❖ Pain and pressure are other stimulations.
  - *Vasoconstriction below the level and vasodilation above the level of injury* with bradycardia.
  - Hypertensive crisis complications like myocardial infarction, cardiac dysrhythmias, intracranial haemorrhage, stroke, seizures, retinal haemorrhage, pulmonary oedema may occur.
  - Severe headache, nasal obstruction, anxiety, flushed skin, diaphoresis, and piloerection above the level of injury.
  - Catheterize a patient in retention or relieve faecal impaction.
  - **Oral nifedipine and prazosin** can be used prophylactically to prevent attack.
  - Prompt reduction of BP will include nitrates, labetalol, hydralazine.
  - Atropine or Glycopyrrolate for bradycardia.

✓ **Radiological assessment**
  - **Canadian C-spine rule (CCR)**[Q]: The fully conscious, sober, cooperative patient, involved in low-energy trauma, with no neck pain or midline tenderness, can actively rotate head 45 degrees in both directions with no distracting injuries is highly unlikely to have a cervical spine injury and can be cleared on clinical examination alone.
  - The fully conscious, sober, cooperative trauma patient with neck pain or tenderness can have upright[Q] plain radiography including flexion/extension films.
  - **High-resolution CT images** of the whole cervical spine should be done to clear cervical spine (4.3% of patients have false-negative rate) in the situations written below. The image should be reviewed by consultant radiologist.
    ❖ Age ≥65 yr
    ❖ Dangerous mechanism
    ❖ Paraesthesia in extremities
  - **MRI** is the gold standard for imaging spinal cord and should be performed in all patients when a patient's neurological examination does not match the fracture pattern seen on CT scan.

- Ultimately, clearing of spine is based on local policy and some trusts will clear the C-spine radiologically and some will clear it clinically only.

Prevention and Treatment

✓ **Prehospital management:** From the scene of accident, complete spinal immobilization with *rigid cervical collar*[Q], **head blocks and tape**, and body straps to secure the patient to a *backboard.*
  - The need is to balance between the risks of a missed cervical spine injury (5% of blunt trauma victims, of which only a small proportion will require surgery) against risk of hard collar immobilization.
  - Spinal boards are for patient transfer only and they should be removed as soon as patient is in hospital.
  - Use **log rolls** for turns[Q] and **30° reverse Trendelenburg position** for unstable thoracic/lumbar spine.

✓ **Resuscitation:** Airway (A), Breathing (B), Circulation (C), Disability (D), and Exposure (E) according to ATLS protocols and in-line manual stabilization for intubation.
  - *Prevention of secondary injury.*
  - *Documentation of focal neurological deficit.*
  - **Suxamethonium**[Q] is safe to use in the first 72 h and can cause dangerous hyperkalaemia afterwards.

✓ **Neuroprotective measures:** Maintain a MAP of at **least 85** mmHg to optimize blood flow to the spinal cord for first 7 d. Initial fluid resuscitation is followed by vasopressor support (norepinephrine).
  - **Steroids are not recommended** in acute spinal cord injury because of concerns about rates of sepsis.

✓ **Operative management:** *Unstable injuries should be reduced and stabilized within the first 72 h once the patient is stable.*
  - Other indications for surgery are progressive neurological deficits and patients who can not tolerate bracing (obesity, skin lesions, multi-extremity injuries)

✓ **Pharmacological thromboprophylaxis** with LMWH should be started within 48 h after discussing with surgeons.
  - IVC filter in patients who are not candidates for anticoagulation.

✓ **Respiratory dysfunction prevention: Especially for high cervical injuries**
  • Intensive physical therapy and breathing exercises
  • Abdominal strap
  • Mechanical insufflation–exsufflation device promoting cough
✓ **Pressure sore prevention** should start from day 1.
  • Adequate patient positioning and nutrition along with skin examination several times a day.

THORACIC TRAUMA

Epidemiology

✓ Motor vehicle collisions account for 70–80% of all thoracic injuries.
  • Two-thirds of thoracic-related deaths occurs in the prehospital setting due to tracheo-bronchial tree, cardiac and great vessels.
  • Rib fractures are the commonest finding followed by haemothorax.

Presentations

✓ **Pulmonary contusion:** Present with hypoxaemia which worsens in the first 48 h.
  • **Chest X-ray:** Focal or diffuse consolidative process that doesn't typically follow anatomical segments or lobes.
  • **CT scans** help to diagnose it early and quantify it. A contusion affecting more than 28% of total lung volume is an indication for need of mechanical ventilation and predictive of ARDS.
  • *Chest physiotherapy, high-flow oxygen therapy and non-invasive ventilation is recommended in cases of hypoxaemia.*
  • If no improvement within one hour, endotracheal intubation should be done.
✓ **Flail chest**[Q]: *Rib fractures are the most common injuries in chest trauma.* Flail chest happens when two or more contiguous ribs are broken at two points. Pulmonary contusions below cause major morbidity and mortality.
  • Segment of ribs moves independently of the rest of the chest wall leading to paradoxical respiration. Pain due to fracture leads to alveolar hypoventilation.
  • Elderly patients are at risk of higher mortality. May require non-invasive ventilation to avoid intubation.

• Most patients are treated conservatively with effective analgesia (thoracic epidural and paravertebral catheter).
  ❖ Paracetamol[Q], NSAIDs, and opioids can also be used. Short prescription of NSAIDs can be given in elderly as well.
  ❖ **Serratus anterior block**[Q]**:** Anterior rib fracture, **Erector Spinae block**[Q]**:** Posterior rib fracture.
• *Surgical repair may be considered in the presence of any costal segment that may damage the lung parenchyma and patients on invasive ventilation*[Q].
  ❖ May lead to chronic pain issues[Q].
• Mortality increases with increasing number of rib fractures.
✓ **Sternal fractures:** Possibility of blunt cardiac injury with sternal fractures, so patients should undergo testing to rule out heart damage.
  • **Managed conservatively** if the injury is not of the high-velocity impacts, fracture is not severely displaced, no clinically significant injury and complex analgesia is not required.
  • **Surgery** may be considered for displaced for unstable fractures.
✓ **Pneumothorax:** Decreased breath sounds, resonance on percussion, hypotension and neck veins distended in tension pneumothorax which is an emergency.
  • Anterior pneumothorax can be missed on chest X-ray and detected only on FAST and confirmed by CT scan.
  • *Treatment for an open pneumothorax involves dressing over the wound with **taping on three sides allowing to act as a one-way valve** and a chest tube drainage at a separate site.*
✓ **Tracheobronchial injury:** 30–80% of patients will die before reaching the hospital.
  • **Bronchoscopy** is gold standard for identifying tracheobronchial injuries and ideally intubation should be done over a fibre-optic bronchoscope.
  • *Approach through collar bone (cervical trachea), sternotomy (mediastinal injury) or thoracotomy (bronchial injury) may be needed.*
✓ **Oesophageal injury:** Iatrogenic injuries are the most common cause. Cervical tear may present with crepitus in the neck. Pleural effusions are

present in >50% of cases of perforations of the thoracic oesophagus.

- **Chest X-ray** can show subcutaneous emphysema, pneumomediastinum, pleural effusion, or pneumothorax. Contrast studies are done to confirm the diagnosis and define the exact site.
- A conservative approach (nil by mouth and broad-spectrum antibiotics) may be considered for patients with minimal symptoms and a small self-contained leak.
- **Surgery** for a communicating leak or patient appears septic. **Primary repair with drainage is the preferred method.**

✓ **Diaphragmatic rupture**: Blunt trauma on the left side is more common due to congenital deficiencies.

- Nasogastric tube in thorax after chest X-ray can help in diagnosis.
- **Laparoscopic exploration** can help in diagnosis and as well help in repair.

✓ **Blunt cardiac injury**: Seen in violent deceleration and mostly right ventricle is involved. Normal ECG and serum troponin levels at presentation and 8 h later rules out significant myocardial contusion.

- Arrhythmias and low cardiac output state are seen in moderate injury. Echocardiography is the technique of choice.
- *Cardiac rupture presents with cardiac tamponade and is repaired in theatre with cardiopulmonary bypass support nearby but not necessarily in use.*

✓ **Traumatic aortic injury (TAI)** in blunt trauma happens most commonly in the **proximal descending aorta**^{Q} at the site of ligamentum arteriosum. Aorta is fixed here, and rapid deceleration can cause tears here.

- 80% of TAIs die at the scene and mortality rate for patients that reach the hospital is 10–30%.
- **Chest X-ray**: Left-sided haemothorax, displacement of mediastinal structures to the right, widened mediastinum, abnormal aortic arch silhouette.
- ECG-gated contrast CT can help in diagnosis.
- Control BP and heart rate to reduce the risk of injury.
- *Surgical management can be either an open repair or thoracic endovascular aneurysmal repair (TEVAR).*

✓ **Blast injury:** Complex type of physical trauma resulting from direct or indirect exposure to an explosion.

- **Spectrum of blast injuries**
  - ❖ **Primary:** Direct effect of high-pressure blast wave. Blast lung, ruptured tympanic membrane, bowel perforation.
  - ❖ **Secondary:** Propelled debris causing penetrating trauma and lacerations.
  - ❖ **Tertiary:** Persons are themselves displaced by the blast wind and get bony fractures.
  - ❖ **Quaternary:** Injuries caused by explosive products such as burns, asphyxiation.
  - ❖ **Quinary:** Radiation exposure and bacterial infections.
- **Blast lung:** Forces propagate through the lung parenchyma, disrupting the alveolar capillary membrane leading to alveolar haemorrhage, pneumothorax, bronchoalveolar fistula, and ARDS.

Diagnosis

✓ **Chest X-ray:** Initial investigation of choice. 98% negative predictive value and hence useful when normal.

- Mediastinal widening can indicate major aortic disruption.

✓ **CT scan:** Highly sensitive for detecting blunt chest trauma and for visualization of lung contusions, pneumothorax, haemothorax, haemopericardium, sternal fractures, pneumomediastinum, bronchial rupture, and tracheal rupture.

- Useful for major intrathoracic aortic injury and diaphragmatic ruptures as well.
- CT angiogram is gold standard for **diagnosing thoracic injuries in stable patients.**

✓ **Ultrasound: Focused abdominal sonogram for trauma (FAST)** can identify pneumothorax, haemothorax, haemopericardium and tamponade.

- Combination of FAST, CXR, and physical exam is extremely helpful in immediately life-threatening injuries.

✓ **VATS:** Main indications are diagnosis and treatment of diaphragmatic injuries, persistent haemorrhage, retained thoracic collections, diagnosis of bronchopleural fistula, and persistent post-traumatic pneumothorax.

- Not suitable for unstable patients and those who can't tolerate thoracotomy.

Indications for Urgent Surgery[Q]

✓ **Haemothorax:** Intercostal or mediastinal vessels rupture causing haemothorax.
  - Decreased breath sounds and dullness on percussion.
  - **Small to moderate-sized haemothorax** that stop bleeding during tube thoracostomy (large bore 32–36F tube anterior to midaxillary line at the fifth or sixth intercostal space) can usually be managed conservatively.
  - **Surgery (Thoracotomy)[Q]** if bleeding >200 mL/h for 3 h, accumulation of >1500 mL of bleed after placement of chest drain and haemodynamic instability.
  - Video-assisted thoracoscopy surgery (VATS) can be considered for the stable patient.
✓ **Massive air leak:** Persistent pneumothorax after chest tube placement, significant subcutaneous emphysema, pneumomediastinum are warning signs for major tracheobronchial injury.
✓ **Cardiac tamponade:** Seen more in left-sided trauma. **Beck's triad[Q]:** hypotension, muffled heart sounds and raised JVP. Echocardiography helps in diagnosis. Resuscitation and decompression of the pericardium.
  - Needle[Q] is inserted immediately below and to left of xiphisternum, between the xiphisternum and the left costal margin.
✓ **Cardiovascular collapse:** Resuscitative thoracotomy. Survival better in penetrating thoracic trauma compared to blunt trauma.
  - **Resuscitative endovascular balloon occlusion of the aorta (REBOA)** has been used as a temporizing measure for penetrating thoracic trauma. A balloon is passed up the femoral artery to occlude aorta. This technique is still under investigation for its role.

Additional Questions

✓ A right-sided raised hemi-diaphragm may be seen in right phrenic nerve palsy[Q]. It can also be seen in right-sided pneumonectomy and subphrenic abscess.

ABDOMINAL TRAUMA

Epidemiology and Aetiology

✓ Abdominal trauma can be categorized as blunt and penetrating.
  - **Blunt trauma:** Managed non-operatively frequently.
  - **Penetrating:** Requires operative intervention frequently.
✓ **Mechanisms of injury[Q].**
  - **Compression:** Seatbelt causing subcapsular haematomas to solid organs.
  - **Deceleration:** Shear off between free and fixed structure (e.g. mesenteric tears).

Clinical Features and Diagnosis

✓ **FAST USG:** Performed in the unstable patient with suspected abdominal haemorrhage.
  - If patient is haemodynamically stable or if FAST scan is positive, then CT scan should be performed as soon as possible.
  - Patient who are too unstable should go directly to the operating theatre[Q].
✓ **CT scan with contrast:** Only 75% of organ perforations are diagnosed with CT-scan. Can still be possible in haemodynamically instable patients.
  - Best modality to see retroperitoneal organ injury in blunt trauma abdomen patients.
  - Better than USG for therapeutic interventions.
✓ **Diagnostic peritoneal lavage:** More sensitive than CT scan for detection of hollow viscous injuries.
  - In lower chest stab wounds, RBC count >5000–10,000/mm³ is considered positive.
  - It can lead to negative laparotomy.
✓ **Amylase:** Apart from pancreas, can be increased in injury to salivary glands, bowel ischaemia, perforation, or obstruction.
  - Its elevation is not an indication for exploratory laparotomy.
✓ **Diaphragm injuries:** 10% of penetrating chest trauma patients. Diagnosis only in 30% of patients preoperatively.
  - Trauma anterior to anterior axillary lines is associated with an incidence of visceral injury approaching 70% whereas flank injuries are associated with a 30% risk.
  - *Gunshot wound has 95% chance of requiring surgery whereas stab wound will require surgery in 30% of cases.*

- Diaphragmatic rupture in blunt trauma is more common on the left as right side is protected by the liver[Q].
- ✓ **Splenic injury:** Splenic injury can happen and is managed conservatively or surgically depending upon factors like active bleeding and size of spleen involved.

American Association for the Surgery of Trauma (AAST) grade of splenic injury is used

Grade	Parenchymal Laceration Depth	Haematoma
I	<1 cm	Subcapsular haematoma <10% of surface area, capsular tear
II	1–3 cm	Subcapsular haematoma 10%–50% of surface area, intraparenchymal haematoma <5 cm
III	>3 cm	Subcapsular haematoma >50% of surface area, intraparenchymal haematoma >5 cm, ruptured subcapsular/intraparenchymal haematoma
IV	• 25% devascularization • Splenic vascular injury or active bleeding confined within splenic capsule	
V	• Splenic injury with active bleeding beyond spleen into peritoneum • Shattered spleen	

- Failure rates with non-operative approach increases as grade of injury increases.
- Any sign of ongoing bleeding should lead to immediate surgery.
- Patients with higher-grade (III to V) splenic injury should get all the vaccinations even with the spleen in situ.
- ✓ **Liver injury:** Like spleen, non-operative management of liver injured has a high success rate (80%).
  - Unstable patients should be taken to theatre for cauterization and suture repair. Perihepatic packing is also done ± IR guided angioembolization.
    - ❖ Contrast extravasation into peritoneum on CT scan is also an indication for surgery.

- Biliary complications: They occur later in course and biliary fistula is common and can lead to biliary peritonitis or infected biloma.
  - ❖ Biliary peritonitis requires surgery and infected biloma is managed by percutaneous drainage or ERCP.
- ✓ **Pancreatic injuries:** Trauma to pancreas occurs in 10% of all injuries related to blunt abdominal trauma.
  - Due to high-impact injury to the epigastrium. Happens rarely in isolation and **missed injuries are common.**
  - Management strategy depends upon injury to the main pancreatic duct injury with high grade injuries (III-V) including main duct injury. Ductal injury calls for surgical intervention.
  - ERCP and MRCP can be done in stable patients to diagnose duct injury.
  - Isolated pancreatic contusions or superficial lacerations are treated conservatively with bowel rest, NG suction, and nutritional support.
- ✓ **Kidney injury:** Haemodynamic instability due to renal injury is typically due to a high-grade injury (grade V) and normally results in nephrectomy.
  - Haemodynamic stable patients with high grades IV and V are also managed non-operatively.
  - Rupture of the collecting system can lead to persistent urine leak or urinoma with risk of infection.
    - ❖ Double J catheter is used initially, and surgical drainage may be needed sometimes.
- **Fluid surrounding solid organs is mostly from a bowel injury or rupture of bladder.**
- ✓ **Bladder injuries:** Mostly associated with pelvic injuries.
  - **CT cystogram:** To rule out bladder injury in case of gross haematuria. Differentiates intraperitoneal from extraperitoneal urine leakage.
    - ❖ Intraperitoneal leakage requires operative repair whereas extraperitoneal leakage can be managed with a urinary catheter for 2 wk.
  - **Retrograde urethrogram:** If blood is noted at meatus to rule out urethral injury.

✓ **Small bowel injuries:** 80% of small bowel injuries occur from the ligament of Treitz to the terminal ileum.
- Trauma to small bowel is the third most common intra-abdominal injury following liver and spleen.
- Duodenal injury presents with signs of gastric outlet obstruction and is managed NG tube decompression and nutritional support by TPN.
- Intra-abdominal bleeding can cause bowel paralysis initially.
- **Missed bowel Injuries are always a concern as complications are severe if hollow viscus injuries are detected later than 24 h.**
- Delayed consequences of abdominal trauma are intestinal perforation, mesenteric ischaemia, haematoma rupture.

✓ **Rectal injuries:** Should be considered in all pelvic fractures and blood on rectal examination calls for rigid sigmoidoscopy.
- Diverting colostomy may be needed in these cases.

Treatment

✓ **Blunt injury:** Non-operating management of abdominal solid organ injury only for haemodynamically stable patients in whom the injuries are identified by imaging.
- Hollow viscus injuries are managed with intervention except extraperitoneal rupture of the bladder or intramural haematoma of the duodenum.

✓ **Penetrating injury:** Any haemodynamic instability or peritoneal signs mandates exploration.
- **Stab wounds** are managed conservatively more frequently than **gunshot wounds.**

✓ **Abdominal trauma needs immediate laparotomy^Q in case of**
- Severe continuous bleeding
- Hollow organ perforation
- Rupture of diaphragm causing displacement of abdominal contents into thorax
- Penetrating abdominal trauma in most cases
- Abdominal compartment syndrome

✓ **Damage control surgery**
- It should be undertaken in the following circumstances.
  - If more than 10 units of blood has been transfused.

- Base excess of less than −18 mmol/L if patient is less than 55 yr old or less than −8 mmol/L if patient is greater than 55 yr old
- Lactate acidosis >5 mmol/L.
- Hypothermia of less than 35°C
- **Three phases of damage control surgery**
  - Limited operative intervention aimed at controlling haemorrhage.
  - Resuscitation in ICU with blood products and active rewarming to current coagulopathy, hypothermia, and acidosis
  - Planned return to theatre for definite surgical procedure
- Aortic cross-clamping may be required in an exsanguinating patient.

✓ **Angiographic coiling** of bleeding sites should be considered.
✓ **Tranexamic acid** should be administered in the bleeding trauma patients.
✓ **VTE prophylaxis** within 24 h with haemodynamic stability and bleeding ceased in case of solid organ injuries. Consultation with surgeon is recommended.
✓ **Add antifungals** if patient not improving over days. In case of peritonitis, cover anti-pseudomonal activity like piperacillin/tazobactam.

ORTHOPAEDIC INJURIES

✓ **Open fractures:** Infection is a big concern.
- **Gustilo–Anderson fracture classification**
  - **Type I:** Clean wounds <1 cm in length with simple fracture pattern.
  - **Type II:** Laceration >1 cm but <10 cm with moderate soft tissue damage.
  - **Type IIIa:** Laceration >10 cm with extensive soft tissue damage.
  - **Type IIIb:** Type IIIa + Periosteal stripping and bone exposure.
  - **Type IIIc:** Vascular injury.
- **Treatment:** Antibiotics for infection prevention and should be given early, ideally within one hour of injury.
  - Gram-positive coverage usually for 24 h.
  - Addition of Gram-negative coverage for type III Gustilo–Anderson fractures for 72 h.
  - Wound debridement and irrigation.
  - Fracture stabilization: External fixation of the fracture.

❖ Early wound closure.

❖ Amputation in selected patients.

✓ **Pelvic fracture:** Haemorrhage expanding in the retroperitoneal space. Patients with unstable pelvic fracture doesn't mean that patient is haemodynamically unstable.

- **Arterial bleeding:** 20% of cases, **Venous bleeding:** 80% of cases.
- **Clinical features:** Abnormal limb rotation or shortening of limb.
  ❖ Blood coming from urethral meatus[Q], anus or vagina can be a sign of open pelvic fracture.
  ❖ Neurovascular examination of both legs along with checking of sphincter tone and bulbocavernosus reflex should be done.
- **Young and Burgess system** classifies fracture on four impact patterns.
  ❖ Anterior-posterior compression
  ❖ Lateral compression
  ❖ Vertical shear
  ❖ Combined/complex pattern
- **Tile classification**
  ❖ A: Stable
  ❖ B: Rotationally unstable, vertically stable
  ❖ C: Rotationally and vertically unstable
- **Management[Q]:** Avoid log roll if possible.
  ❖ Pelvis binder is used initially to limit blood diffusion space, restore part of bone continuity and limit venous bleeding by applying pressure at **greater trochanters.**
  ❖ Remove pelvic binders as soon as possible with maximum after 24 h.
  ❖ Resuscitation with crystalloids and blood products.
  ❖ **Haemodynamic unstable patient[Q]:** E-FAST scan has good positive predictive value but high false-negative rate for intraperitoneal fluid.
    - Diagnostic peritoneal lavage (DPL) if negative or equivocal E-FAST.
    - If too unstable[Q], *angiographic arterial embolization or pelvic packing for venous bleeding may be necessary.*
  ❖ **Haemodynamic stable patient:** Abdomin-pelvic CT scan with IV contrast[Q] (most effective in evaluating the degree of internal bleeding).

❖ **Retrograde cystourethrogram** for suspected genitourinary injuries.

- **ICU complications:** Ileus, abdominal compartment syndrome, thromboembolism, urogenital injuries.

✓ **Extremity injury:** Femur (17%) and tibia (13%) are more commonly involved in major trauma. CT angiography[Q] may be required in case of joint dislocation and lack of pulse.

- **Femoral shaft injury:** Traction device is applied in the field to stabilize.
  ❖ Portable traction devices should be removed as soon as possible as they cause sciatic nerve pressure injury or skin ulceration.
  ❖ *Intramedullary nailing is the gold standard for treatment.* Plate fixation is done in selected cases.
- **Tibial shaft injury:** Higher chances of open injury due to thin, soft tissue surrounding it.
  ❖ *Treated with intramedullary nailing as well.* Plating done for fractures involving the articular joints.
- **Humeral shaft injury:** Can be complicated by injury to brachial artery and radial nerve injuries.
  ❖ Fracture cast, brace, or operative management (polytrauma) have all been used.
  ❖ Nailing or plating done for operative management.

✓ **Fat embolism syndrome (another exam favourite topic):** Clinical syndrome due to release of fat into circulation.

- **Risk factors:** Pelvis fracture, long bone fracture, pancreatitis, alcoholic liver disease.
- **Pathophysiology**
  ❖ **Mechanical theory:** Obstruction of vessels by emboli.
  ❖ **Biochemical theory:** Fat is broken down by lipases and free fatty acids cause release of proinflammatory cytokines leading to ARDS.
- **Clinical features**
  ❖ Presents 24–72 h post-insult. Pulmonary dysfunction is the first to manifest as hypoxaemia.
  ❖ **Triad[Q]** of hypoxia, petechiae, and neurological dysfunction.
  ❖ **Complications:** ARDS, biventricular failure, seizures, coma, renal failure, liver dysfunction, DIC.

❖ **Scoring systems:** Clinical diagnosis of exclusion. Schonfeld's criteria, Lindeque's criteria, and Gurd's criteria.
- **Gurd's criteria**[Q]: one major and 4 minor criteria.
  - ❖ **Major:** Hypoxaemia, axillary or conjunctival petechiae and CNS depression disproportionate to hypoxaemia.
  - ❖ **Minor:** Tachycardia >110 bpm, Pyrexia >38.5°C, emboli present in the retina on fundoscopy, fat present in urine, fat globules in the sputum, thrombocytopaenia, drop in haemoglobin, high ESR.
- **Treatment:** Supportive care of ABCDE.
  - ❖ Early surgical fixation (<24-hour trauma) lowers risk.
  - ❖ External fixation with plating produces lesser lung injuries.
  - ❖ Steroids, aspirin, and heparin have all been tried but not demonstrated reliable efficacy.
  - ❖ Mortality rate of 5–15%.
✓ **Muscle compartment syndrome:** Usually appears 24 h after the trauma and is characterized by pain out of proportion to the clinical findings.
- Pressure differential between intra-compartmental pressure and diastolic pressure of 30 mmHg is diagnostic of compartment syndrome.
- CK levels are raised and myoglobinuria is seen.
- Treatment is surgical fasciotomy within 6 h.
✓ **Peripheral nerve injury:** Most of injuries are neuropraxias which recover on their own. Prognosis of radial nerve injury is better than sciatic nerve injury.
✓ **Deep vein thrombosis:** Patients with pelvis and hip fractures are at higher risk.
- DVT prophylaxis with LMWH should be started within 24 h in patients who do not have contraindications. 4 wk of prophylaxis for patients at high risk of VTE.
- IVC filter in patients with high risk of VTE and contraindications to LMWH.
- Combined pharmacological and pneumatic compression devices should be used where able.

Surgical Treatment Considerations

✓ **Early total care (ETC):** Early definitive fixation of fractures. Intramedullary fixation.

✓ **Damage control orthopaedics (DCO):** Early temporary fixation of fractures with a delayed definitive surgery.
- External fixation is done in patients with severe and multiple injuries to avoid systemic inflammatory response like in patients with concomitant lung and head injuries.
✓ **Safe definitive surgery (SDS):** Combines both ETC and SDS and decision is taken upon patient behaviour in theatre.

Additional Questions

✓ **Winging of scapula**[Q]: Long thoracic nerve: C5–7.

TRAUMA AND PREGNANCY

Physiological Changes in Pregnancy[Q]

Parameter	Value Change
Cardiovascular System[Q]	
Cardiac output at 1st of stage labour	↑ 50%
Cardiac output at 2nd of stage labour	↑ 60%
Cardiac output post-delivery	↑ 80–100%
Stroke volume	↑ 25–30%
Heart rate	↑ 15–25%
SVR	↓ 20%
PVR	↓ 35%
Intravascular fluid volume	↑ 35–45%
RBC volume[Q]	↑ 25%
Plasma volume[Q]	↑ 50%
CVP/PCWP	No change
Respiratory System	
Minute ventilation	↑ **45–50%**
Respiratory rate	↑ 0–15%
Tidal volume	↑ 40–45%
Total lung capacity	↓ 0–5%
Vital lung capacity	No change
Functional residual capacity	↓ **20%**
Residual volume	↓ 15–20%
FEV_1	No change
FEV_1/FVC	No change
Closing capacity	No change
Oxygen Consumption	
At term	↑ 20%
At 1st stage of labour	↑ 40%

Parameter	Value Change
At 2nd stage of labour	↑ 75%
Coagulation System	
Factors that increased	I, VII, VIII, IX, X, XII, and vWF
Factors that decreased	XI, XIII, antithrombin III, and tPA
Platelets	↓ 0–10%
Liver Changes	
ALT/AST/bilirubin	Increases to upper limit of normal
ALP	Double the normal level
Plasma cholinesterase	↓ 25–30%
Total protein	↓ 10%
Albumin	↓ 25%
Colloid osmotic pressure	27–22 mmHg
Renal Changes	
Renal blood flow	↑ 50–60%
GFR	↑ 50–60%
BUN	↓ 50%
Creatinine	↓ 50%
Arterial Blood Gases	
pH	7.42–7.44
$PaCO_2$ᵠ	↓ **to 30** mmHg
PaO_2	>100 mmHg
Bicarbonate	↓ to 20–21 mEq/L
Miscellaneous Changes	
Leucocytes	Up to 13,000/mm³
Minimum alveolar concentration	↓ 28%
Local anaesthetic sensitivity	↑
Total thyroid hormonesᵠ	↑
Thyroid-binding globulinᵠ	↑
Free T_3 and T_4ᵠ	Unchanged

✓ **Mother:** Every female of reproductive age with trauma should be considered pregnant until proven otherwise by a definitive pregnancy test or pelvic ultrasound.
  - Maternal care is always the priority.
  - Hyperdynamic state means that hypovolaemia can be concealed post-trauma. Pregnant woman can lose up to 35% of blood before showing any sign of shock.

- A neurological cause of trauma like eclampsia should be excluded.
- If necessary, X-rays and CT scans should be performed for diagnosis.
- All Rh-negative pregnant women with a history of abdominal trauma should have a prophylactic injection of Rho(D) immune globin within 72 h of traumatic event.

✓ **Fetus:** More than 50% of trauma occur during the third semester of pregnancy. Fetal mortality is up to 60% in severe trauma.
  - Main cause of fetal death is maternal shock and maternal death followed by placental abruption.
  - Fetal heart rate should be assessed on admission. It should be complimented with ultrasound and cardiotocography (CTG).
  - Best treatment for the fetus is to provide optimal resuscitation of the mother.

✓ **Blunt trauma:** 91% of abdominal injuries are blunt injuries.
  - Bowel is somewhat protected in blunt abdominal trauma, but the uterus and fetus are more vulnerable.
  - Pelvic fracture in the late gestation can cause skull fracture of the fetus.
  - Unrestrained pregnant women have a higher risk of premature delivery and fetal death.
    ❖ Using a shoulder restraint along with a lap belt compared to a lap belt alone reduces the likelihood of fetal injury.
    ❖ Airbags in motor vehicles do not increase pregnancy associated risks.
  - Placenta is not elastic and can result in injury at the uteroplacental interface.

✓ **Penetrating trauma:** 9% of abdominal injuries are penetrating injuries.
  - In case of chest tube placement, it should be positioned higher to avoid intra-abdominal placement due to elevation of the diaphragm.
  - Bowel injury can happen during penetrating trauma.
  - Signs of peritoneal irritation may be less evident in pregnancy.

✓ **Treatment**
  - Manual displacement of the uterus to the left side should be done to relieve pressure on the inferior vena cava.
  - A normal fibrinogen level may indicate DIC as fibrinogen levels are doubled during pregnancy.

- Presence of amniotic fluid in the vagina (pH of 4.5) represents ruptured membranes.
- An abdominal/pelvis CT scan radiation dose is mostly 25 mGy and fetal radiation doses less than 50 mGy are generally not associated with fetal anomalies.

BURNS

Epidemiology and Aetiology

✓ **Anatomy:** Epidermis is the superficial thin layer but capable of regenerating without a scar.
  - Dermis is thick layer below the epidermis but forms scars while healing.

✓ **Classification of burns**[Q].
  - **Superficial (First degree):** Damage to epidermis only.
    ❖ Painful erythema. No blisters.
    ❖ Heals within a week.
  - **Partial thickness (Second degree):** Damage to **epidermis plus part of underlying dermis.**
    ❖ *Painful blisters.*
    ❖ Heals between 10 and 21 d.
  - **Full thickness (Third degree):** Damage to **epidermis, dermis plus subcutaneous fat** and muscle.
    ❖ Painless because of loss of hair follicles and nerve endings.
    ❖ White and leathery appearance
    ❖ **Escharotomy:** Surgical excision of the burn and superficial fascia in order to permit the cut edges to separate and restore blood to unburned tissue distal to eschar.

✓ **Pathological changes**
  - **Zone of coagulation:** Central zone of irreversible damage.
  - **Zone of stasis:** Area of impaired blood flow and potentially salvageable.
  - **Zone of hyperaemia:** Perfusion increased due to vasodilation.

✓ **Flame burns** most frequent cause of burns in adults and overall.
  - Coagulative necrosis at the site of entry, surrounded by zone of stasis with vascular damage and vessel leakage. Outermost layer is zone of hyperaemia caused by vasodilation from inflammation.
  - Flame burns often cause deep or full thickness burns.
  - **Scalds are more common in children.**

Clinical Features and Diagnosis

✓ **Burns assessment:** Rule of nines and Lund–Browder charts for contiguous burns and palmar methos for non-contiguous burns. Assessment should include only partial and full-thickness burns and is done as part of the secondary survey[Q].
  - **Wallace's rule of nines**[Q] overestimates the size of burn and is more accurate in adults than children and obese.
    ❖ **Adults**[Q]: Head and neck total for front and back is 9%, thorax and abdomen front is 18%, thorax and abdomen back is 18%, each upper limb total for front and back is 9%, each lower limb total for front and back is 18%. Perineum becomes 1%.
    ❖ **Paediatrics**[Q]: Head and neck total for front and back is 18%, thorax and abdomen front is 18%, thorax and abdomen back is 18%, each upper limb total for front and back is 9%, each lower limb total for front and back is 13.5%. Perineum becomes 1%.
  - **Palmar method:** Palm accounting for 1% of surface area.
  - **Lund–Browder charts** take age into account and change body surface area according to the age and hence are useful in the paediatrics age group. Most widely used tool.

✓ **Inhalational injury:** Damage due to breathing of harmful gases and particulate matter and respiratory failure[Q] is the primary reason for mortality following an inhalational injury.
  - **Supraglottic airway injury (thermal injury):** Singed nasal hair, lip/tongue swelling, hoarseness, difficult swallowing, and stridor.
    ❖ Nasal fibre-optic endoscopy by ENT surgeons can help access the severity.
  - **Infra-glottic airway injury (smoke):** Cough with carbonaceous sputum, breathlessness, wheeze, and hypoxia.
    ❖ Bronchoscopy is done for diagnosis and treatment.
  - Risk of carbon monoxide (CO) and Cyanide poisoning[Q].
    ❖ More in enclosed spaces. Less with flash burns.
    ❖ Loss of consciousness at scene.

- **Carbon monoxide poisoning**: It will over-estimate the oxygen saturation. Co-oximetry is needed. Lethal carbon monoxide levels are >60% carboxyhaemoglobin.
- **Cyanide toxicity**: Suspected in smoke with plastics or synthetic polymers burn. 20 times more toxic than carbon monoxide.
  - ❖ *Refractory acidosis with high lactates is seen*[Q]. Lethal cyanide levels are 1 μg/mL.
- **Inhalation of particulate matter can cause obstruction of airways and lead to inflammation causing ARDS.**
- Hoarseness, stridor, and a swollen uvula are concerning signs and calls for urgent prophylactic intubation.
- Independent risk factor for mortality in burns.

✓ **Burns shock**: Fever or high temperatures are common in first 24–48 h and do not signify infections.
- Burns shock is vasodilatory shock and is seen in burns **exceeding >20% TBSA.**
- Patients will develop tachycardia to counter the hypovolemic shock and maintain it for weeks after the burns.
- Sepsis may be difficult to diagnose in a burns case as tachycardia and high temperature is already present. The **American Burn Association suggests that sepsis may be present if at least 3 of the following are present.**
  - ❖ Temperature >39°C or <36.5°C
  - ❖ Heart rate >110/min
  - ❖ Ventilatory frequency >25 breaths/min or minute ventilation >12 L/min
  - ❖ Platelets <100 × 10^9 L/min (>3 d after initial resuscitation)
  - ❖ Hyperglycaemia >11.1 mmol/L or insulin infusion requirements >7 units/h
  - ❖ Intolerance of enteral feed

✓ **Stress ulcers**: MC causes are mechanical ventilation for 48 h and coagulopathy. **Burns,** traumatic brain injury, and renal failure can also cause it.

✓ **Hypermetabolic stage**: From 48 h to 1 yr post-injury.

Treatment

✓ **Airway and breathing:** Patients with inhalational injury[Q] should be intubated prophylactically after checking and observing for increasing swelling. Swelling peaks in first 12 h.

- Uncut tube must be used for intubation.
- **Suxamethonium**[Q] **is safe to use within first 24 h and after 1 yr post-burn.**
  - ❖ Proliferation of extra-junctional acetylcholine receptors can cause dangerous hyperkalaemia[Q] between this period.
- **Early bronchoscopy** to diagnose and lavage to reduce effects of inhaled toxins.
- Nebulized[Q] heparin, N-acetylcysteine, and salbutamol with regular **bronchoscopic** washout might be needed.
- Give maximal FiO$_2$ initially till carboxyhaemoglobin becomes less than ≤3%.
- Extubation should be done after doing *air leak test.*
- *Regular chest physiotherapy would be needed.*

✓ **Circulation: Parkland formula**[Q] for initial resuscitation: 4 × TBSA % × kg over 24 h
- Fluid replacement should be from time of injury. Half of the volume in first 8 h and rest delivered over the subsequent 16 h. Ringer lactate is recommended.
- *For major burns >15% only (10% in children and elderly) or over 10% burns with inhalational injury, fluid resuscitation is used.*
  - ❖ *Erythematous regions are omitted unless additional blistering or evidence of partial thickness burn can be seen.*
- For children under 20 kg of weight, an additional glucose-based maintenance fluid is recommended.
- Monitor urine output in adults (0.5–1 mL/kg/h) and children (1–2 mL/kg/h).
- Urine output and not advanced monitoring for fluid responsiveness. Give fluid bolus of 250 mL up to 3 boluses/h rather than diuretics for increasing urine output.
- Excess fluid can lead to fluid creep and cause intra-abdominal hypertension. If fluid volumes given exceeds 6 mL/kg/h at 12 h, 4.5 % Albumin can be given. Replace one-third of crystalloids with albumin.
- Vasopressors only for refractory hypotension to crystalloids and albumin and haemodynamic monitoring for patients with renal failure and congestive heart failure.
- *By third post-burn day, the inflammation starts coming down and the patient can be started on diuresis.*

✓ **Nutrition:** Early enteral nutrition should be started early within 24 h to counter catabolism.
- **Resting energy expenditure is increased 2–3 times** the normal and 1.5–2 times the calories intake is given to the patients depending upon TBSA of burns.
  - ❖ Glucose should contribute not more than 60% of the calories and significant burn injuries require 2g/kg/day protein.
- **Oxandrolone** can be given from around day 5 at a dose of 0.2 mg/kg/day (max dose 20 mg) into two divided doses for protein anabolism in patients with ≥30% TBSA. Recombinant human growth hormone has been used.
- **Hypothermia is common and temperature of the room should be kept warm (28–33°C)** to prevent calories being used for temperature maintenance.
- **Glutamine** use hasn't shown any mortality benefit in **RE-ENERGIZE trial (2022).**
- **Vitamin C** in high doses reduced oxidative stress. Doses as high as 10 gram a day were used.
- **Beta-blockers like Propranolol** have been used to attenuate the hypermetabolic response.

✓ **Infection:** *Systemic prophylactic antibiotics are not recommended until cultures are positive or florid infection is suspected.*
- **Topical silver sulfadiazine** (broad spectrum against both Gram-positive and negative organisms) can help decrease the incidence of burn wound infections.
- Early wound infections are caused Gram-positive organisms while later, *Pseudomonas aeruginosa* infection will predominate and have blue-green pigment and smell like grapes.
- Lung infection and wound infections are the commonest causes of death due to sepsis.
- Consider tetanus vaccination.

✓ **Surgical management: Escharotomy** is performed for patients with full-thickness burns to release pressure from swelling and prevent compartment syndrome.
- Early excision and grafting (within 5 d) for full-thickness burns.

✓ **Cyanide poisoning:** Hydroxocobalamin[Q] 5 g IV can be given in suspected poisoning or haemodynamic instability. Treatment is Sodium thiosulphate, Sodium Nitrite, Amyl Nitrite.
- Hydroxy cobalamin causes orange-red discolouration of skin and body fluids.

✓ **Carbon monoxide poisoning**
- **Colourless odourless gas.** Poisoning seen in fire in enclosed spaces.
- CO have 250 times affinity for haemoglobin compared to O2. Left shift of Oxyhaemoglobin dissociation curve (ODC). CO also inhibits mitochondrial enzymes.
  - ❖ CO binds avidly to cardiac myoglobin.
- **Standard pulse oximeter overestimates the true arterial oxygen saturation. Co-oximetry should be used.**
- **Carbon monoxide toxicity features**
  - ❖ <10% COHb: Mostly asymptomatic
  - ❖ 10–20% COHb: Non-specific symptoms
  - ❖ 20–40% COHb: Headache, nausea/vomiting, confusion, metabolic acidosis
  - ❖ 40–60% COHb: Seizures, Coma, dysrhythmias, respiratory disease
  - ❖ >60% COHb: Cardiovascular collapse
- Carbon monoxide (CO) causes tissue hypoxia leading to rhabdomyolysis[Q].
- Half-life of CO is **6 h** which is shortened to **90 min by 100% oxygen. It is reduced to 23 min with hyperbaric oxygen**[Q].
- Hyperbaric oxygen for patients who had COHb levels >20%, loss of consciousness, neurologic and cardiac insult and in pregnant female. Best within 6 h of exposure.

✓ **Pain control:** Adequate pain control is needed to prevent long-term psychiatric effects like post-traumatic stress disorder (PTSD) on burns patients.
- Background pain can be controlled by IV paracetamol, opioid infusion, and ketamine infusion whereas breakthrough pain or procedural pain can be managed by IV opioids bolus.

Specialized burn services: All full-thickness burns, all circumferential burns, all burns ≥2% TBSA in children, all burns ≥3% TBSA in adults, all burns not healed in 2 wk should be referred to a specialized burn service.

✓ Discussion with consultant and referral should be done for following injuries.
- All burns to hands, feet, face, perineum, or genitalia
- Any chemical, electrical or friction burn

- Any cold injury
- Any unwell child with a burn
✓ **Specialized burn services are divided into three levels**
  - **Burns centres:** Highest level. Critical care units and immediate operation theatre access
    - ❖ Paediatric: Any burn of ≥30% TBSA should be referred.
    - ❖ *Adults: **Any burn >40% TBSA**[Q] should be referred or >25% TBSA with inhalation injury.*
  - **Burn units:** Separately staffed, discrete ward for burns.
    - ❖ Paediatric: Any burn of ≥5% but <30% TBSA should be referred.
    - ❖ Adults: Any burn of ≥10% but <40% TBSA should be referred or <25% TBSA with inhalation injury.
  - **Burn facilities:** Standard plastic surgical ward for the care of non-complex burn patients.
    - ❖ Paediatric: Any burn of ≥2% but <5% TBSA should be referred.
    - ❖ Adults: Any burn of ≥3% but <10% TBSA should be referred.

Prognosis

✓ **Baux score:** Score that combines age and TBSA and gives mortality for burns greater than 15% TBSA.
  - Score >75 indicates "almost certain death".
  - In modified Baux score an additional 17% is added to TBSA for inhalational injury.
✓ Mortality is around 15% in hospitalized patients.
  - Mortality is high in patients >30% TBSA.

ELECTRICAL INJURY

Electrical Injury

✓ **UK electricity:** Alternating current (AC), 50 Hz, 240 V.
✓ **Types of injuries:**
  - **Low-voltage injury** (<600 V) causes thermal burns and injures tissues superficially. Induces ventricular fibrillation.
  - **High-voltage injury** (>1000 V) causes injury to underlying muscle and bone and cutaneous injury might not be obvious. Induces ventricular fibrillation.

✓ **Severity of injury:** Depends on current type, amplitude, density, duration, and path followed.
✓ **Mechanisms of injury from electricity**
  - Electrocution
  - Burns
  - Traumatic complications like fall
✓ **Pathophysiology:** External current disrupts the intrinsic electrical currents like nerve impulse transmission and myocardial conduction.
  - Pathway of the current through the body from the entry to the exit point is important to find out to know the number of organs affected.
  - Electrical energy condensed at a single point can cause thermal injury.

Electrical Injury Due to Devices Used in ICU[Q]

✓ **Macroshock:** Macroshock occurs when current passes through the body via contact with the skin.
  - Resistance of skin is between 40,000 and 100,000 Ω.
  - Impedance of wet skin is 100 times less than the dry skin[Q].
  - At low voltages, alternating current (AC) will produce greater injury than a shock caused by direct current (DC) of the same amperage as DC causes a single muscle contraction that throws the victim away from the power source.
  - At high voltages they both have the same effect.
    - ❖ 1 mA → Tingling
    - ❖ 5 mA → Pain
    - ❖ 15 mA → Severe pain and muscle spasm (No let go)
    - ❖ 50 mA → Respiratory muscle spasm
    - ❖ **100 mA → Ventricular fibrillation**
    - ❖ **1000 mA → Extensive burns and charring**
✓ **Microshock:** Microshocks[Q] occur when invasive patient connections are placed across or in close proximity to myocardial tissue.
  - 50–100 µA of current directly to the ventricle can induce ventricular fibrillation.
  - Pulmonary artery catheters are type CF electrical equipment that can be directly connected to the heart.
✓ **Electrical safety devices**[Q]
  - **Fuses**
  - **Earth leakage circuit breakers (ELCB)**

- **Isolating transformer (Floating circuit)**
- **Line isolation monitor (LIM)**

Clinical Features of Electrical Injury

✓ **Respiratory effects:** Laryngospasm, aspiration, and respiratory failure.
✓ **Cardiovascular effects:** Direct necrosis of the myocardium and cardiac arrhythmias.
  - ECG should be monitored in first 24 h after high-voltage injury.
  - *Direct current required to cause VF is much higher than the alternating current.*
✓ **Neurological injuries:** Peripheral nerve injury, autonomic dysfunction, and coma.
  - CT head in all severe cases of lightening injury and injuries due to fall.
✓ **Spinal column fracture:** From direct injury or fall and can lead to spinal cord injury.
✓ **Compartment syndrome:** Muscle necrosis is common, and patient should be monitored for 24 h with daily CPK monitoring.
  - Serial evaluation of LFTs and KFTs along with CT scan to determine injury.
✓ **Gastrointestinal injury:** Bowel contusion, ileus, bowel necrosis.
✓ **Other injuries:** Cataracts and tympanic membrane rupture.

Prevention and Treatment

✓ Cardiopulmonary resuscitation based on ATLS ABCDE algorithm.
✓ Aggressive fluid management to prevent renal shutdown because of **muscle necrosis**[Q].
✓ **Burns** management.
✓ **Tetanus** management.

Lightning

Lightning: Involves voltage of $>30 \times 10^6$ V.
✓ Spider-like appearance (ferning or arborescent rash)[Q] of entrance and exit wounds.
  - Damage is mostly due to heat energy produced from high-voltage current.
  - Can cause asystole and direct neurological injury.
  - Severe muscular contraction can throw a person as well.
  - Prognosis good with 80–90% survival.

FIRE IN ITU

✓ **Fire:** *Arson is the commonest cause of fire in ITU*[Q]. Triad[Q] of the following elements must be present for fire to occur.
  - **Oxygen supply:** Air, Oxygen cylinders, open windows and doors, chemicals with oxidizing materials.
  - **Heat:** Electrical equipment, cooking equipment, boilers, and engines.
  - **Fuel source:** Patient gowns and bedding, dustbin contents, alcohol-based skin preparations, papers, and cards.
✓ **Fire prevention**
  - **Oxygen:** Store cylinders away from combustible materials.
    ❖ Upright position for **cylinders in unit and in designated holders**
    ❖ Oxygen cylinder valves should be opened slowly in the unit
    ❖ Setting the cylinder up for use before placing it close to the patient
    ❖ Not placing the cylinders on the beds
    ❖ Staff members should have knowledge of shutting off valves of **pipeline oxygen (area valve service units) and cylinders**
  - **Training and maintenance:** *Mandatory fire training for all the staff on induction.*
    ❖ *Fire extinguisher training for selected individuals.*
    ❖ Regular maintenance of electrical equipment and not use faulty equipment.
    ❖ Keep hospital *clutter free* as it can block fire exits and disrupt access for the fire fighters.
    ❖ Minimized use of *emollients and oil/ alcohol-based products.*
    ❖ Extinguish cigarettes properly in the bins provided.
  - **Unit design:** Division into clinical vs non-clinical areas, small bays rather than open areas.
    ❖ *>10 air changes of ventilation per hour in high-risk areas.*
    ❖ Fire signages, fire *refuge points*, fire doors (minimum 30 min protection) and emergency lighting.

❖ Each bed should have an *evacuation box* (propofol, neuromuscular blocker, neuromuscular reversal, intravenous fluids, painkillers, vasopressors).

❖ *Evacuation aids* like sheets, chairs and mats should be available.

❖ A *computerised fire alarm handler system* should be installed in hospital switchboards to make it quicker and easier to liaise with the Fire and Rescue Services.

❖ **Laminated fire action cards** explaining evacuation plan should be placed next to **fire call points**.

Fire Extinguishers[Q] (You will hate getting a question wrong on this one, so do revise a day before the exam)

	Water	Foam Spray	Carbon Dioxide	ABC Powder
Wood, paper, and textiles	√	√	✗	√
Flammable liquids	✗	√	√	√
Flammable gases	✗	✗	✗	√
Electrical[Q] contact	✗	✗	√	√
Cooking oil and fats	✗	✗	✗	✗

✓ **ICU evacuation measures**[Q]
  • **Immediate measures**
    ❖ Rapidly remove all patients and staff from immediate danger area and *stop open circuit delivery of oxygen through masks to patients.*
    ❖ *Raise alarm through switchboard and state location and nature of fire.*
    ❖ *Escalate to senior staff.*
    ❖ Shut all doors and windows.
    ❖ Trained staff to use **fire extinguisher and fire blankets.**
    ❖ **If fire is uncontrolled, start evacuation of the patients via the fire exits.**
  • **Fire containment**
    ❖ *Shut off oxygen pipeline supply and use transport oxygen cylinders.*
    ❖ Do not use lift and *shut all doors and windows as you leave areas.*
  • **Evacuation to safe areas**
    ❖ Follow orders from the fire warden.
    ❖ *Evacuation to designated assembly points on the same floor.*
    ❖ Horizontal and then vertical evacuation to floors below[Q].
    ❖ Follow internal major incident policy.
✓ **Reverse triage principle**[Q]
  • It means the one closest to the fire and visitors of the patients go first followed by the least unwell ones followed by the most unwell and then those in the side rooms.

12

Toxicology

GENERAL TOXICOLOGY

✓ **History:** Including collateral history from friends, families, and paramedics.
- Identification of ingested agent, timing and quantity of it, co-ingestion of alcohol.
- Poisoning should be a differential in a patient with altered conscious level or seizures.
- **Repeated vomiting:** Higher chances of oesophageal injury or partial self-elimination of drugs.
- In poisonings such as lithium and salicylate poisoning, lower serum concentrations in patients are required to cause poisoning in patients who chronically ingest these medications.
- *Normally drug dosing more than 10 times the therapeutic dose is required to cause symptoms of poisoning.*

✓ **Examination**
- **CNS: Coma:** Hypoglycaemia, sedatives/hypnotics, opioids, anticonvulsants, antidepressants, anticholinergics. Failure to improve in GCS after 12–18 h should raise the possibility of another cause of coma.
  - ❖ **Hyperreflexia and myoclonus:** *Serotonergic,* anticholinergic, sympathomimetic drugs.
  - ❖ **Convulsions:** *Neuroleptics,* antidepressants, anticholinergics, sympathomimetics, opioids, salicylates, theophylline, carbon monoxide, cyanide, lithium.
  - ❖ **Delirium and hallucinations:** Anticholinergic, sympathomimetics, Phencyclidine, LSD.
  - ❖ **Pupils:** *Pinpoint:* Opioids, phencyclidine, pesticide. *Dilated:* Anticholinergics or sympathomimetic drugs, pethidine, LSD.
- **Respiratory: Cyanosis** Methaemoglobinaemia.
  - ❖ **Sputum production:** Irritant gases like ammonia, chlorine, smoke, and non-inhalation agents like paraquat.
  - ❖ **Bronchospasm:** Cholinergic drugs.
  - ❖ **Hyperventilation:** Salicylates, organophosphate pesticides.
  - ❖ **Non-cardiac pulmonary oedema:** Heroin, cocaine, ethylene glycol, methanol, and salicylates.
- **Cardiovascular: QT prolongation:** Neuroleptics, antidepressants, organophosphates.
  - ❖ **Hypertension:** Sympathomimetics, anticholinergics, phencyclidine, MAO inhibitors (MAOIs).
- **Gastrointestinal: Ulceration around mouth:** Alkali, acid, paraquat poisoning.
  - ❖ **Ileus:** Anticholinergics and opioids.

Toxidromes

Syndrome	Causes	Signs
Anticholinergic	Antihistamines, antipsychotics, antidepressants, antiparkinsonian agents, antispasmodics, muscle relaxants, *Amanita muscaria*	Tachycardia, dry mouth and flushing, **sedation, mydriasis, urinary retention**, ileus, **hyperpyrexia**, delirium, seizures

DOI: 10.1201/9781003476214-12

Syndrome	Causes	Signs
Cholinergic	Organophosphate^Q and carbamate insecticides, nerve gases (sarin), **pyridostigmine**, edrophonium	**Bradycardia**, salivation, **lacrimation**, bronchorrhoea, miosis, **urinary and faecal incontinence**, gastrointestinal cramping, emesis, seizures
Sympathomimetic	Cocaine, amphetamines, synthetic cannabinoids, over-the-counter decongestants (ephedrine, pseudoephedrine), phencyclidine, caffeine, aminophylline	Tachycardia, dysrhythmias, hypertension, **hyperpyrexia**, mydriasis, hyperreflexia, diaphoresis, agitation, delusions, paranoia, seizures
Serotoninergic	SSRIs, tramadol, synthetic opioids like fentanyl	**Muscle fasciculation**, **myoclonus**, hyperreflexia, hyperpyrexia, tachycardia, diaphoresis, confusion, agitation, tremor
Sedative	Ethanol, ethylene glycol, methanol, benzodiazepines, barbiturates, valproic acid	Depressed level of consciousness, respiratory depression, **hypotension**, **hypothermia**, hyporeflexia
Opiates	Opioids, tramadol	**Miosis**, depressed level of consciousness, **respiratory depression**, hypotension, bradycardia hypothermia, hyporeflexia, ileus

✓ **Investigations:** 12-lead ECG.
- **Toxicology screen:** Qualitative urine and quantitative blood tests. *Acetaminophen and salicylate poisoning.*
- **ABG:** To check anion gap and look for causes of high anion gap metabolic acidosis. Methaemoglobinaemia.
- **Plasma osmolality and osmolar gap:** For osmotically active substances like alcohols.
- **Liver function tests:** Paracetamol poisoning
- **Creatine kinase:** Cocaine, long lies.

✓ **Immediate management**
- **A (airway) and B (breathing):** Patients are at increased risk of aspiration. Endotracheal intubation may be needed.
- **C (circulation):** Vasodilatation is the most common cause of haemodynamic instability.
  - Direct acting vasopressors like norepinephrine should be used.
  - **Sodium bicarbonate:** Treat QRS prolongation as well as effect of AV block due to drugs.
- **D (CNS depression):** Although not validated in these patients, Glasgow Coma Scale (GCS) score is used.
- **E (Expose):** Remove clothing and wash skin to prevent topical route of absorption.

- **Prevent absorption of the poison**
  - **Gastric lavage:** Gastric lavage doesn't change the clinical course of illness in mild and moderate poisonings. It is absolutely contraindicated in people who have ingested petroleum distillates and corrosive substances.
  - **Multiple dose-activated charcoal (MDAC):** MDAC involves repeated administration (>2 doses) of activated charcoal. 50 g within one to two hours after ingestion of the poison and repeat dose of 25 gram every 2 h. Clinical benefit hasn't been demonstrated. MDAC is used for theophylline, carbamazepine, quinine, dapsone, anti-depressants, paracetamol, salicylate, and digoxin. Not^Q used for iron, lithium, alcohols, hydrocarbons, electrolytes, cyanide, strong acids and bases.
  - **Whole bowel irrigation:** Administration of 1–2 L/h of **polyethylene glycol** by NG tube or orally until rectal effluent becomes clear. Can be used for **lithium or iron.** Contraindications are ileus, GI perforation, haemodynamic instability, and intractable vomiting.

- **Increased elimination of the poison**
  - ❖ **Alkaline diuresis:** Salicylate and barbiturate poisoning. Forced diuresis is not recommended.
  - ❖ **Haemodialysis:** Salicylates, ethylene glycol, methanol, lithium, carbamazepine, theophylline, metformin, and potassium.
  - ❖ **Plasmapheresis:** Amanita phalloides.
- **Specific antidotes**
  - ❖ Opioid overdose: Naloxone
  - ❖ Benzodiazepine Flumazenil
  - ❖ Alcohol: Fomepizole
  - ❖ Iron: Desferrioxamine
  - ❖ Amanita phalloides: Silibinin
- ✓ **Additional management principles**
  - Seek advice from pharmacist or specialist database like TOXBASE.
  - Report any safeguarding concerns.
  - Refer to mental health team if applicable.
  - Forensic examination if suspected sexual assault.

Miscellaneous Toxicities

- ✓ **Hyperoxia[Q]:** Tissues and organs are exposed to an excess supply of oxygen.
  - **Pathophysiology of oxygen toxicity:** Reactive oxygen species[Q] generated causes damage to DNA/RNA, cell membranes and proteins.
  - **Effects on specific populations**
    - ❖ **Neonates:** Retinopathy of prematurity, bronchopulmonary dysplasia.
    - ❖ **Type 2 respiratory failure in patients with COPD, neuromuscular disease, morbid obesity:** Hypercarbia.
  - **Pulmonary complications**
    - ❖ **Acute tracheobronchitis is the earliest manifestation followed by diffuse alveolar damage like in ARDS.**
    - ❖ *Acute tracheobronchitis is seen after 24 h in patients having high level (50%) of normobaric oxygen therapy.*
    - ❖ It can start as early as 4 h after starting >95% oxygen.
    - ❖ It can be seen in 3 h in patients with hyperbaric oxygen.
    - ❖ *Tickling sensation to throat, substernal pain, cough, retrosternal burning sensations.*
  - **CNS Complications**
    - ❖ Seen in **hyperbaric conditions:** Dizziness, headache, tinnitus, seizures, and coma.

- **Ocular complications**
  - ❖ Ophthalmic effects like **reversible myopia** and **cataract[Q].**
- *Acute tracheobronchitis and CNS oxygen toxicity are usually reversible.*
- **Other side effects of hyperoxia**
  - ❖ Increases **peripheral vascular resistance**
  - ❖ *Impaired hypoxic pulmonary vasoconstriction*
  - ❖ **Decreased mucociliary clearance**
  - ❖ *Absorption atelectasis*
  - ❖ **Pulmonary fibrosis post–bleomycin chemotherapy**
  - ❖ *Exacerbation of paraquat toxicity*
- **Avoid hyperoxia** in patients with stroke[Q], myocardial infarction[Q] and post-cardiac arrest[Q].
  - ❖ Target SpO_2 of 94–98% or PO_2 of 10–13 kPa in post-cardiac arrest patients.
- **Advantages of high oxygen**
  - ❖ **Hyperbaric oxygen** at 2–3 atmospheres dissolves oxygen up to 60 mL/L in contrast to dissolved oxygen of 3 mL/L at 1 atmosphere. Used for *decompression sickness*, gas embolism, *necrotizing fasciitis*.
  - ❖ **Normobaric oxygen:** Pneumothorax, carbon monoxide poisoning, during CPR, preoxygenation for induction of anaesthesia, post-extubation.
  - ❖ **HOT-ICU Trial (2021):** In patients with hypoxaemic respiratory failure (>10 L/min O2 or FiO2 50%), no mortality difference between conservative PaO2 (8kPa) vs liberal PaO2 (12kPa) targets.
  - ❖ **BOX trial (2022):** Among patients with out of hospital cardiac arrest, a more restrictive oxygenation goal (PaO2 9–10 kPa) did not reduce mortality compared to a liberal oxygenation goal (PaO_2 13–14 kPa).
- ✓ **Paraquat poisoning[Q]**
  - Herbicide. More common in the developing world.
  - Exposure to skin can lead to systemic toxicity.
  - Paraquat damages cells and inhibits essential enzymes.
  - Irritant to eyes and mucosa, oesophageal ulceration.

- **Diffuse alveolar damage.**
- Severe poisoning: 20–40 mg/kg. Fulminant poisoning: >40 mg/kg.
- Activated charcoal, RRT.
- **Oxygen can worsen lung injury[Q].**

✓ **Baclofen toxicity**
- Acts on GABA$_B$ receptors. Given in multiple sclerosis.
- Hypotension, bradycardia, and comatose patient.
- Paradoxical seizures, delirium, fixed dilated pupils, flaccid paralysis with no tendon reflexes areflexia, and absent brainstem reflexes.
- Patient can appear brain dead.
- Supportive treatment.

✓ **Chemical ingestion**
- Alkalis damages oesophagus more and acid causes more severe stomach injury.
- Acid injury has a worse prognosis.
- Upper GI endoscopy should be done in first 24 h to assess the degree of damage.
- Late complications are strictures, SCC of stomach.
- Steroids do not decrease the risk of stricture.

ACETAMINOPHEN POISONING

Epidemiology and Aetiology

✓ One of the most common agents associated with both incidental and accidental poisoning.

✓ **Acetaminophen** is 95% eliminated by hepatic conjugation. Cytochrome P450 converts 5% of Acetaminophen to toxic metabolite NAPQI (N-acetyl p-benzoquinoneimine).
- NAPQ-I is conjugated with glutathione sulfhydryl to non-toxic metabolite.
- Patients with depleted levels of Glutathione are at risk of toxicity.

✓ Toxic dose after single ingestion is 150 mg/kg. Paracetamol: 8–10 gram is toxic dose but can be 4 grams in patients with pre-existing liver disease.

Diagnosis

✓ **Risk factors[Q]:** Cystic fibrosis, chronic liver disease, AIDS, alcoholism, malnutrition, enzyme-inducing drugs like carbamazepine, rifampicin.

✓ **Clinical Features**
- **First 24 hr:** Acute GI symptoms: Nausea and vomiting, abdominal pain.
- **24–72 hr:** Rise in ALT and AST concentration. They rise above 1000 IU/L in severe toxicity.
- **72–96 hr:** End-organ renal and hepatic toxicity leading to encephalopathy[Q] and coagulopathy.

✓ Peak levels of paracetamol in blood occur after an overdose occur at approximately 4 h.
- Prothrombin time (PT)[Q] is the most sensitive indicator of impending acute hepatic failure.

✓ **King's College Criteria used for transplantation**

Treatment

✓ **Activated charcoal** can be given within 1 h of overdose of >150 mg/kg paracetamol[Q] (NICE guidelines). Gastric lavage is not recommended.

✓ **N-acetyl cysteine (NAC)[Q]** increases glutathione levels and can directly detoxify NAPQI. It can be given up to 48 h after paracetamol ingestion and even after staggered overdose. When given early, NAC leads to 95% survival.
- Effective by both oral and IV route.
- **12-h SNAP regimen:** 100 mg/kg over 2 h followed by 200 mg/kg over 10 h.
- **21-h protocol:** 150 mg/kg over 1 h, 50 mg/kg over 4 h, 100 mg/kg over 16 h.
- Some physicians give NAC till improvement in patient biochemistry.
- All patients should be treated with NAC irrespective of nomogram-generated risks[Q].
- **Anaphylactoid reactions[Q]** like pyrexia, tachycardia and dyspnoea are also common (20%) which can be treated with slowing the rate of infusion, antihistamine, and fluid resuscitation.

✓ **Management of acute liver failure:** Given in Chapter 1.

ALCOHOL AND RECREATIONAL DRUG POISONING

✓ **Drug Legislations in UK**
- **Medicines Act (1968):** Manufacture and supply of medicines with or without prescription.
- **Misuse of Drugs Act (1971):** Controls drugs to prevent non-medical use.

❖ **Class A:** Cocaine, MDMA, Heroin, LSD, Methadone.

❖ **Class B:** Cannabis, codeine, ketamine, barbiturates.

❖ **Class C:** Anabolic steroids, benzodiazepines.

- **Psychoactive Substances Act (2016)**

  ❖ Restricts production, sale and supply of new psychoactive substances which were originally termed as legal highs.

  ❖ Exemptions are food, alcohol, nicotine, caffeine, medicine, and drugs already under the Misuse of Drugs Act (1971).

✓ **Toxic alcohols:** Methanol, ethylene glycol, isopropyl alcohol, and propylene glycol. (Latest research has shown that even a glass of wine is harmful. Damn.)

- All alcohols except **propylene glycol** cause an initial presentation like ethanol consumption.

- Traumatic brain injuries (TBIs) are more common in patients who are intoxicated with ethanol, but outcome is same in both intoxicated and non-intoxicated patients.

- In burn patients however, intoxication at time of injury means six times more chances of death.

- Metabolic acidosis[Q] due to lactic acidosis is the commonest acid-base abnormality seen.

  ❖ **Ethanol and isopropyl alcohol do not produce metabolic acidosis.**

- Alcoholic ketoacidosis is seen in chronic alcoholics. These patients are already suffering from malnutrition.

  ❖ **Dextrose and saline are treatment of choice for alcoholic ketoacidosis instead of insulin and dextrose.**

- **All ingested alcohols produce osmolar gap but that gap can be normal if patient presents late.**

  ❖ Osmolal gap raised[Q] in sugars like mannitol and sorbitol, hypertriglyceridemia and Waldenström macroglobulinaemia as well.

✓ **Methanol**

- Used in antifreeze, as an industrial solvent, embalming fluid, and in windshield washing fluid.

  ❖ Lethal dose: 1.2 mL/kg

- *Alcohol dehydrogenase converts methanol into formaldehyde and converts formaldehyde into formic acid[Q].*

  ❖ Formic acid causes the ocular toxicity and the metabolic acidosis.

  ❖ Raised anion gap metabolic acidosis and increased osmolar gap.

- **Clinical stages of illness**

  ❖ **First 6 hr:** Ethanol poisoning symptoms like GI upset, nausea, vomiting.

  ❖ **After 6 hr:** Ocular toxicity, reduced consciousness, seizures, basal ganglia haemorrhage.

- Supportive treatment with Ethanol/Fomepizole for **methanol concentration >200 mg/L, osmolar gap >10 mOsm, arterial pH <7.30.**

  ❖ Fomepizole dose: 15 mg/kg followed by 10 mg/kg every 12 h until acidosis is resolved.

  ❖ Ethanol is given as 50 g (50 mL of absolute alcohol in 1000 mL of 5% dextrose).

- **Haemodialysis** removes both methanol and its toxic metabolites. Indications for use are ingestion of large amounts (>0.5 mL/kg), **initial methanol concentration >500 mg/L,** pH <7.15 and anion gap >24 mmol/L.

  ❖ Ethanol and Fomepizole are still required to inhibit its metabolism.

- **Folinic acid** enhances metabolism and elimination of formic acid.

✓ **Ethylene glycol[Q]** (A viva favourite question).

- Used in antifreeze and radiator fluid and is sweet in taste. Odourless and colourless.

  ❖ Lethal dose: 1–1.5 mL/kg

- *Alcohol dehydrogenase[Q] metabolizes Ethylene glycol to glycolaldehyde and then to glycolic acid and glycolate oxidase metabolizes it to oxalic acid. Oxalic acid chelates calcium and forms calcium oxalate that cause cerebral oedema and AKI.*

  ❖ Glycolic acid may cause a spuriously high lactate[Q].

  ❖ **Raised anion gap metabolic acidosis and increased osmolar gap.**

- **Clinical stages of illness:**

  ❖ **First 2 hr:** Ethanol poisoning symptoms like GI upset, nausea, vomiting.

  ❖ **12–24 hr:** Cardiopulmonary symptoms like myocardial dysfunction and ARDS.

❖ **24–72 hr:** Renal-like AKI.

❖ **>72 hr:** Neurological sequelae like cranial nerve defects, external ocular paralysis.

- *Fluorescence of urine under a wood's lamp which detects sodium fluorescein from antifreeze.*
    - ❖ *Oxalates are seen under microscopy[Q].*
- **Treatment** is supportive and Fomepizole/Ethyl alcohol may avoid the need for haemodialysis.
    - ❖ *Haemodialysis is indicated in severe acidosis and removes ethylene glycol and its metabolites except oxalate.*
    - ❖ Symptomatic hypocalcaemia should be treated with calcium but not otherwise as it can precipitate calcium stones.
- *Pyridoxine and thiamine[Q] should be given alongside.*

✓ **Isopropyl alcohol**

- Used in rubbing alcohol and hand sanitizers.
- Fruity odour in their breath due to it getting metabolized to acetone and **hence no metabolic acidosis but osmolar gap is there.**
    - ❖ Falsely elevated creatinine levels can be seen due to interference of acetone.
- Potent CNS depression that causes altered level of consciousness and respiratory depression.
    - ❖ Ketonuria and ketonaemia is seen.
- **Treatment** is supportive and haemodialysis need is not common.

✓ **Propylene glycol**

- Used as industrial solvent and solvent for medications (lorazepam, **diazepam,** etomidate, phenobarbital, phenytoin)
- **Raised anion gap metabolic acidosis and increased osmolar gap.**
- Haemolysis, arrhythmias, seizure, renal, or hepatic dysfunction.
- Discontinue offending medication.
- **Fomepizole and haemodialysis** are normally not required although haemodialysis may be necessary in the setting of AKI.

✓ **MDMA (3,4-methylenedioxymethamphetamine) or ecstasy**

- Class A illegal drug[Q]. Causes increased release and reduced uptake of Serotonin, dopamine, and norepinephrine in the brain.
- **Symptoms[Q]:** Improved mood and euphoria, mydriasis, tachycardia.
    - ❖ Hyperthermia, DIC, **Rhabdomyolysis, hyponatraemia[Q] due to ADH secretion.**
- Long-term effects: Dilated cardiomyopathy, pulmonary hypertension.
- Peak body temperature >42°C is associated with poor outcome.
    - ❖ Serotonin syndrome can also be precipitated with MDMA.
- **Treatment:** Activated charcoal. Benzodiazepines[Q] for violent behaviour and acute psychosis.
    - ❖ **Alkalinization of urine[Q] to protect kidneys from myoglobinuria.**

✓ **Cocaine toxicity**

- Inhibits presynaptic reuptake of norepinephrine, dopamine and serotonin and enhances catecholamine release.
- **Sympathomimetic effects[Q]:** Agitation, delirium, euphoria, hallucinations, dilated pupils, tachycardia, hypertension.
    - ❖ Repeated ingestion can lead to choreoathetosis, dystonias, and akathisia due to accumulation of dopamine in basal ganglia.
    - ❖ Can cause ischaemic and haemorrhagic stroke and can cause seizures.
    - ❖ Bowel ischaemia[Q] due to severe vasoconstriction.
    - ❖ ECG shows ST elevation in V1–3 and T wave inversion in V1–2.
- **Treatment:** Activated charcoal. Benzodiazepines for violent behaviour and acute psychosis.
    - ❖ GTN[Q] for hypertensive crisis over betablockers as it prevents unopposed alpha receptor stimulation.

✓ **Gamma-hydroxybutyrate (GHB) toxicity[Q] (cherry meth, fantasy, liquid ecstasy)**

- Precursor of gamma-aminobutyric acid (GABA).
- Initially induces euphoria followed by CNS depression. Alcohol dehydrogenase mediates its metabolism.
- Low GCS, hypothermia, bradycardia, and emesis.
- No specific antidote. Supportive management.

SEDATIVE POISONING

Opioid

✓ One of the most common severe poisonings seen.

✓ CNS depression, respiratory depression, **miosis** are the three main symptoms.

- Non-cardiogenic pulmonary oedema (diamorphine, methadone), status epilepticus, and cardiotoxicity.

✓ Paracetamol toxicity should be considered together as well.

✓ **Treatment:** Oxygenation and ventilation, manage hypotension, and naloxone.

- Activated charcoal is the decontamination method of choice.
- **Naloxone (opioid antagonist)** 100–400 mcg IV every 1–2 min for a controlled reversal with a maximum dose of 2 mg.
  - ❖ Goal is to restore spontaneous respirations and complete arousal. Maximal effect is for 5–10 min.
  - ❖ Naloxone can be given intranasally, intramuscularly, or subcutaneously.
  - ❖ IV naloxone infusion may be needed with one-half to one-third the full reversal dose as a drip rate per hour.

Benzodiazepines

✓ CNS depression, respiratory depression, bradycardia, hypotension, hypothermia, and hyporeflexia.

✓ Screen for paracetamol and alcohol toxicity as well.

✓ **Treatment:** Flumazenil is antidote. Activated charcoal is not of much use as drugs are already absorbed.

- **Flumazenil** is a reversible competitive inhibitor of benzodiazepines.
  - ❖ Administered slowly (0.2 mg/min up to 3–5 mg) as large doses may cause agitation and withdrawal.
  - ❖ Flumazenil has a short half-life (0.7–1.3 h) and re-sedation is common.
  - ❖ *A risk of seizure exists in patients taking cyclic antidepressants or with chronic use of benzodiazepines.*
  - ❖ Contraindicated in patients with increased ICP and history of epilepsy.

Barbiturates

✓ Hypotension, respiratory depression, ataxia, incoordination, nystagmus, slurred speech, hyporeflexia, altered level of consciousness, coma.

✓ **Treatment:** Airway management and ventilation.

- Alkaline diuresis for long-acting barbiturates. Haemodialysis for phenobarbital poisoning.

CARDIAC MEDICATION POISONING

✓ **Calcium channel blocker (CCBs) toxicity**

- CCBs affect L-type channels in cardiac myocytes, vascular smooth muscle and beta islet cells.
- Bradycardia, AV block, junctional rhythm, hypotension, ***profound hyperglycaemia.***

✓ **Beta-blockers**

- Toxic dose is two to three times the recommended daily dose.
- Bradycardia, AV heart block, hypotension, ***bronchospasm,*** *hypoglycaemia*, altered mental status, seizure, and coma.

✓ **Common treatment for CCBs and beta-blockers**[Q]: *GI decontamination with activated charcoal.*

- **Early use of vasoactive medications** like noradrenaline, adrenaline, isoprenaline and vasopressin.
- ***Calcium chloride:*** *10 mL of CaCl2 over 2 to 3 min with additional boluses every 5 to 10 min along with infusion of 10% CaCl2 at 10 mL/h.*
- **Glucagon** (3–5 mg stat IV) increases intracellular cAMP and has inotropic and chronotropic effect independent of beta-receptors.
- **Haemodialysis is not a good option as CCBs are highly protein bound with a large volume of distribution.**
  - ❖ Haemodialysis is not beneficial for beta-blockers as well. Hydrophilic agents like sotalol or atenolol can be haemodialyzed.
- **Hyperinsulinaemic euglycaemia therapy (HIET)**[Q]: Indicated in myocardial dysfunction.
  - ❖ **Mechanism of action:** It allows the heart to overcome the metabolic starvation. CCBs prevent blockage of insulin

release. Insulin release is important for better uptake of carbohydrates by heart during stress instead of normally used free fatty acids.

- ❖ **Insulin:** Bolus of 1 U/kg followed by infusion of 1 U/kg/h. Titrated to rates of 10 U/kg/h.
- ❖ **Glucose:** 50 mL of 50% dextrose is given followed by infusion of 1 mL/kg/h of 50% dextrose.
- **Pacing,** IABP in refractory cases.
- **20% Lipid emulsion has also shown good effect.**
- **VA-ECMO has been used as well.**

Digoxin Toxicity

- ✓ **Narrow therapeutic index.** Acute GI upset precedes neurological symptoms.
- ✓ Neurological symptoms: Colour alteration, blurred vision, diplopia, delirium.
- ✓ *ECG Changes*^{Q}: Classic presentation is **supra-ventricular tachycardia and slow ventricular response**.
  - All kind of ECG changes are seen with PVCs (ventricular bigeminy/trigeminy) being the commonest abnormality.
  - Sinus bradycardia, slow AF, AV block, junctional rhythm, and ventricular tachycardia.
  - Down sloping ST segment with **reverse tick appearance,** inverted or biphasic T waves and shortened QT interval.
- ✓ *Risk factors:* Hypokalaemia^Q, hypomagnesaemia, hypercalcaemia, increased sympathetic activity.
  - ❖ Hyperkalaemia happens as a result of toxicity.
- ✓ Toxic side effects at plasma levels >2.5 µg/L.
- ✓ **Digoxin-specific antibody fragments**^{Q} indicated when
  - At levels >20 µg/L
  - Acute digoxin ingestion >10 mg
  - Bradyarrhythmia not responsive to atropine
  - VT/VF/Cardiac arrest
  - Potassium >5–6 mmol/L
- ✓ **Treatment:** Correct Potassium and discontinue Digitalis.
  - **If haemodynamically unstable:** Use phenytoin or digitalis antibodies if available. No need to check digoxin levels post–use of antibody^Q as the assay measures both digoxin bound to fragments and free digoxin.

- Phenytoin may suppress tachycardia and result in asystole and hence pacing should be kept on standby.

Salicylate Poisoning

- ✓ Causes direct central stimulation of the respiratory centre and uncouples the oxidative phosphorylation inhibiting ATP-dependent reactions.
- ✓ **Levels of toxicity.** Measured after 4 h of ingestion.
  - Mild: 300–500 mg/L
  - Moderate: 500–700 mg/L
  - Severe: >700 mg/L
- ✓ **Tinnitus is an early sign of overdose and indicates mild toxicity.**
  - Tachypnoea, hyperthermia, sweating, dehydration, restlessness, convulsions, cerebral oedema, oliguria, renal failure.
  - **Initial respiratory alkalosis due to direct stimulation of the respiratory centre followed by high anion gap metabolic acidosis^Q.**
  - **Doses and features^Q**
    - ❖ **<150 mg/kg:** No clinical features.
    - ❖ **150–300 mg/kg:** Respiratory alkalosis, tinnitus, sweating.
    - ❖ **>300 mg/kg:** Metabolic acidosis, seizures, coma.
- ✓ **Activated charcoal can be given in first hour.**
  - **Forced urine alkaline diuresis^Q** with urine pH maximum up to 8.
  - **Haemodialysis** should be considered in all patients and is the most effective method. Specific indications^Q are severe metabolic acidosis and levels >700 mg/L.
  - Upper GI endoscopy if enteric coated tablets as they peak up to 12 h.

PSYCHIATRIC AGENT POISONING

- ✓ **TCA Toxicity**
  - **Mechanism of actions^Q**
    - ❖ Inhibits the reuptake of norepinephrine and serotonin
    - ❖ Central and peripheral anti-muscarinic effects
    - ❖ Peripheral alpha-1 adrenergic blockade
    - ❖ Histamine-1 receptors (H-1) blockade
    - ❖ Anti GABA$_A$ receptors blockade
    - ❖ Sodium and L-type calcium channel blockade

- *Block fast-acting Na channels. Heart is affected early in overdose and life-threatening effects are seen early in poisoning (2–6 h).*
- Atropine like anticholinergic effects: Tachycardia, dry mouth, dilated pupils, ataxia, **convulsions,** and drowsiness.
- Vasodilation and orthostatic hypotension.
  - ❖ ECG[Q]: Increased PR interval, broad QRS interval (>100 ms seizure risk, >160 ms VT risk), prolonged QT interval, Brugada type 1 (large coved ST-segment elevations, T wave inversions in leads V1–3, dominant R wave >3 mm in lead aVR and ventricular arrhythmias.
- Increase in plasma pH to achieve alkalosis reduces the free fraction of TCA by up to 20%.
- Treatment[Q]: Oral-activated charcoal within 1 h.
  - ❖ Early intubation and ventilation for compromised GCS.
  - ❖ Cardiac monitoring.
  - ❖ Seizures are terminated with benzodiazepines.
  - ❖ **Sodium bicarbonate[Q]** should be started if seizures, haemodynamic instability, and pH <7.20 or QRS >100 ms or QTc >430 ms.
    - It provides a large amount of sodium to overcome sodium blockade, buffers acidosis and causes urinary alkalinization[Q].
    - Multiple 1–2 mmol/kg boluses f/b 150 mEq of NaHCO3 in 1 L of D5W at 2–3 mL/kg/h.
    - Goal should be pH 7.50–7.55.
  - ❖ **Hypertonic saline in refractory cases of hypotension.**
  - ❖ **Magnesium** if arrythmias persist despite bicarbonate.
  - ❖ **Lidocaine and lipid emulsion** can be used for refractory arrythmias.
  - ❖ Type 1a and 1c antiarrhythmics[Q] should be avoided as they act on sodium channels.
- ✓ **Acute SSRI toxicity**
  - Often benign overdose.
  - SSRIs in excess can themselves cause symptoms due to anticholinergic effects like dizziness, dilated pupils, tremors, and agitation.

- ❖ Citalopram and escitalopram can cause QRS and QT prolongation and seizures.
- ❖ Symptoms of hyponatraemia due to SIADH-like effects.
- **Treatment:** Activated charcoal. Supportive management.
- ✓ **Acute neuroleptic toxicity**
  - CNS depression and coma. These agents can cause seizures.
    - ❖ Extrapyramidal effects such as acute dystonic reactions can occur.
    - ❖ Prolonged QT interval, AV block, sinus and ventricular tachycardia and asystole.
    - ❖ Hypotension can happen due to the alpha-adrenergic blocking effect.
  - **Treatment:** Activated charcoal.
    - ❖ Benzodiazepines for agitation. Anti-delirium drugs like dexmedetomidine or clonidine.
- ✓ **Lithium toxicity**
  - Recommended levels: 0.6–1.5 mEq/L.
    - ❖ Severe toxicity: >3.5 mEq/L.
  - 100% absorption via gastrointestinal tract.
  - **Long-term therapy with lithium causes:** Goitre, leucocytosis, nephrogenic DI.
  - **Risk factors for chronic lithium toxicity[Q]:** Dehydration, renal impairment, DI, hypothyroid, thiazide diuretics, ACE inhibitors, ARBs.
  - **Acute intoxication**
    - ❖ Neurological: Fine tremor, fasciculations, muscle weakness, ataxia, delirium, hyperthermia.
    - ❖ Gastrointestinal tract: Ileus, diarrhoea.
    - ❖ Cardiovascular: Bradycardia, hypotension, long QT.
  - **Haemodialysis if levels >4 mEq/L or levels >2.5 mEq/L in patients with renal impairment.**
    - ❖ Activated charcoal is ineffective.

LOCAL ANAESTHETIC SYSTEMIC TOXICITY

- ✓ Local anaesthetic systemic toxicity (LAST): Local anaesthetics block sodium channels leading to conduction disturbances in neurons.
- ✓ **Clinical features:** Neurological symptoms precede cardiovascular symptoms.
  - **Neurological:** *Perioral tingling*, metallic taste, tinnitus, agitation, seizures.

- **Cardiovascular:** Hypotension, brady-cardia, AV blocks, asystole, ventricular tachycardia.
✓ **Risk factors**
  - **Local anaesthetic related:** Bupivacaine is more toxic than levobupivacaine. Bupi-vacaine has a cardiovascular collapse/induction of seizures (CC/CNS ratio) of 2 compared to 7.1 for lidocaine.
  - **Block related:** Topical anaesthesia and intercostal blocks > caudal > epi-dural > brachial plexus > subcutaneous injection^Q.
    ❖ Continuous infusion can lead to LAST.
  - **Patient related:** Comorbidities of liver and kidney can decrease metabolism. Elderly and paediatric patients have low metabolism.
✓ **Prevention**
  - **Pre-procedure:** Thorough risk assessment of patient's comorbidities.
    ❖ Correct dose calculation.
  - **Intra-procedure:** Stop before you block, frequent aspiration.
  - **Post-procedure:** Clear labelling of catheters and non-luer lock connections.
✓ **Treatment**
  - Stop the injection.
  - **Airway:** Immediate oxygenation to prevent hypoxia and acidosis can reduce the pro-gression to seizures.
  - **Breathing:** Hyperventilation to correct acidosis temporarily.
  - **Circulation:** Prolonged CPR may be required in these cases.
    ❖ Large doses of adrenaline are avoided.
    ❖ Vasopressin is avoided as it can cause pulmonary haemorrhage.
    ❖ Amiodarone for ventricular arrhyth-mias as well.
  - **Disability:** Seizures managed with benzodiazepines.
✓ **Intralipid^Q:** 20% Lipid emulsion used in LAST.
  - Dose: 1.5 mg/kg bolus followed by infu-sion at 0.25 mL/kg/min. 2 more boluses at 5-minute intervals (Total 3 boluses). Increase infusion rate to 0.5 mL/kg/min.
  - Propofol is not a suitable substitute as it can cause cardiovascular toxicity.

METHAEMOGLOBINAEMIA

✓ **Methaemoglobinaemia:** (So many questions from this topic that I decided to create a sepa-rate section for it to emphasize its importance.)
  - **Methaemoglobin (MetHb)** is produced when ferrous (Fe^{2+}) is oxidized to ferric (Fe^{3+})^Q. MetHb does not bind oxygen and leads to tissue hypoxia.
  - **Causes:** Nitrates, local anaesthetics, aniline dyes, dapsone, antimalarials, **sulpha drugs, valproic acid, and phenytoin.**
    ❖ Topical EMLA cream with lignocaine and **prilocaine^Q** has been implicated as well.
  - Saturation fixed at 85%^{Q}. **Co-oximetry** is needed to find the real saturation levels. **Cyanosis** develops unresponsive to 100% oxygen. Blood samples are chocolate brown in colour.
    ❖ **<20%** asymptomatic
    ❖ **20–30%:** Headache and weakness
    ❖ **30–50%:** Dyspnoea, nausea, chest pain and anxiety
    ❖ **>60%:** Reduced consciousness, metabolic acidosis, arrhythmias, and seizures
    ❖ **>70%:** Lethal
  - **Methylene blue^Q** is antidote, 1 mg/kg. Methylene blue is c/I in G-6 PD deficiency.
    ❖ Exchange transfusion is one of the options if methaemoglobinaemia >35%.
  - High dose of riboflavin.

SNAKEBITE

Epidemiology and Aetiology

✓ Majority of snakebites are by non-venomous snakes.
✓ In UK the only indigenous venomous snake is the adder^Q or *Vipera berus*.
  - Mortality from adder bites is low but is more common in children.
  - Males have been bitten more than females by snakes.

Clinical Features and Diagnosis

✓ Venom can be having multiple effects.
  - **Tissue destruction:** Local tissue necrosis and muscle necrosis.
  - **Neurotoxic:** Neuromuscular blockade lead-ing to cardiac and respiratory failure.

- **Thrombogenic:** Clot formation and plasmin activation.
✓ **Local envenoming:** Venom injection into skin and subcutaneous tissues leading to pain, paraesthesia, erythema, and lymph nodes enlargement.
  - **Systemic envenoming**: Venom in blood. Fever, rash, vomiting, tachycardia, angioedema, and bronchospasm.

Treatment

✓ **Prehospital:** Limb should be immobilized with splints. Tourniquets should be avoided.
✓ **Hospital:** Observe the patient in hospital for local swelling for at least 2 h.
  - Clean the bite site.
  - Give anti-tetanus prophylaxis as required.
✓ **Indications for anti-snake venom (ASV)** are hypotension, signs of systemic envenoming.
✓ **Anti-snake venom (ASV):** Local infiltration isn't recommended as it can cause necrosis. Early reaction to ASV is by anaphylaxis. Late reaction is like serum sickness (lymphadenopathy). Steroids may not be useful to early reaction and adrenaline might be needed.
  - ASV is polyvalent refined immunoglobin.
  - Venom bound to tissue will have no effect by ASV.

Specific Snakes

✓ **Krait bite:** Neurotoxic: Venom has effect on pre- as well as post-synaptic site.
  - Patient has no swelling or bite mark. Hence patient brought in the morning after being bitten at night.
  - Neostigmine is of no use as pre-synapses involved as well.
  - Paralysis of flexors of muscles of the neck giving the broken neck sign.
    - ❖ **It can cause fixed, dilated non-reactive pupils simulating brainstem death, however, can recover fully^Q.**
    - ❖ Ptosis is one of the early manifestations of Krait bite. Causes diplopia and dysphagia.
  - Requires smaller doses of ASV.
✓ **Cobra bite:** Sharp burning pain at the bite site and neurological complications like ptosis.
  - Visible fang marks.
  - Low doses of ASV are required.

✓ **Viper bite:** Vasculo-toxic complications
  - Incidence of renal failure is higher with viper bite.
  - Viper requires higher doses of ASV.
  - Vasculo-toxic cases have multisystem involvement, but they present late to hospital.
  - Late ASV can be given if features are still present at a week.
  - Viper requires higher doses of ASV.
  - Spontaneous bleeding by viper bite will stop in an hour and coagulation reverts to normal within 6–12 h.

ENVIRONMENTAL POISONS

Chemical agents: Accidental poisoning or used for warfare.
✓ **Classification:** Classified based on their mechanism of actions and physiological effects.
  - **Nerve agents:** Most toxic. Organophosphorus compounds
  - **Vesicants/blistering agents:** Sulphur mustard, lewisite
  - **Cyanide/blood agents**
  - **Pulmonary/choking agents:** Phosgene and chlorine
  - **Non-lethal incapacitating agents:** 3-quinuclidinyl benzilate (BZ), 2-chloro-1-phenylethanone (CN)
✓ **Organophosphate poisoning**
  - Apart from weapons, they are used in insecticides as well.
  - Absorbed through skin, lungs, and GIT. They bind to acetylcholinesterase^Q and increases the amount of acetylcholine at receptors.
  - **Acute cholinergic toxicity**
    - ❖ **SLUDGE^Q:** Salivation, lacrimation, urination, defecation, gastric distress, and emesis.
    - ❖ Bradycardia, miosis, bronchospasm is also seen.
  - **Treatment:** Decontamination of the patient.
    - ❖ Early intubation and ventilation is needed for respiratory failure.
    - ❖ Use **atropine** initially with 1–2 mg intramuscularly and double every 5 min until secretions and bronchospasm is cleared. Atropine doesn't bind to nicotinic receptors.

❖ **Pralidoxime**[Q] reactivates acetylcholinesterase and should be given early.

❖ AChE aging is rapid with dimethyl phosphate compounds and oximes therapy may not be beneficial.

❖ Diethyl organophosphate poisoning benefits from oxime up to 5 d.

❖ If Oxime therapy terminated early, it can lead to intermediate syndrome (neck flexion and proximal muscle weakness, cranial nerve abnormalities).

❖ **Diazepam** should be given for seizures.

✓ **Sulphur mustard**

- Oily liquid that is yellow to dark brown in colour. Evaporates at temperature above 100° F and causes damages.

- Mustard alkylates and cross links DNA leading to cell death.

- **Presentation:** Causes vesicae and bullae on contacting the skin, conjunctivitis, necrosis of mucus membranes of airway, gastrointestinal tract, and bone marrow.

- **Treatment:** Decontamination and ABCDE approach.

  ❖ Supportive treatment with calamine lotion and topical steroids for skin, bronchodilators, N-acetyl cysteine and systemic corticosteroids for respiratory care.

✓ **Cyanide toxicity**

- Apart from being a chemical warfare agent, it is found in pesticides, tobacco smoke, burning of vinyl or polyurethane (plastic furniture burning in a closed room) and sodium nitroprusside (5 cyanide groups per molecule).

- Binds to cytochrome oxidase within the mitochondria and blocks aerobic respiration.

- **Clinical features:** Abdominal pain, delirium, muscle spasms and restlessness, metabolic acidosis with lactate production (HAGMA), low arterio-venous oxygen gradient, and haemodynamic deterioration.

- **Treatment:** 100% oxygen.

  ❖ Hydroxy cobalamin[Q] (5g over 15 min) binds cyanide to produce cyanocobalamin which is renally excreted.

  ❖ Sodium thiosulphate (150 mg/kg) given can convert cyanide to thiocyanate which is excreted renally.

✓ **Phosgene**

- Colourless gas at room temperature but become a volatile liquid on cooling or compression.

- **Presentation:** Causes irritation of the eyes, oropharynx and lower airways causing non-cardiogenic pulmonary oedema and bronchospasm.

  ❖ Irritation is due to formation of hydrochloric acid when phosgene reacts with water.

- **Treatment** is decontamination and supportive management.

Radiation agents: Accidental or warfare due to radiologic dispersion devices (dirty bombs) or nuclear weapons.

✓ **Acute radiation syndrome:** Acute illness caused by radiation exposure of the entire body by a high dose of penetrating radiation in a very short period of time.

- **Pathophysiology:** Immature parenchymal stem cells are destroyed.

- **Preconditions**

  ❖ Large dose: >70 rads
  ❖ Source external to body
  ❖ Penetrating: X-rays, gamma rays, and neutrons
  ❖ Entire body
  ❖ Short time

- **Syndromes**

  ❖ **Bone marrow syndrome:** >70 rads. Anorexia, fever, and malaise. Infections and haemorrhage. Dose dependent increase in mortality.

  ❖ **Gastrointestinal syndrome:** >1000 rads. Diarrhoea, fever, dehydration, and electrolyte imbalance. Death within 2 weeks.

  ❖ **CVS/CNS syndrome:** >5000 rads. nervousness, confusion, convulsions, and coma. Death within 3 d mostly.

- **Stages**

  ❖ **Prodromal (Minutes to several days):** NVD stage (nausea, vomiting and diarrhoea).

  ❖ **Latent (hours to weeks):** Patient feels generally healthy.

  ❖ **Manifest illness (hours to months):** Specific symptoms as mentioned above.

  ❖ **Recovery or death:** Die within months or recover over years.

- **Management**
  - ❖ ABC resuscitation with external decontamination.
  - ❖ Treat other traumatic burn and respiratory injuries.
  - ❖ Symptomatic treatment for nausea and vomiting.
  - ❖ **Check lymphocyte count every 2 to 3 h during the first 8 h and every 4–6 h for first 2 d. Haematopoiesis by growth factors/stem cell transplant may be needed.**
  - ❖ Check HLA typing prior to any transfusion.
  - ❖ Supportive care in an environment that is suitable for **neutropenic patients.**
  - ❖ Psychological support.

Biological agents: Accidental release or used as biological weapons of mass destruction.

✓ Centers for Disease Control and Prevention (CDC) categorizes potential bioterrorism agents based on their severity, availability, and potential for widespread harm. Category A has the highest potential for mass casualties.

Category A	Category B	Category C
• *Bacillus anthracis* (anthrax)	• *Coxiella burnetii*	• Nipah virus
• *Yersinia pestis* (plague)	• (Q fever)	• Hantavirus
• Variola virus	• *Brucella species*	• Tickborne haemorrhagic fever viruses
• (smallpox)	• (brucellosis)	• Yellow fever
• *Clostridium botulinum*	• *Burkholderia mallei*	• MDR TB
• (botulism)	• (glanders)	
• *Francisella tularensis* (tularaemia)	• Ricin	
	• *Clostridium perfringens*	
	• Epsilon toxin	
	• Staphylococcal enterotoxin B	

✓ **Smallpox:** Although eradicated, remains a potential biological warfare agent and vaccination of military personnel is done.

✓ **Anthrax:** Gram-positive, spore-forming bacillus.
  - • Three manifestations mainly
    - ❖ **Cutaneous:** 95% of cases. Painless pruritic papule followed by ulceration.
    - ❖ **Gastrointestinal:** Ingestion of contaminated meat. Fever, mucosal ulcers, GI bleeding, and sepsis.
    - ❖ **Inhalational:** Fever, cough, chest pain, and dyspnoea.
  - • **Treatment:** Fluroquinolones plus carbapenem combination is used for systemic anthrax.

✓ **Plague:** Zoonosis with rats as natural reservoirs. Transmitted by a plague-infected flea.
  - • Secretes endotoxin like other Gram-negative bacilli and causes sepsis, acute respiratory distress syndrome and multiorgan failure.
  - • Three manifestations mainly
    - ❖ **Bubonic:** Lymphadenitis and local swelling called bubo.
    - ❖ **Septicaemic:** Haematogenous spread with seeding of spleen, liver, and mucus membranes.
    - ❖ **Pneumonic:** Inhalation of droplets. Pneumonia-like features.
  - • **Treatment:** Doxycycline is the first line of treatment for bubonic plague. Fluroquinolones for pneumonic and septicaemic version.

✓ **Ricin:** Toxin that inhibits ribosomes and is extracted from castor plant, Ricinus communis.
  - • Routes of administration are parenteral, gastrointestinal, and inhalational.
  - • **Presentation:** Symptoms are flulike illness with fevers, myalgias, arthralgia along with pulmonary oedema, hallucinations, and seizures.
    - ❖ Ricin can cause type I and IV hypersensitivity syndromes as well.
  - • **Treatment:** Decontamination by removing all clothing and washing. Treatment is mostly supportive.

Heavy metal toxicity: Occupational exposure or consuming food that contains these elements.

✓ **Pathophysiology:** DNA damage, peroxidation of cell membrane lipids, protein denaturation due to free radical generated by them.

✓ **Arsenic:** Poisoning due to industrial processes or accidental ingestion or due to suicidal or homicidal intent.
  - • Enters in human body by ingestion and inhalation. Arsenic is bound to proteins in the blood. Metabolized by liver and kidney.
  - • **Symptoms:** GI tract affected mostly. Burning sensation in the mouth and throat.

Metallic taste and garlicky odour.

❖ Haemorrhagic gastroenteritis can lead to hypovolemic shock.

❖ Arrhythmias with QTc prolongation, bone marrow suppression (has been used for treatment of leukaemias), confusion, delirium, convulsions, encephalopathy, stocking and glove neuropathy, and coma.

- **Treatment:** Gastric lavage. Supportive therapy. Dimercaprol also known as BAL (British anti-lewisite) is used for chelation. Dimercaptosuccinic acid (DMSA) can be used as well.

✓ **Lead:** Poisoning due to vehicle exhaust, paint, food, and water.

- Enters in human body by ingestion and inhalation. All lead in the blood is located within RBCs and from RBCs transferred to soft tissues and bones.

- **Symptoms:** Acute ingestion of large dose causes **abdominal pain**^{Q}, toxic hepatitis, and anaemia^Q.

  ❖ Chronic exposure leads to fatigue, arthralgias, decreased libido, depression, weight loss, insomnia.

  ❖ **Encephalopathy** and peripheral nerve involvement causing lead palsy.

- **Treatment:** Gastric lavage. Supportive therapy.

  ❖ BAL and Calcium EDTA are used for lead encephalopathy.

  ❖ DMSA can be used as well.

✓ **Mercury:** Poisoning due to occupational hazards like battery makers, miners, explosive makers.

- Inhalation is the main form of entry. Elemental mercury ingestion in patients with bowel abnormality mostly. Organic and inorganic compounds absorbed from GIT.

- **Symptoms:** Inhaled mercury acts like an irritant and a cellular poison. Fever, chills, headache, dyspnoea, metallic taste, chest tightness, and abdominal cramping.

  ❖ Neuropsychiatric disturbances like tremors.

- **Treatment:** Supportive therapy.

  ❖ BAL, DMSA, and D-penicillamine are used as chelators.

✓ **Iron:** Poisoning due to overdose of iron tablets.

- Ingestion is the main form of toxicity. Tablets are radiopaque and can be confirmed by chest/abdominal X-ray.

- **Symptoms:** Severe abdominal pain, metabolic acidosis, hepatic dysfunction, and CVS instability.

- **Treatment:** Activated charcoal isn't helpful^Q and whole bowel irrigation is recommended.

  ❖ **Desferrioxamine** is used for severe toxicity and when levels >90 mmol/L.

  ❖ PPIs increase stomach pH and decrease absorption of iron.

WITHDRAWAL SYNDROMES

✓ **Withdrawal:** Group of symptoms that occur upon abrupt discontinuation or decrease in the intake of the drug.

- Withdrawal can be physical or psychological.

✓ **Ethanol withdrawal**

- Ethanol produces its behavioural effects (euphoria, disinhibition) and physiological effects (slurred speech, ataxia, sedation) by increase in endogenous opiates, potentiating the inhibitory GABA receptor and inhibiting NMDA receptors.

  ❖ Alcohol also increases the affinity of 5-HT receptors to the agonists.

- **Classification of withdrawal symptoms**

  ❖ **Mild withdrawal:** Hyperadrenergic state with↑ HR,↑ BP and tremors seen 6–8 h after the last ethanol intake. Peak between 24 and 36 h and 80% patients recover uneventfully.

  ❖ **Moderate withdrawal:** Seizures are very common. Short, generalized, tonic–clonic seizures. Status epilepticus is uncommon and suggests another diagnosis.

  ❖ **Severe withdrawal:** *Delirium tremens:* Life-threatening late manifestation of ethanol. Starts 3 to 5 d later and characterized by hallucinations (mainly visual, auditory in 20% cases), delusions, tremors, psychomotor disturbances (like picking at bedclothes, agitation).

- **Diagnostic evaluation:** Hypoglycaemia, hyponatraemia, hypomagnesaemia needs to be ruled out as potential causes of seizures.

  ❖ Differentials: Meningitis, intracranial bleeds, thyroid storm, pheochromocytoma, serotonin syndrome, neuroleptic malignant syndrome, sympathomimetic agent poisoning, anticholinergic agents, MAO inhibitors.

- **Management**
  - ❖ Initial ABCDE approach.
  - ❖ IV 100 mg Thiamine[Q] and 50 grams glucose.
  - ❖ Sedation with benzodiazepines like diazepam, chlordiazepoxide and lorazepam. High doses may be required.
  - ❖ Short-acting benzodiazepine like lorazepam and oxazepam should be used in patients with severe liver dysfunction[Q].
  - ❖ Second GABAergic agent may be needed in cases requiring high doses of diazepam (like 40 mg in first hour). Phenobarbital and propofol have been used.
  - ❖ Ketamine (NMDA antagonist), Dexmedetomidine and clonidine (alpha-2 agonists) have been used as agents as well.
  - ❖ Phenytoin is ineffective for the prevention or treatment of ethanol withdrawal seizures.
- ✓ **Benzodiazepine withdrawal**
  - Seen more commonly in patients who have been taking higher than recommended doses.
    - ❖ Short-acting agents like lorazepam or alprazolam may present with withdrawal symptoms after 24 h of cessation whereas diazepam withdrawal may present with up to 8 d after stoppage of drug.
    - ❖ Acute withdrawal symptoms for up to 1–2 wk.
    - ❖ **Flumazenil[Q]** can lead to seizures due to reversal of anticonvulsant effect of benzodiazepines in the presence of proconvulsive drugs or other predispositions to seizures.
  - Signs of symptoms of CNS excitation and autonomic hyperactivity like ethanol withdrawal are seen with **sympathetic hyperactivity.**
  - **Treatment:** Reintroduction of the drug is needed with slower withdrawal over 2 to 4 wk.
    - ❖ Longer-acting agents like diazepam are preferred during withdrawal reactions.
    - ❖ Barbiturates, beta-blockers, clonidine have been used as well.
- ✓ **Opioid withdrawal**
  - Stimulation of opioid receptors decreases catecholamine release. Hence withdrawal leads to increased sympathetic discharge.
    - ❖ However, manifestations of opioid withdrawal are rarely life-threatening.
  - ❖ Withdrawal from heroin occurs around 12 h later whereas withdrawal from methadone happens around 48 h later. Withdrawal symptoms are more intense with shorter-acting agents.
  - ❖ Iatrogenic withdrawal in ICU patients on prolonged opioid infusions can prolong weaning from ventilators.
- **Signs and symptoms:** Mydriasis, lacrimation, rhinorrhoea, diaphoresis, yawning, piloerection, and anxiety.
  - ❖ Fever, seizures, and altered mental status are uncommon symptoms.
  - ❖ Cognitive effects like dysphoria may persist for weeks.
- **Prevention**
  - ❖ Use paracetamol or gabapentin for pain.
  - ❖ Slow (10–20%) reduction in dose rather than abrupt stoppage.
- **Management**
  - ❖ Buprenorphine (partial acting opioid μ receptor agonist and κ receptor antagonist) is used for opioid detoxification and withdrawal.
  - ❖ Methadone has been used for withdrawal of heroin addiction.
  - ❖ Clonidine has been used to treat autonomic hyperactivity symptoms of opioid withdrawal.
- ✓ **Nicotine withdrawal**
  - Nicotine binds nicotine acetylcholine receptors and induces their upregulation.
  - **Signs and symptoms:** Agitation, anxiety, insomnia, and bradycardia. Symptoms start 1–2 d after last use, peak within first week and persist for 2–4 wk.
  - Role of nicotine replacement therapy in withdrawal is controversial as some studies have shown increased mortality.
- ✓ **Stimulant withdrawal**
  - Cocaine and amphetamines work by increasing the activity of dopamine, norepinephrine, and serotonin in the body.
    - ❖ Withdrawal symptoms are mostly due to depletion of these neurotransmitters.
  - Fatigue, sleepiness, depression, anxiety are seen 6–12 h after the last dose. Symptoms are not life-threatening.
  - **Treatment:** Symptomatic management with benzodiazepines for anxiety and restlessness.

13

Obstetrics

HYPERTENSIVE DISEASE OF PREGNANCY

Epidemiology

✓ **Hypertension:** American College of Obstetricians and Gynecologists (ACOG) define hypertension in pregnancy as systolic blood pressure (SBP) ≥140 mmHg and diastolic blood pressure (DBP) ≥90 mmHg or both, ideally confirmed on two occasions or at least 4 h apart.

- **Chronic hypertension:** Hypertension presenting before 20 wk gestation.
- **Gestational hypertension:** New onset hypertension that develops after 20 wk gestation without any features of pre-eclampsia.
- **Pre-eclampsia[Q]:** Hypertension (140/90 mmHg) developing after 20 wk of gestation with presence of significant proteinuria [a urine protein/creatinine ratio of ≥30 mg/mmol, albumin: creatinine ratio (ACR) ≥8 mg/mol or both].
  - ❖ **Severe pre-eclampsia[Q]:** Pre-eclampsia with **BP ≥160/110** mmHg along with signs of end organ damage.
    - **Liver derangement** (ALT or AST >70 IU/L, right upper quadrant, vomiting, liver tenderness)
    - *Renal insufficiency* (doubling of the serum creatinine concentration in the absence of other renal disease)
    - **Neurological issues:** Severe headache, visual disturbance, papilledema, clonus
    - *Haematological impairment* (platelets <100 × 109/L)
    - **HELLP syndrome**

- **Eclampsia:** Seizure occurs because of preeclampsia.

Pathophysiology: Abnormal placental implantation in the first trimester.

✓ **Risk factors[Q]**
- Prior pre-eclampsia
- Chronic hypertension
- Maternal BMI >30
- Pregestational DM
- Antiphospholipid syndrome
- Primigravida
- Advanced maternal age ≥40 yr
- Multigravidas with a new partner
- Multiple gestation

Clinical Features and Diagnosis

✓ **Clinical features:** Frontal headache, nausea and vomiting, abdominal pain, visual disturbances, shortness of breath, sudden swelling of face and limbs.

✓ **HELLP (Haemolysis, elevated liver enzymes, low platelet) syndrome:** Presents with gastrointestinal symptoms.
- Headache and visual disturbances may also be present.
- HELLP syndrome is normally a mild variant.
- Normally occurs after 28 wk of gestation but can happen as early as 22 wk in patients with antiphospholipid syndrome. TTP can present anytime during pregnancy.
- Schistocytes and elevated LDH. It can occur without proteinuria or hypertension.
- Dexamethasone or plasma exchange may be needed in severe cases.

DOI: 10.1201/9781003476214-13

✓ Patient can present straight with eclampsia without preceding preeclampsia.
  • Eclampsia describes grand-mal seizures. Seizures are usually short-lived and self-terminate.

Prevention

✓ **Aspirin:** NICE recommends that women at high risk of developing pre-eclampsia should be given aspirin 75–150 mg daily from 12 wk until the birth of the baby.
✓ **Calcium:** Calcium supplementation (>1 g/day) can lower the chances of developing pre-eclampsia.

Treatment

✓ **Delivery of baby**^{Q} is definitive management and neuraxial anaesthesia is the preferred mode.
✓ **Pre-eclampsia:** A sustained BP ≥140/90 mmHg, warrants treatment, targeting a BP ≤135/85 mmHg.
  • Main aim of controlling the maternal BP is the prevention of intracerebral haemorrhage.
  • Oral labetalol^Q initially to control blood pressure, followed by Nifedipine^Q and then Methyldopa^Q as alternatives.
  • Women with severe pre-eclampsia should be admitted to hospital.
✓ **Severe pre-eclampsia:** Treatment in high dependency unit (HDU).
  • **Intravenous labetalol** starting with 20 mg IV given over 2 min and increasing incrementally up to 80 mg IV.
  • **IV Hydralazine** 5–10 mg IV over 2 min can be given followed by a further 10 mg IV after 20 min if the BP remains high.
  • **IV infusion of glyceryl trinitrate (GTN):** 5–100 µg/min can be used for acute pulmonary oedema.
  • **Fluid restriction** (80 mL/h), urine output (>100 mL/4 h), and invasive haemodynamic monitoring. Pulmonary oedema can happen even with small fluid boluses.
  • **Diuretics (Furosemide) should be considered in patients with euvolemic oliguria.** RRT may be needed. Kidneys improve following delivery.
  • **HELLP:** If no rupture of liver haematoma, don't do laparotomy or drainage. Give blood and blood products.

✓ **Eclampsia:** Eclamptic seizures are usually self-limiting.
  • In a pre-eclamptic woman with persistent neurological symptoms or signs like (severe headache, signs of cerebral irritability, clonus, or visual disturbance), **magnesium sulphate** is the first line of treatment for prevention of eclamptic seizures^Q.
    ❖ Magnesium antagonizes calcium channels^Q and prevents cerebral vasospasm.
    ❖ It inhibits platelet aggregation by increasing release of prostacyclin from endothelium.
    ❖ Side effects^Q of magnesium therapy are bradycardia, areflexia^Q (at levels of 4–6 mmol/L), and respiratory depression.
  • Load with magnesium^Q 4 g bolus over 5 min followed by infusion of 1 g/h and deep tendon reflexes should be monitored throughout treatment as they can get diminished.
    ❖ Any further seizures should be treated with a bolus dose of 2 gram over 5 min.
  • Target serum magnesium range is 2–4 mmol/L.
  • Deliver the baby once patient stabilized and steroids have been given.

Prognosis

✓ Post-partum hypertension can persist for up to 6–8 wk.
✓ Lifelong follow-up as they are at increased risk of hypertension.

MAJOR OBSTETRIC HAEMORRHAGE

Aetiology

✓ Uterine blood flow at term is 600–900 mL/min and uncontrolled bleeding from the uteroplacental bed is the commonest cause (27%) of maternal death worldwide and the most common cause of admission to critical care.
  • Blood loss ≤500 mL after a vaginal delivery or ≤1000 mL after caesarean section is normal.
✓ **Antepartum haemorrhage (APH):** Bleeding from the genital tract after the 24th week of pregnancy.
  • **Major APH:** Bleeding of 50–1000 mL with no signs of shock (RCOG).

- **Massive APH:** Bleeding ≥1000 mL and/or bleeding of any volume with clinical signs of shock (RCOG).
✓ **Causes of APH:** Placenta previa, placental abruption, uterine rupture, and bleeding from the vulva.
✓ **Post-partum haemorrhage (PPH):** American College of Obstetricians and Gynecologists (ACOG) defines PPH as being ≥1000 mL blood loss within 24 h with or without associated clinical signs of hypovolaemia.
  - **Primary post-partum haemorrhage:** Within the 24 h after delivery. *The commonest cause of primary post-partum haemorrhage is uterine atony.*
  - **Secondary PPH:** From 24 h after delivery to 12 wk post-partum. It is caused by infection or retained products of conception.
✓ **Causes for post-partum haemorrhage:** 4Ts.
  - **Tone:** Uterine atony, haematoma
  - **Trauma:** Laceration, uterine rupture/inversion
  - **Tissue:** Retained tissue, invasive placenta
  - **Thrombin:** Coagulopathy
✓ **Risk factors:** Emergency caesarean section, prolonged labour, multiple pregnancy, polyhydramnios, macrosomia, obesity, intrapartum sepsis, and uterine inversion.

Clinical Features

✓ **Antepartum haemorrhage:** Obvious vaginal bleeding, concealed vaginal bleeding, shock in mother, abnormal/pathological CTG, haematuria.
✓ **Post-partum haemorrhage:** Vaginal bleeding and signs and symptoms of shock.
✓ **Kleihauer–Betke test:** Blood test used during pregnancy to screen maternal blood for the presence of fetal blood cells. A positive test indicates a risk for stillbirth.

Prevention and Treatment

✓ **Blood loss ≥1000 mL ± signs of hypovolaemia:** Major obstetric haemorrhage call
  - Lie the woman flat and 100% oxygen through a non-rebreathing mask. Alert haematologist, blood transfusion laboratory and consultant obstetrician on call.
✓ **Resuscitation:** 2 wide bore 14/16-gauge cannulas with blood taken or full blood count, renal

function, clotting (including fibrinogen) and cross matching.
  - Rapid resuscitation by 2 L of warm fluids followed by blood products (RBCs, fresh frozen plasma, and platelets).
  - Set up a rapid blood infuser.
  - O-negative blood in cases of life-threatening haemorrhage.
  - **Fresh frozen plasma (FFP):** 12–15 mL/kg and two packs of cryoprecipitate can be given for every 4 units of red blood cells.
  - **Transfusion targets:** Hb >70 g/L, Platelets >75 × 10^9/L, PT/INR <1.5, **Fibrinogen >2 g/L^Q**, Ca^{2+} >1.13 mmol/L.
  - **Point of care testing:** ROTEM or TEG are very helpful in guiding treatment of coagulopathies.
  - **Tranexamic Acid (TXA)** 1 gram b bolus followed by another 1-gram bolus after 30 min.
✓ **Uterotonic drugs:** First-line management is IV oxytocin 5 IU bolus followed by 5 IU bolus. Infusion @ 40 IU over 4 h.
  - Ergometrine 250–500 µg IM. Carboprost (prostaglandin F$_{2\alpha}$ agonist) 250 µg IM to a maximum of 2 mg.
  - Misoprostol (Prostaglandin E$_1$ agonist) 600 µg PR.
✓ **Surgical interventions:** Manual massage, manual removal of placenta, uterine packing with Bakri balloon, B-lynch compression sutures, and hysterectomy as last resort.
✓ Interventional radiology for uterine artery ligation.
✓ Antibiotic prophylaxis may need to be repeated if blood loss >1500 mL.

MATERNAL SEPSIS

Epidemiology and Aetiology

✓ **WHO definition:** Life-threatening condition characterized by organ dysfunction resulting from infection during pregnancy, childbirth, after abortion or the post-partum period.
  - Incidence is 0.04%–0.1% in pregnant and post-partum patients.
  - **Sepsis^Q** is one of the leading causes of direct maternal death in developed nations with up to a quarter of maternal deaths are caused by sepsis or complications of sepsis.

❖ **Thrombosis and thromboembolism**[Q] was the leading cause of maternal death during and up to six weeks after pregnancy in 2021–2023.

  ❖ **Cardiac disease** is the leading indirect cause.

✓ **Causes:** Pneumonia, (MC in pregnant women), infections of the genital or urinary tracts (MC in post-partum women), chorioamnionitis, endometritis.

✓ **Pathogens:** *Escherichia coli*, Staphylococcus, **Group A *Streptococcus* (GAS)**, and other Gram-negative bacteria found in gastrointestinal tract.

✓ **Risk factors**

- **Obstetric factors:** Preterm delivery, premature rupture of membranes, multiple gestation, induction of labour, instrumental vaginal delivery, caesarean delivery, postpartum haemorrhage.
- **Medical factors:** Anaemia, congestive heart failure, chronic liver and kidney disease, obesity.
- **Demographic factors:** African American race, deprivation.

Clinical Features and Diagnosis

✓ Physiological changes associated with pregnancy mimic the haemodynamic shifts cause by sepsis.

- Maternal early warning systems are more effective tools to evaluate maternal sepsis than qSOFA and SIRS.
- Fetal heart monitoring may serve as an important physiological monitor.

✓ **UK Obstetric Surveillance System (UKOSS):** Diagnosis of sepsis if two or more of the following.

- Ventilatory frequency >20 bpm, twice with measurements at least 4 h apart.
- Heart rate >100 beats/min, twice with measurements at least 4 h apart.
- Temperature <36°C or >38°C, twice with measurements at least 4 h apart.
- WBCs >17 × 10⁹/L or <4 × 10⁹/L or with immature bands, with measurements on two different blood samples.

✓ **Genital tract sepsis:** Fever, diarrhoea, vomiting, abdominal pain, vaginal discharge, and wound infection.

- Puerperal sepsis caused by GAS is commonly preceded by a sore throat.

- Typical rash of GAS develops over 12–48 h.
- Erythematous rash appears on chest and axillae followed by spread to the trunk and extremities.
- Rash disappears with pressure unlike the petechial rash typical of meningococcal septicaemia.

✓ **Non-obstetric sepsis:** Urinary tract infections or pyelonephritis, pneumonia, appendicitis, cholecystitis, meningitis.

✓ **Imaging:** Abdominal ultrasound for retained products of conceptions or abdominal collection, chest X-ray, CT scan of the chest, abdomen, and pelvis.

Management

✓ **Multi-professional approach:** Intensive care specialists, anaesthetists, obstetricians, microbiologists, and haematologists.

✓ **Surviving Sepsis Campaign (SSC 2021)** recommends early diagnosis using a ***standardized screening tool.***

✓ 100% Oxygen to keep saturation above 94%, blood cultures and wound swabs, serum lactates and monitoring of urine output.

✓ **Fluid resuscitation:** 30 mL/kg within first 3 h from the diagnosis of sepsis. Vasopressor administration should be used for hypotension.

✓ ***Broad-spectrum antibiotics*** should be administered within the first hour as with sepsis in non-pregnant female.

- **Community-acquired pneumonia:** Ceftriaxone 1–2 g IV q24h.
- **Urinary tract infections:** Ceftriaxone 1–2 g IV q24h.
- **Endometritis:** Gentamicin 1.5 mg/kg bolus followed by 1 mg/kg IV q8h + Clindamycin 900 mg IV q8h.
- **Chorioamnionitis:** Ampicillin 2 g IV q6h + gentamicin 1.5 mg/kg IV q8h.
- **Skin and soft tissue infections (necrotizing fasciitis):** Vancomycin 15 mg/kg IV bolus followed by infusion + Piperacillin and tazobactam 4.5 g IV q6h + Clindamycin 900 mg IV q8h.
- **Piperacillin and Tazobactam** provides good cover (except MRSA) and should be used for severe disease.
  - ❖ **Co-amoxiclav** doesn't cover MRSA and *Pseudomonas* and concerns about risk of necrotizing enterocolitis in neonates exposed to co-amoxiclav in uterus.

❖ Tetracycline, Tigecycline, and quinolones should be avoided.
❖ **IVIg** is recommended for invasive
streptococcal and staphylococcal
infection.

✓ **Source control:** Within 6–12 h of the diagnosis
of sepsis.

✓ **ECMO:** Rescue therapy for refractory septic
shock complicated by left ventricular dysfunction or failure.

Prognosis

✓ **Group A *Streptococcus* is the reason for 50%
of maternal deaths.**

Additional Questions

✓ New-onset tonic–clonic epilepsy[Q] in female of
childbearing age is treated by Lamotrigine and
folic acid supplementation.

AMNIOTIC FLUID EMBOLISM

Epidemiology

✓ 2 per 100,000 maternities. Case fatality rate
of 19%

✓ **Risk factors:** Maternal age >35 yr, eclampsia,
placenta previa, multiple pregnancy, polyhydramnios, induction of labour by any method,
assisted delivery, caesarean section.

Pathophysiology

✓ **Mechanical theory:** Amniotic fluid containing
fetal squamous cells, meconium, and vernix
caseosa can block the major blood vessels.

✓ **Immune theory:** Immunological activation
secondary to exposure to fetal antigens.

Clinical Features and Diagnosis

✓ Occurs during labour (70% of cases), caesarean
delivery (19%) or up to 48 h post-partum (11%
of cases).
• It has been seen during termination of pregnancy in the first and second trimester.

✓ Acute onset of **obstructive shock (hypotension) leading to cardiac arrest**[Q], hypoxaemia
due to pulmonary oedema, encephalopathy in
the mother.
• **Phase 1**[Q]: Amniotic fluid and fetal cells
enter the maternal circulation. V/P

mismatch because of pulmonary artery
spasm is the commonest cause of hypoxia.
This causes RV failure.
• **Phase 2**[Q]: LV failure follows RV failure.
**Disseminated Intravascular Coagulation
(DIC)**[Q] is very common.

✓ **Diagnosis of AFE** is mainly clinical and that of
exclusion. C3 and C4 complement fractions are
found to be low in these patients.

✓ Fetal distress is seen if it happens before delivery. Babies born to women who had AFE are at
increased risk of hypoxic ischaemic encephalopathy and cerebral palsy.

Prevention and Treatment

✓ Urgent decision to deliver the baby may be needed.

✓ **Supportive management:** Early intubation may
be needed.
• Inotropic support should be started immediately even with concerns of fetal toxicity
or placental hypoperfusion.
• Peripartum evacuation of the uterus must
be performed by the 5th minute.
• Patient may require intra-aortic balloon pump
counter pulsation or ECMO may be needed.

✓ **Haemorrhage control:** Uterine tone by oxytocin, ergometrine and prostaglandins. Intrauterine balloon may be needed. Hysterectomy
should not be delayed if bleeding persists.

✓ **Treatment of coagulopathy** guided by
thromboelastography.
• Massive obstetric haemorrhage protocol
should be activated.
• Hypofibrinogenaemia should be corrected,
and tranexamic acid has been shown to reduce
mortality in post-partum haemorrhage.

Prognosis

✓ High mortality of 60–80%.

ACUTE FATTY LIVER OF PREGNANCY

Aetiology

✓ **Incidence:** 1: 7000 to 1: 20,000 pregnancies.
• Due to deficiency of long-chain 3-hydroxy-
acyl-coenzyme A dehydrogenase.
• Occurs late in pregnancy or first few days
post-partum.

✓ **Risk factors:** Male fetal sex, multiple gestation,
and low BMI.

Clinical Features and Diagnosis

✓ Patients present with non-specific symptoms of nausea and vomiting.
- Raised aminotransferases (5–10 × normal range). *LDH is elevated but not as high as compared to in TTP.*
- Signs and symptoms of acute liver failure like jaundice[Q], ascites, encephalopathy, disseminated intravascular coagulopathy, **hypoglycaemia**[Q], AKI (90% of patients), and multiorgan failure.
- Thrombocytopaenia in early stage and DIC in late stages but is severe. Schistocytes are absent.
- Platelet function remains stable unlike in HELLP syndrome.

✓ **Swansea criteria**[Q]: 6 of the following 14 features are required.

History	Abdominal pain	Polydipsia/ polyuria	Vomiting			
Examination	Encephalopathy					
Biochemistry	Ammonia >47 mmol/L	AST/ALT >42 IU/L	Bilirubin >14 mmol/L	Creatinine >150 mmol/L	Glucose <4 mmol/L	Urate >340 mmol/L
Haematology	Leucocytes >11 × 10⁹/L	PT >14 s or APTT >24 s				
Imaging	Ascites or bright liver echotexture					
Histology	Micro-vesicular steatosis					

	Acute Fatty Liver of Pregnancy	HELLP Syndrome	Intrahepatic Cholesta-sis of Pregnancy
Signs and symptoms	Non-specific (nausea/ vomiting), followed by signs of acute liver failure	Headache, abdominal pain, hypertension, pulmonary oedema	Pruritus, right upper quadrant pain; jaundice rare
Liver biochemistries[Q]	↑ ALT (3–15 times) ↑ bilirubin (4–15 times)[Q]	↑ ALT (3–30 times) ↑ bilirubin (1.5–10 times)	↑ ALT (1.5–8 times) ↑ bile acids (1.5–15 times); normal GGT
Prognosis	Maternal and fetal mortality low if diagnosed, stabilized, and delivered early; can recur in subsequent pregnancies	Low maternal mortality but can have high morbidity; fetal mortality can be high (20–35%); recurs in 3–27% of subsequent pregnancies	No maternal mortality; fetal mortality (1–2%); recurs in 60–70% of subsequent pregnancies

Treatment

✓ **Primary treatment: Delivery of child** must be expedited once the patient is stabilized
- Correct hypoglycaemia and coagulopathy before delivery.

✓ Rapid and dramatic reversal of both clinical condition and laboratory abnormalities following delivery.

✓ **Liver transplant** may be considered in cases of liver failure despite intensive medical support.

14

Paediatrics

PAEDIATRIC LIFE SUPPORT

- ✓ Children are much more likely to collapse due to respiratory distress.
  - Non-shockable rhythms are most common.
  - More susceptible to hypothermia due to high surface area-body mass ratio[Q].
- ✓ **Initial step** is check for a response and shout for help. If two responders, one of them can go to call EMS.
  - PLS advises to open the airway and assess for breathing and signs of life.
  - After this, provide 5 rescue breaths if no breathing[Q].
  - In the absence of signs of life, start chest compressions and ventilation @ 15:2.
  - For single responders with a collapsed child give 5 rescue breaths and then use the phone to call EMS while putting the phone on speaker.
  - If no phone available, then give 1 min of CPR and then call EMS.
- ✓ **Weight calculation for drugs**[Q]
  - 1–12 months: (0.5 × age in months) + 4
  - **1–5 yr**[Q]**: (2 × age in years) + 8**
  - **6–12 yr**[Q]**: (3 × age in years) + 7**
- ✓ **Blood volume**
  - Up to 2 yr: 80 mL/kg
  - After 2 yr: 70 mL/kg
- ✓ **Systolic blood pressure**
  - Age × 2 + 80 mmHg
- ✓ **Drug dosages**
  - Defibrillation energy: 4J/kg
  - **Endotracheal tube (ET) size**[Q]**: Uncuffed = Age/4 + 4, Cuffed = Age/4 + 3.5**
  - Straight blade laryngoscope[Q] like Miller blade is used and epiglottis is lifted with it

- ET length = Age/2 + 12 at the mouth
- Fluids: 10 mL/kg bolus in trauma (max 20 mL/kg), 20 mL/kg in non-trauma
- **Adrenaline**[Q]**: 10 µg/kg of 1: 10,000 solutions**
- **Glucose: 2–5 mL/kg of a 10% dextrose solution**
- Paracetamol: 15 mg/kg for those above 10 kg
- Fentanyl: 1–5 µg/kg
- Ketamine: 1–2 mg/kg
- ✓ Initial resuscitation fluids should always contain sodium between 130–154 mmol/L.
- ✓ **Holliday and Segar formula**[Q] for daily maintenance. Maintenance fluids should be hypotonic. 0.45% Saline + 5% dextrose.
  - 4 mL/kg/h for the first 10 kg
  - 2 mL/kg/h for the second 10 kg
  - 1 mL/kg/h thereafter
- ✓ **Paediatric airway**[Q]
  - Oral cavity is relatively small compared to tongue.
  - Cricoid ring is the narrowest part of a child's upper airway.
  - Cuffed endotracheal tube can be used keeping a cuff pressure <30 mmHg.
  - Large occiput. Need a shoulder bolster to avoid airway obstruction lying flat.
  - Mapleson F circuit[Q] is used for neonates.
- ✓ **Paediatric bradycardia**
  - Compensated: Treat the cause, consider oxygenation and vagal tone.
  - Decompensated: <1 yr is <80/min, >1 yr is <60/min.
    - ❖ Oxygenation and ventilation.
    - ❖ If signs of vagal stimulation: Give atropine 20 µg/kg.

DOI: 10.1201/9781003476214-14

❖ If no response to oxygenation and atropine: Give adrenaline 10 μg/kg.

❖ If unconscious and HR <60/min despite oxygenation. Start chest compressions.

✓ **Paediatric tachycardia**

- **Compensated:** If SVT consider vagal manoeuvres and adenosine

- **Decompensated:** Narrow complex (sinus tachycardia/SVT) or broad complex (VT)

  ❖ Sinus tachycardia: Infant: 180–220/min, Child: 160–180/min

    • Treat the cause like crying, fear, anxiety, and identify precipitant like hypovolaemia

  ❖ SVT: Infant: >220/min, Child: >180/min

    • Synchronized cardioversion with analgesia: Start with 1 j/kg, then 2 j/kg and then up to 4 j/kg

    • **Adenosine:** Up to 1 yr, give 150 μg/kg. Increase by 50–100 μg/kg every 1–2 min. Maximum dose in neonate is 300 μg/kg and infant is 500 μg/kg. In children between 1–11 yr give 100 μg/kg and increase by 50–100 μg/kg every 1–2 min. Maximum dose is 500 μg/kg. In children between 12–17 yr. Give 3 mg, then 6 mg and then12 mg.

    • Consider Amiodarone before third shock: 5 mg/kg over >20 min

  ❖ VT: Could be SVT or VT. If unsure treat as VT

    • Synchronized cardioversion with analgesia: Start with 1 j/kg, then 2 j/kg and then up to 4 j/kg

Additional Questions

✓ **Congenital paediatric anomalies**

- **Acyanotic heart disease**[Q]**:** Atrial septal disease, ventral septal disease, patent ductus arteriosus, coarctation of the aorta, aortic or pulmonary stenosis.

- **Cyanotic heart disease**[Q]**:** Tetralogy of Fallot, transposition of great vessels, total anomalous venous drainage, truncus arteriosus, tricuspid atresia.

- **Tetralogy of Fallot**[Q]**:** VSD, Pulmonary valve stenosis, overriding aorta and right ventricular hypertrophy.

- **Turner's syndrome**[Q]**:** Coarctation of aorta, bicuspid aortic valve.

- **Eisenmenger syndrome**[Q]**:** Right-to-left shunt in a patient with long-standing left-to-right shunt leading to cyanosis.

- **Patent ductus arteriosus**[Q]**:** Prostaglandins are used to maintain the patency and indomethacin to close the duct.

PAEDIATRIC INFECTIONS

Respiratory distress: Most common cause of paediatric attendance in emergency departments. ABCDE stepwise approach with simultaneous assessment and therapy. *Call for consultant help and referral to tertiary care paediatrics centre for transfer.*

✓ **Causes of respiratory distress**[Q]

- **Upper airway:** Uvulitis, epiglottitis, croup, retropharyngeal abscess, foreign body, tumours.

- **Lower airway:** Tracheitis, bronchiolitis, asthma.

- **Pulmonary:** Pneumonia, Empyema, pulmonary oedema.

✓ **Uvulitis:** Infection caused by group A *Streptococcus. Inflammation can be caused by trauma, allergic reaction, and thermal injury as well.*

- Fever, pain, dysphagia, and drooling is seen but **respiratory distress is not that common.**

- Intubation if needed and antimicrobials if infective causes are suspected.

✓ **Acute epiglottitis:** Oedema beneath the loosely adherent anterior surface of the epiglottis resulting in stridor.

- Most caused by *Haemophilus influenzae* **type B**. *Streptococcus* species can also cause it. Vaccinated children can develop epiglottitis due to non-type B H. *influenzae* otherwise acute epiglottitis[Q] is seen more commonly in adults now due to vaccination.

- Short history of **respiratory distress, drooling, stridor,** and sniffing posture in a child with high fever and odynophagia.

- Enlarged epiglottis (**thumb sign**) can be seen on X-ray.

- Difficult intubation with ENT surgeon on standby if **tracheostomy needed**.

- **Venous cannulation itself can cause additional respiratory distress.**

- Antimicrobial therapy should be started as soon as possible when venous cannulation is taken. **IV co-amoxiclav** 30 mg/kg is a good initial agent.

- Mechanical ventilation is needed for 2–3 d before extubation is permissible and done after establishing cuff leak, apyrexia, and ability to swallow.
- Inhalation induction of anaesthesia for intubation may be needed.

✓ **Croup: Viral laryngotracheobronchitis** due to swelling and oedema of the epithelial layer of the upper airway.
  - **Parainfluenza virus (types 1–3)** is most commonly responsible for croup epidemics. RSV, adenovirus, and human coronavirus may also be responsible for croup.
  - Seen in children between **6 months to 3 yr.**
  - *Fever, stridor, barking cough, and hoarseness seen after a bout of nasal congestion and coryza.*
  - **Stridor** causes severe airway obstruction and suprasternal and intercostal recessions may be seen.
  - Inhalational induction of anaesthesia for intubation may be needed.
  - *Dexamethasone (oral/intramuscular 0.15 mg/kg)* or **nebulized budesonide (2 mg)** *are helpful in reducing inflammation.*
  - **Nebulized adrenaline (0.5 mL/kg of 1:1000)** also gives transient clinical improvement.

✓ **Retropharyngeal abscess:** Infections of the tonsil and surrounding structures is caused by group A *Streptococcus*, staphylococcus, and respiratory anaerobes such as *Fusobacteria* and *Prevotella*.
  - Retropharyngeal space extends from the skull base to the posterior mediastinum.
  - Fever, dysphagia, change in voice, drooling, trismus, and torticollis is seen.
  - Surgical drainage of abscess and antibiotics are needed.
  - Difficult intubation with ENT surgeon on standby if **tracheostomy needed.**

✓ **Tracheitis:** *Staphylococcus aureus* is the most common organism involved.
  - Cough, stridor, and fever are seen with child looking toxic.
  - Difficult intubation with ENT surgeon on standby if **tracheostomy needed.**
  - Endoscopy is important for both diagnosing and treatment by removing pseudo-membranous exudates.
  - Antibiotics to cover Gram-positive bacteria.

✓ **Bronchiolitis:** Acute viral infection of the lower respiratory tract and *leading cause of hospital admission in infants.*
  - The most common cause is **Respiratory Syncytial Virus (RSV)**[Q]. Other causes are Rhinovirus, human metapneumovirus, influenza, parainfluenza, enterovirus, and adenovirus.
  - *Clinical diagnosis with upper respiratory tract infections progressing to lower respiratory tract symptoms like cough, wheeze, and laboured breathing in 1 to 3 d.*
  - **Criteria for hospital referral**
    ❖ Respiratory distress (RR >70/min, nasal flaring, grunting, chest wall recession)
    ❖ Poor feeding (<50% of usual intake over preceding 24 h)
    ❖ Apnoeic episodes
    ❖ Oxygen saturations <92%
    ❖ Toxic-looking child (temperature >40°C)
  - **Risk factors for severe viral bronchiolitis**
    ❖ Prematurity <32 wk
    ❖ Young age <3 months
    ❖ Small weight
    ❖ Male sex
    ❖ *Adenovirus*
    ❖ *Immunodeficiency, neuromuscular disorders, chronic lung disease, heart disease*
  - **Treatment:** Supportive management including supplemental oxygen, tube feeding, and gentle nasal suctioning.
    ❖ A trial of non-invasive ventilation to avoid the need for invasive ventilation.
    ❖ *NICE guidelines recommend against use of systemic steroids and inhaled bronchodilators.*
    ❖ Antibiotics shouldn't be started unless there is clear evidence of a bacterial infection.

Paediatric Sepsis

✓ Definition of paediatric sepsis is still an immense challenge and without consensus. **International Paediatrics Sepsis Consensus Conference (IPSCC), 2005** guidelines are still widely used. *Paediatric sepsis is still discussed in relation to systemic inflammatory response syndrome (SIRS) criteria, defined as presence of two of the following criteria.*
  1. Temperature >38.5°C or <36°C.

2. Tachycardia, defined as a **mean HR >2 standard deviations (SD) above normal for age** in the absence of external stimulus, chronic drugs or painful stimuli or unexplained persistent or otherwise unexplained persistent increase in HR over a 0.5–4-hour time period.
3. **Mean ventilatory frequency >2 SD above normal for age** or mechanical ventilation for an acute process not related to underlying neuromuscular disease or general anaesthesia.
4. Leucocyte count increased or decreased for age or >10% immature neutrophils.

✓ **Sepsis:** SIRS in the presence of a known or suspected infection is considered diagnostic of **sepsis.** *When cardiovascular organ dysfunction exists in the presence of sepsis, the child is considered to be in* ***septic shock.***
 • **Cardiovascular dysfunction:** Presence of the following features below despite giving isotonic IV fluid bolus ≥40 mL/kg in 1 h.

1. Decrease in BP (hypotension) <5th percentile for age or systolic BP <2 SD below normal for age, or
2. Need for vasoactive drug to maintain BP in normal range (dopamine >5 µg/kg/min, or dobutamine, adrenaline, or noradrenaline at any dose).
3. Two of the following
 • Unexplained metabolic acidosis: base deficit >5 mEq/L
 • Increase arterial lactate >2 times upper limit of normal
 • Oliguria: urine output <0.5 mL/kg/min
 • Prolonged capillary refill >5 s
 • Core to peripheral temperature gap >3°C

✓ **Current status:** The SIRS Criteria may under-identify children with infection at the highest risk of mortality and **an age-adapted SOFA scale may demonstrate more accurately children at risk.**
 • **Abnormal vital signs for recognition of sepsis in paediatrics**

Age	Heart Rate	Mean Arterial Pressure (mmHg)	Systolic Blood Pressure (mmHg)	Respiratory Rate
0 d–1 wk	>205 <100	<46	<60	>50
>1 wk–1 month	>205 <100	<55	<60	>40
>1 month–1 yr	>190 <90	<55	<70	>34
2–5 yr	>140 <60	<62	<70+ (age in years × 2)	>22
6–12 yr	>130 NA	<65	<70+ (age in years × 2)	>18
13–18 yr	>110 NA	<67	<90	>14

Worrisome Features

Heightened concern if >2 features or 1 feature with comorbid condition	
Core temperature	>38.5°C, or <36°C
Altered mental status	Decreased conscious level, irritable, confused, lethargic, inappropriate cry
Altered peripheral perfusion	Prolonged capillary refill >3 s (cold shock); flash capillary refill (warm shock)
Inappropriate tachycardia	For the age
If strong clinical suspicion → start resuscitation	

✓ **Management**
 • **Oxygen therapy:** 100% via a non-rebreather mask or high-flow oxygen device.
 ❖ CPAP and BiPAP can be tried initially.

Children are at increased risk of pulmonary oedema. Appropriate fluid resuscitation and vasopressor support should be started before intubation.
 • **Monitoring:** Vital monitors monitored

continuously or checked at every 5 min. Urine output and glucose concentration should also be monitored.

- **Vascular access:** IV or IO access should be attained within 5 min of sepsis recognition. In children under 3 kg, IO access is contraindicated.
  - ❖ All IV medications can be given through IO access including adrenaline, antibiotics, and blood.
  - ❖ All medications should be flushed, and fluids should be given continuously through the IV cannula via an infusion pump to avoid clotting and loss of access.
- **Fluids:** Initial fluid bolus (balanced crystalloids) of 20 mL/kg^Q should be given. 40–60 mL/kg in the first hour of resuscitation may need to be given before normal BP is attained.
  - ❖ *5–10 mL/kg bolus in those who have signs of cardiogenic shock, hepatomegaly, or crackles.*
  - ❖ If fluid resuscitation has been ongoing for more than 15 min and a child is not responding to rapid fluid boluses, consider fluid refractory shock and start adrenaline as recommended by the American College of Critical Care Medicine as the initial inotrope in paediatric cold shock. *Peripheral adrenaline can be started at 0.05–0.3 kg/min until central access is attained.*
  - ❖ Hypoglycaemia should be corrected with 2 mL/kg bolus of 10% dextrose followed by maintenance.
  - ❖ Hypocalcaemia is also common and should be corrected with calcium chloride 10 mg/kg or calcium gluconate 30 mg/kg.
- **Antibiotics:** Broad-spectrum antibiotics within 1 h of presentation. Combination therapy of two antibiotics should be given in septic shock.
  - ❖ Ceftriaxone 50 mg/kg, vancomycin 15 mg/kg, Metronidazole 10 mg/kg.
- **Fluid refractory shock:** If fluid resuscitation has been ongoing for more than 15 min and a child is not responding to rapid fluid boluses, consider fluid refractory shock.
  - ❖ Start adrenaline as the initial inotrope in **paediatric cold shock.** Peripheral

adrenaline can be started at 0.05–0.3 µg/kg/min until central access is attained. Noradrenaline or milrinone can be added depending upon parameters.
  - ❖ Noradrenaline is the preferred inotrope in vasodilatory or **warm shock.** Dose is 0.05–0.3 µg/kg/min. Add vasopressin 0.002–0.2 units/kg/min.
- **Catecholamine-resistant shock:** Septic shock responding poorly to both fluids and inotropic/vasopressor support.
  - ❖ *Rule out pneumothorax, cardiac tamponade, blood loss.*
  - ❖ Source control may be needed.
  - ❖ *Clindamycin and IV immunoglobin should be added for suspected toxic shock.*
  - ❖ Metronidazole to cover anaerobic organisms if gastrointestinal infection suspected or CNS doses of antibiotics if meningitis is suspected.
  - ❖ Consider steroid replacement if adrenal suppression suspected.
  - ❖ Consider ECMO.

Diabetic ketoacidosis: British Society for Paediatrics Endocrinology and Diabetes (BSPED) guidelines 2021

- ✓ **Definition:** Acidosis (bicarbonate$^-$ <15 mmol/L or pH <7.30) and ketonaemia >3 mmol/L (beta-hydroxybutyrate is tested). Blood glucose may be normal in children who develop DKA.
  - • Children with very high blood glucose (>33 mmol/L) with little or no acidosis or ketones have **hyperosmolar hyperglycaemic state (HHS)** and require different treatment.
  - • *DKA may be precipitated by sepsis and fever and lactic acidosis should increase concern about sepsis.*
- ✓ **Fluid bolus**
  - • All children who are not shocked and are felt to require IV fluids should receive 10 mL/kg 0.9% NaCl bolus over 30 min. This bolus should be subtracted from total fluid deficit.
  - • All children who are shocked and are felt to require IV fluids should receive 10 mL/kg 0.9% NaCl bolus over 15 min. This bolus should not be subtracted from total fluid deficit.

❖ **Bolus up to a total of 40 mL/kg**. Vasopressors may be needed after that.

✓ **Insulin:** *Blood glucose falls rapidly after rehydration. Hence insulin is started after 1–2 h of therapy.*

  ❖ *0.05–0.1 units/kg/h fixed-dose regimen.*

✓ **Blood glucose <14 mmol/L:** *Add 5% glucose as maintenance* and reduce insulin rate to 0.05 units/kg/h. Once ketones are <1 mmol/L, switch intravenous to subcutaneous insulin.

✓ **Cerebral oedema:** Children are more susceptible to cerebral oedema. Headache, irritability, reduced conscious level.

  • **Treat cerebral oedema** with 3% hypertonic saline (2.5–5 mL/kg) or 20% mannitol (0.5–1 g/kg) over 15 min.

  • **Rule out other diagnoses by CT scan once patient is stable.**

✓ **Fluid management:** Requirement is deficit + maintenance. 0.9% NaCl with 20 mmol potassium chloride in 500 mL until blood glucose levels are less than 14 mmol/L.

  • **Fluid deficit** is calculated based on blood pH and should be replaced over 48 h along with maintenance fluids.

    ❖ **Mild DKA:** 5% dehydration. Venous pH 7.2–7.29 or HCO_3^- <15 mmol/L.

    ❖ **Moderate DKA:** 7% dehydration. Venous pH 7.1–7.19 or HCO_3^- <10 mmol/L.

    ❖ **Severe DKA:** 10% dehydration. Venous pH less than 7.1 or HCO_3^- <5 mmol/L.

  • **Maintenance fluid** by Holliday Segar formula for 24-hour fluid requirement.

    ❖ 100 mL/kg/day for first 10 kg body weight

    ❖ 50 mL/kg/day for the second 10 kg

    ❖ 20 mL/kg/day for each additional kg

PAEDIATRIC TRAUMA

✓ **Injury** is the most common cause of death and disability in childhood.

  • Other causes of deaths are drowning, house fires, homicides, and falls.

  • *Multiple organ system injury should be assumed until proven otherwise.*

✓ **Unique characteristics of paediatric patients**

  • *Greater force of trauma being imparted per unit of body area, hence multiple injuries in the paediatric population.*

  • **Child's head is proportionately larger than an adult's resulting in higher frequency of blunt brain injuries in paediatric age group.**

  • Child's skeleton is less calcified and hence bone fractures are less likely in children.

✓ **Airway**[Q]

  • Occiput is prominent in children.

  • Tongue and tonsils are relatively large compared to the tissues in the oral cavity[Q], which may compromise visualization of the larynx.

  • Larynx and vocal cords are more cephalad and anterior in the neck.

  • Plane of the midface is maintained parallel[Q] to the spine board in a neutral position, rather than in the sniffing position by placing 1 inch layer of padding beneath the infant or toddler entire torso.

  • The practice of inserting the airway backward and rotating it 180 degrees is not recommended for children.

  • Concerns about cuffed endotracheal tubes causing tracheal necrosis are no longer relevant and cuff pressure <30 mmHg is considered safe.

  • Atropine pretreatment should be considered for infants requiring drug assisted intubation as they have stronger vagal response to endotracheal intubation.

  • Etomidate 0.1–0.3 mg/kg or midazolam 0.1 mg/kg can be used for intubation and rocuronium 0.6 mg/kg for muscle paralysis.

  • In case of failed intubation and bag mask ventilation, *needle cricothyroidotomy is recommended.* **Surgical cricothyroidotomy for children older than 12 yr.**

✓ **Breathing**

  • Use of paediatric bag and mask is recommended for children under 20 kg.

  • Needle decompression just over the top of the third rib in the midclavicular line for tension pneumothorax.

  • Site of the chest tube insertion is the same in children as in adults, the fifth intercostal space, just anterior to the midaxillary line.

✓ **Circulation**

  • Infant's blood volume: 80 mL/kg, child age 1–3 yr: 75 mL/kg, children over 3 yr: 70 mL/kg.

- Up to a 30% decrease in circulating blood volume may be required to cause a decrease in child's systolic blood pressure.
  - ❖ **Paediatrics major haemorrhage:** Severe ongoing, often non-compressible bleeding requiring immediate blood product resuscitation.
  - ❖ **Paediatric massive transfusion:** >40 mL/kg transfusion.
- Tachycardia and poor skin perfusion often are the only early features of hypovolaemia.
- **Normal systolic blood pressure:** 90 mmHg + twice the child's age in years.
  - ❖ **Lower limit of systolic blood pressure:** 70 mmHg + twice the child's age in years.
- *Hypotension in a child represents a state of decompensated shock and indicate severe blood loss of greater than 45% of the circulating volume.*
  - ❖ *This hypotension may be accompanied by change of tachycardia into bradycardia.*
- If venous access is unsuccessful after two attempts[Q], consider intraosseous infusion via a bone marrow needle. 18 gauge in infants, 15 gauge in young children.
  - ❖ Sites for IO are proximal anteromedial tibia followed by distal femur.
- Initial 20 mL/kg bolus of isotonic crystalloid followed by weight-based blood product resuscitation with 10–20 mL/kg of packed red blood cells and 10–20 mL/kg of fresh frozen plasma and platelets.
  - ❖ Cryoprecipitate of 10 mL/kg and TXA 15 mg/kg.
- **Urine output** goal in infants is 1–2 mL/kg/h, children up to adolescence is 1–1.5 mL/kg/h and 0.5 mL/kg/h for teenagers.

✓ **Chest trauma**
- Children with chest injuries have multiple injuries.
- Vast majority of chest injuries in childhood are due to blunt mechanisms, most commonly caused by motor vehicle injury or falls.
- **Rib fractures if present indicate a severe impacting injury and as ribs are relatively pliable, serious injuries can happen even without fracture.**

- The mobility of mediastinal structures makes children more susceptible to tension pneumothorax which is the most common immediately life-threatening injury in children.
- Screening chest X-rays can diagnose most chest injuries.
- Most paediatric thoracic injuries can be successfully managed by using an appropriate combination of supportive care and tube thoracostomy.

✓ **Abdominal trauma**
- Most paediatric abdominal injuries result from blunt trauma that involves motor vehicles and falls.
- Most infants and young children who are stressed and crying will swallow large amounts of air and orogastric tube decompression is preferred in infants.
- **Diagnosis:** The presence of intraperitoneal blood on CT scan, focused assessment sonography in trauma (FAST) or diagnostic peritoneal lavage (DPL), the grade of injury and the presence of vascular blush does not necessarily mandate a laparotomy.
  - ❖ **CT scan:** CT scan with contrast in children with blunt trauma and no haemodynamic instability.
  - ❖ **FAST:** FAST should not be relied upon as a sole diagnostic test to rule out the presence of intra-abdominal injury.
  - ❖ **DPL:** May be used in haemodynamic unstable patients to detect intra-abdominal bleeding.
- Bleeding from an injured spleen, kidney and liver is generally self-limited.
  - ❖ Bladder is intra-abdominal and more exposed.
- *If the child's haemodynamic status can't be normalized and diagnostic procedure is positive for blood, a laparotomy (damage control surgery) should be performed to control haemorrhage.*

✓ **Head trauma**
- Outcome in children who suffer severe brain injury is better than that in adults.
- *Although infrequent, hypotension can occur in infants following significant blood loss into subgaleal, intraventricular, or epidural spaces because of the infants open cranial sutures.*

- **An infant who is not comatose but has bulging fontanelle should be assumed to have a severe injury.**
- They are prone to cerebral oedema.
- Rapid restoration of normal blood volume is critical to maintain cerebral perfusion pressure as uncorrected hypovolaemia can worsen outcome.
- **Indications of CT scan in paediatric age group <16 yr with any one of these risk factors.**
  - ❖ On initial ED assessment, for babies less than 1 yr GCS 14, GCS ≤13 otherwise for older kids
  - ❖ At 2 h, GCS score of ≤14
  - ❖ Post–traumatic seizure.
  - ❖ Focal neurological deficit.
  - ❖ *Suspicion of non-accidental injury (NAI)*
  - ❖ Suspected open or depressed skull fracture or tense fontanelle
  - ❖ Basal skull fracture.
  - ❖ Swelling or laceration of more than 5 cm on the head for babies under 1 yr
- **Indications of CT scan in paediatric age group <16 yr with more than one of these risk factors**
  - ❖ *Loss of consciousness >5 min.*
  - ❖ *Amnesia (antegrade or retrograde) >5 min.*
  - ❖ Abnormal drowsiness.
  - ❖ *3 or more discrete episodes of vomiting.*
  - ❖ *Dangerous mechanism of injury with fall from height >3 m, high-speed injury.*
  - ❖ Any current bleeding or clotting disorder.
- ✓ **Spinal cord injury**
  - Around 40% of children younger than 7 yr of age show anterior displacement of C2 on C3 and 20% of children up to 16 yr show this phenomenon.
    - ❖ Hence subluxation seen on a lateral cervical spine X-ray can be pseudo-subluxation or a true cervical spine injury.
    - ❖ True subluxation will not disappear after taking the X-ray by putting the child's head in a neutral position using a 1-inch layer of padding beneath the entire body except the head.
  - The growth centre of the spinous process can resemble fractures of the tip of the spinous process.

- Children sustain spinal cord injury without radiographic abnormalities (SCIWORA) more commonly than adults.
- When in doubt about the integrity of the cervical spine or spinal cord, assume that an unstable injury exists and limit spinal motion along with a neurosurgical consultation.
- ✓ **Musculoskeletal trauma**
  - Blood loss associated with long bone and pelvic injuries is proportionately less in children than in adults and an isolated femur fracture should prompt evaluation for other sources of blood loss, usually abdomen.
  - The immature, pliable nature of bones in children can lead to greenstick fractures.
  - Injuries to areas where the physis hasn't closed yet can alter the development of the bone.
- ✓ **Considerations of whole-body CT scan in paediatric trauma patients**
  - Injury >1 body region
  - Fractured pelvis
  - Haemodynamic instability
  - High mechanism of injury (high-speed RTC >30 mph, prolonged entrapment >30 mins, ejection from vehicle)
- ✓ **Child maltreatment (non-accidental injury)**[Q]: Clinicians should suspect child maltreatment in the following situations.
  - Discrepancy between the history and degree of physical injury
  - History of repeated traumas
  - History of hospital or doctor shopping
  - Parents do not comply with medical advice
  - Prolonged interval between the time of the injury and presentation for medical care
  - Multicoloured bruises
  - Perioral injuries
  - ***Injuries to the genital or perianal area***
  - **Fractures of long bones in children younger than 3 yr of age**
  - Ruptured internal viscera without antecedent major blunt trauma
  - Multiple subdural haematomas, especially without a fresh skull fracture
  - ***Retinal haemorrhages***
  - Bizarre injuries like bites, cigarette burns, and rope marks
  - Sharply demarcated second- and third-degree burns
  - **Skull fractures seen in children less than 24 months of age**

Miscellaneous Organ Problems

15

DERMATOLOGICAL MANIFESTATIONS

Drug Eruptions

✓ **Mild drug eruptions**
- 90% of adverse drug reactions presents with a classical morbilliform/maculopapular rash (**macule:** flat non-palpable lesion <1 cm, **papule:** elevated, solid, palpable lesion <1 cm).
- Common drugs involved are penicillin, NSAIDs, allopurinol and antiepileptics.
- Seen after **4 to 14 d** of starting the drug.
- **Most reactions are mild and resolve when the drug is stopped.**
- **Symptomatic relief** with *topical corticosteroids*, emollients and antihistaminic.

✓ **Severe drug reactions:** Life-threatening reactions.
- Stevens–Johnson syndrome (**SJS**), Toxic epidermal necrolysis (**TEN**), Drug rash, eosinophilia, and systemic symptoms (**DRESS**).
- **Signs and symptoms of severe cutaneous drug reaction.**
  - ❖ Fever >39°C
  - ❖ Widespread rash
  - ❖ Mucosal involvement
  - ❖ Lymphadenopathy
  - ❖ Fatigue, arthralgia, sore throat
  - ❖ Abnormal liver or kidney function tests
  - ❖ Eosinophil count >1 × 10⁹/L
- **General management of life-threatening dermatoses**
  - ❖ Any patient with *epidermal loss of >10% body surface area* should be referred to a specialist burns centre.
  - ❖ Severity of illness score for TEN should be calculated within the first 24 h of admission.

- ❖ Strict barrier nursing for preventing nosocomial infections.
- ❖ IV lines through non-lesioned skin.
- ❖ Take swabs for bacterial and candida culture from three areas of lesioned area on alternate days.
- ❖ Systemic antibiotics only if clinical signs of infection
- ❖ Good pain and sedation.
- ❖ Early patient-specific nutrition.
- ❖ Regular multidisciplinary team review for need for surgical intervention.

- **Drug rash, eosinophilia, and systemic symptoms (DRESS)/drug hypersensitivity syndrome.**
  - ❖ *Life-threatening adverse drug reaction.* Type 4 delayed hypersensitivity[Q].
  - ❖ **Causes:** *Antiepileptics like phenytoin and carbamazepine (MC),* antibiotics, antivirals, NSAIDs, allopurinol, ranitidine, fluoxetine.
  - ❖ **Lag phase of 4–6 wk after trigger. Fever and facial oedema** followed by erythematous rash from head descending towards lower limbs.
  - ❖ Rash is painful, diffuse, and pruritic.
  - ❖ *Eosinophilia, atypical lymphocytes, deranged LFTs and abnormal serum creatinine.*
  - ❖ Lymphadenopathy, hepatosplenomegaly, pulmonary infiltrates, and interstitial nephritis.
  - ❖ Autoimmune thyroiditis and type 1 diabetes are late sequelae.
  - ❖ **Registry of severe cutaneous adverse reaction (RegiSCAR) scoring system is used to diagnose DRESS.**

DOI: 10.1201/9781003476214-15

- ❖ **Treatment** is immediate cessation of the drug and *high-dose steroids with withdrawal of steroids over 8–12 wk.*
- ❖ Mortality rate is 10%.
- **Stevens–Johnson Syndrome (SJS)/Toxic Epidermal Necrolysis (TEN):**
  - ❖ SJS and TEN form a spectrum of disease with drugs as causative agents in up to 85% of cases.
  - ❖ **SJS** <10% BSA, **TENS:** >30% BSA, 10–30% **overlapping SJS/TEN**[Q]
  - ❖ **Type IV reaction:** *Dermatological emergency because of an immune reaction leading to destruction of keratinocytes expressing foreign antigen.*
  - ❖ Caused[Q] mostly by drugs (90%) like anticonvulsants, antibiotics (sulphonamide, penicillin), antivirals (nevirapine), and NSAIDs.
  - ❖ *Infections like HIV, CMV, and Mycoplasma can also cause it.*
  - ❖ **Presentation:** Fever, sore throat, and myalgia followed by painful erythematous lesions across the trunk, face, and limbs.
  - ❖ **Nikolsky's sign**[Q]: Dislodgement of epidermis by direct pressure.
  - ❖ Mucosa of eyes, oropharynx, respiratory tract, gastrointestinal tract and genitalia will get involved.
  - ❖ **Treatment:** Cessation of the drug, Vaseline impregnated gauze dressing.
    - *IV immunoglobins, corticosteroids and ciclosporin are commonly used.*
    - **Multidisciplinary care with involvement of ophthalmologists, urologists, and gynaecologists.**
  - ❖ Death is mostly due to sepsis and multiorgan failure. 5–30% mortality.
  - ❖ Score of TEN (**SCORTEN**) and ABCD-10 criteria can be used to predict mortality at the time of admission for TEN and SJS.
  - ❖ **SCORTEN:** Uses heart rate >120/min, Serum glucose >14 mmol/L, age >40 yr, initial epidermal detachment >10%, serum urea nitrogen >10 mmol/L, bicarbonate <20 mmol/L and presence of malignancy.

- ❖ **ABCD-10 criteria:** Age >50 yr (1), Bicarbonate level <20 mmol/L (1), Cancer (2), Dialysis (3), Epidermal detachment >10% (1).
- ✓ **Acute generalized exanthematous pustulosis (AGEP)**
  - Rare reaction with **widespread erythema in the folds of skin, trunk, and extremities.**
  - 90% of cases are drug related with beta-lactam antibiotics most commonly involved.
  - Patients will present with fever, leucocytosis, and **multiple sterile pustules on a background of generalized erythema.**
  - If there is no resolution within 15 d of drug withdrawal, the diagnosis should be questioned.
  - Mortality is <5% due to multiple organ dysfunction.
- ✓ **Erythroderma (exfoliative dermatitis)**
  - Inflammatory condition causing widespread erythema and oedema affecting over 90% of the skin surface.
  - **Peeling and scaling of the skin** is seen followed by **widespread erythema** within 2 to 6 d.
  - Seen in patients with a pre-existing dermatological condition that has worsened example psoriasis or atopic dermatitis.
  - Also seen in drugs like ACEIs, anticonvulsants, antifungals, and barbiturates.
  - Admission to critical care for multiple organ failure and infections.
  - **Treatment** is immunosuppressants.
- ✓ **Acute generalized pustular psoriasis**
  - Sudden onset of widespread **sterile pustules on a background of erythematous tender skin.**
  - Fever, headache, loss of appetite, nausea, malaise.
  - 10% of cases have a preceding history of plaque psoriasis[Q].
  - Linked to abrupt withdrawal of steroid therapy, drugs (NSAIDs/Rituximab), and infections (EBV, VZV).
  - Admission to critical care for multiple organ failure and infections.
  - **Treatment** is immunosuppressants.

Infections

✓ **Toxic shock syndrome: (TSS)**[Q] Exotoxin released from Gram-positive infections.
- Cause: *Streptococcus pyogenes* (group A *Streptococcus*/GAS) and *Staphylococcus aureus*.
  - ❖ *Streptococcus*[Q]: Burns, necrotizing fasciitis.
  - ❖ *Staphylococcus*[Q]: Tampons, nasal packing, intrauterine devices.
- Toxins act as superantigens. Preexisting antibody to the bacterial toxin is a critical host factor for prevention of TSS.
- Streptococcal infection patients have more propensity of bacteraemia and less of rash with higher mortality.
- **Diagnostic criteria for Streptococcal Toxic Shock Syndrome (STSS)**
  - ❖ **Clinical criteria**
    - Hypotension
    - Diffuse erythematous rash
    - Multisystem involvement: At least 2 out of the following: renal impairment, coagulopathy, liver involvement, acute respiratory distress syndrome, soft tissue necrosis.
  - ❖ **Laboratory criteria:** Isolation of group A *Streptococcus*.
- **Complications:** Haemolytic anaemia disseminated intravascular coagulation and multiorgan failure.
- Rule out Rocky Mountain spotted fever, leptospirosis, and measles.
- **Treatment**
  - ❖ Aggressive fluid resuscitation.
  - ❖ Broad spectrum antibiotics[Q] + antitoxin[Q] (clindamycin, linezolid).
  - ❖ Surgical debridement[Q] may be required in streptococcal TSS.
  - ❖ Role of IVIg[Q] and hyperbaric oxygen is unclear but should be given in life-threatening cases.
- *Mortality of 50% in streptococcal infections and 5% in staphylococcal infection.*
✓ **Staphylococcal scalded skin syndrome (SSSS):** Caused by an exfoliative toxin produced by roughly 5% of *Staphylococcus aureus*.
- Fever, red rash, and separation of the epidermis.
- Infants and young children are most commonly affected.
- *Mucosal involvement is not seen in comparison to TEN.*
  - ❖ Skin biopsy differentiates it from TEN as SSSS shows cleavage in the mid-epidermis with no associated inflammation whereas TEN shows cleavage at the dermo-epidermal junction and there is cellular necrosis of the epidermis.
- **Treatment** is IV antibiotics targeting *S. aureus. Steroids are contraindicated.*
✓ **Cellulitis and erysipelas:** Cellulitis is a bacterial infection in the lower dermis and subcutaneous fat.
- **Erysipelas** is a superficial form of cellulitis affecting the upper dermis and superficial lymphatics with clearly demarcated borders.
- **Cellulitis** presents as **unilateral spreading erythema** that may not be well demarcated along with **pyrexia and lymphadenopathy.**
- They typically present affect the lower limbs.
- Cellulitis can lead to septic shock and hence admission into critical care.
- Commonly caused by MSSA, MRSA and GAS. Purulent cellulitis is likely to be *S. aureus*.
- If a patient presents with flu-like illness and necrotizing skin infection, Panton-Valentine-leucocidin *S. aureus* should be suspected.
- **Treatment:** Antibiotics covering Gram-positive bacteria should be used.
✓ **Necrotising fasciitis:** Bacterial infection affecting the soft tissue and fascia.
- Explained in detail in the chapter on necrotizing fasciitis.

Vasculitis

✓ **Cutaneous small vessel vasculitis**
- Affects arterioles and venules and presents with purpura and petechiae that can form haemorrhagic bullae.
- Can be secondary to infections like HIV, hepatitis viruses or drugs like NSAIDs, diuretics, antibiotics, anticonvulsants, antipsychotics.
- **Complications:** Ulceration, wound infection, cellulitis.
- **Treatment:** Discontinue the trigger, treat infection, compress affected limb, and dress the ulcer.

✓ **Purpura fulminans**
- Symmetrical peripheral gangrene in two or more extremities without large vessel obstruction or vasculitis.
- Seen in patients with disseminated intravascular coagulation, septic shock, and high doses of vasopressor drugs.
- Amputation and skin grafting should be delayed until full demarcation of the necrotic area has occurred, and the patient's condition has improved.
- **Treatment:** If infection happens, antibiotics and early surgical intervention may be needed.

Immune Mediated

✓ **Erythema multiforme**
- Widespread polymorphous lesions that erupt over 24 h.
- Target lesions: Dark centre and a red erythematous ring around it.
- Most common causes are infections (90%): HSV and *Mycoplasma pneumoniae*. 10% of cases are due to drugs.
- Self-limiting condition usually.

✓ **Pemphigus vulgaris**
- IgG mediated destruction of desmosomal proteins in the epidermis causes widespread intraepithelial and mucocutaneous blistering.
- Presents with blistering of the oral mucosa in the third and sixth decade of life.
- Cutaneous blistering on the upper chest, back, scalp and face and develop over weeks to months.
- Admission to ITU may be needed for infection.
- **Treatment:** Corticosteroids, plasma exchange, and IV immunoglobulin therapy.

Common Skin Conditions Seen in ITU

✓ **Intertrigo:** Skin folds become inflamed, tender, and erythematous leading to fissures and peeling.
- Due to increased moisture levels, lack of ventilation to the skin fold and rubbing of opposing skin.
- Can lead to secondary bacterial and fungal infections.
- **Treatment:** Daily cleansing and drying of the patient's skin folds along with the use of barrier creams or talc.
  - ❖ Topical antifungal or antibacterial creams.

✓ **Miliaria:** Sweat rash is caused by the obstruction of eccrine sweat gland ducts.
- Red, non-follicular papules or vesicles seen in critical care when fever, dressings, or prolonged bed rest leads to blockage of ducts in the epidermis.
- Rash is generally erythematous and itchy and found on the trunk, neck, and flexures.
- **Treatment:** Cool the skin, emollients and topical steroids.

✓ **Pressure ulcers:** *Acute skin failure due to hypoperfusion of skin.*
- Skin receives one-third of the circulating blood volume.
- Areas affected are over a bony prominence such as sacrum, calcaneus, and ischium.
- **European Pressure Ulcer Advisory Panel classification of pressure ulcers**
  - ❖ **Grade 1:** Intact skin with non-blanchable redness of a localized area usually over a bony prominence.
  - ❖ **Grade 2:** A shallow open ulcer with a red, pink wound bed.
  - ❖ **Grade 3:** Full thickness tissue loss. *Subcutaneous fat* may be visible but bone, tendon or muscle are not exposed.
  - ❖ **Grade 4:** Full thickness tissue loss with exposed bone, tendon, or muscle.
- **Regular skin assessment** should be performed with repositioning of the patient at least every 4 h.
- **Treatment:** Redistributing mattresses to relieve pressure on bony prominences.
  - ❖ If the skin is still intact the ulcer will usually heal by itself.
  - ❖ If the skin has broken, dressings should be used that promote a warm, moist healing environment.

✓ **Extravasation injuries**
- Accidental injection or leakage of fluid into the subcutaneous or perivascular tissues.
- Drugs that can cause local damage are as follows.
  - ❖ Vasoconstrictors
  - ❖ Hyperosmolar agents (calcium, magnesium sulphate, parenteral nutrition, sodium bicarbonate, potassium chloride)

❖ Acid or alkalis (amiodarone, erythro-mycin, phenytoin, vancomycin)
- Fluid should be aspirated from the cannula and it be left in place.
  ❖ Limb should be elevated to promote venous drainage.
  ❖ Analgesia and heat to local area to improve drug reabsorption.
  ❖ **Spread and dilute method**[Q]: Used when risk of tissue necrosis is high. Stab wounds are created around the affected area and a cannula is inserted into one of these wounds. Flushing of cannula is done with saline to exit through the other stab wounds.

Confusion Buster

✓ **Beta-haemolytic Group A streptococci (GAS)** *Streptococcus pyogenes*[Q]
- Asymptomatic carriage in up to 30% of the population.
- **Non-invasive infections:** Impetigo, phar-yngitis/tonsillitis, **scarlet fever**[Q] (notifiable disease).
- **Invasive infections:** Necrotizing fasciitis, Toxic shock syndrome[Q].
- Post–streptococcal glomerulonephritis.
- Can lead to **rheumatic fever** indirectly.
✓ **Beta-haemolytic Group B streptococci** (*Strep-tococcus agalactiae*)
- Causes neonatal pneumonia and meningitis.
✓ **Alpha-haemolytic Streptococci is** *S. viridans*: Endocarditis.
✓ **Gamma-haemolytic streptococci:** *Enterococcus faecalis* and *E. faecium*

RHEUMATOLOGICAL PROBLEMS

Rheumatological conditions: Can present in ICU with end organ sequelae of the primary disease or infectious complications of the immunosuppressive therapy for these diseases.
✓ Three-fourths of patients[Q] admitted to ITU because of rheumatological diseases have rheu-matoid arthritis, systemic lupus erythematosus (SLE), or scleroderma.
✓ Female preponderance and multiorgan system involvement is common.
✓ ICU mortality can be between 15–55%.

Vasculitides

✓ **Classification:** Group of disorders character-ized by *destructive inflammation in vessel walls.*
- **Primary:** *Idiopathic or immune complex mediated* (Goodpasture's, Henoch Schoen-lein purpura, cryoglobulinaemia). *Primary idiopathic* can be classified as
  ❖ **Large vessels:** Giant cell arteritis, Takayasu's arteritis.
  ❖ **Medium vessels:** Polyarteritis nodosa, Kawasaki disease.
  ❖ **Small vessels:** Granulomatosis with polyangiitis (**GPA**) or formerly called as Wegener's granulomatosis, Eosinophilic granulomatosis with polyangiitis (**EGPA**) or formerly called as Churg Strauss syn-drome, microscopic polyangiitis (**MPA**).
- **Secondary**
  ❖ Autoimmune disease (rheumatoid arthritis, *lupus*)
  ❖ Malignancy (lymphoma, **leukaemia**)
  ❖ Infection (endocarditis)
  ❖ Drug related (*hydralazine*, penicilla-mine, carbimazole)
✓ **Differential diagnosis:** Embolism due to endocarditis, hypercoagulable disease due to antiphospholipid syndrome, radiation arteriopathy.
✓ **Takayasu's arteritis:** Affects *aortic arch* and branches in women up to the age of 50.
- Fatigue, weight loss, and limb claudication.
- Patient can present with stroke and aortic dissection.
- **Treatment** involves immunosuppressants and steroids.
✓ **Kawasaki disease:** Inflammation of the blood vessels seen in children under 5 yr old.
- Fever that lasts for more than 5 d, swollen glands in the neck, swollen red tongue, and rash.
- Leading cause of **acquired heart disease (coronary artery aneurysms and myocar-ditis)** in children in Western nations.
- **Treatment** is aspirin and IVIg.
✓ **Polyarteritis nodosa:** *Systemic necrotizing vasculitic* lesions occur at the bifurcations or branches of vessels.
- Skin, *peripheral nerves (60% cases),* kid-neys, GI tract, and joints are main organs involved.

- Sudden onset paraesthesia and motor deficits is a common presentation.
- Malaise, *arthralgia (50% of cases),* weight loss, fever, abdominal pain, hypertension, and azotaemia with proteinuria. *Glomerulonephritis is rare.*
  - PAN is associated with hepatitis B.
- ↑ ESR,↑ CRP and thrombocytosis. *Antineutrophil cytoplasmic antibody (ANCA) and antinuclear antibody (ANA) are typically not present in PAN.*
- **Treatment** is oral steroids for moderate to severe disease and IV methylprednisolone 1 mg/kg for 3 d followed by oral corticosteroids for the fulminant disease.
  - Azathioprine, cyclophosphamide, and mycophenolate are second-line drugs.
  - Plasmapheresis with antiviral therapy in patients with hepatitis B.

✓ **Microscopic polyangiitis**Q: Presents with alveolar haemorrhage and *rapidly progressive glomerulonephritis.*
- Renal involvement is seen in 90% of cases.
- Pulmonary involvement in 50% of cases.
- *Cutaneous lesions and neuropathy* are seen in 30–50% of cases.
- ANCA positivity is found in 75% of cases with **myeloperoxidase (MPO) positivity** seen more than proteinase-3 (PR3).
- Diagnosis is by biopsy of lung, kidney, skin, or nerve along with ANCA positivity.
- **Treatment** is corticosteroids and Rituximab/cyclophosphamide.
  - Plasmapheresis is not of much use.

✓ **Eosinophilic granulomatosis with polyangiitis/Churg–Strauss syndrome**Q: *Nasal polyps with an eosinophilic asthma.*
- Presentation is a patient with asthma having *weight loss and malaise* along with peripheral neuropathy and **cardiomyopathy** (myocarditis, pericarditis, and myocardial infarction).
- **Pulmonary involvement in 70% of cases.**
  - Pulmonary infiltrates and peripheral eosinophilia are seen.
- Renal involvement is seen in 45% of cases.
- *ANCA positivity is found in 60% of cases with mostly myeloperoxidase (MPO) positivity.*
- **Treatment** is corticosteroids and Rituximab.

✓ **Granulomatosis with polyangiitis (GPA)/Wegener's granulomatosis**Q: Granulomatous vasculitis causing diffuse alveolar haemorrhage and segmental necrotizing glomerulonephritis.
- Pulmonary involvement in 90% of cases. All parts of the respiratory tract from nasal mucosa to pleura and pulmonary artery are involved.
  - Subglottic stenosis might be seen leading to difficult intubation.
  - *Multiple, nodular, bilateral cavitary infiltrates in lungs without sharp margins.*
  - Cavitating lesions that are fleeting in nature.
  - Clinically apparent haemoptysis is absent in about one-third of the patients.
- Renal involvement is seen in 80% of cases.
- *c-ANCA positivity with predominant PR3 positive.*
- Diagnosis is with clinical findings and ANCA positivity.
- **Treatment** is induction with Rituximab/cyclophosphamide + steroids followed by maintenance phase by Rituximab/azathioprine/mycophenolate.

✓ **Goodpasture syndrome**Q: Rapidly progressive renal and pulmonary disease.
- *Auto antibodies against type IV collagen found in both glomerular and alveolar basement membrane*Q. Small vessel vasculitis.
- Two peaks, one in patients aged 20–30 yr and again in older patients (60–70 yr).
- Fever, malaise, and weight loss.
- Diagnosis is with positive immunology and renal biopsy.
- **Treatment** is immunosuppression like steroids and cyclophosphamide and plasma exchange.

✓ **Cryoglobulinemic vasculitis:** Cryoglobulins are immunoglobins that precipitate below 37°C.
- **Type I:** Seen in myeloproliferative disorders, **type II:** mixed essential cryoglobulins, **type III:** mixed polyclonal.
- Type II and III are most commonly involved with hepatitis C infection.
- *Cutaneous vasculitis, arthritis, and peripheral neuropathy.*
- C4 levels are decreased.
- **Treatment** is Rituximab + steroids. Plasmapheresis or cryofiltration for patients with progressive glomerulonephritis.

✓ **Drug-induced vasculitis:** Propylthiouracil, Allopurinol, hydralazine, phenytoin, minocycline, cefaclor, d-penicillamine, and methotrexate are common drugs involved.

- ANCA positivity with MPO positive.
- Skin involvement can present as purpura, bowel, nervous system, and renal involvement can happen as well.
- **Treatment** is withdrawal of the medication and corticosteroids.

✓ **CNS vasculitis:** Primary angiitis of the CNS or secondary to other systemic illness.

- Subacute memory loss, acute encephalopathy, seizures, cranial nerve abnormalities, and focal deficits.
- Disease generally involves small and medium vessels.
- **CSF shows increased protein levels and elevated cell counts, mainly of lymphocytes.**
  - ❖ Angiographic changes show stenosis and ectasia. MRI shows ischaemic lesions.
  - ❖ Biopsy may be needed for diagnosis.
  - ❖ Treatment is corticosteroids and cyclophosphamide/Rituximab.

Scleroderma Renal Crisis

✓ **Scleroderma:** Autoimmune disease characterized by fibrosis and inflammation of internal organs.

✓ **Scleroderma renal crisis (SRC):** Life-threatening complication of scleroderma seen in 5–10% of cases.

- Rapidly progressive hypertension^Q, microangiopathic haemolytic anaemia (MAHA)^Q with AKI^Q.
- Male: Female incidence is 1:3 and average age of presentation is 53 yr.
- **Clinical features:** Patient presents with headache, visual disturbance, encephalopathy, seizures, pulmonary oedema, and myocarditis.
- Acute deterioration in renal function with >30% decrease in eGFR.
- Treatment is **ACE inhibitors**, calcium channel blockers, labetalol, nitrates, plasma exchange (if extensive microangiopathy).
- **25% of patients will require renal replacement therapy.**

- Overall renal recovery is slow and 5-year survival for systemic sclerosis with SRC is 65%.

Antiphospholipid Syndrome

✓ **Epidemiology and aetiology**

- Antiphospholipid syndrome (APS) is an autoimmune hypercoagulable state characterized by presence of antiphospholipid antibodies.
- **Primary:** No immediate underlying autoimmune disorder.
  - ❖ **Secondary:** Associated with systemic lupus erythematosus (SLE), systemic sclerosis, rheumatoid arthritis.
- Higher incidence in *women of reproductive age and Afro-Caribbean populations*.

✓ **Clinical features and diagnosis**

- History of vascular thrombosis, recurrent pregnancy loss and thrombocytopaenia.
  - ❖ **Both arterial and venous thrombosis seen similar to** hyper-homocysteinaemia and polycythaemia vera.
  - ❖ Factor V Leiden, Protein C deficiency, and anti-thrombin deficiency will cause just venous thrombosis.
- Low blood pressure, hyponatraemia, hyperkalaemia,↑ **aPTT**^{Q} are seen.
- Cardiac involvement is common and patients under the age of 40 are at increased at the risk of myocardial infarction.
- **Diagnosis:** *Anti-cardiolipin antibody*, lupus anticoagulant antibody, anti-β2 glycoprotein-I antibody.
  - ❖ Diagnosis is made in the presence of one or more antibodies at the time of event and 12 wk later in the presence of vascular thrombotic event or pregnancy-related morbidity.
- Anti-lupus antibody and IgG anti-β2 glycoprotein-I antibody confer the greatest risk of thrombosis.
- *Patient with VTE and baseline prolonged VTE should be evaluated for APS.*

✓ **Catastrophic antiphospholipid antibody syndrome (CAPLA)** also known as Asherson's syndrome.

- Less than 1% of APLS patients, 50% cases won't have APLS background. 3–5% of SLE patients.
  - ❖ Infections are precipitating factor in about half of the cases.

❖ Anticoagulation withdrawal or sub-therapeutic anticoagulation is one of the causes.

• *Small vessel occlusion* leads to multiorgan failure. Large vessel involvement in 10% of cases.

❖ Acute-onset renal failure is the commonest clinical manifestation in about 75% of patients.

❖ *Libman-sacks endocarditis,* myocardial infarction.

❖ ARDS, pulmonary haemorrhage, pulmonary hypertension.

❖ Brain infarcts, encephalopathy, seizures

❖ *Coombs positive haemolytic anaemia.*

❖ Adrenal insufficiency in 15% of cases^Q.

❖ *Digital ischaemia, skin necrosis, livedo reticularis.*

✓ **Management**

• Unfractionated Heparin is the most important treatment as it has effect on complement activation as well.

❖ LMWH is used in patients with **raised baseline APTT^Q.**

❖ Titrate against anti-Xa level as lupus anticoagulant artificially increases aPTT.

• Heparin should be transitioned to oral anticoagulation to warfarin. Lupus anticoagulant interferes with PT/INR as well and monitoring should be done using chromogenic factor × activity assay.

• If venous thrombus and antibody negative, then only we can use DOACS.

✓ **CAPLA treatment:** Anticoagulation and immunosuppression with steroids and cyclophosphamide should be used.

• *Plasmapheresis and IVIG have been used as well.*

• **Rituximab:** CD20 inhibitor, prevents B-cell activation

• **Eculizumab:** Prevents conversion of C5. Can be used earlier in disease. Increases risk of meningococcal meningitis. Vaccines and antibiotics should be given.

✓ **Prognosis**

• 90–94% survival over next ten years.

• More than 30% of patients develop permanent organ damage and more than 20% develop severe disability.

• Poor prognostic features include CAPLA, pulmonary hypertension, nephropathy, CNS involvement and gangrene of extremities.

• Lupus patients with antiphospholipid antibodies carry a high risk of neuropsychiatric disorders.

• Survival rate of catastrophic APS is about 50%.

• Anti-Ro (SSA) antibodies^Q can cross placenta and cause congenital complete heart block in female with SLE during pregnancy.

Haemophagocytic Lympho-Histiocytosis (HLH)

Epidemiology and Aetiology

✓ **Haemophagocytic lympho-histiocytosis (HLH):** Syndrome of dysregulated immune function characterized by fever, cytopaenia, and organ dysfunction.

✓ **Classified** as **Familial/Primary** (seen in children) or **acquired/secondary** (mostly in adults)

• **Macrophage activation syndrome (MAS)** is HLH in patients with rheumatological diseases like systemic juvenile idiopathic arthritis, adult-onset still's disease.

✓ **Infections** are the most common causes of secondary HLH with **EBV** as the most common cause. Other common causes are tuberculosis, malaria, *Pneumocystis jirovecii*, HIV.

• **Malignancies** like *lymphomas and chemotherapy* can also cause HLH.

✓ **Pathogenesis:** Uncontrolled immune stimulation post-infection leading to a cytokine storm and hyperinflammation causing end organ damage.

Clinical Features and Diagnosis

✓ High index of suspicion in a seriously sick patient with unexplained fever, cytopaenia, and organ dysfunction.

✓ **HLH 2004 (Both adult and children)^Q:** Diagnosis of HLH can be established if either 1 or 2 below is fulfilled.

1. Molecular diagnosis consistent with HLH

2. Diagnostic criteria with 5 out of 8 criteria below.

❖ Fever

❖ Splenomegaly

❖ Cytopaenia (≥2 lineages, Hb <90 g/L, Neutrophils <1000/μL, Platelets <100000/μL)

❖ Haemophagocytosis in bone marrow or spleen or lymph nodes

❖ Ferritin: >500 μg/L

❖ Hypertriglyceridemia: ≥265 mg/dL

❖ Soluble CD25 ≥2400 U/L

❖ Fibrinogen ≤1.5 g/L

✓ Haemophagocytosis is neither sensitive nor specific for HLH. It's a late finding.

✓ **HScore:** Bedside probability scoring tool. Score >169 has 93% sensitivity and 86% specificity.

✓ **ESR is low as is fibrinogen. NK cells are low in HLH.**

Treatment[Q]

✓ Treat the underlying cause, infection, or tumour.

✓ Dexamethasone, Anakinra (IL-1 antagonist), Etoposide, Intrathecal methotrexate.

✓ **Allogenic stem cell transplantation** isn't first-line therapy and should be considered: If malignancy is the trigger, refractory disease, HLH with genetic mutations or CNS involvement.

✓ ATG, Cyclophosphamide, **IVIG for refractory disease**

✓ **HLH-94 regimen (only children):** Dexamethasone, Etoposide, Cyclosporine A and intrathecal methotrexate in patients with neurological involvement followed by Stem cell transplantation.

✓ In Covid-19, **Tocilizumab (IL-6 Blockade)** can be used. It itself can lead to Macrophage activation syndrome.

• MAS and Covid-19 are treated by **JAK inhibitors like Baricitinib as well.**

✓ **MAS:** High-dose methylprednisolone, Cyclosporine, Anakinra, Tocilizumab.

Prognosis

✓ 55% survival rate of 3 years and 5-year survival rate of 22%.

✓ Primary HLH, ITU admission carries a high mortality of around 60%.

✓ Malignancy associated HLH mortality will be 80%.

✓ High Ferritin means high mortality. Rapid fall in ferritin is associated with favourable short-term outcome.

Disease-Modifying Anti-Rheumatic Drugs (DMARDs) for Treating Rheumatoid Arthritis

✓ **Conventional synthetic DMARDs:** Methotrexate, Hydroxychloroquine, Sulfasalazine, Leflunomide.

✓ **Biologic DMARDs**

• **Anti-TNF agents:** Infliximab, adalimumab, etanercept.

❖ They suppress the immune system and predispose the patients to infections like tuberculosis, *Listeria*, *Salmonella*, *Varicella*, *Pneumocystis jirovecii*, and *Aspergillus*.

• **B-cell depletion:** Rituximab is a monoclonal antibody against CD20, a protein found on the surface of B-lymphocytes.

❖ Predisposes to tuberculosis and JC virus leading to progressive multifocal leucoencephalopathy.

• **T-cell co-stimulators:** Abatacept binds to CD80 and CD86 receptors on the surface of T cells.

• **IL-6 antagonists:** Tocilizumab

✓ **Targeted synthetic DMARDs:** Janus kinase inhibitors like Baricitinib, Tofacitinib.

Methotrexate Pneumonitis

✓ Methotrexate can cause pulmonary toxicity by increasing pulmonary fibrosis.

• Clinical features are breathlessness, cough, fever, bibasal lung crackles.

• Gas transfer is decreased, eosinophilia is seen and patchy ground-glass opacities.

• The Searles and McKendry criteria is used for diagnosis.

• Differential diagnosis is Pneumocystis infection.

• Treatment is discontinuing methotrexate and start methylprednisolone if needed.

• Antibiotic cover may be needed if Pneumocystis infection can't be ruled out.

• Patients are put on methotrexate are started after screening with pulmonary function tests and chest X-ray.

OPHTHALMOLOGICAL DISORDERS

✓ **Lagophthalmos:** Incomplete closure of the eyelids.

• **Grade 0:** Lids completely closed.

• **Grade 1: Conjunctival exposure:** *Lubrication with ointment*[Q] (not drops) every 4 h.

• **Grade 2: Corneal exposure:** Lubrication and taping along lash margin with micropore tube.

✓ **Exposure keratopathy:** *Dryness of the cornea* due to incomplete lid closure allows tear evaporation and the subsequent failure of the tears to spread adequately across the eye surface.

✓ **Corneal abrasion: Superficial scratch** removing the surface epithelium.
- Fluorescein dye eye drops, and a blue light is used. Epithelial defect glows bright yellow.
- In ITU, 60% of patients sedated for >48 h develop corneal epithelial defects.
- Treatment of a simple corneal abrasion without secondary infection can be with *chloramphenicol ointment four times daily 5–7 d.*

✓ **Keratitis (Corneal infection)**
- Red sticky eye with ulceration
- Bacterial, HSV (Dendritic ulcer)
- Urgent ophthalmology review

✓ **Chemosis**
- *Conjunctival oedema* causing bulging due to *impaired venous return* (positive pressure ventilation), *generalized oedema* (fluid overload), gravitational causes of increased hydrostatic pressure (prone ventilation) and **increased capillary leak** (SIRS).
- Chemosis can cause impaired eyelid closure.

✓ **Conjunctivitis**
- *Red and sticky eye*
- Bacterial and infectious
- **Send swab for culture**
- Remove eye discharge with warm water, using separate gauze for each eye
- *Chloramphenicol ointment four times a day for 5–7 d.*
- If the eye becomes dull or a white patch appears, an urgent ophthalmological opinion should be sought

✓ **Acute glaucoma**
- Sudden rise in intra-orbital pressure in those nursed prone.
- Retinal/optic nerve ischaemia.

✓ **Endogenous endophthalmitis:** Emergency[Q]
- Red eye due to haematogenous spread.
- Hypopyon with white pus fluid level in anterior chamber.
- Risk of vitreous haemorrhage with tap or injection of antimicrobials.

✓ **Ischaemic optic neuropathy**
- Severe/recurrent hypotension
- May involve central *retinal artery occlusion[Q] (painless loss of vision).*

✓ **Orbital compartment syndrome**
- Raised intraocular pressure leading to reduced retinal an optic nerve perfusion.
- **Causes:** Trauma, thrombosis, haemorrhage, infection.
- **Signs:** Rapid, progressive vision loss, pain, swelling around the eyeball.
- **Treatment:** Immediate decompression: Lateral canthotomy and cantholysis.
  - ❖ Local anaesthesia at lateral canthus.
  - ❖ Surgical exposure and severing of lateral canthal tendon at the outer corner of the eye.

General Treatment Measures

✓ Allow ideally 5 min difference between each medication in the eye.
- Always put drops before ointment. Ointment is water repellent and prevents the drops from getting into the eye tissues.
- Clean off old ointment before putting in new one.
- Always check corneal clarity with bright light: If not clear: Alert medical staff.

✓ All patients with a positive blood culture[Q] or "line tip" for candida, *aspergillus* (cystic fibrosis) or any other fungal organism should be referred for urgent ophthalmological assessment[Q].
- Antifungal of choice is fluconazole for albicans species or voriconazole for non-albicans species.

16

Airway and Resuscitation

DIFFICULT AIRWAY

Difficult Intubation

✓ **NAP4 audit:** 20% of all airway incidents occurred in the ICU.
  • **Position for intubation**[Q]: Sniffing the morning air: C-spine flexion and atlanto-occipital extension.
✓ **Difficult bag mask ventilation if ≥2 of 5 factors**
  • Obese (BMI >26 kg/m²)
  • Bearded
  • Edentulous
  • Snoring
  • Elderly (>55 yr)
✓ **Difficult Intubation in ICU**[Q]: MACOCHA score >2 predicts difficult airway.
  • Mallampati 3/4: 5 points.
  • Apnoea (Obstructive sleep): 2 points.
  • Cervical spine movement limitation: 1 point.
  • Opening of mouth <3 cm: 1 point.
  • Coma: 1 point.
  • Hypoxaemia (<80%): 1 point.
  • Anaesthetist absence for intubation: 1 point.
✓ **LEMON Tool**[Q]
  • **Look:** Assess for large incisors, tongue, moustache, beard, or facial trauma
  • **Evaluate 3–3–2:** Inter-incisor distance: 3 fingers, Hyo-mental distance: 3 finger breadths, Thyromental distance: 2 finger breadths.
  • **Mallampati:** Class I to IV.
  • **Obstruction:** Stridor, abscess, and foreign bodies.
  • **Neck mobility:** Ability to touch chin to chest and extend neck to ceiling.

✓ **Difficult intubation guidelines**[Q]
  • **Plan A:** Tracheal intubation: 3 + 1(experienced colleague) intubation attempts. Cricoid pressure may be reduced to improve the view.
  • **Plan B:** Oxygenation using SAD insertion: 3 attempts using a second-generation SAD.
  • **Plan C:** Facemask Ventilation: Use 2-person technique.
  • **Plan D:** (CICO): **Front of neck access (FONA):** Adequate NMB, Scalpel (number 10 blade), bougie and tube (cuffed 6.0mm ID) required.
✓ **Can't intubate, can't oxygenate (CICO)**[Q]: Emergency situation.
  • **Surgical cricothyroidotomy only.** Needle or Seldinger cricothyroidotomy is no longer recommended.
  • **Laryngeal handshake** and palpate cricothyroid membrane.
  • **Transverse stab incision** through skin and cricothyroid membrane and turn the blade 90° with sharp edge towards feet. Insert bougie. Railroad tube over it and remove bougie.
  • In less emergent situation, vertical skin incision from below the laryngeal prominence, blunt dissection, and then a horizontal incision through the cricothyroid membrane.
  • Definite airway (tracheostomy) after a period of stability.
✓ **Capnography is gold standard for confirmation of ETT placement**[Q].
  • It works on the principle of infrared analyzer[Q]. Molecules with two or more dissimilar atoms will absorb infrared radiation[Q] (4.28 μm).

DOI: 10.1201/9781003476214-16

- **Phases of capnography**[Q]
  - ❖ **Phase 1:** Start of expiration with expiration of CO_2 free gas from anatomical dead space.
  - ❖ **Phase 2:** Represents the mixed gas from alveoli and airway with a progressive increase in CO_2.
  - ❖ **Phase 3:** Expiration of pure alveolar gas. Alveoli with longer time constants empty later and have a higher concentration of CO_2 and causes the slopping.
  - ❖ **Phase 4:** Absence of CO_2 during inspiration.
- $ETCO_2$ is normally 0.5–1 kPa less than $PaCO_2$[Q]. Increase in dead space like in pulmonary embolism can lead to increase in gap between $PaCO_2$ and $ETCO_2$.
- In bronchospasm, saw tooth appearance[Q] of capnography is seen.
  - ❖ Rapid decrease in $ETCO_2$[Q] over the course of few breaths can be seen in oesophageal intubation or large air embolism.

Stridor

- ✓ **Stridor:** High pitched, musical sound that occurs during breathing due to partial airway obstruction.
  - Three types of stridor.
    - ❖ **Inspiratory:** Obstruction above the level of larynx (e.g. acute epiglottitis, anaphylaxis).
    - ❖ **Expiratory:** Obstruction at the level of tracheobronchial tree (e.g. inhaled foreign body).
    - ❖ **Biphasic:** Glottic/subglottic obstruction (e.g. subglottic stenosis, recurrent laryngeal nerve damage).
- ✓ **Causes of stridor for admission to ITU.**
  - **Infections:** Acute epiglottitis, laryngotracheobronchitis, bacterial tracheitis.
  - **Oedema:** Anaphylaxis, post-extubation.
  - **Foreign body:** Nuts, coins.
  - **Nerve damage:** Iatrogenic recurrent laryngeal nerve damage.
  - **Acute exacerbation of chronic conditions:** Tumour, goitre.
- ✓ **Post-extubation stridor:** Laryngeal oedema is the most common cause. Other causes are laryngospasm, laryngeal nerve palsy.

- **Risk factors**[Q]: Large tube size, prolonged intubation (>48 h), high cuff pressure, multiple intubations, gastro-oesophageal reflux.
- **Cuff leak test:** Difference in inspiratory and expiratory tidal volumes after deflating the cuff should ideally be more than 10% of tidal volume or 110 mL.
  - ❖ Record the expiratory tidal volumes over six breathing cycles after deflation of cuff and average the lowest three values.
- **Management**
  - ❖ 100% oxygen by non-rebreathing mask.
  - ❖ IV corticosteroids (dexamethasone) for 24–48 h.
  - ❖ **Nebulized adrenaline:** 5 mg (5 mL of 1:1000) undiluted in single dose. May be repeated as needed.
  - ❖ **HFNO/NIV:** Helps in preparing for reintubation of the patient.
  - ❖ Avoid nasal endoscopy as can cause bleeding and further complicate the airway.

TRACHEOSTOMY

- ✓ **Trachea**
  - Starts at level of cricoid cartilage (C6)[Q] and extends till T4.
  - 16 to 20 C-shaped trachea cartilage rings and 10–12 cm long.
  - Isthmus of the thyroid overlies 2nd to 4th tracheal rings anteriorly.
- ✓ **Indications of elective tracheostomy**
  - **Prolonged ventilatory support:** Most common indication in ICU.
  - **Upper airway obstruction**
    - ❖ Vocal cord paralysis
    - ❖ Trauma of face
    - ❖ Burns
    - ❖ Infections: epiglottitis, croup, Ludwig angina
    - ❖ Neoplasms
  - **Clearance of secretions**
    - ❖ Excess secretions
    - ❖ Neuromuscular disease
- ✓ **Indications of emergency tracheostomy**
  - ❖ Transected trachea
  - ❖ Severe facial trauma
  - ❖ Acute laryngeal obstruction

- ❖ Paediatric patients <12 yr requiring emergency surgical airway as cricothyrotomy is not advised

✓ **Contraindications**
- No absolute contraindications
- Relative contraindications
  - ❖ Uncorrected coagulopathy
  - ❖ High levels of ventilatory support
  - ❖ Abnormal anatomy of upper airway

✓ **Timing of tracheostomy**
- **TracMan trial (2013)**[Q]: In patients who will require at least 7 d of mechanical ventilation, early tracheostomy (day 4) didn't improve mortality but was associated with a higher rate of unnecessary tracheostomy compared to late tracheostomy (after day 10).
- *Early tracheostomy is beneficial in multi-organ trauma patients, patients with head trauma with poor Glasgow Coma Scale, acute spine trauma, or facial injuries.*

✓ **Advantages of tracheostomy**[Q]
- Reduced need for sedation
- Increased patient comfort
- Reduced pressure/injury to lips, teeth, tongue
- Vocalization
- Oral feeding
- Decreased nursing requirement

✓ **Tracheostomy procedures**
- **Open surgical tracheostomy**
  - ❖ **Indications:** Severe respiratory failure (FiO2 >0.60, PEEP >10), obese patients, patients with large goitres, abnormal airway, abnormal bleeding diathesis.
  - ❖ **Procedure:** Horizontal skin incision. Strap muscles are separated, thyroid isthmus is mobilized. Vertical incision in 2nd or 3rd tracheal ring[Q]. Tracheal stoma matures in 7–10 d.
- **Percutaneous dilational techniques**
  - ❖ Performed using Seldinger's technique with tracheal dilation done over guidewire.
  - ❖ Bronchoscope used for direct visualization of tracheal puncture.

✓ **Tracheostomy care**
- Careful observation and handling to avoid **tracheostomy emergencies** like tube displacement, haemorrhage, surgical emphysema, pneumothorax, pneumomediastinum.

- Dressing changes should be done twice a day or when the dressings are soiled.
- Inner cannulas should be used at all times for most tracheostomy tubes during critical illnesses.
- Warm humidified gases should be used to prevent complications.
- Routine suctioning is not indicated and should be only on demand.
- A tracheostomy should not be changed until the first 7–10 d after its initial placement and should be changed approximately 30 d after placement[Q].
- Pressure in the cuff is **checked every 8–12 h** and should be kept below **20–25 cm H₂O**[Q].

✓ **Oral feeding and swallowing dysfunction with tracheostomies**
- Tracheostomy tethers the larynx and prevents its normal upward and anterior movement needed to assist in glottic closure and cricopharyngeal relaxation.
- Cuffed tubes also compress the oesophagus and interferes with deglutition.
- 40–65% of patients with tracheostomy aspirate while swallowing.
- **Speech and language therapists (SALT)** review assessment is recommended before starting oral feeding in these patients.
  - ❖ They do bedside fibre-optic endoscopic evaluation of swallowing (FESS) to detect silent aspiration and create individualized plans for the patient.
- **Excessive salivation** is managed by hyoscine patch, glycopyrrolate, sublingual atropine and botulinum toxin to the salivary glands.

✓ **Complications**[Q]
- **Immediate complications (0–24 h)**
  - ❖ Tube displacement
  - ❖ Arrhythmia
  - ❖ Pneumothorax
  - ❖ Pneumomediastinum
  - ❖ Acute surgical emphysema
  - ❖ Haemorrhage
- **Intermediate complications (Day 1 to 7)**
  - ❖ *Persistent bleeding*
  - ❖ *Tube displacement*
  - ❖ Tube obstruction
  - ❖ Wound infection
- **Late complications (> Day 7)**
  - ❖ *Tracheo-innominate artery fistula*[Q]
  - ❖ Tracheomalacia

❖ Tracheal stenosis[Q]: Commonest late complication. Use high-volume, low-pressure cuff. Asymptomatic until 75% narrowing

❖ Tracheo-oesophageal fistula

❖ Major aspiration

❖ Tracheo-cutaneous fistula

❖ Dysphagia and aspiration

✓ **Emergency tracheostomy dislodgement management: National Tracheostomy Safety Project (NTSP)[Q]**

- **Call for help** and look, listen, and feel for signs of breathing. (Mapleson C circuit and capnography will help in assessment).

  ❖ The NTSP tracheostomy/laryngectomy algorithm should be present at the head of the bed and if not available, ask for it (in OSCE exam as well).

- **Breathing check no 1:** If patient is breathing apply high flow oxygen to **both the tracheostomy and face**. If patient is not breathing, check for pulse and if no pulse, start CPR.

- **Assess tracheostomy patency**

  ❖ Remove any speaking valve, inner tube and use a suction catheter down the tracheostomy to assess patency.

  ❖ If unsuccessful, deflate the tracheostomy cuff.

- If patient doesn't improve, remove tracheostomy tube and *reassess patency by look, listen and feel at the mouth and tracheostomy.*

- **Breathing check no 2:** If patient is breathing continue ABCDE assessment. If patient is not breathing, check for pulse and if no pulse, start CPR and start oxygenation plan.

- **Primary oxygenation plan: Attempt bag ventilation** through oral airway (using mask/LMA) first by covering the tracheostomy site followed by tracheostomy stoma ventilation with paediatric mask/LMA.

- **Secondary oxygenation plan:** Try **oral Intubation** first and advance the tube beyond the stoma and if not possible, try securing the tracheal stoma (smaller tracheostomy tube/ETT size 6 mm ID).

- **In case of laryngectomy[Q], no oral route is there, so only laryngectomy stoma oxygenation and intubation is there, rest all the steps are the same.**

✓ **Bleeding tracheostomy**

- **Classification**

  ❖ **Early (≤4 d):** Skin-related, thyroid vasculature, anticoagulant/platelets.

  ❖ **Late (>4 d):** Granulation, trachea-innominate artery fistula, mucosal trauma.

- **General management of bleeding tracheostomy**

  ❖ Sit the patient up.

  ❖ Minor bleeding by TXA or adrenaline-soaked gauze pieces.

  ❖ High flow oxygen.

  ❖ Urgent anaesthetic and ENT support.

  ❖ Anticoagulant reversal.

- **Specific management of bleeding tracheostomy**

  ❖ If the tube cuff is inflated, do not deflate the cuff until expert help has arrived.

  ❖ Hyperinflate the tube cuff to augment any tamponade effect.

  ❖ Bronchoscopy to access the source and severity of bleeding.

  ❖ Endotracheal intubation if ongoing bleeding.

  ❖ Direct digital pressure manoeuvre by inserting a finger in stoma after oral intubation only.

- **Trachea-innominate artery fistula:** Rare but dreaded complication with massive haemorrhage and high mortality rate. A pulsating tracheostomy might give a clue about it.

  ❖ **Risk factors:** high pressure of cuff causing pressure necrosis, use of steroids or immunosuppressants, tracheostomy below the third tracheal ring, prolonged intubation.

✓ **Tracheostomy tube with an adjustable flange[Q]:** Obese patients, low lying tracheostomy stomas, and anatomical abnormalities

✓ **Speaking valves**

- **Montgomery valve:** Open position speaking valve that requires exhalation to close which means that some expiratory airflow is through the tracheostomy opening as well.

  ❖ Valve with a diaphragm that opens on inspiration and closes on expiration.

  ❖ Doesn't require patients to occlude using finger for vocalization.

  ❖ Can be used with a mechanical ventilator.

- **Passy–Muir valve (PMV)**[Q]: Closed position speaking valve that closes at the end of inspiration automatically, redirecting exhalation through the vocal cords.
  - ❖ Valve with a diaphragm that opens on inspiration and closes automatically on expiration.
  - ❖ Doesn't require patients to occlude using finger for vocalization.
  - ❖ Can be used with a mechanical ventilator.
- **Tracheo-oesophageal puncture valve (TEP):** Valve that allows one way passage of gas from trachea to oesophagus to allow for vocalization. Used in patients with laryngectomy.
  - ❖ Patient needs to occlude using finger for vocalization during expiration.
  - ❖ These valves shouldn't be removed during resuscitation as this can damage the fistula.

ADULT ALS

- ✓ *Advanced Life Support (ALS): 25% of initial cardiac arrest rhythms are shockable.*
  - *23.6% survival to hospital discharge if in hospital cardiac arrest.*
  - *10% of patients survive to hospital discharge after out of hospital cardiac arrest.*
- ✓ **Chain of survival**
  - Early recognition and call for help.
  - Early, uninterrupted, good quality CPR
  - Prompt defibrillation.
  - Good quality post-resuscitation care.
- ✓ Early bystander CPR, uninterrupted high-quality CPR and **early defibrillation** have been shown to have mortality benefit[Q].
  - No drugs or advanced airway techniques have been shown to improve survival.
- ✓ **Adult Advanced Life Support (RCUK guidelines)**
  - Defibrillation should be done as soon as possible, and pulse check is done after 2 min of CPR.
  - Give **Epinephrine 1 mg**[Q] as soon as possible in patients with non-shockable rhythm. Atropine is no longer recommended for **asystole/PEA.**
  - Epinephrine (1 mg)[Q] and **amiodarone (300 mg)**[Q] are used after the third shocking **refractory VF/VT.**

- Repeat Epinephrine 1 mg every 3–5 min during CPR.
- Amiodarone 150 mg IV can be given after 5th shock in patients with refractory VF/VT.
- Lidocaine 100 mg IV can be given if amiodarone is not available. An additional bolus of 50 mg IV can be given after 5 defibrillation attempts.
- Three shocks can be given if shockable rhythm is present and temperature is <30°C, further defibrillation should not be attempted until the temperature is >30°C.
- Drug boluses should be avoided until the temperature exceeds 30°C and double the dose frequency until the temperature is above 35°C.
- In witnessed, monitored arrests in post-cardiac surgery patients, three stacked shocks may be given before commencing compressions.
- **Calcium chloride 10 mL 10% (6.8 mmol):** Arrest due to hyperkalaemia, hypocalcaemia or CCBs overdose.
- **Sodium Bicarbonate 50 mL 8.4%:** TCA overdose and hyperkalaemia.
- **Alteplase 50 mg:** In pulmonary embolism. Bolus followed by another dose of 50 mg if CPR >30 min.
- **PARAMEDIC2 Trial (2018):** Adrenaline arm had higher rates of return of spontaneous circulation but the proportion of alive patients with severe neurological impairments increased.
- ✓ **Chest compressions:** 100–120/minute, depth of 5–6 cm[Q].
  - Achieves only up to 25% of normal brain flow. Interruption should be minimal <10 s.
  - Increases the likelihood of VF being successfully defibrillated.
  - Hand placement[Q] might require adjustment to a higher position on the sternum.
- ✓ **Precordial thump:** Given if witnessed and monitored pulseless VT arrest.
  - Clenched fist with the ulnar side down from a height of 20 cm on the lower sternal border.
  - Shouldn't be used post–cardiac surgery.
  - Patient can get into VF from sinus rhythm and sinus rhythm from asystole.
- ✓ **Traumatic cardiac arrest (TCA):** Condition where heart ceases to beat due to blunt trauma

or penetrating trauma. Managed differently from a medical cardiac arrest.

- **Indications**
  - ❖ Penetrating injury + arrest + previous signs of life
  - ❖ Blunt injury + arrest + previous signs of life
- **Withholding resuscitation**
  - ❖ Massive trauma incompatible with survival (decapitation)
  - ❖ No signs of life in the preceding 15 min.
  - ❖ Signs of prolonged cardiac arrest (rigor mortis)
- **Resuscitation process**[Q]
  - ❖ **Deprioritize** external chest compressions, vasopressors, and defibrillation.
  - ❖ **Airway:** Intubation to reverse hypoxia.
  - ❖ **Breathing:** Bilateral thoracostomies are done.
  - ❖ **Circulation:** Rapid blood transfusion is done, and pelvic binders applied for external haemorrhage.
  - ❖ **Circulation:** Point of care ultrasonography to check for presence of any cardiac contractility.
  - ❖ **Circulation: Resuscitative emergency thoracotomy**[Q] **where indicated should be done in first 10 minutes post-arrest. Bilateral thoracostomies** are joined by clamshell incision in fourth intercostal space and attach self-retaining rib spreader.
  - ❖ **Cardiac tamponade:** Vertical incision on tent of anterior pericardium.
  - ❖ **Cardiac rupture:** Finger occlusion/suture/staple.
  - ❖ **Cardiac massage:** Two handed massage.
- Once circulation is restored, patient should be transferred to theatre for CT scan and damage control surgery.
- **Indications to stop resuscitation in traumatic cardiac arrest.**
  - ❖ Cardiac standstill on ultrasound with tamponade excluded.
  - ❖ Lack of response to life saving interventions.
  - ❖ Persistently low-end tidal carbon dioxide
  - ❖ Long duration of cardiac arrest.
- Survival rates are better in penetrative trauma than blunt trauma.

- ❖ Unlikely to be successful if penetrating trauma with CPR >15 min or blunt trauma with CPR >10 min.
- ✓ **E-CPR:** Use of VA-ECMO as an additional measure to the conventional CPR.
  - Femorofemoral cannulation.
  - Preferred if short no flow (<5 min) and low flow (<100 min) time and initial shockable rhythms and the cause is reversible.
- ✓ **Prolonged resuscitation**
  - Hypothermia
  - Drowning
  - Local anaesthetic systemic toxicity
  - Drug intoxication like calcium channel and beta-blockers
  - Refractory anaphylaxis
  - Pulmonary embolism requiring thrombolysis
- ✓ **Intraosseous (IO) access**[Q] is recommended after two unsuccessful attempts at cannulation (ATLS). *Endotracheal route is no longer recommended.*
  - Short-term alternative to intravenous access only and speed of drug onset is comparable to it. Drug dosages are the same[Q].
  - Manual IO needles: 14, 16, and 18 gauge.
  - EZ-IO needles: Battery operated. Proximal tibia, distal tibia, proximal humerus.
    - ❖ BIG device: Spring-loaded. Proximal tibia, proximal humerus.
    - ❖ FAST 1 device: Sternum. Manually activated.
  - Complication rate is 1% and no long-term effects on bone growth.
- ✓ **Obstetric cardiac arrest**[Q]**:** High-survival group in this subgroup
  - Manual displacement of uterus.
  - Perimortem caesarean section within 5 min of cardiac arrest is indicated after 20 wk gestation to improve maternal and fetal outcome by relieving aortocaval compression.
- ✓ **ALS guidelines for bradycardia (RCUK guidelines)**
  - *If haemodynamically unstable* (shock, syncope, myocardial ischaemia, heart failure) or *risk of asystole* (Mobitz type II block, *complete heart block*, recent asystole, or ventricular pauses >3 s).
  - Initial treatment is atropine, 6 doses of 0.5 mg IV each.

- Adrenaline (2–10 mcg/min), Isoprenaline infusion (5 mcg/min), or transcutaneous pacing.
- **Glucagon** in case of beta-blocker/calcium channel blocker poisoning.
- Dopamine or Aminophylline are the alternative drugs.
- Ultimately transvenous pacing needs to be done.

✓ **ALS guidelines for tachycardia (RCUK guidelines)**
  - *If haemodynamically unstable^Q (Shock with SBP <90 mmHg, Syncope, myocardial ischaemia, and heart failure).*
    ❖ Synchronised DC shock (70–120 J)^Q, up to three attempts.
    ❖ Amiodarone 300 mg iv over 10–20 min, repeat synchronized DC shock.
  - **If haemodynamically stable**
    ❖ If QRS <0.12 s and regular, use vagal manoeuvres, Adenosine 6mg, 12 mg, 18 mg. If ineffective give verapamil or beta-blocker.
    ❖ If QRS <0.12 s and irregular, control rate by beta-blocker or diltiazem. If heart failure, consider Digoxin or amiodarone. Anticoagulate if duration >48 h.
    ❖ If QRS >0.12 s and regular, If VT, use amiodarone 300 mg IV over 10–60 min. If previous SVT with BBB, treat as regular narrow complex tachycardia.
    ❖ If QRS >0.12 s and irregular, If AF with BBB, treat as irregular narrow complex tachycardia. If Polymorphic VT give magnesium 2g over 10 min.
    ❖ If still ineffective, give synchronized DC shock up to 3 attempts for both regular or irregular QRS complexes.
    ❖ **Confusion buster: VT with pulse, give cardioversion. Pulseless VT give shock.**

✓ **Pacing**
  - **Non-invasive:** Transcutaneous or percussion
    ❖ **Percussion:** Used in peri-arrest situation or where there is P-wave asystole. From a height of 10 cm onto the pericardium at the lower left sternal edge.
    ❖ **Transcutaneous:** Average current required is 50–100 mA.

- **Invasive:** Temporary or permanent intravenous pacing

✓ **Choking:** Partial or complete airway obstruction by a foreign body.
  - **BLS guidelines for adults**
    ❖ Encourage coughing.
    ❖ If coughing not effective, 5 back blows.
    ❖ If back blows not effective, 5 abdominal thrusts (Heimlich manoeuvre).
    ❖ Alternate back blows and abdominal thrusts till the time patient either becomes better or becomes unresponsive.
    ❖ If unresponsive, start CPR.
  - **BLS guidelines for infants**
    ❖ Child in prone position, head pointing down on rescuer's lap.
    ❖ 5 back blows between shoulder blades.
    ❖ Child in supine position, **5 chest thrusts.**
  - **BLS guidelines for child >1 yr**
    ❖ Child leaning forward.
    ❖ 5 back blows between shoulder blades.
    ❖ Child in supine position, **5 abdominal thrusts.**

✓ **Gas embolism**
  - **Gas embolism:** Entrapment of gas into circulation. Can be arterial or venous.
    ❖ Gases involved can be air, oxygen, **$CO2$ (laparoscopy)** and **helium (IABP).**
    ❖ In arteries even 0.02 mL/kg can be potentially fatal.
  - **High-risk procedures for gas embolism.**
    ❖ Laparoscopy
    ❖ Posterior fossa surgery
    ❖ Sitting position craniotomy
    ❖ CVC insertion/removal
  - **Pathophysiology of gas embolism**
    ❖ **Mechanical obstruction:** Blood vessels, heart chambers.
    ❖ **Biochemical activation:** Activation of complement, platelets, coagulation pathway.
  - **Clinical features of venous gas embolism**
    ❖ **CVS:** Chest pain, dyspnoea, mill wheel murmur, signs of right heart failure, **cardiac arrest.**
    ❖ **CNS:** Anxiety, seizures, drowsiness, focal neurological deficits, stroke (paradoxical right to left shunt).
    ❖ **Respiratory:** Wheezing, haemoptysis, cyanosis, apnoea.

- **Management**
  - ❖ Notify surgeon to occlude entry sites (saline flooding).
  - ❖ Lower surgical field to below the level of the heart.
  - ❖ 100% oxygen.
  - ❖ **Durant manoeuvre:** Left lateral decubitus position.
  - ❖ CPR may actually break the gas bubble and relieve right ventricular outflow tract.
  - ❖ Early vasopressors/inotropes.
  - ❖ Transoesophageal echocardiography.
  - ❖ **Hyperbaric oxygen.**

Additional Questions

✓ **Defibrillator[Q]:** Delivers DC shock to heart as AC causes myocardial damage.
- A **rectifier** is used to derive DC power from AC power.
- A **step up transformer** increases the mains voltage from 240V to 5000V.
- A capacitor is used to store charges. They have low reactance to AC but high resistance to DC.
- An inductor is used to prolong the duration of current discharge. A magnetic flux is induced whenever a current flows through the coils causing back EMF and prolongs the charge. Inductor has high reactance to AC but low resistance to DC.
- During charging, current just flows through the capacitor plates which store the charge.
- When discharging, the stored charge from the capacitor is now delivered to the patient. The inductor prolongs the effective delivery of current to myocardium.
- Biphasic waveform[Q] defibrillate more effectively at lower energies compared to their monophasic counterparts.

CARDIAC-ALS

✓ **Causes of cardiac arrest in the early post-operative period post-cardiac surgery**
- **Preload reduction (Hypovolaemia):** Mostly because of bleeding (medical or surgical).
- **Afterload reduction (Vasodilation):** Prolonged bypass time, preoperative infection.
- **Low cardiac output state**
  - ❖ **Tamponade:** Emergency re-sternotomy
  - ❖ **Ischaemic cardiac failure:** IABP/Cath lab/re-operate.

- ❖ **Valvular failure:** Re-operate. IABP for MR prior to going back to theatre.
- ❖ **Ventricular impairment:** Inotropes + mechanical support.
- ❖ **Tachyarrhythmias:** Amiodarone/Magnesium/DC cardioversion.
- ❖ **Bradyarrhythmias:** Atropine/adrenaline/pacing.

✓ **C-ALS: Algorithm for cardiac arrest in patients with sternotomy**
- **Cardiac arrest: Access rhythm**
  - ❖ **Ventricular fibrillation:** Give 3 DC shocks, start BLS support with amiodarone 300 mg via central venous line. Prepare for emergency re-sternotomy and continue CPR with single DC shock every 2 min until re-sternotomy.
  - ❖ **Asystole/severe bradycardia:** Pace if wires available, start BLS support and consider external pacing. Prepare for emergency re-sternotomy and continue CPR until re-sternotomy.
  - ❖ **Pulseless electrical activity (PEA):** If paced turn off pacing to exclude underlying VF. Start BLS support and prepare for emergency re-sternotomy and continue CPR until re-sternotomy.

✓ **Simultaneous ongoing management**
- If patient is ventilated turn FiO2 to 100% and take patient on bag/valve circuit otherwise give bag mask ventilation at ratio of 30 compressions to 2 breaths.
- Check the position of endotracheal tube and that the cuff is inflated.
- Rule out pneumothorax and haemothorax.
- Once adequate airway and breathing is confirmed, reconnect to the ventilator, and remove PEEP.
- Do not give EPINEPHRINE unless a senior doctor advises.
- All pre-arrest infusions should be stopped.
- If an IABP is in place, change to pressure trigger.
- **Do not delay Basic Life Support (BLS) for defibrillation or pacing for more than one minute.**
- **Automated external defibrillators (AEDs)** should not be used in cardiac surgical patients in the ICU when manual defibrillator is available as AED can deliver 3 shocks.

- **Re-sternotomy** should be done within 5 min and should be used in all patients till 10th post-operative day.
- ✓ **Re-sternotomy**
  - Sternal wires are cut, and sternal retractor used to open the chest.
  - Pericardial cavity is opened and clot overlying the heart is removed using Yankauer sucker. If tamponade was the cause, there should be return of cardiac activity.
  - If no return of cardiac activity, start intra-cardiac massage at the rate of 40–60 compressions/minute and if there is a shockable rhythm give 3 back-to-back 20 J shocks with internal defibrillator pads.

ANAPHYLAXIS

Epidemiology and Aetiology

- ✓ **Anaphylaxis:** Severe, life-threatening, generalized, or systemic hypersensitivity reaction.
  - **Allergic:** IgE antibodies involved. IgG or complement also might be involved.
  - **Non-allergic (anaphylactoid reaction):** No IgE antibodies involved. Atracurium and mivacurium can cause non-allergic anaphylaxis.
- ✓ **Causes**
  - **NAP6 report:** Antibiotics (47%), Muscle relaxants (33%), Chlorhexidine (9%).
  - Incidence of perioperative anaphylaxis is 1 in 10,000. Female preponderance. Mortality of 3–6%.
  - Prior drug exposure is not necessary. Prior history of atopy and asthma may be present.
  - Rocuronium[Q] is the most likely muscle relaxant that can cause anaphylactic reaction.
- ✓ **World Allergy Organization (WAO) diagnostic criteria:** Any one of the following two are fulfilled. (Imagine trying to remember a criteria while diagnosing something as serious as an anaphylaxis, what the hell).
  - Acute onset of an illness with involvement of **skin, mucosal tissue, or both** (pruritus, swelling) and at least one of the following.
    - ❖ **Airway/breathing:** Dyspnoea, bronchospasm, stridor.
    - ❖ **Circulation:** Reduced BP or associated signs of end-organ dysfunction.
    - ❖ **GIT:** Abdominal pain, vomiting.
  - Acute onset of **hypotension or bronchospasm or laryngeal involvement** after exposure to a known allergen **even in the absence of typical skin involvement.**
- ✓ **Pathophysiology**
  - Distributive shock leading to vasodilation and fluid extravasation due to capillary leak.

Clinical Features and Diagnosis

- ✓ **Medical emergency and clinical diagnosis**
  - **Hypotension** (commonest feature). Can have both **bradycardia** and tachycardia.
- ✓ **Grading of anaphylaxis (WAO classification)[Q]** (Again, what the hell)
  - **Grade 1:** 1 Organ involved.
    - ❖ **Conjunctiva:** Erythema, pruritus
    - ❖ **Skin:** Urticaria, angioedema.
    - ❖ **Upper respiratory tract:** Rhinitis.
  - **Grade 2:** 2 of the above organs involved and **gastrointestinal:** Vomiting, diarrhoea.
  - **Grade 3:** Any 1 of the following.
    - ❖ **Lower airway:** Mild bronchospasm: cough, wheeze responding to treatment.
    - ❖ **Gastrointestinal:** Vomiting, diarrhoea.
    - ❖ **Uterine cramps ± bleeding.**
  - **Grade 4**
    - ❖ **Lower airway:** Severe bronchospasm: Not responding to treatment.
    - ❖ **Upper airway:** Severe stridor
  - **Grade 5:** Respiratory failure, cardiovascular collapse, loss of consciousness.
- ✓ Usually resolves in 2–8 h but may be biphasic, so observations of the patients for 24 h may be needed.

Resuscitation (RCUK Guidelines)

- ✓ Call for help and remove the trigger.
- ✓ **A/B:** High 100% oxygen and raise the legs.
- ✓ **C:** Adrenaline.
  - **Perioperative (in specialist settings like operating theatre or critical care department).**
    - ❖ **Adult and child >12 yr[Q]:** 50 micrograms IV [0.5 mL of 1 mg/10 mL (1:100000)]
    - ❖ Child <12 yr: 1 microgram/kg, titrate to effect.
    - ❖ If no IV access: 10 micrograms/kg IM (Max 500 micrograms IM) of 1 mg/mL (1:1000) and secure IV/IO access.

- **In non-specialist settings like ward:**
  Adrenaline 1 mg/mL (1:1000)
  - ❖ **Adult and child >12 yr[Q]:** 500 micrograms Adrenaline IM (0.5 mL)
  - ❖ Child 6–12 yr: 300 micrograms Adrenaline IM (0.3 mL)
  - ❖ Child 6 months to 6 yr: 150 micrograms Adrenaline IM (0.15 mL)
  - ❖ Child <6 months: 100–150 micrograms Adrenaline IM (0.1–0.15 mL)
  - ❖ Repeat IM adrenaline after 5 min and if no response after 2 doses of IM adrenaline, follow the refractory anaphylaxis algorithm

✓ **C:** Intravenous fluids.
- Adult and child >12 yr: 500–1000 mL.
- Child <12 yr: 20 mL/kg.
- Multiple fluid boluses may be needed. (3–5 L in adults, 60–100 mL/kg in children)
- Avoid colloids.

✓ If poor response to adrenaline boluses, start IV infusion and involve ICU team early.
- Peripheral low-dose IV adrenaline: 0.5 mg [0.5 mL of 1 mg/mL (1:1000)] in 50 mL and start at the rate of 0.5–1 mL/kg/h.

✓ If systolic BP <50 mmHg or cardiac arrest, start CPR.

Further Management

✓ **Airway/Breathing**
- **Severe bronchospasm:** Exclude oesophageal intubation, check airway patency, nebulized salbutamol/ipratropium, and IV bronchodilator.
- For stridor nebulize with adrenaline 5 mL of 1mg/mL (1:1000).

✓ **Circulatory**
- Refractory to adrenaline: Add noradrenaline or vasopressin.
  - ❖ Consider Glucagon 1 mg in adults on beta-blockers.
  - ❖ **Consider steroids for refractory shock[Q].**
  - ❖ Consider extracorporeal life support.

Immediate Follow-Up

✓ If surgery is urgent or time critical and patient is stable, proceed with surgery but avoid suspected triggers.

✓ A **mast cell tryptase[Q]** should be sent as soon as possible and again at 1 to 2 h and then 24 h after the event.
- During anaphylaxis, tryptase peaks at 1 h and half-life is 2 h. Normal tryptase level do not exclude anaphylaxis.
- The assay for tryptase includes A-tryptase and B-tryptase. High specificity but low sensitivity. Even post-mortem samples are valid.
- Intravenous fluid replacement dilutes the blood and therefore the tryptase concentration.
- B-tryptase is specific for anaphylaxis. May be raised in trauma and myocardial infarction.

✓ **Referral to local allergy clinics** for testing of trigger.

✓ **Alert the general practitioner** and complete a **yellow form** if a drug reaction is considered likely.

✓ Report reaction to the anaphylaxis registry and adrenaline injector to be carried as an interim measure.

Refractory Anaphylaxis Algorithm

✓ **Refractory anaphylaxis:** No improvements in respiratory or cardiovascular symptoms despite 2 doses of IM adrenaline.

✓ **Management**
- Establish dedicated peripheral IV or IO access.
- Give IV fluid bolus and start peripheral adrenaline infusion.
- Give IM adrenaline every 5 min until adrenaline infusion has been started. (IV adrenaline in specialist settings)
- High flow oxygen to maintain SpO2 above 94%.
- Monitor HR, BP, pulse oximetry and ECG. Take blood sample for mast cell tryptase.

Angioedema

Angioedema: Painful swelling due to leakage of small blood vessels in the deeper layers of the skin and mucous membrane.

✓ **Causes**
- **Idiopathic:** Stress or infection
- **Medications:** ACE inhibitors, Aspirin
- **Allergic:** Food or environmental allergens like milk, nuts, shellfish
- **Hereditary:** C1 esterase deficiency

- ✓ **Symptoms:** Puffy or swollen lips, tongue, eyes, abdominal pain, diarrhoea, swollen hands, feet, or genitals
- ✓ **Treatment**[Q]
  - Injectable adrenaline, corticosteroids, and antihistamines.
  - C1 inhibitor concentrate.
  - Fresh frozen plasma may be given.
- ✓ **Prognosis:** Mild cases last up to 3 d and go on their own most of the times. Severe cases can be life-threatening and require immediate medical attention.

17

Monitoring

CARDIAC MONITORING

✓ Cardiac output (CO) = Heart rate × stroke volume. Normal = 4–6 L/min.
- **Cardiac index**[Q] = Cardiac output/body surface area. Normal = 2.5–4 L/min.

✓ $CaO_2 = (1.39 \times Hb \times SaO_2) + (0.0225 \times PaO_2)$ where CaO_2 is oxygen content[Q].
- $DO_2 = CO \times CaO_2$ where CO is cardiac output and DO_2 is oxygen delivery[Q].

✓ **MAP** = CO × SVR where SVR is systemic vascular resistance. CO = HR × SV where HR is heart rate and stroke volume. *So, it depends upon preload, contractility, and afterload.*
- **Neural control:** Baroreceptors in the carotid sinus and aortic arch.
- **Hormonal control:** Adrenaline/noradrenaline, vasopressin, and angiotensin II cause vasoconstriction. Histamine and Nitric oxide cause vasodilation.
- *Heart, brain, and kidney have autoregulation of their blood pressure[Q].*

✓ **Shock:** Globally impaired tissue and organ perfusion inadequate for the metabolic needs of the body.
- **Types of shock**
  - ❖ **Distributive shock:** Sepsis, anaphylaxis, neurogenic shock. Cardiac Index (CI) >2.2 L/min/m² initially. *CVP low.* Most common type of shock.
  - ❖ **Hypovolemic shock:** Haemorrhage, Diarrhoea and vomiting. CI <2.2 L/min/m². *CVP low.*
  - ❖ **Cardiogenic shock:** Myocardial infarction, arrhythmias. CI <2.2 L/min/m². *CVP high.*
  - ❖ **Obstructive shock:** Pulmonary embolism, cardiac tamponade, tension pneumothorax. CI <2.2 L/min/m². *CVP high.*

Method	Monitoring System
Pulmonary thermodilution	• Pulmonary artery catheter
Transpulmonary thermodilution	• PiCCO • VolumeView
Transpulmonary indicator dilution	• LiDCO
Arterial pressure waveform derivation	• PiCCO • LiDCO • Flotrac • Finapres
Applied Fick method	• NICO
Doppler	• Oesophageal Doppler
Transthoracic electrical bioimpedance	• Bioimpendance

✓ **Pulmonary artery catheter (PAC)**
- **Gold standard for cardiac output:** Change in temperature measured using thermistor[Q].
  - ❖ Stewart–Hamilton equation is used to measure cardiac output.
- **Four lumens:** Proximal, distal, inflation balloon, and thermistor lumen.
- **Directly measured variables**[Q]: Temperature, Cardiac output (CO), CVP, right atrial pressure (RAP), pulmonary artery pressure (PAP), pulmonary artery occlusion pressure (PAOP), and mixed venous saturations[Q].
- **Indirectly measured variables**[Q]: Stroke volume, Cardiac index, SVR, PVR, LVEDP, and SVV.

DOI: 10.1201/9781003476214-17

- **PAC-MAN** trial (2005) showed no mortality difference in patients with PAC vs no PAC in critically ill patients.
- **Cardiac output measurement:** Measures CO intermittently.
  - ❖ A bolus of extremely cold[Q] saline is injected into the right atrium via a PAC port and change in blood temperature at the PAC tip is measured.
  - ❖ **Over estimation of cardiac output:** A small volume of injectate, tricuspid regurgitation with intact right ventricle function, cardiac index <2.5 L/min/m^2 and in right to left shunt.
  - ❖ **Under estimation of cardiac output:** Tricuspid regurgitation (yes, it can lead to both under and over estimation)
  - ❖ Continuous CO measurement is available and uses a thermal filament that warms blood in SVC and change in blood temperature at the PAC tip is measured.
- **Pulmonary capillary wedge pressure (PCWP)[Q]:** Used interchangeably with pulmonary artery occlusion pressure (PAOP).
  - ❖ Measured by advancing a pulmonary artery catheter into a small pulmonary artery branch.
  - ❖ Balloon is then inflated to allow a continuous column of blood between catheter tip and the left atrium.
  - ❖ **Normal range is 4–12** mmHg.
  - ❖ Normally mean Pulmonary artery pressure should be more than pulmonary capillary wedge pressure.
  - ❖ High PCWP[Q] seen in hypervolaemia, tamponade, or myocardial dysfunction.
  - ❖ **In acute LVF, LVEDP be greater than PCWP. In pulmonary embolism, LVEDP will be less than PCWP[Q].**
  - ❖ Pulmonary artery systolic pressure >55 mmHg shows chronicity.
- **Other parameters**
  - ❖ Equalization of the RA, RV and PA diastolic and PAOP pressures indicates cardiac tamponade.
  - ❖ **PEEP elevates the PCWP by 50% of the amount applied.**
- **PAC Trace: Expected depth:** Right atrium: 10–15 cm, right ventricle: 25–30 cm, pulmonary artery: 35–40 cm and PCWP: 45 cm.
  - ❖ Position of the catheter is confirmed by chest X-ray and the catheter tip should not extend beyond the pulmonary hilum[Q].
  - ❖ PAC tip should be in West zone 3[Q]. Catheter tip location should be below the level of the left atrium on lateral chest X-ray[Q].
  - ❖ Blood saturation at SVC: 70%, RA: 75%, RV: 75%, PA: 75%, Wedged position: 100%
  - ❖ **Difficult PAC insertion:** Low cardiac state (can't float), Dilated RV (can get kinked), Pulmonary HTN and tricuspid regurgitation.
  - ❖ Continuous increase in pressure with the balloon inflated, consistent with an over wedged position. Seen due to eccentric inflation or the balloon being trapped against the vessel wall. Pulling the catheter back is the treatment[Q].
  - ❖ If the RV waveform doesn't transition[Q] to a PA waveform after advancing for long, withdraw the PA catheter.
- **Complications:** Colonization of the catheter is the most common complication of PAC insertion[Q].
  - ❖ Carotid artery puncture is next common complication. Overall, 10% complication rate.
  - ❖ Pulmonary artery infarction or rupture may happen because of wedged catheter.

✓ **Oesophageal Doppler**
- **Principle:** Measures shifts in reflected sound waves to estimate flow velocity[Q] in the descending thoracic aorta.
  - ❖ It assumes all red blood cells flow in the same velocity[Q] and assumes aorta is a uniform cylinder.
  - ❖ Minimal or no blood flow in the descending aorta will be detected by the oesophageal Doppler probe during diastole[Q] is also assumed.
  - ❖ Nomogram[Q] is used to extrapolate true aortic cross-sectional area and cross-sectional area remains constant throughout systole.
  - ❖ Uses age, height, and weight of the population to calculate aortic cross-sectional area.
  - ❖ It is also assumed that 70% of total cardiac output passes the probe[Q].

- **Procedure:** Length is up to 40–45 cm through nose or 35–40 cm through the mouth[Q].
  - ❖ Angle of incident between ultrasound beam and aortic blood flow should be 45°–60°.
  - ❖ Poor probe position leads to underestimation of SV and CO.
  - ❖ It can be used in children as well.
- Mortality benefit in perioperative settings but not in ICU patients.
- **Parameters**
  - ❖ **Flow time corrected (FTc)[Q]:** Indicates preload. 0.33–0.36 s.
  - ❖ **Peak velocity (PV)[Q]:** Indicates Contractility. 90–120 cm/sec.
  - ❖ **Mean acceleration[Q]:** Indicates contractility.
  - ❖ **Stroke volume (SV)[Q]:** Measured by stroke distance × aortic root diameter.
- **Actions for deranged findings**
  - ❖ *High FTc:* Increased afterload. Give vasodilation.
  - ❖ *Low PV + Low FTc:* Increased afterload. Decrease afterload.
  - ❖ *Low SV:* Low preload. Give fluid.
  - ❖ *Low PV:* Low contractility. Give inotrope.
- ✓ **Pulse contour analysis (PCA):** Uses information from the waveform of **arterial pressure trace** to calculate stroke volume (SV) and cardiac output (CO). Knowledge of compliance and SVR is also required for calculation of SV and CO. **Some are calibrated with indicator dilution methods (PiCCO/LiDCO) and some use demographic and physical data method (FloTrac).** Accuracy is dependent upon arterial trace.
  - **Volume view**
    - ❖ Calibrated
    - ❖ **Principle:** First reading by pulmonary thermodilution (femoral artery used), followed by second reading by pulse contour analysis.
      - A drop in temperature is measured over time. Measures temperature change in the femoral artery compared to pulmonary artery for PAC for calculating cardiac output.
      - Uses a CVC and a femoral artery catheter.

- Works on Stewart-Hamilton algorithm.
- ❖ If all parameters of perfusion are normal, no need to give extra fluid.
- ❖ **Intrathoracic blood volume (ITBV):** Includes volume in the four cardiac chambers and thoracic vasculature.
  - Normal range: **850–1000 mL/m^2**
- ❖ **Global end diastolic volume (GEDV)** indicates preload and includes volume in the four cardiac chambers.
  - GEDV = ITBV/1.25
  - Normal range: **600–800 mL/m^2**
- ❖ **Extra vascular lung volume Index (EVLW):** All the fluid within the lung but outside of the vasculature compartment.
  - Normal range is 3–7 mL/kg.
  - Uses predicted body weight for calculation.
  - Water at 4°C for calibration as saline at room temperature overestimates the value.
  - Increase in EVLWI by 14% has sensitivity of 70% and specificity of 99% about weaning failure due to cardiac origin.
  - Increase in EVLWI doesn't always talk about pulmonary oedema. Pneumonia can also cause it.
  - EVLWI underestimates pulmonary oedema only in total occlusion of pulmonary vessel.
  - EVLWI doesn't show any mortality benefit.
- ❖ **Pulmonary vascular permeability Index (PVPI)**
  - **PVPI** = EVLW/0.25 × GEDV
  - Normal value: 1–3
  - **Increased EVLWI with PVPI less than 3 indicates pulmonary** oedema is cardiogenic in nature
  - **PVPI greater than 3 indicates leaky capillaries** irrespective of value of EVLWI
- **PiCCO[Q]**
  - ❖ **Principle:** First reading by pulmonary thermodilution (femoral artery used), followed by continuous cardiac output readings by pulse contour analysis.
    - A drop in temperature is measured over time. Measures temperature

change in the femoral artery compared to pulmonary artery for PAC for calculating cardiac output.

- Uses a CVC and a femoral artery catheter.
- Analyses area under systolic portion of the curve is analyzed to determine SV recognizing the dicrotic notch.
  ❖ ITBV, GEDV, and EVLW can be calculated as well.

- LiDCO[Q]
  ❖ **Principle:** First reading by pulmonary indicator dilution followed by continuous cardiac output readings by pulse contour analysis.
    - The first reading is used to calibrate the device and then used every 8 h to calibrate it.
    - A change in indicator concentration is measured over time.
    - PVC or CVC can be used to inject the indicator (2 mL, 0.3 mmol of lithium). Peripheral arterial line is required.
    - Assumes that complete mixing of blood and indicator happens without any loss of indicator between site of injection and detection.
  ❖ Limited utility in intra cardiac shunt or in patients on IABP.
  ❖ Analyzed the arterial waveform using pulse power analysis.

- FloTrac
  ❖ Provides continuous CO monitoring using the arterial waveform monitoring.
  ❖ Uncalibrated
  ❖ Analyses the waveform 100 times/ second over 20 s (dynamic tone technology)

✓ **Fick method:** Fick principle states that total amount of a substance produced or taken up by the body is equal to cardiac output multiplied by the arteriovenous concentration difference.

- Using pulmonary artery and peripheral arterial oxygen measurements and assuming a value of oxygen consumption of 125 mL/min/m[2], cardiac output can be estimated.
- $CO = VO_2/C_a-C_v$ where VO_2 is measurement of oxygen concentration with a closed

loop spirometer, C_a is oxygen concentration of artery, C_v is oxygen concentration of vein.
- It assumes no intracardiac shunt.
- **Non-invasive cardiac output (NICO)** uses **Indirect Fick method** that is CO_2 instead of O_2.
  ❖ Compares $EtCO_2$ measured during normal ventilation and during periods of partial CO_2 rebreathing.

✓ **Invasive arterial blood pressure**
- **Principle:** The arterial line is connected to pressurized fluid in rigid tubing. Intra-arterial pulsations travel to the pressure transducer[Q] which is made of a sensitive diaphragm and strain gauge arranged in a Wheatstone[Q] bridge setup.
  ❖ Pulsations due to blood flow deform the diaphragm alter strain gauge resistance.
  ❖ Electronic device detects the changes in resistance and Fourier analysis processes the data to display the blood pressure waveform.
  ❖ Natural frequency[Q] of the system should be ten times the frequency of primary harmonic. System should be a little over damped.
  ❖ A heart rate of 60 bpm will have a frequency of 1 Hz. So, for a heart rate of 120 bpm (2 Hz), a resonant frequency of 20 Hz of the system will be needed.
- **Zero referencing[Q]** is done at the level of right atrium[Q] (4th intercostal space, midaxillary line).
  ❖ Transducer height above heart: Falsely low BP
  ❖ Transducer height below heart: Falsely high BP
- **Parameters** that can be derived from IABP[Q].
  ❖ **Stroke volume and cardiac output[Q]:** Area under the curve of the systolic part of pressure:
    - **Contractility:** Slope of the pressure waveform at the onset of systole.
    - **Intravascular filling:** Changes in arterial pressure over the respiratory cycle.
    - **Systemic vascular resistance:** Slope of the diastolic pressure decay.
    - **Arterial compliance:** Dicrotic notch[Q] represents closure of the aortic valve and in sepsis

(vasodilation) there is a downward shift of the dicrotic notch[Q].

- **Damping:** A fast flush test (square wave test) helps in determination of damping coefficient and natural frequency of the transducer system.
  - ❖ **Wide, stiff, and short cannula makes a normal wave**[Q] where natural frequency of measuring system is higher than the frequency of arterial blood pressure.
  - ❖ **Optimal damping:** Rapid return to zero with a minimal overshoot. **The optimal damping value is 0.64. Damping where real-time accuracy is greatest.**
  - ❖ **Under damped**[Q]**:** Underdamped signals resonate around a step change.
    - If natural frequency of the transducer system is nearer to the frequency of the monitored arterial waveform.
    - High SBP, low DBP, multiple dicrotic notches.
    - Excessive tubing length, aortic regurgitation and atherosclerosis can cause this.
    - **MAP isn't affected.**
  - ❖ **Overdamped**[Q]**:** Overdamped signals take a long time to respond to a step change.
  - ❖ Clots, air bubbles, arterial spasm, kinking of the tube, underinflated pressure bag, fluid of high viscosity and loose connections can cause overdamping of tracing.
  - ❖ **MAP isn't affected.**
  - ❖ Heparin use in flush system isn't mandatory and flush system should be pressurized to 300 mmHg and infusion should be at the rate of 2–4 mL/h[Q].
- **Arterial line swing:** During mechanical ventilation, right atrium gets lower venous return during inspiration while left atrium gets increased venous return.
  - ❖ So, the left ventricle output increases during inspiration followed by a decrease in stroke volume during expiration.
  - ❖ This interaction is increased in hypovolaemia, and we can see a "swing" on the arterial pressure waveform.

- **Complications:** Temporary radial artery occlusion and bleeding/haematoma formation are the common ones.
- ✓ **Finapres:** Non-invasive technique. Penaz technique[Q].
  - Inflatable finger cuff (bladder with an infrared plethysmograph) is put on middle phalanx of the finger.
  - The cuff pressure is continuously adjusted counteract changes in arterial diameter due to blood pressure fluctuations.
  - The pressure within the cuff, which is equal to the intra-arterial pressure at the clamped diameter is measured and used to determine the blood pressure.
  - Basically, the Finapres mimics the conditions of an invasive arterial measurement by clamping the finger artery at its natural diameter and using the counteracting cuff pressure as a proxy for blood pressure.
  - Continuous stroke volume and cardiac output is calculated using systolic pressure area.
- ✓ **Transthoracic electrical bioimpendance:** Based on the principle that during systole, ejection of blood from the heart is associated with change in electrical impedance of the thoracic cavity due to increased blood volume.
  - Rate of change of this impedance is proportional to cardiac output (CO).
  - Four electrodes are placed on the neck and thorax and a low current is passed between them.
  - Blood volume and velocity within the aorta changes from beat to beat and this leads to changes in thoracic impedance.
  - Device measures the changes in impedance and signifies Cardiac output.

Additional Questions

- ✓ **Non-invasive blood pressure (NIBP):** Korotkoff sounds.
  - Korotkoff method: Auscultation over the brachial artery.
    - ❖ Phase I: Tapping sound: SBP is when first sound is heard
    - ❖ Phase II: Muffling sound: Auscultatory gap
    - ❖ Phase III: Reappearing of tapping sound
    - ❖ Phase IV: Muffling sound again: DBP
    - ❖ Phase V: Sound disappears

✓ **Transpulmonary indicators:** Thermodilution using **cold fluid**, e.g. PiCCO (CVC and femoral artery catheter) or Pulmonary artery catheter and **Lithium** e.g. LiDCO (PVC and peripheral artery can be used)

FLUID RESPONSIVENESS

✓ **Fluid responsiveness:** Increase in stroke volume or cardiac output after giving a bolus of fluid.
- **Fluid challenge:** Definitive test for checking fluid responsiveness.
  - ❖ Give 500 mL of crystalloid over 10–15 min and stroke volume increases by ≥10%.
  - ❖ A marked rise in CVP with fluid challenge indicates a failing ventricle.
  - ❖ Only 50% of patients with septic shock are fluid responsive and the response can be short lived as most of the fluid leaks into tissues.
- **Mini-fluid challenge:** 100 mL of colloid over 1 min. Real time cardiac output monitoring is needed. >6% change in CO is predictive of fluid responsiveness.

✓ **Significance**
- Fluid responsiveness doesn't mean that a patient should be given fluids.
- It means patients are on the ascending portion of the starling curve.
- However, the fluid administered may not stay in the circulation for long and can cause tissue or pulmonary oedema.

✓ **Static indicators**
- Central venous pressure (CVP)
- Pulmonary capillary wedge pressure (PCWP)
- Left ventricular end-diastolic volume (LVEDV)
- Global end diastolic volume (GEDV)
- IVC diameter
  - ❖ PCWP is explained in chapter on cardiac output monitoring.
  - ❖ LVEDV is measured by echocardiography.
  - ❖ GEDV is measured by PiCCO and volume view (explained in chapter on cardiac monitoring).

✓ **Dynamic indicators**
- Passive leg raising test (PLR)
- End-expiratory occlusion test (EEOT)

- Tidal volume challenge (TVC)
- Pulse pressure variability (PPV)
- Stroke volume variability (SVV)
- Systolic pressure variability (SPV)
- Pleth variability index (PVI)
- Point of care ultrasound (POCUS)

✓ **Central venous pressure (CVP)**
- Assesses right atrial pressures.
- CVP isn't a good predictor of fluid responsiveness.
  - ❖ Predictive value of extreme values of CVP (like <4 or >16) give a bit of safety margin.
  - ❖ Two-thirds of patients with CVP less than 8 mmHg but one-third of patients with CVP >12 mmHg will respond to fluids.
- One should try to maintain lowest possible CVP to maintain organ pressure.
- Monitoring trends in CVP over time is more important than single measurements.
- **CVP Waves[Q]:** "**a**": Atrial contraction, "**c**": Right ventricular contraction, "**v**": passive atrial filling.
  - ❖ **Absent "a" wave:** Atrial fibrillation.
  - ❖ **Cannon "a" wave:** Complete heart block, ventricular tachycardia.
  - ❖ **Giant "C-V" wave[Q]:** Severe tricuspid regurgitation.
  - ❖ **Large "a" wave** with **slow "y" descent:** Tricuspid stenosis.
  - ❖ *Exaggerated "x" and "y" descent:* constrictive pericarditis (Friedrich's sign[Q]).
  - ❖ *Exaggerated "x" descent:* Cardiac tamponade.

✓ **Passive leg raising test[Q] (PLR)**
- **Method:** Patient should be in semi-recumbent position (45°).
  - ❖ Patient's upper body is lowered to horizontal, and legs are raised passively at 45° up.
  - ❖ Real time cardiac monitoring should be available as we need to capture that cardiac output in 90 s. TTE might be cumbersome to do.
  - ❖ CO >10%, predicts fluid responsiveness.
- Reliable in spontaneously breathing patient.
- Unreliable in patients with hypovolaemia and intra-abdominal hypertension.

✓ **End expiratory occlusion test (EEOT)**
- **Method:** Occluding the circuit at end-expiration stops the cyclic effect of inspiration

of reducing left cardiac preload and acts like a fluid challenge.

❖ A 15 s expiratory occlusion is done; patient must be able to tolerate a 15 s pause in ventilation.

❖ Increase in cardiac output by more than 5% will be considered as fluid responsiveness.

• Can be done in patients with arrythmias and low tidal volumes.

• Can't be done in spontaneously breathing patient.

✓ **Pulse Pressure Variability (PPV)**

• Pulse pressure is the difference between systolic and diastolic blood pressure.

• **Method:** PPV refers to the difference between the maximum and minimum pulse pressure during a single mechanical breath.

❖ During spontaneous breathing, systolic blood pressure fluctuates by 5–10 mmHg with higher systolic blood pressure during expiration.

❖ **Pulsus paradoxus:** Systolic blood pressure fluctuates by more than 10 mmHg during spontaneous breathing.

❖ **Reverse pulsus paradoxus[Q]:** Occurs during mechanical ventilation where arterial blood pressure falling during expiration.

❖ Change in pulse pressure during mechanical ventilation >**13** % predicts fluid responsiveness[Q].

• **Prerequisite[Q]**

❖ Sinus rhythm

❖ Sedated patient with absence of spontaneous breathing efforts (complete paralysis not necessary)

❖ TV >8 mL/kg

❖ Absence of right heart failure

• **PPV is better than SPV in fluid responsiveness.**

• Measured by PiCCO and LIDCOplus.

✓ **Stroke Volume Variability (SVV)**

• Change in stroke volume over one mechanical breath.

• Same prerequisites as PPV.

• Change >10 % predicts fluid responsiveness.

• Measured by PiCCO and LIDCOplus.

✓ **Systolic Pressure Variation (SPV)**

• Change in systolic pressure over one mechanical breath.

• Same prerequisites as PPV.

• Less sensitive and specific than PPV.

• Measured by PiCCO and LIDCOplus.

✓ **Tidal Volume Challenge (TVC)**

• **Method:** Test involves changing TV for controlled ventilation from 6 mL/kg to 8 mL/kg for 1 min and observing the change in PPV

❖ Change >3.5% predicts fluid responsiveness.

• Useful to overcome tidal volume or grey zone limitations in PPV/SVV.

✓ **Pleth Variability Index (PVI)**

• Non-invasive measurement using pulse oximetry to check the dynamic changes in the perfusion index during a respiratory cycle.

• Change >20% is a weak predictor of fluid responsiveness in patients receiving norepinephrine.

✓ **Point of Care Ultrasound (POCUS)**

• **Echocardiography**

❖ Stroke volume is calculated using velocity time index (VTI) at left ventricular outflow tract (LVOT).

❖ Changes in stroke volume can be calculated after giving a fluid bolus.

❖ Increase in LVOT VTI of >10% suggests fluid responsiveness.

• **Lung ultrasound**

❖ **Three or more than three B-lines between rib spaces are considered pathological[Q] and** signifies accumulation of interstitial fluid in lungs.

• **IVC/SVC compressibility**

❖ IVC compressibility during inspiration is measured during inspiration.

❖ IVC diameter variation >12% predicts fluid responsiveness.

❖ **SVC diameter variation is better than IVC in predicting volume responsiveness with cut off of >36%[Q].**

• **VEXUS (Venous Excess Ultrasound)**

❖ Combines IVC measurements with Doppler assessments of hepatic, portal, and intrarenal veins to quantify venous congestion.

❖ **Hepatic vein Doppler**

• **Normal:** Systolic wave > diastolic wave

• **Mildly abnormal:** Systolic < diastolic wave

- **Severely abnormal:** Systolic wave reversal
- ❖ **Portal vein Doppler**
  - **Normal:** <30% pulsatility index
  - **Mildly abnormal:** 30–49% pulsatility index
  - **Severely abnormal:** >50% pulsatility index
- ❖ **Renal vein Doppler**
  - **Normal:** Continuous monophasic flow
  - **Mildly abnormal:** Discontinuous biphasic flow with systolic/diastolic phases
  - **Severely abnormal:** Discontinuous monophasic flow with only diastolic phase
- ❖ **Grading**
  - **Grade 0:** IVC <2 cm, **no congestion**
  - **Grade 1:** IVC >2cm and any combo of normal or mildly abnormal patterns, mild congestion
  - **Grade 2:** IVC >2cm and one severely abnormal pattern, **moderate congestion**
  - **Grade 3:** IVC >2 cm and ≥2 severely abnormal patterns, **severe congestion**

BIOMARKERS

Organ System	Biomarker	Significance
Cardiac		
	Troponins	Marker for perioperative myocardial infarction
	B-type natriuretic peptide (BNP) and NT-proBNP	Elevated levels indicating heart under stress or heart failure
Infection/Inflammation		
	Procalcitonin	Marker to differentiate bacterial infections from non-bacterial ones

Organ System	Biomarker	Significance
	C-reactive protein	Non-specific biomarker of inflammation
	Interleukin-6 (IL-6)	Established role in paediatric cases
	Presepsin	Early indicator of sepsis
Fungal		
	Galactomannan	Aspergillus
	1,3-beta D glucan	Pan-fungal marker
Renal		
	Creatinine	Marker for renal dysfunction
	Neutrophil gelatinase–associated lipocalin (NGAL)	Early indicator for post-operative acute kidney injury (AKI)

Cardiac Biomarkers

✓ **BNP and NT-proBNP:** BNP and NT-proBNP are derived from proBNP which is synthesised by myocytes and fibroblasts in heart in response to the ventricular filling pressures and wall stress.
- BNP inhibits sympathetic axis in the body and reduces secretion of renin, angiotensin, and aldosterone.
- BNP also decreases blood pressure, increases diuresis and vasodilation. BNP is degraded by endopeptidases with a half-life of 5–10 min.
- European Society of Anaesthesia and Intensive Care (ESAIC) 2023 guidelines recommend that they can be used post-operatively based on clinical suspicion of symptoms like dyspnoea and hypoxia in high-risk patients.
- Canadian Cardiovascular Society suggests preoperative measurement of BNP or NT-proBNP, followed by post-operative troponin surveillance with 92 ng/L as cut off for BNP and 300 ng/L as cut off for NT-proBNP in patients with known cardiovascular disease undergoing non-cardiac surgery[Q].

- A normal NT pro-BNP is useful for ruling heart failure in ITU[Q].
✓ **Troponins:** High-sensitivity cardiac troponins (hs-cTns) are sensitive, quantitative markers of myocyte injury, and increased levels of these biomarkers are suggestive of myocardial injury.
  - Acute cardiac events should be excluded by ECG or symptoms post-operatively with troponins >99th of upper range limit among patients with high cardiovascular risk according to ESAIC 2023 guidelines.

Sepsis Biomarkers

✓ **Procalcitonin (PCT)[Q]**
  - Pro-peptide of calcitonin and is produced by C cells in the thyroid gland during normal circumstances (<0.05 ng/mL).
    ❖ It is raised when neuroendocrine cells in the lung and intestine are triggered by bacterial endotoxin and inflammatory cytokines PCT concentrations begin to rise in 4 to 6 h in blood and peak after 12–24 h.
  - PCT levels may rise post-surgery, trauma or burns. In these conditions, levels fall to normal within 24–48 h. Failure to fall within normal may indicate infection.
  - **Higher levels of PCT were associated with Gram-negative sepsis and mortality.**
  - PCT was found to be more reliable in identifying the infection than CRP in a systemic review done by Hassan et al in 2022.
  - PCT value corelates better with severity of illness, APACHE-II and SOFA score than CRP.
  - **Procalcitonin levels help in limiting antibiotic duration in respiratory tract infections but no mortality benefit.**
  - **Detection of infection:** >0.5 ng/mL suggestive of bacterial infection. Sensitivity: 80–90%, Specificity: 65–90%
✓ **C-reactive protein (CRP)**
  - Pentraxin protein and an acute phase reactant **synthesized in the liver[Q]** and is increased in conditions with inflammation like arthritis, myocardial infarction.
  - Hepatic synthesis of CRP starts within 6–8 h of onset of infection and peak concentrations are seen in 36–48 h after infection.

- It activates complement system by binding to phosphocholine on surface of dead cells.
- Half-life of CRP is 19 h and is cleared by liver.
- **Detection of infection:** >10 mg/L. Sensitivity: 55–75%, Specificity: 55–75%
✓ **Interleukin-6 (IL-6)**
  - IL-6 is released by inflammatory cells, fibroblasts, and endothelial cells.
  - Fastest biomarker as it reaches peak levels within 2 h of the infection.
  - Its use in paediatrics population is well established.
  - **Detection of infection:** >25 ng/mL.
  - Sensitivity: 80%, Specificity: 85%.
✓ **Presepsin**
  - Presepsin is a 13 kDa fragment of CD14 receptor available on surface of macrophages.
    ❖ CD14 is a high affinity receptor for lipopolysaccharide (LPS), a crucial component of cell membrane of Gram-negative bacteria.
  - Short half-life (4 h) and can be detected early during onset of sepsis.
  - Can differentiate Gram-negative sepsis from Gram-positive infection.
  - Elevated in connective tissue disorders as well.
  - A meta-analysis showed that presepsin had some superiority in early diagnosis of sepsis.
  - Sensitivity: 85%, Specificity: 78%.

Fungal Infections

✓ *Galactomannan* **(GM):** *Aspergillus.*
  - BAL GM is better compared to serum GM in all kinds of patients.
  - **False positive GM:** Patients on piperacillin-tazobactam, gut malabsorption.
  - Neither GM is suitable for detecting mucor mycosis nor 1,3-beta-D-glucan.
  - **Detection of infection:** BAL >1 ODI (Optical density index), Sensitivity: 80%, Specificity: 95%.
    ❖ Serum >0.5 ODI. Sensitivity: 75%, Specificity: 90%.
✓ **1,3-beta D glucan (Pan fungal marker)**
  - Component of fungal cell wall of major fungi including Candida, *Aspergillus,*

and *Pneumocystis jirovecii* species and is released into the blood during systemic infection.

- Positive in *Fusarium* as well.
- Values greater than 80 pg/mL are interpreted as positive.
- **Detection of infection:** >80 pg/mL. Sensitivity: 50–70%, Specificity: 80–90%.

Acute Kidney Injury

✓ Biomarkers for acute kidney injury are given in section in Chapter 6 on acute kidney injury.

MICROCIRCULATION

Microcirculation: A dense network of arterioles, capillaries, and venules with diameter less than 150 µm.

✓ **Physiology**
- Local factors like nitric oxide (NO), prostaglandins and systemic mechanisms like renin-angiotensin system control microcirculation.
- **Vasoconstrictors:** Thromboxane A2, Endothelin, Platelet activating factor.
- **Vasodilators:** Prostacyclin, Nitric Oxide.
- **Nitric Oxide:** Generated from L-Arginine by Nitric Oxide Synthase (NOS). NO increases cGMP^Q.
  ❖ During normal time, constitutive NOS works with use of calcium. During sepsis, inducible NOS works in a calcium independent process.
  ❖ Arteriolar vasodilation and microcirculatory dysfunction.
- In resting conditions only 20–30% capillaries are functioning. Venules have role in immune and act as capacitance vessels.
- Sepsis causes microcirculation dysfunction by arteriolar hypo-responsiveness, decrease in capillary density and endothelial dysfunction.
- **Clinical methods^Q** of assessing microcirculation include capillary refill time and central-peripheral temperature gradient.

✓ **Assessment of microcirculation**
- **Direct method:** Laser Doppler flowmetry, Video microscopic techniques like Orthogonal polarization spectral (OPS) imaging, incident dark-field (IDF) imaging CytoCam, and sidestream dark-field (SDF) imaging.
- **Indirect method:** Transcutaneous tissue PO2, Near infrared spectroscopy, SvO2, Tissue CO2 (gastric pCO2 gap and venous-arterial CO2 gap) and lactate.
- **Dynamic methods:** Vascular occlusion tests.

✓ **Video microscopic monitoring:** Uses highly sensitive video microscopes.
- Visualization of capillary density, perfusion, and flow dynamics. CytoCam is a handheld microscope.
- Variables used are total vessel density (TVD), perfused vessel density (PVD), microvascular flow index (MFI), Proportion of perfused vessels (PPV), and heterogeneity index (HI).
- Microcirculatory shock occurrence in acutely ill patients (microSOAP) study showed that 17% of 501 patients had an abnormal MFI. Out of those with abnormal MFI, HI was increased whereas PPV and PVD were decreased. TVD was not affected. Abnormal MFI along with tachycardia was associated with increased mortality.

✓ **Near Infrared Spectroscopy (NIRS)**
- Near infrared light wavelength: 700–1000 nm.
- Utilizes the decrease in wavelength of both infra-red and near-infra-red light by oxygenated and de-oxygenated haemoglobin and works on Beer-Lambert Law
- Non-invasive and assesses tissue saturation.
- Spot value of tissue oxygenation saturation (StO2) <70% at presentation to the emergency department was associated with increase in ICU admission.
- Not able to differentiate sepsis of different severity.

✓ **Mixed venous oxygen saturation (SvO$_2$):** O$_2$ saturation of blood returning to the right side of the heart. Calculated using Pulmonary artery catheter (PAC).
- **Normal SvO$_2$:** 65–70%. **Normal ScvO$_2$ (from CVC)** is normally 2–5% lower than SvO$_2$ because it contains predominantly SVC blood from the upper body which has a higher oxygen extraction ratio.
- **Low SvO$_2$** means tissues are extracting more oxygen from the blood.
  ❖ **Decreased O$_2$ delivery:** Anaemia, decreased cardiac output, hypovolaemia.

❖ **Increased O_2 utilization:** Hyperthermia, pain, seizures.

- **High SvO_2** means oxygen delivery is high, or extraction is low which can be due to
  - ❖ **Increased O_2 delivery:** Hyperoxia.
  - ❖ **Decreased O_2 utilization:** Hypothermia, neuromuscular blockade, shunting away from peripheries due to septic shock, cyanide poisoning.
- No evidence of any mortality benefit.

✓ **Venoarterial CO_2 gap (PCO_2 GAP):** Partial pressure of CO_2 in Venous blood ($PvCO_2$)—arterial blood ($PaCO_2$).
- Determining the PCO_2 gap during resuscitation of critically ill patients helps in deciding when to stop resuscitation despite persistent evidence of organ ischaemia and an $ScvO_2$ of greater than 70%.
- In patients with lactic acidosis and signs of circulatory shock.
  - ❖ **When $ScvO_2$ >70%,** PCO_2 gap <6 mmHg can signify cytopathic hypoxia. PCO_2 gap >6 mmHg suggests shock that may be due to hypovolaemia or decreased contractility.
  - ❖ **When $ScvO_2$ <70%,** PCO_2 gap <6 mmHg can signify anaemic hypoxia. PCO_2 gap >6 mmHg suggests shock that may be due to hypovolaemia or decreased contractility.
- Elevated PCO_2 gap showed good correlation with poor outcome among medical (septic) and surgical ICU patients who had circulatory shock.
- Bicarbonate in arterial and venous samples have no difference. Venous pH is 0.03–0.05 units lower than arterial pH.

✓ **Gastric PCO_2 gap:** Gastric mucosal CO_2 ($PgCO_2$) is measured using tonometry.
- Splanchnic hypoperfusion occurs early in septic shock which leads to intramucosal acidosis and increased CO_2.
- Increased Gastric PCO_2 gap (Gastric mucosal CO_2 – arteriolar CO_2) >25 mmHg may denote decreased perfusion. No convincing evidence that it improves outcome.
- Feeding can interfere with it and should be stopped for 2 h before measurement.

✓ **Vascular occlusion tests:** Dynamic measures of microcirculation can be obtained by using NIRS to obtain StO_2 along with brief periods of arterial occlusion by means of a blood pressure cuff.

Lactate

✓ Normal plasma concentration is 0.3–1.3 mmol/L. Levels depend upon production and clearance. Doesn't help in differentiating between different causes of shock.
- In humans, lactate exists in levorotatory isoform.

✓ **Metabolism**
- Lactate is generated via pyruvate→ lactic acid under anaerobic conditions. Pyruvate to lactate uses NADH to NAD^+ and is catalyzed by lactate dehydrogenase (LDH).
- Supply of NADH determines conversion of pyruvate to lactate.
- Glycolysis requires NAD^+. "Ox-phos" shuttle[Q] (**malate-aspartate** and glycerol-phosphate shuttles) converts NADH to NAD to keep the NADH levels low.
- Lactate released by muscle is taken up by the liver to enter the Cori cycle, converted into pyruvate[Q] and generates glucose.
- **Periportal hepatocytes** in liver causes clearance of 60% of lactates mostly by gluconeogenesis[Q] (inhibited by biguanides and alcohol).
- **Mitochondrial-rich tissues** like skeletal muscle, cardiac muscle cells and proximal tubule cells remove the rest of lactate by converting it to pyruvate.
- **Kidneys** excrete up to 5% of total lactates.
- In brain, lactate is a source of energy, transported from astrocytes to neurons and then converted into pyruvate.
- With severe exercise, type II myocytes produce large amounts of lactates which are utilized by heart.

✓ **Types of hyperlactataemia: Hyperlactataemia:** Plasma lactate >2 mmol/L. **Lactic acidosis:** Hyperlactataemia plus acidosis.
- **Type A[Q]:** Tissue hypoxia and anaerobic respiration leads to faster production than removal.
  - ❖ Reduction in blood flow to liver to 25% of normal will result in reduction in lactate clearance.

- **Type B[Q]:** Causes other than tissue hypoxia.
  - ❖ **B1:** Disease such as phaeochromocytoma.
  - ❖ **B2:** Metformin, Salbutamol, Adrenaline, linezolid, HIV Reverse transcriptase, Cyanide.
  - ❖ **B3:** Inborn errors of metabolism like pyruvate carboxylase deficiency, thiamine deficiency.

✓ **In sepsis, main cause of hyperlactataemia is due to increase in glycolysis and impaired pyruvate dehydrogenase[Q].**
  - Hepato-splanchnic ischaemia can cause hyperlactataemia.
  - Lactate is a buffer in peritoneal dialysis and can be increased in these patients.
  - Patient on long-term beta-blocker therapy have decreased lactate levels in patients with sepsis.
  - D-lactate[Q] forms a small fraction of tissue lactate and is seen in short bowel syndrome. This causes a rise in anion gap but lactate levels are normal by the usual lactate assay.
  - Adrenaline induces glycolysis and pyruvate generation via β-2 receptors and causes lactic acidosis.

✓ **Management**
  - Venous lactates can be used to monitor lactates as they are same as arterial lactates.
  - Treatment of type A hyperlactataemia is restoration of local and systemic perfusion.
  - Treatment of type B hyperlactataemia is removal of an offending agent.
  - No mortality benefit of administering bicarbonate to the patient[Q].
  - **Lactates are not removed efficiently by CVVH[Q].**
  - Hartmann's fluid is not absolutely contraindicated. The lactate in Hartmann's solution will lead to transient acidosis and will be ultimately metabolized. By the liver.

✓ **Prognosis**
  - Lactate level >10 mmol/L is associated with >80% mortality. Lactate >2 mmol/L for 48 h after injury in trauma patients has a mortality of 86%.

LUNG ULTRASOUND

✓ **Different types of ultrasound probes[Q]**
  - **Linear:** 5–15 MHz: Used for vascular access and see pleural sliding

- **Curvilinear:** 2–5 MHz: Thorax and abdomen USG
- **Phased array:** 1–5 MHz: Echo and inferior vena cava.

✓ **Ultrasound terminology**
  - **Gain[Q]:** Modifies the amplification of reflected ultrasound waves.
  - **Doppler effect[Q]:** Change in frequency or pitch of a sound wave when the source of the sound is in motion in relation to an observer.

✓ **Lung ultrasound** has higher diagnostic accuracy than physical examination and chest radiography combined.
  - Examination is done above and below the level of nipple and are classified as superior and anterior.
  - Anterior and the posterior axillary lines divide the hemithorax into anterior, lateral, and posterior zones.
  - So, there are 6 zones per hemithorax with zones 1 and 2 are superior and inferior anterior areas. Zones 3 and 4 are superior and inferior lateral areas and zones 5 and 6 are superior and inferior posterior areas.
  - **Diaphragm**

✓ **A Lines:** Horizontal lines generated between the ultrasound waves bouncing back and forth between the pleura and the transducer.
  - The **pleural line** is a horizontal, 2.5 cm long hyperechoic line located 0.5 cm below the rib line in the adult.
    - ❖ Two upper ribs with a lower pleural line in between gives *"the bat sign"*.
    - ❖ **M-mode in a normal pleural sliding shows** *"seashore" sign*[Q]
  - A-lines are the **repetitive horizontal hyperechoic lines** generated by the ultrasound waves bouncing back and forth between the pleura and the transducer.
    - ❖ **A-lines** demonstrate the presence of air below the pleura, they are present both in normal lungs and in pneumothorax.
    - ❖ **They are multiple in number and are equidistant from each other.**
    - ❖ **On a normal lung ultrasound, only A-lines are seen**[Q].
  - **Pneumothorax[Q]:** *Lung appears to slide with normal respiration. M-mode shows this as seashore sign.*
    - ❖ **Lung sliding will be absent** in pneumothorax. **M-mode in a**

pneumothorax shows horizontal straight lines *"barcode/stratosphere" sign*[Q].

❖ *Lung point* is diagnostic for pneumothorax[Q]. It is a transition point between the normal sliding lung and no sliding due to collapsed lung.

❖ *Absence of B lines*[Q].

- **Pleural effusion:** They are seen on dependent area caudally and posteriorly due to gravity.
  - ❖ Ultrasound identifies pleural effusion between the diaphragm and lung at the **posterolateral point**. Lung will float on top of an effusion.
  - ❖ USG will reveal septations and can distinguish transudates and exudates.
  - ❖ **Quad sign:** A static sonographic four-sided figure made by visceral pleura, pleural line, and shadows from the rib.
  - ❖ **Sinusoid sign:** A dynamic M-mode sign that shows a movement of the lung line toward the pleural line on inspiration.
  - ❖ **Spine sign:** A large pleural effusion creates an acoustic window that allows visualization of the vertebral bodies below known as the spine sign.
  - ❖ **Anechoic (total black)** effusion indicates transudate origin of clear fluid.
  - ❖ **Fluid with hypoechoic (less black)** content is usually an exudate.

✓ **B Lines:** Injured lung is characterized by increasing tissues density with fluid replacing air.
- B-lines are **vertical hyperechoic** "comet tails" which move with lung sliding.
- Generated by the juxtaposition of alveolar air and septal thickening.
- **Three or more than three between rib spaces are considered pathological**[Q].
- Presence of multiple B-lines separated by **7 mm** result from **interstitial syndrome.**
- Presence of coalescent B-lines **less than 3 mm** apart signifies severe decrease in lung aeration due to filling of alveolar spaces by **pulmonary oedema or bronchopneumonia**[Q].
- **Shred sign:** The interface between consolidated abnormal lung and aerated normal lung is seen as an irregular hyperechoic line known as Shred sign.

- **Tissue-like sign:** Appearance of liver-or spleen-like structure on the ultrasound above the diaphragm is called a "tissue-like sign".
- **Dynamic air bronchogram:** Pea sized, small hyperechoic artefacts that move during respiratory cycle. Air trapped in distal airway.
- **Fluid bronchogram:** Tubular hyperechoic structures that are generated by the inflammatory fluid trapped in the distal airway.

✓ **Combining A and B lines**
- **Cardiogenic pulmonary oedema**[Q]**:** Homogenous distribution, regular pleura, small pleural effusion in dependent zones.
- **ARDS**[Q]**:** Inhomogeneous distribution, pleural irregularities, subpleural consolidation, spared areas, posterior consolidation.
- **Recruitment:** Lung ultrasound has been used for confirming the efficacy of the recruitment manoeuvre. Coalescent B-lines change into separated B-lines and separated B-lines change into A-lines.

✓ **Normal lung signs: Bat sign, lung sliding, A-lines.**

✓ **C-lines**[Q]**:** Vertical lines that originate from sub pleural consolidations but not from pleura itself. They have the appearance of B-lines but they do not cut A-lines. Seen in viral illnesses.

Other Modalities for Monitoring

✓ **Chest X-ray**
- **Carina**[Q] **at the level of T 5–7.**
- Normal chest X-ray has right-sided diaphragm higher than left-sided diaphragm. Left-sided hilum is higher than right-sided hilum.
- Chest radiography gives a background natural radiation of approximately 28 d.
  - ❖ CT scan gives a background natural radiation of approximately 4 yr.
- **Collapse of lobes**
  - ❖ **Right upper lobe collapse** is associated with golden s sign[Q].
  - ❖ **Right middle lobe collapse** leads to obscuration of right heart border.
  - ❖ **Right lower lobe collapse** is associated with loss of right medial hemidiaphragm.
  - ❖ **Left upper lobe collapse:** Veiling opacity due to anterior collapse within left hemithorax.

❖ **Left lower lobe collapse:** Sail sign[Q] or the double cardiac contour is seen.
- **Bilateral/unilateral hilar lymphadenopathy**[Q]
  ❖ Tuberculosis
  ❖ Sarcoidosis
  ❖ Malignancy like lymphoma, metastasis.
  ❖ Silicosis (mostly bilateral)

ELECTROENCEPHALOGRAM

✓ **Electroencephalogram (EEG):** Continuous graphic display over time of spatial distribution of changing voltage fields at the scalp surface.
- Main signal generators are pyramidal neurons.
- Measured as µV (normal is 20–100 µV) compared to millivolts in ECG[Q].

✓ **Indications for EEG monitoring in ITU**
- Patients with acute brain injury and unexplained and persistent altered consciousness
- Status epilepticus monitoring in known epilepsy
- Diagnosis of non-convulsive status epilepticus (NCSE)
- Post–cardiac arrest neuromonitoring: at 24 and 72 h
- **Encephalopathies:** EEG can't distinguish between different aetiologies, but it can help to rule out treatable causes like NCSE.
  ❖ It can also give the degree of severity of encephalopathy.
  ❖ Earliest changes are usually slowing or fall out of the alpha rhythm[Q].
- Monitor effects of escalating anaesthetic medications to get and maintain a burst suppression

✓ **EEG monitoring system**
- Cup electrodes, needle electrodes or cap with integrated electrodes can be used.
- **Spot EEG** are normally of 30–60-minute recording. It is used in post-cardiac arrest patients. **Continuous EEG** (cEEG) is used for non-convulsive seizures.
- **10–20 system:** These numbers denote that the actual distances between adjacent electrodes are either 10% or 20% of the total front-back or right-left distance.
  ❖ **21 Electrodes.** Odd numbers on left hemisphere and even numbers on the right hemisphere while z (zero) represents midline. The letters F, T, C, P and O stand for areas of brain like frontal, temporal, central, parietal, and occipital, respectively.

✓ **EEG Assessment**
- **Background activity:** Assessed by frequency, continuity, and reactivity.

Frequency[Q]

Wave	Frequency (Hz)	Characteristics
Alpha	8–13	Awake and resting. Located in posterior regions
Beta	14–30	Awake with mental activity. Predominant on frontal regions.
Theta	4–7	Sleeping. Normal in children up to 13 yr. Abnormal in awake patients.
Delta	1–3	Deep sleep (stage 3 or 4). Dominant rhythm in infants.

Continuity[Q]

Pattern	Characteristics
Continuous	Normal EEG
Nearly continuous	<10% suppressed (<10 µV) or attenuated (>10 µV but <50% of background amplitude)
Discontinuous	10–49% of the record attenuated or suppressed
Burst suppression	>50% suppressed or attenuated
Suppression	Entire EEG suppressed (<10 µV)
Electrocerebral inactivity	Entire EEG totally suppressed (<2 µV)

❖ **Reactivity:** An EEG tracing that is reactive to visual, noxious or auditory stimulus is predictor of good neurological outcome.
- **Transients:** Isolated waveforms seen on background activity.
  ❖ **Spikes:** High frequency, high amplitude sharp wave seen in patients with epilepsy.
  ❖ **Sharp waves:** Slower than spikes, high amplitude waves with slower return to baseline. Seen in epilepsy.

❖ **Poly spikes:** Multiple spikes coming together and seen in generalized epilepsy.

❖ **Spike and wave:** Combination of spikes and slow waves.

✓ **Basic principles**

- **Normal sleep[Q]:** Awake patient with eyes closed has an alpha rhythm in posterior brain regions which moves to frontal regions as beta waves when eyes are open.

  ❖ **Non-REM sleep:** Theta and delta waves. Sleep spindles and K complexes seen.

  ❖ **REM sleep:** Mix of low voltage fast activity as in wakefulness and bursts of theta and delta waves.

- **Burst suppression[Q]:** Seen in general anaesthesia, status epilepticus and hypoxic ischaemic encephalopathy. Patients that will evolve from burst suppression to less malignant trace will have good prognosis. Patients with burst suppression in absence of confounders at will represent poor neurological outcome.

- **Effect of pharmacological agents on EEG[Q]**

  ❖ Ketamine can lead to theta rhythms.

  ❖ Dexmedetomidine can lead to slow-wave sleep spindles.

  ❖ Volatile anaesthetics, propofol and thiopental lead to progressive slowing and burst suppression.

Additional Questions

✓ **Bispectral index (BIS)[Q]:** Processes EEG data to calculate a BIS value.

- 40–60 for general anaesthesia. Total range is between 0 to 100 with 0 indicating complete suppression of the brain activity.

18

Nutrition

NUTRITIONAL ASSESSMENT

✓ **European Society for Parenteral and Enteral Nutrition (ESPEN)** 2019 guidelines identify three phases in the intensive care unit.
  - Acute early phase: 1–2 d
  - Acute late phase: 3–7 d
  - Recovery phase: >7 d

✓ **Concepts: Bed rest** can lead to the loss of 20% muscle mass within a week even with nutritional support.
  - Around 35–40% of weight loss from ideal body weight can lead to malnutrition-related death.
  - *Feeding during resuscitation is inappropriate and may be detrimental.*
  - **Basal Metabolic Rate (BMR):** Amount of energy expended per unit time during a period of rest. BMR is normally around 40 Kcal/m²/h℃.
  - **Energy expenditure:** It is the sum of *internal heat produced and external work.*
    ❖ It increases by 10% for each 1°C above 37°C.
    ❖ Greatest elevations in resting energy expenditure in seen in patients with sepsis, burns and ARDS by as high as 80%.
  - The **Faisy equation** corrects for minute ventilation and body temperature and hence can be used for calculating energy expenditure in ventilated patients.
  - **Harris–Benedict** for calculating basal energy expenditure. *Can be inaccurate in ventilated patients.*
    ❖ For men, BMR = 66.5 + (13.75 × weight [kg]) + (5.003 × height [cm]) − (6.775 × age [years])

  ❖ For women, BMR = 655.1 + (9.563 × weight in kg) + (1.850 × height in cm) − (4.676 × age).

✓ **Nutritional screening:** To determine patients at risk of developing nutrition-related complications.
  - NICE recommends **Malnutrition Universal Screening Tool (MUST)**: 5 steps.
    ❖ Measure height and weight: **BMI score.**
    ❖ % Unplanned weight loss and **Weight loss score** using tables.
    ❖ **Acute disease effect score**.
    ❖ Add these three scores to obtain overall risk of malnutrition.
    ❖ Use management guidelines and local policy to develop care plan.
  - Nutrition risk screening 2002 (**NRS 2002**): High risk ≥5, At risk >4. Majority of ICU patients will score 3 on this score.
  - Nutrition risk in the critically ill score (**NUTRIC**): High risk ≥6.
  - A 10% or 10-pounds weight loss over the previous 12 months are an indicator of protein calorie malnutrition.
  - All patients admitted to ICU>48 h should be considered at high risk of malnutrition.

✓ **Nutrition assessment**
  - **Body composition:** Subjective Global Assessment (SGA) tool
    ❖ SGA looks for signs of fat loss (triceps and fat pads of the eye) and muscle wasting (clavicle and deltoid)
  - **Biochemistry:** Low serum albumin is associated with poor prognosis, but it has a long half-life (20 d) and falls immediately after fluid resuscitation.

DOI: 10.1201/9781003476214-18

❖ Albumin is not a sensitive indicator as it is an acute marker of inflammation as well.
- **Biomarkers:** Serum urea to creatinine ratio for guiding nutritional interventions.
- **Clinical assessment:** Abdominal drains can have up to 6 g/L of protein.
  - ❖ Citrate anti coagulation and propofol are a source of energy.
  - ❖ Amino acids and micronutrients are lost in CRRT.
  - ❖ Fats are not lost in dialysis.
✓ **Respiratory quotient[Q]:** Ratio of CO_2 released to O_2 used during respiration.
- Carbohydrate: 1, Protein: 0.8, Fat: 0.7.
✓ **Energy targets[Q]:** Most accurate method to calculate the energy expenditure in mechanically ventilated patients is to measure it by **indirect calorimetry (impractical though).**
- Energy requirements: 25–30 kcal/kg/day
- Carbohydrate: 2–4 g/kg/day
- Fluids: 25–30 mL/kg/day
- Protein: 0.8–1.5 g/kg/day
- Lipid: 1–1.5 g/kg or 15–20% of total calories per day
- Nitrogen: 0.2 g/kg/day
- Na$^+$: 2 mmol/kg/day
- K$^+$, Cl$^-$: 1 mmol/kg/day
- Magnesium: 0.1 mmol/kg/day
- Calcium: 0.1 mmol/kg/day
- Phosphate: 0.4 mmol/kg/day
- Glucose: 50–100 g/day
- Selenium: 100 µg
- Zinc: 10 mg
- Vitamin B1: 100 mg
- NICE recommends 2 L of "0.18% NaCl with 4% glucose and 27 mmol/L Potassium" for the first 24 h of maintenance fluids
✓ **Energy targets** can be increased to 35 kcal/kg for burns and trauma patients.
✓ **Fat targets:** Omega-6 polyunsaturated fatty acids should be provided in doses adequate to prevent essential fatty acid deficiency.
- Medium chain triglycerides are more water soluble and require less lipase activity and bile salt for absorption. Patients with malabsorption, pancreatic enzyme insufficiency and chronic liver disease can absorb them more easily.

✓ **Protein targets**
- **Increased requirements:** Burns, RRT, necrotizing fasciitis, BMI >30 kg/m², open abdomen
- **Decreased requirements:** Hepatic encephalopathy
✓ **Micronutrients:** Supplementation needed in
- Burns
- High-output intestinal fistulae
- ARDS
- Multiple trauma
- Severe inflammatory and septic diseases
✓ **Role of trace elements**
- **Selenium deficiency can lead to acute cardiomyopathy.**
- Ascorbic acid deficiency can cause scurvy[Q].
  - ❖ Vitamin C ↑ Catecholamine sensitivity and ↑ wound healing.
- Thiamine deficiency[Q] can lead to Korsakoff syndrome and Wernicke's encephalopathy.
- Vitamin B1 deficiency can lead to lactic acidosis.
- Copper deficiency can lead to arrhythmias and altered arrhythmias.
- Vitamin A, C, E, and selenium are anti oxidants[Q].

ENTERAL NUTRITION

✓ Gut has been described as MOTOR of multiple organ failure (MOF). Translocation of bacteria, fungi, viruses, and parasites is an important mechanism for sepsis and MOF.
- **Enteral nutrition:** Method of feeding that uses the gastrointestinal tract to deliver nutrients directly into the stomach or the small intestine bypassing the need for oral intake.
- Enteral nutrition stimulates splanchnic and hepatic circulations, improve mucosal blood flow, prevents intramucosal acidosis and eliminates the need for stress ulcer prophylaxis.
✓ **Advantages of EN:** More physiological than parenteral nutrition (PN).
- No need of CVC and hence catheter-related sepsis
- Less costly feeding solutions
✓ **Contraindications of EN:** Adequate oral intake (80% of the energy target).
- Anatomic disruption of the GIT (perforation, bowel ischaemia or obstruction)

- Severe shock
- Abdominal compartment syndrome
✓ **Start of enteral feeding**
  - *Initiation of enteral feeding doesn't require active bowel sounds or passage of flatus or stool*[Q].
  - EN can be given in prone positioning, post–abdominal aortic surgery, absence of bowel sounds.
✓ **European Society for Clinical Nutrition and Metabolism (ESPEN) guidelines 2019 recommend.**
  - Assess patients on admission to the ITU for nutrition risk and calculate both energy and protein requirements to determine goals of nutrition therapy.
  - Oral diet shall be preferred over enteral or parenteral nutrition in critically ill patients who are able to eat.
  - Initiate enteral nutrition (EN) within 48 h following the onset of critical illness and admission to the ICU if oral intake is not possible.
  - **If EN is not tolerated, supplemental parenteral nutrition (PN) should be initiated EARLY after the acute phase of critical illness (within the first 3–7 d).**
  - **Early and progressive parenteral nutrition can be started in case of contraindications for enteral nutrition in severely malnourished patients.**
  - Feed should be started within 48 h of ICU admission[Q].
    - ❖ Start EN at 50% of estimated target. Advance EN by 10–25 mL/h/day. Increase to 70% of target over 48 h. Full nutritional goal to be reached in 7 d[Q].
  - Continuous rather than bolus EN should be used.
  - Take steps to reduce the risk of aspiration[Q] or improve tolerance to gastric feeding[Q] (prokinetic agents, continuous infusion, chlorhexidine mouth wash, elevate the head end).
  - Intravenous erythromycin is the first-line prokinetic therapy.
✓ **Routes of enteral nutrition**
  - **Nasogastric/Naso-jejunal:** Tube length estimated by placing the tip at the xiphisternum, take tube to back of the ear and then across to the nostril.

- ❖ Tube length varies according to site stomach (60 cm), duodenum (110 cm) and jejunum (120 cm).
- ❖ Contraindicated in a patient with base of skull fracture.
- ❖ NG tube[Q] is confirmed if an aspirate is obtained and a pH between 1 and 5.5 is detected. If an aspirate can't be obtained or if pH is not between 1 and 5.5, a chest X-ray should be done. A pH indicator paper rather than litmus paper should be used.
- ❖ A correctly placed NG tube[Q] should bisect the carina, stay in midline, and descend below the diaphragm.
- ❖ If no aspirate is obtainable the NG tube should never be flushed.
- ❖ Failure to detect misplacement of NG tube is a never event and misinterpretation of chest X-ray images is the leading cause for it.
- ❖ Tubes need to be flushed regularly to avoid clogging with medications or tube feedings.
- ❖ Naso-jejunal tubes may be used in patients at risk of aspiration associated with reflux.
- **Percutaneous endoscopic gastrostomy (PEG):** When prolonged EN support (>4–6 wk).
  - ❖ Percutaneous endoscopic jejunostomy (PEJ) can also be put by putting tube into the stomach and then guiding it into the duodenum under endoscopic control.
  - ❖ Insertion should be avoided in patients with uncontrolled infection, poor gastric emptying, and ascites.
✓ **Enteral nutrition formulas:** Iso-osmotic 300 mOsm/L polymeric solutions containing 1–2 kcal/mL, 45–60% carbohydrates, 20–35% lipids and 15–20% as proteins.
- **Elemental:** Free amino acids, glucose, and medium-chain triglycerides
- **Semi-elemental:** Peptides, oligosaccharides, and medium-chain triglycerides. Indicated in intestinal malabsorption or diarrhoea.
- *Polymeric:* Whole protein, polysaccharides, and long-chain triglycerides and fibres. **Standard of care.**
✓ **Permissive underfeeding**: Deliberate energy administration below 70% of calorie targets.

- **PermiT Trial (2015):** No mortality difference from standard enteral feeding was seen with permissive enteral feeding among a predominant non-surgical mechanically ventilated ICU population.
- ✓ **Trophic feeding:** Small volumes of enteral feeding which are not enough for the patient's nutrition but are used for positive gut benefits. <500 Kcal/day.
  - **EDEN Trial (2012):** Either Trophic or full nutrition by enteral route is appropriate in patients with ARDS and no mortality difference was seen.
- ✓ **Gastric residual volumes (GRV):** Gastric juices are produced per hour at the rate of 60–80 mL/h. **Used as a marker of gastrointestinal tolerance.**
  - *Do not use gastric residual volumes as part of routine care to monitor ICU patients receiving EN.*
    - ❖ However, worsening abdominal distention or diarrhoea more than 1000 mL/d requires a medical evaluation.
  - High gastric residue up to 500 mL/6 h shouldn't stop the feed.
    - ❖ Reduce feeding rate by 50%. If GRV remains >500 mL in three consecutive measurements, consider jejunal feeding.
  - **NUTRIREA-1 Trial (2013):** In non-surgical mechanically ventilated patients, not monitoring gastric residuals was not inferior to monitoring them regarding development of ventilator associated pneumonia.
  - Jejunal feeding can cause small bowel dilatation and perforation.
  - If enteral contrast media needs to be given by post–pyloric tube, use smaller amounts and slower administration (<100 mL/h).
- ✓ **Bowel sounds:** Normal is 5–35 sounds/min. Auscultation for at least one minute in four quadrants.
  - Bowel sound may be decreased or absent in half of ICU patients.
  - Lack of bowel sounds should not be the reason to delay enteral nutrition.
- ✓ No role of **Glutamine, Arginine** (wound healing) and **Selenium** in sepsis patients.
- ✓ **Propofol infusion provides a significant part of daily calorie intake and should be taken in account.**
- ✓ **Prokinetic drugs/Motility agents:** Used for gastroparesis and act on stomach and small bowel.

- **Erythromycin:** Motilin receptor agonist. Dose: 250 mg q6h IV.
  - ❖ Limited effect on small intestine.
  - ❖ It can cause arrhythmias (QT prolongation). Effectiveness is decreased to one-third after 72 hr[Q].
  - ❖ Increased risk of minor episodes of GI bleeding.
- **Metoclopramide:** Dopamine D2 antagonist, 5-HT3/4 agonist. Dose: 10 mg q8h IV.
  - ❖ It may increase ICP and is contraindicated in head injury patients.
  - ❖ Effectiveness is decreased to one-third after 72 hr[Q]. Can cause dyskinesias.
  - ❖ Metoclopramide doesn't reduce the risk of pneumonia.

PARENTERAL NUTRITION

- ✓ **Parenteral nutrition:** Method of feeding a patient intravenously, bypassing the gastrointestinal tract, when they cannot eat or absorb enough nutrients.
  - **EPaNIC Trial (2011)[Q]:** Compared early (day 3) vs late (day 8) parenteral nutrition in critically ill adults. No difference in mortality.
  - **CALORIES Trial (2014)[Q]** showed no difference in mortality between enteral and parenteral nutrition and *no increase in risk of infection in PN group* with short-term administration of PN (up to 7 d).
  - **NUTRIREA-2 Trial (2018):** In mechanically ventilated patients in shock and on vasopressors, early initiation of parenteral nutrition didn't improve or worsen clinical outcomes in comparison to enteral nutrition.
- ✓ *Ideal timing, dose, and composition of PN remains unclear.*
  - Better if started later at day 8.
- ✓ **Indications of parenteral nutrition[Q]**
  - If enteral feeding is not possible and patient is having malnutrition or at risk of malnutrition.
    - ❖ Malnutrition: BMI <18.5 or weight loss of 10% over 6 months or a BMI of <20 with 5% weight loss over 6 months.
    - ❖ Risk of malnutrition: Grossly inadequate oral intake for 5 d or more,

poor absorption, hypermetabolism or increased loss of nutrients.

- If patient's caloric requirements are not adequately met (>60% of requirements by enteral route) within 7–10 d of enteral feeding, supplementation by TPN should be considered.
- Common indications include Crohn's disease, short bowel syndrome, chemotherapy, and acute pancreatitis.

✓ **Advantages of parenteral nutrition**
- Avoids EN-associated risk of gastro-oesophageal reflux and aspiration.
- Avoids EN associated risk of GI intolerance.
- Avoids risk of bowel ischaemia in patients with severe shock.

✓ **Contraindications to parenteral nutrition**
- Adequate oral intake, enteral nutrition meeting nutritional targets
- Absence of central venous access.

✓ **Parenteral nutrition routes:** Majority of PN solutions are hyperosmotic and requires central venous administration.
- Tubing connecting the PN bag to the patient's catheter should be changed once a day to avoid bacterial contamination.
- Tunnelled subclavian vein access is recommended for long-term PN (>30 d).
- Peripherally delivered PN requires 2.5–3.5 L of iso to slightly hyperosmotic (<900 mOsm/L) solutions.
- A PVC can be used for short-term PN (<14 d) if a CVC isn't needed for other reason.

✓ **Parenteral nutrition formulas:** Majority of PN solutions are hyperosmotic.
- **Content of bag**[Q]: Energy: 25 kcal/kg/day. Carbohydrate as glucose **2g/kg/day.** Lipids as soyabean oil **1–2 g/kg/day.** Protein as balanced amino acid mixtures @ 1.3–1.5 g/kg/IBW.
- Balanced mixture of amino acids. No benefit of use of branched chain amino acids. No Glutamine used because of stability issues and no mortality benefits.
- Glucose should be less than 6g/kg/day as excess glucose can cause hyperglycaemia, hypertriglyceridemia, and liver steatosis.
- Lipid emulsions are contained in a small volume (9 kcal/g) and reduces the osmolarity of nutritional mixtures. Lipids <30% of total energy as fat reduce infection rates.

- Propofol 1% solution contains 1.1 kcal/ml[Q] and should be counted in calories.
- PN solutions do not contain trace elements or vitamins in contrast to enteral feeds and these micronutrients should be co-administered parenterally till the patients receives sufficient enteral feeding.
  ❖ Trace elements include thiamine, ascorbic acid, copper, selenium, zinc, chromium, and iron.

✓ Continuous administration is preferred method specially if the patient is significantly unwell. For those with longer term requirements, intermittent TPN should be used.
- If TPN is required for >30 d, a tunnelled line is used[Q].

✓ **Complications**
- **Catheter-related sepsis:** If no signs of local or systemic sepsis, routine CVC changes are not recommended.
  ❖ Low grade fever or inflamed or purulent insertion site may be a site of catheter infection.
  ❖ If mild infection, either guide wire exchange for culture of catheter tip or taking cultures "in situ" and "wait and watch".
  ❖ If signs of severe sepsis, PN should be interrupted, and catheter removed immediately.
- **Liver abnormalities:** AST, ALT and Bilirubin should be checked twice weekly[Q].
  ❖ Biliary tract sludge and stasis in the biliary tract may cause chronic acalculous cholecystitis may be associated with prolonged PN.
- **Pancreatic disorders:** Pancreatitis can happen. Lipid infusion need to be modified if plasma triglycerides exceed 4 mmol/L.
  ❖ Check amylase or lipase regularly[Q].
- Lipids and glucose levels are also checked[Q].

REFEEDING SYNDROME

Aetiology and Pathophysiology

✓ **Refeeding syndrome:** Potentially life-threatening metabolic syndrome due to re-introduction of feeding after a period of starvation.
- **Thiamine deficiency** is the most common vitamin deficiency (Wernicke's encephalopathy-partially reversible).

✓ **Pathophysiology:** Macronutrients restarted after prolonged period of food restriction → Insulin ↑ → Intracellular entrance of phosphate, potassium, and Vitamin B1 → Electrolyte disturbances.
- Even 5% glucose may be enough to start the process.
- Refeeding syndrome can be seen in patients on both TPN and enteral nutrition[Q].

Risk Factors for Refeeding Syndrome[Q]

	Major	Minor
BMI (kg/m²)	<16	<18.5
Weight loss in 3–6 months	15%	10%
Days without food	10	5
Other	Low Mg^{2+}, K^+, PO_4^{3-}	Alcohol abuse, diuretics, insulin, **chemotherapy**

- Patients with one major or two minor risk factors are more likely to develop refeeding syndrome on initiation of feeding.

Clinical Features and Diagnosis

✓ Seen in patients on **diuretics, anorexia nervosa**, alcohol abuse, post–bariatric surgery, antacid use (phosphate chelation) and elderly.
✓ **Presentation:** Hyperglycaemia, **hypokalaemia, hypophosphataemia** (commonest), hypomagnesaemia.
- **Hypophosphataemia can lead to global muscle weakness** including respiratory muscle weakness presents as tachypnoea, extraocular muscle weakness as double vision.
- Diarrhoea, rhabdomyolysis, haemolytic anaemia, Wernicke's encephalopathy, and seizures.
- Pulmonary oedema, cardiac failure, cardiac arrhythmias (sudden cardiac death).

Treatment[Q]

✓ Identify patents at risk using nutritional risk and assessment.
✓ Supply electrolytes and thiamine before start of feed even if in normal range depending on the risk.
- **IV 200 mg Thiamine from day 1–5.**

- Vitamin B complex and supplemental multivitamins from day 1–10.
✓ **Permissive underfeeding[Q]: Feeding less than 40–60%** of calories required for daily energy needs. Start at 5–10 kcal/kg/day and increase gradually to full requirements by day 7.
- That normally means calorie restriction at 10–20 Kcal/h for 2 d, followed by 2–3 d progressive return to normal return.
- Calorie and not protein restriction is needed[Q].
- Concurrent correction of electrolytes (potassium, phosphate, and magnesium) along with start of feeding is done.
- No significant difference in risk between enteral and parenteral routes[Q].
✓ **Check laboratory for phosphate, potassium, magnesium, sodium, calcium, glucose, urea, and creatinine.**
- **Day 1–3:** Daily
- **Day 4–6:** Every 2 d
- **Day 7–10:** 1–2 times/week

DISEASE-SPECIFIC NUTRITION

✓ **Renal failure**
- **Energy requirements in AKI:** 25–30 kcal/d
- **Protein requirements without stress**
  ❖ CKD patient not on HD: 0.6–0.8 g/kg/day
  ❖ CKD patient on intermittent HD: 1.2 g/kg/day
  ❖ AKI on intermittent HD: 1.5 g/kg/day
- **Protein requirements with stress**
  ❖ AKI on HD: 1.2–2 g/kg/day
  ❖ AKI on CRRT: 1.8–2.5 g/kg/day
- **Fluid** is restricted to 1 to 1.5 L/day in non-dialysis anuric or oliguric patients.
  ❖ Concentrated enteral formulas (1.5–2 kcal/mL) are often needed.
- CRRT allows for a liberalization of fluid provisions.
- Phosphorus will need replacement as it is effectively cleared by CRRT.
✓ **Liver failure**
- Hepatic reserve functional capacity is high and hepatic dysfunction is not seen unless 80–90% of the liver cells have been injured.
- **Energy requirements in liver disease:** 25–30 kcal/d

- **Protein requirements without hepatic encephalopathy**
  - ❖ Alcoholic steatohepatitis and cirrhosis, unstressed: 0.8–1.2 g/kg/day
  - ❖ Acute and subacute liver failure: 0.8–1.2 g/kg/day
  - ❖ Alcoholic steatohepatitis and cirrhosis, stressed: 1.2–1.5 g/kg/day
- **Protein requirements with hepatic encephalopathy**
  - ❖ Alcoholic steatohepatitis and cirrhosis: 0.8 g/kg/day
  - ❖ Fulminant hepatic failure: 0.8 g/kg/day
- Branched-chain amino acid preparations for liver disease may be considered in grade III or IV hepatic encephalopathy.
- **IV glucose** at a dose of 2 to 3 g/kg/day should be given when EN cannot be given for 12 or more hours due to risk of hypoglycaemia.
- *Infusion of 10% dextrose solutions should be given prophylactically to patients with fulminant hepatic failure to prevent hypoglycaemia until full feeding by EN or PN may be started.*

✓ **Pulmonary failure**
  - Trophic feeding (10–20 kcal/h) for up to 6 d is as effective as full enteral nutrition and has fewer gastrointestinal complications and is recommended in patients with low to moderate nutrition risk.

✓ **Trauma:** Start nutritional support within 24 h and increase gradually to full nutrition within 5–7 d.
  - **Energy:** Catabolic phase: 20–30 kcal/kg/day, Anabolic phase: 30–35 kcal/kg/day
  - **Protein:** 1.2–2 grams/kg/day
  - **Carbohydrates:** 2–5 gram/kg/day
  - **Fat:** 0.7–1.5 grams/kg/day

19

ITU Issues

DELIRIUM

✓ **Definition:** Acute and fluctuating disorder of attention and awareness along with consciousness and cognition.
- **Incidence rate of 29%** during an ICU stay. **Happens in up to 80%** of mechanically ventilated cases in ITU.
- Median duration of delirium is 2–3 d.

✓ **Risk factors**
- **Predisposing risk factors**[Q]: Age >70 yr, **dementia, alcoholism** (>3 units/day), smoking history (>10/day), pre-existing malnutrition, **hypertension/hypotension**, visual and hearing impairment, and **severity of illness** at admission.
- **Precipitating risk factors:** Multiple traumas, sepsis, need for ventilatory support, pain, benzodiazepines, anticholinergic drugs, opioids, corticosteroids, increased noise, lack of daylight.

✓ **Pathophysiology**
- Neurotransmitter imbalance: Increased dopamine, low acetyl choline, fluctuating serotonin.
  - ❖ Neuroinflammation and alterations in neural network due to stress and sepsis can also lead to delirium.

✓ **Clinical presentation:** Mixed-type delirium is the most common type (45%), then hypoactive (45%), and then hyperactive (10%).
- Impaired ability to focus and steady slow decline in cognitive function.
- Fragmented sleep/wake cycle and sleeplessness.
- Disorientation in time, place, and person.
- **Hypoactive delirium:** reduced alertness, motor activity, and speech.

- ❖ **Hyperactive delirium:** Restlessness and agitation.
- Hallucinations and delusions.
- May be first sign of underlying severe critical care illness.

✓ **Diagnosis:** Several tools have been developed for diagnosis, but still up to 60% of cases can be missed.
- EEG changes are diffuse, slowing of background activity, electrographic seizures, and periodic epileptiform discharges.

✓ **Confusion assessment method for ICU (CAM ICU):** High sensitivity 80%.
- **Criteria 1:** First, consider whether the patient has shown an **acute mental status change** in the last 24 h.
- **Criteria 2:** Check for **inattention.** If patient makes **more than two errors**[Q], go on to check altered levels of consciousness with the RASS score.
  - ❖ Patient is asked to squeeze the hand or blink on hearing letter A and SAVEAHAART is read before the patient.
- **Criteria 3:** Check the RASS score of the patient.
- **Criteria 4:** If RASS score is other than zero, check **disordered thinking** with four questions, like, "Will a stone float on water?" "Are there fish in the sea?" "Does one pound weigh more than two pounds?" "Can you use a hammer to pound a nail?" Then, patient is told to hold two fingers with the other hand and then told to do the same with the other hand.
  - ❖ Score of more than one error on the questions or commands means there is delirium.

- Positive CAM-ICU is criteria 1 plus 2 and either 3 or 4. Can be performed on patients who are **intubated or sedated (RASS <−3)**.
- Either altered level of consciousness or disorganized thinking are the criteria.
✓ **The Intensive Care Delirium Screening Checklist (ICDSC):** High sensitivity 74%.
  - More subjective than the CAM-ICU, but CAM-ICU is more specific and is better in predicting outcome than the ICDSC.
  - It requires a nurse to assess the patient over the course of the nursing shift.
✓ **Delirium prediction models:** *Early predictions of delirium ICU (E-PRE-DELIRIC) and PRE-DELIRIC tools are made using the two models.*
✓ Sedative-related delirium had better hospital outcomes.
  - Long-term delirium put patients on higher risk for long-term cognitive impairment after critical illness.
  - The longer the duration of delirium in the ICU, the higher the chances of cerebral atrophy and cerebral white matter disruption.
✓ **Prevention measures**[Q]
  - **Non-pharmacological**
    ❖ Repeated orientation with 24-hour clocks, glasses, and hearing aids
    ❖ Earplugs
    ❖ Reduction of nighttime noise and light
    ❖ Increase exposure to sunlight
    ❖ Minimal sleep disturbances
    ❖ Early mobilization and physiotherapy
    ❖ Timely removal of catheters/lines and physical restraints
    ❖ Correction of dehydration and physiological derangements
    ❖ Family involvement
  - **Pharmacological**
    ❖ Stop benzodiazepines, opiates, anticholinergics.
    ❖ Daily sedation holds and pain management.
    ❖ Prophylactic melatonin.
    ❖ **Dexmedetomidine** (reversal by atipamezole)[Q] has shown promise for preventive management. Can be used in patients with prolonged QT syndrome.

❖ Haloperidol and ketamine shouldn't be used for prevention[Q].
✓ **Treatment of delirium**[Q]
  - Sedation with **dexmedetomidine** (α-2 agonist). Used for agitation during delirium.
    ❖ **Dexmedetomidine to lessen ICU agitation (DahLIA Trial 2016):** In patients with agitated delirium on mechanical ventilation in ITU, dexmedetomidine resulted in a shorter duration of mechanical ventilation at 7 d but no mortality benefit.
    ❖ Atipamezole is a selective α-2 antagonist and a reversal agent.
  - **Haloperidol** to treat psychosis (hallucinations and delusions) in delirium[Q].
    ❖ **MIND-USA Trial (2018):** In critically ill patients with hypoactive and hyperactive delirium, haloperidol, and ziprasidone didn't reduce the duration of delirium.
  - **BZDs shouldn't be used** except in alcohol withdrawal.
  - **Quetiapine**[Q]: Has been used for delirium.
    ❖ 5-HT2A antagonism, D2 antagonism, and 5-HT1A partial agonism.
    ❖ Can drop blood pressure and have sedative effects and cause weight gain.
✓ **Prognosis**
  - 10% increase in the relative risk of death for each day of delirium.
  - Patients with hypoactive delirium have worse prognosis[Q].
  - Sedative-related delirium had better hospital outcomes.
  - Delirium also puts patients on higher risk for long-term cognitive impairment after critical illness.
  - The longer the duration of delirium in the ICU, the higher the chances of cerebral atrophy and cerebral white matter disruption.

Additional Questions

✓ **Critical Care Pain Observational Tool**[Q]: Validated 8-point scale tool to assess pain in ICU.
  - Can we assess pain in both intubated and sedated patients?

SEDATION

✓ **Sedation:** Depression of a patient's awareness to the environment and reduction of patient's responsiveness to external stimulation.

✓ **Indications of sedation in ITU**
  * Analgesia for invasive procedures.
  * Mechanical ventilation initiation and maintenance.
  * As treatment in its own right (e.g. seizure control, increased ICP).
  * To decrease oxygen consumption, like in a patient with myocardial infarction.
  * Anxiety.
  * Dyspnoea.
  * Delirium.
  * To facilitate nursing care.

✓ **Undersedation**[Q]: Patient discomfort, hypercatabolism, increased sympathetic activity leading to myocardial ischaemia, post-traumatic stress disorder (PTSD).
  * **Oversedation**[Q]: Hypotension, prolonged recovery, increased need for tracheostomy, critical illness myopathy, increase in delirium, ileus, immunosuppression, increases risk of nosocomial pneumonia, deep vein thrombosis.

✓ **Agents available**
  * **Intravenous agents:** Propofol, ketamine
  * **Opioids:** Alfentanil, fentanyl, remifentanil
  * **Benzodiazepines:** Midazolam, lorazepam
  * **Neuroleptics:** Haloperidol
  * **α-2 agonists**[Q]: Dexmedetomidine, clonidine
  * **Inhalational agents:** Sevoflurane, isoflurane

	Propofol	Alfentanil	Remifentanil	Midazolam[Q]	Dexmedetomidine	Clonidine
Onset	1–5 min	Rapid, 1 min	Rapid, 1 min	0.5–5 min	5–10 min	10 min
Offset	5–10 min after bolus, but up to 60 min after infusions	30–60 min	<10 min, even after long infusions	2 h after bolus, but effects may be for days after infusions	Distribution half-life of 6 min, and terminal half-life of 2 h	3–7 hr
Titrability	Easily titratable	Easily titratable as short CSHT	Easily titratable as shortest CSHT	**Accumulates after infusions**	Easily titratable	Can be titrated
CVS effect	Hypotension and bradycardia	Stable as doesn't cause histamine release	Stable as doesn't cause histamine release but can cause hypotension and bradycardia at higher doses	Minimal effect in euvolemic patients	Hypotension and bradycardia	Hypotension and bradycardia
Respiratory depression	Dose-dependent respiratory depression	Dose-dependent respiratory depression	Dose-dependent respiratory depression	Dose-dependent respiratory depression	Minimal	Minimal
Analgesia	Not an analgesic	Excellent analgesia	Excellent analgesia	Not an analgesic	Good analgesic	Good analgesic
Hepatic dysfunction	Not affected	Elimination dependent on liver metabolism	Metabolized by tissue esterases, hence not affected	Elimination dependent on liver metabolism[Q]	Prolonged effect	Not affected

	Propofol	Alfentanil	Remifentanil	Midazolam^Q	Dexme-detomidine	Clonidine
Renal dysfunction	Not affected	Renal dysfunction prolonging its effects	Metabolized by tissue esterases, hence not affected	1-Hydroxy midazolam an active metabolite and can accumulate^Q	Not affected	Renal dysfunction prolonging its effects
Drug interactions	Minimal	Serotonin syndrome with MAOIs	Serotonin syndrome with MAOIs	Increased respiratory depression with opioids	Increased respiratory depression with opioids	Hypertensive crisis with MAOIs
Dependence	None	Dependence and tolerance	Physiological dependence seen	Withdrawal reactions after prolonged infusions	None	Used for weaning patients off other sedating agents

✓ **Inhalational agents:** Used in paediatrics age group in patients on multiple infusions and severe asthmatic patients for bronchodilation.
  - Can be given by a stand-alone device into the ventilator circuit (AnaConDa) or by anaesthetic machine.
  - Methoxyflurane (Penthrox) is used as analgesic in pre-hospital trauma.
✓ **Depth of sedation:** *Richmond Agitation–Sedation Scale^Q is the most validated* and widely used tool to assess depth of sedation. Sedation–Agitation Scale (SAS) can also be used.

	Criteria	
+4	Combative	Violent and immediate danger to staff
+3	Very agitated	Pulls or removes tubes or catheters immediately
+2	Agitated	Frequent non-purposeful movements and fights ventilator
+1	Restless	Anxious but not aggressive
0	Alert and calm	
−1	Drowsy	Not fully alert, but sustained awakening (eye opening/eye contact >10 s)

	Criteria	
−2	Light sedation	Briefly awakens (eye opening/eye contact <10 s)
−3	Moderate sedation	Movement or eye opening to voice, but no eye contact
−4	Deep sedation	No response to voice, but movement or eye opening to physical stimulation
−5	Unarousable	No response to voice or physical stimulation

- RAAS score of −2 or higher is indicated in most patients in ITU, with RASS of −3 or −4 only for severely sick patients like those with ARDS or raised ICP.
  - ❖ Greater depth of sedation was associated with higher duration of mechanical ventilation and in-hospital mortality.
- Sedation agitation score (SAS) can also be used.
✓ **Muscle relaxants:** Should be used only if needed as they contribute to ICU-acquired weakness (ICUAW).
  - **Indications**
    - ❖ Endotracheal intubation
    - ❖ Transfer of patients
    - ❖ ARDS

- ❖ Ventilator asynchrony
- ❖ Raised ICP
- ❖ Abdominal compartment syndrome
- **Side effects of commonly used agents**
  - ❖ **Rocuronium:** Anaphylaxis, prolonged action in liver, and kidney dysfunction
  - ❖ **Atracurium:** Bronchospasm due to histamine release
  - ❖ **Suxamethonium:** Risk of hyperkalaemia in burns patient after 24 h and spinal cord injury patient after 72 h; contraindicated in GBS patient and patients with malignant hyperthermia predisposition

✓ **Sedation strategies in ICU**
- **Daily sedation interruption**[Q]**:** Short-term suspension of sedative medications.
  - ❖ Prevents accumulation of drug.
  - ❖ Gauges tolerance of patient for complete cessation of sedation.
  - ❖ Identifies the smallest effective dose of drug to be used.
- **Protocolized sedation:** Titration of sedative and analgesic drugs by nurses using a standardized algorithm and sedation assessment scale.
  - ❖ Common goal is to achieve light sedation.
- **Analgesia-based sedation:** Achieve adequate analgesia while avoiding the use of sedative drugs.

✓ **Evidence and key trials for sedation**
- **Kress et al., NEJM (2000):** Amongst medical ICU patients, patients with daily sedation interruption were liberated from mechanical ventilation quicker and left the ICU earlier.
  - ❖ However, there was no difference in hospital length of stay or mortality.
- **ABC (2008) (Awake and Breathing Trial):** Combination of a sedation awakening trial (SAT) and spontaneous breathing trial (SBT) was superior to SBT alone and reduced duration of mechanical ventilation and 90 d mortality.
  - ❖ The combination of SAT and SBT was associated with more self-extubation, but not more reintubation after self-extubation.
- **SLEAP (2012):** Amongst mechanically ventilated patients with light sedation goal, daily interruption of sedation didn't improve patient outcomes.
  - ❖ Daily interruption was associated with higher opioid and benzodiazepine requirements.
- **SPICE III (2019):** There was no difference in mortality between dexmedetomidine and propofol as sedation for patients requiring mechanical ventilation.
  - ❖ Patients with dexmedetomidine required additional sedatives to achieve sedation goals and were associated with more bradycardia and hypotension.
- **NONSEDA (2020):** In mechanically ventilated patients, a non-sedation strategy (IV morphine for analgesia only) in comparison to a light sedation strategy (propofol for 48 h and then midazolam) didn't reduce mortality or mechanical ventilation.
- **MENDS2 (2021):** In mechanically ventilated patients with sepsis, no difference between number of days alive without delirium or coma during the first 14 d between patients receiving dexmedetomidine and those with propofol.
  - ❖ There was no difference between dexmedetomidine and propofol for 28 d ventilator-free days, death at 90 d, or cognition at 6 months.

✓ **Propofol infusion syndrome**[Q]
- Rare life-threatening condition characterized by **refractory bradycardia, along with one or more of the following:**
  - ❖ Metabolic acidosis
  - ❖ Rhabdomyolysis
  - ❖ Hypertriglyceridaemia
  - ❖ Hepatomegaly
- **Pathophysiology**
  - ❖ Imbalance of energy demand and utilization.
  - ❖ Mitochondrial oxidative phosphorylation and free fatty acid utilization are impaired, leading to lactic acidosis and muscle necrosis.
  - ❖ Propofol itself has a negative inotropic effect on the heart.
- **Risk factors**
  - ❖ Children[Q]: Low glycogen storage and high dependence on fat metabolism
  - ❖ >48 h of infusion
  - ❖ Dose >4 mg/kg/h

- ❖ Acute neurological injury
- ❖ Catecholamine infusion
- ❖ Glucocorticoid infusion
- • **Diagnosis**
  - ❖ High index of suspicion, clinical diagnosis
  - ❖ Increased lactates, CK, hyperkalaemia, urinary myoglobin
  - ❖ ECG[Q]: Brugada-like changes, heart blocks, bradycardia progressing to asystole, AF, SVT
- • **Management**
  - ❖ Stop propofol infusion and use alternative sedative agent.
  - ❖ Minimize lipid intake and adequate carbohydrate intake[Q].
  - ❖ **Cardiovascular support:** Chronotropic agents, pacing, VA ECMO.
  - ❖ **Renal support:** RRT for AKI.

SLEEP ISSUES IN ICU

- ✓ **Normal sleep architecture**
  - • Adults recommended 7–9 h of sleep a day.
  - • Sleep can be divided into non–rapid eye movement (NREM) and rapid eye movement (REM) stages, and they alternate over 4 to 6, 90-min cycles.
  - • NREM accounts for 75% of sleep, whereas REM accounts for 25% of sleep.
  - • **NREM** consists of three stages: N1 (5%), N2 (50%), and N3 (20%).
    - ❖ Minute ventilation decreases during NREM sleep.
    - ❖ Blood pressure and heart rate decrease during NREM sleep.
  - • **REM sleep** is characterized by muscle atonia, but autonomic activity dominates the latter half of the sleep.
    - ❖ Respiration increases during REM sleep.
    - ❖ Blood pressure and heart rate increase during NREM sleep.
- ✓ **Circadian rhythm**
  - • **Sleep homeostat:** It regulates sleepiness and is dictated by adenosine. The longer you are without sleep, the sleepier you become.
  - • **Circadian pacemaker:** It regulates wakefulness and is dictated by melatonin, with lowest values between 7:00 a.m. and 9:00 a.m.

- ✓ **Sleep architecture of the critically ill**
  - • Sleep in the ICU is dominated by N1 and N2. **N3 and REM are near absent.**
- ✓ **Sleep measurement in the ICU**
  - • **Polysomnography:** EEG, electromyogram, electrooculogram.
  - • **Actigraphy:** Non-invasive accelerometer-based sleep estimation tool with a wrist-watch-like interface. Validated only for healthy adults.
  - • **Bi-spectral index:** Single forehead sensor containing multiple EEG electrodes.
- ✓ **Causes of ICU sleep disruption**
  - • **Noise:** Normal ICU limits are 35 dB and 45 dB during night and morning time.
  - • **Light and melatonin:** Melatonin secretion disrupted by bright lights in ICU, sepsis, and delirium.
  - • **Mechanical ventilation:** Worse sleep quality in those who are mechanically ventilated. Modes that improved patient–ventilator synchrony improved sleep quality.
  - • **Patient care interactions:** Blood sampling and vital signs check are the most disruptive ICU factors.
  - • **Medications**
    - ❖ **Benzodiazepines:** Lower the sleep latency and increase N2 sleep and total sleep time while decreasing N3 and REM sleep.
    - ❖ **Zolpidem and zopiclone:** Decrease sleep latency and increase total sleep time without affecting sleep architecture.
    - ❖ **Opioid:** Decreases N3 and REM sleep.
    - ❖ **Propofol:** Suppresses REM and sequential progression of sleep stages.
    - ❖ **Dexmedetomidine:** Increases N3 sleep and decreases REM sleep.
    - ❖ **Melatonin:** Conflicting data currently, but they appear safe with no major side effects.
    - ❖ **Haloperidol:** Decreases sleep latency and increases total sleep time. Increases N3.
    - ❖ **Quetiapine:** Increases total sleep time but decreases REM sleep.
    - ❖ **Norepinephrine:** Decreases N3 and REM sleep.
    - ❖ **Beta-blockers:** Decrease REM sleep, nightmares, insomnia.

❖ **Drug withdrawal:** Can cause sleep disruptions and insomnia.

✓ **Effects of disrupted sleep in the ICU**
- Decreased FEV1 and FVC.
- Increased oxygen consumption and CO_2 production.
- Increased blood pressure and heart rate.
- Increased rebound REM, causing autonomic instability.
- Release of inflammatory cytokines like TNF-α, IL-1, IL-6.
- Increased catabolism and stress.
- Cortisol and catecholamine release.
- Increased delirium.

✓ **Methods to promote sleep in ITU**
- Lower alarm volumes.
- Minimize non-relevant speech at the bedside.
- Turn off hallway and room lights.
- Earplugs.
- Eye masks.
- Discourage benzodiazepines, opioids, and antihistamines.
- Melatonin (improved outcomes not shown yet).
- Targeted music therapy.

DISORDERS OF TEMPERATURE CONTROL

✓ **Primary thermoregulatory control area:** Preoptic and posterior hypothalamus.
- **Core temperature** 36.1–37°C, with peak temperature around 6:00 p.m.
- IL-1, IL-6, IL-8, and TNF-α lead to activation of hypothalamus, which releases **PGE2.**
- Hypothalamus receives temperature increase signals from skin, deep viscera, and spinal cord and modulates autonomic tone to cause an increase in evaporative heat loss through sweat glands, cutaneous vasodilation, and decreased muscle tone.
- **Gold standard of measuring core temperature is pulmonary artery catheter**
  - ❖ Other core sites are oesophagus, nasopharynx, tympanic membrane, and bladder.
  - ❖ Rectal temperature is 0.4°C higher than core temperature and lags behind changes in actual core temperature.
  - ❖ Axillary and oral methods are less reliable in reflecting core temperature.

Hypothermia: Core Body Temperature Less Than 35°C

✓ **Classification of hypothermia**
- Mild[Q]: 32–35°C
- Moderate[Q]: 28–32°C
- Severe[Q]: <28°C

✓ **Causes**
- **Exposure to cold temperature**
- **CNS-depressant drugs:** Alcohol, phenothiazines, barbiturates, paralytic agents
- **CNS disorders:** Stroke, brain tumours, spinal cord transections
- **Endocrine disorders:** Hypoglycaemia, hypothyroidism
- **Skin disorders:** Burns, psoriasis, erythroderma
- **Trauma**

✓ **Physiological changes[Q]**
- **Metabolism:** Metabolic changes occur in two phases: Shivering (35–30°C) and non-shivering (<30°C).
  - ❖ Shivering reflex[Q] is obtunded at <33.5°C.
  - ❖ *Metabolism reduces by 5–10% for every 1°C* reduction in core temperature.
- **Cardiovascular[Q]:** Increased PR interval, second- or third-degree heart block, broadening of the QRS interval, and prolonged QT interval are seen.
  - ❖ **Osborn waves/J waves** seen in lateral leads on the ECG below 33°C. J-waves may persist for 12–24 h after resuscitation.
  - ❖ AF at 25–34°C, VF occurs at 28°C and asystole at <20°C.
- **Respiratory:** Tidal volume and respiratory rate decline. Loss of cough reflex and bronchorrhoea.
- **Neurological:** Confused during mild hypothermia, verbally responsive but incoherent during moderate hypothermia, and comatose during severe hypothermia.
  - ❖ *Cerebral oxygen consumption decreases by 5–10% for each 1°C decrease in temperature.*
  - ❖ EEG shows decreased α activity and increased β and θ activity.
  - ❖ Visual and auditory evoked potentials show delayed latencies.

❖ *Electromyography is reported to be normal.*
❖ Pupils are fixed and dilated at temperatures <30°C.
- **Renal:** GFR may decrease by 85%; however, urine output is somehow maintained due to defects in tubular reabsorption, and the urine is extremely dilute (cold diuresis).
- **Haematological function:** Haematocrit increased due to haemoconcentration. Platelets count drops as temperature decreases.
  ❖ Coagulopathy may be seen with hypothermia.
- **Gastrointestinal function:** *Ileus*, pancreatitis, and hepatic dysfunction are seen.
- **Endocrine function:** Insulin resistance and hyperglycaemia can be seen.
- **Immune function:** *Infection is a major cause of death among hypothermic patients.*
  ❖ Wound healing is delayed.

✓ **Treatment**
- **Initial field care:** Removal of wet clothes, insulation with blankets.
- **Cardiopulmonary stabilization**[Q].
  ❖ Fluid resuscitation with fluids warmed at least to room temperature should be attempted for all patients.
  ❖ No adrenaline[Q] until patient temperature is above 30°C.
  ❖ Between 30 and 35°C, double the dose intervals[Q] for advanced life support drugs.
  ❖ Shock VF up to three times[Q], if necessary, then no further shocks until the temperature is >30°C.
- **Treat the cause**
  ❖ Correct hypoglycaemia with 25–50 g of 50% dextrose.
  ❖ Thiamine in case of suspected alcohol overdose in chronic alcoholics.
  ❖ IV 0.2–0.5 mg of thyroxine in myxoedematous hypothermic coma.
- **Rewarming**[Q]: Correction rate[Q] of ≤0.5°C per hour to avoid localized temperature differences, as this can lead to cerebral hypoxia.
  ❖ **Passive external rewarming:** Slowest method. Keep the patient dry and covered with blankets. It is helpful only when the patient's core temperature is >30°C.

❖ **Active external rewarming:** Controversial. Raise the skin temperature by hot blankets, electric heating pads, and hot water bottles. Effective for moderate hypothermia. Mortality is higher compared to other methods as rapid active rewarming can cause an "afterdrop"[Q] with vasodilation, leading to movement of cold peripheral blood to the body core.
❖ **Active central rewarming**[Q]: Fastest and most invasive method. Heated IV crystalloids along with heated and humidified oxygen. **In patients in cardiac arrest, active internal rewarming using cardiopulmonary bypass/VA ECMO should be done.**
- **Oesophageal temperature** is the most accurate method to track the progress of rewarming.

Therapeutic hypothermia: Cooling a patient to subnormal body temperatures for therapeutic benefits, like neuroprotection.

✓ **Current indications of therapeutic hypothermia.**
- Neuroprotection in neonatal hypoxic ischaemic brain injury.
- Deep hypothermic circulatory arrest.

✓ **Targeted temperature management (TTM)**
- The term **TTM** replaced the term *therapeutic hypothermia* and has been used specifically for strict temperature control following out-of-hospital cardiac arrest. This has been replaced by a new term, "**temperature control,**" after repeated trials that showed no benefit with hypothermia.
  ❖ **TTM Trial (2013):** No mortality difference in unconscious patients following OHCA for TTM to 33° vs 36°C.
  ❖ **TTM 2 Trial (2021)**[Q]: No mortality difference in unconscious patients following OHCA for TTM to 33° vs 37.5°C.
  ❖ Other trials for use of hypothermia in patients with trauma are given in the chapter on traumatic brain injury.

Hyperthermia: Results from imbalance of heat production, regulation, and loss. Hypothalamic set point is not raised here compared to fever, in which hypothalamic set point is raised. Hyperthermia is less likely to respond to antipyretics like acetaminophen, and extreme elevation of temperature >40°C is common.

Differential diagnosis for hyperthermia is as follows.

✓ **Hyperthermic syndromes**
  • Heat stroke
  • Malignant hyperthermia
  • Neuroleptic malignant syndrome
  • Serotonin syndrome
✓ **Infection**
  • Meningitis, encephalitis, brain abscess
  • Tetanus, typhoid fevers
  • Malaria
✓ **Endocrinopathy**
  • Thyrotoxicosis
  • Pheochromocytoma
  • Diabetic ketoacidosis
✓ **Central nervous system**
  • Hypothalamic stroke
  • Cerebral haemorrhage
  • Status epilepticus
✓ **Oncologic**
  • Lymphoma
  • Leukaemia

Heat stroke: Core temperature above 40.5°C due to failure of heat dissipation leads to hyperthermia. Can be life-threatening.

✓ **Types:** Exertional and non-exertional. **Exertional** seen in young athletes during severe exercise, and **non-exertional** seen in patients with comorbidities who can't compensate.
  • **Causes:** Exercise, fever, thyrotoxicosis, amphetamines, dehydration, beta-blockers, phenothiazines.
  • Genetic predisposition like malignant hyperpyrexia may be there.
✓ **Pathophysiology:** Direct toxicity of temperature above 42°C to mitochondria, enzymes, and cell membranes.
  • IL-1, IL-2, IL-6, Il-8, IL-10, and TNF-α are all increased in heat stroke.
✓ **Clinical features**
  • Cardiac output is increased, and peripheral vascular resistance lowered due to vasodilation. Dehydration occurs, and hypotension can be seen.
  • **Cerebral oedema** and local cranial haemorrhages are seen.
  • Acute kidney injury is seen.

• **Coagulopathy:** Decrease in platelet count and increase in platelet aggregation. DIC is seen.
• Flaccid muscle paralysis is seen. Skeletal muscle necrosis and muscle enzyme elevation are seen.
• Diagnosis is made clinically based on elevated rectal temperature, CNS dysfunction, and exposure to severe environmental heat.
✓ **Treatment**
  • **Resuscitation:** ABCDE approach.
  • **Rapid cooling:** *Starts from cooling in the field first with removing the clothes and constantly wetting the skin.*
    ❖ Evaporative and convective cooling should be done.
    ❖ Cooling should stop as temperature reaches 39°C.
  • Benzodiazepine should be used for agitation.
  • No role of antipyretic agents, such as acetaminophen or aspirin. Dantrolene isn't effective.
✓ **Prognosis:** Mortality between 20 and 60%.

Malignant hyperthermia: Drug- or stress-induced hypermetabolic syndrome characterized by vigorous muscle contractions, an abrupt increase of temperature, and cardiovascular collapse.

✓ **Causes:** Inhaled anaesthetics, succinyl choline[Q].
  • Mutation in ryanodine receptor (**RYR1**), leading to unregulated release of calcium from sarcoplasmic reticulum, leading to muscle contraction and heat generation.
  • Autosomal dominant penetrance and expressivity. Chromosome 19[Q].
  • Incidence: 1:50,000 UK population.
✓ **Physiology**
  • Depolarization of muscle cell happens and spreads in sarcolemma to deeper part of cell through T-tubules.
  • T-tubules cause release of Ca^{2+} from the sarcoplasmic reticulum (ryanodine receptors).
  • **Calcium binds to troponin C**, which releases the tropomyosin from actin and allows binding of actin to myosin-ADP-Pi complex.
  • Defected receptor causes unregulated calcium release, which causes sustained

muscle contraction, causing increased CO_2 production and rhabdomyolysis.

✓ **Clinical features**
  - Masseter spasm[Q] may be the initial feature after succinyl choline administration.
  - Rising carbon dioxide production is the other helpful sign that is seen commonly.
  - High fever >41°C. Temperature raises by 1°C every few minutes. It's a late sign.
  - Metabolic acidosis, DIC, hepatic failure, seizures, ventricular dysrhythmias, renal failure, and cerebral haemorrhage.
  - High CK and muscle rigidity are seen. Muscle contraction is peripherally mediated.
  - Muscle biopsy may appear normal, and caffeine halothane contracture test is the gold standard for diagnosis[Q].

✓ **Treatment**
  - Call for help and halt the surgery. Discontinue the triggering agent.
  - Anaesthesia should be immediately stopped, and all the apparatus, tubing, and ventilation equipment should be changed.
    ❖ Activated charcoal filters should be used.
    ❖ 100% oxygen with TIVA should be used.
  - **Dantrolene** (2–3 mg/kg bolus),[Q] followed by 1 mg/kg every 5 min until the signs of acute MH improve. Avoid going above cumulative doses above 10 mg/kg.
    ❖ The lyophilized powder is a 20 mg vial that is mixed in 60 mL of sterile water and takes a lot of staff to mix it.
    ❖ Aim for ETCO2 <6 kPa, normal minute ventilation, and temperature <38.5°C.
  - **Cooling measures:** Ice packs, cooling blankets, gastric and bladder lavage with cold water, evaporative cooling.
    ❖ Cardiopulmonary bypass may be needed in patients not responding to Dantrolene.
  - **Complications:** *Ventricular fibrillation is the most common cause of death* in early stages and amiodarone, or magnesium should be given to patients.
    ❖ **Hyperkalaemia** with glucose insulin drip; **metabolic acidosis** with bicarbonate; and **myoglobinuria** with forced alkaline diuresis and renal replacement therapy; **DIC** with empirical FFPs, platelets, and cryoprecipitate.

  - **Later actions:** Explanation to family, local incident reporting, notifying GP, and referral for MH susceptibility investigation.

✓ **Prognosis:** Mortality is 6–10%.

Serotonin Syndrome (SS)[Q] (This question is an exam favourite and will be asked in a way to confuse you with neuroleptic malignant syndrome):

✓ **Serotonin:** Neurotransmitter produced by metabolism of **tryptophan**. Metabolized by monoamine oxidase (MAOs) into 5-hydroxyindoleacetic acid (5-HIAA).
  - St John's wort[Q] is both a mild SSRI and a cP450 enzyme inducer.

✓ **Mechanisms of serotonin syndrome**[Q]
  - **Increased release:** MDMA, cocaine, alcohol
  - **Receptor stimulation:** LSD, pethidine, **fentanyl**, TCA, sumatriptans, lithium
  - **Decreased uptake:** SSRIs, **tramadol**, ondansetron
  - **Decreased metabolism:** MAO inhibitors, **linezolid**, methylene blue

✓ **Clinical triad**[Q]
  - **Altered mental status:** Anxiety, agitation, hallucinations, delirium.
  - **Neuromuscular hyperexcitability:** Tremors, **clonus**[Q], **myoclonic jerks**, and hyperreflexia. Ocular clonus and hypertonicity of the lower limbs.
  - **Autonomic hyperactivity:** Labile blood pressure, flushing, **hyperthermia**, and diarrhoea.

✓ Most SS cases present within 6–24 h of a serotonergic agent dose change or introduction of a new substance.
  - SS is much quicker in onset than neuroleptic malignant syndrome (NMS).

✓ **SS is a clinical diagnosis.** *Hunter toxicity criteria decision rules* are used for diagnosis with 84% sensitivity and 97% specificity. It included history of recent exposure to a serotonergic drug plus at least one of the following:
  - Spontaneous clonus
  - Inducible clonus with agitation or diaphoresis
  - Ocular clonus with agitation or diaphoresis
  - Tremors and hyperreflexia
  - Hypertonia and temperature over 38°C with ocular or inducible clonus

✓ **Treatment**
- Resuscitation: ABCDE approach.
- Stop trigger and supportive care.
- **Hypotension:** Use direct-acting agents like noradrenaline.
- Hypertension: Short-acting agents like esmolol.
- **Sedation**[Q] with benzodiazepines and dexmedetomidine.
- Treatment with serotonin antagonists like **cyproheptadine**[Q].
- No evidence of use of **dantrolene.**

Neuroleptic malignant syndrome (NMS)[Q]**:** Life-threatening neurological emergency.

✓ **Idiosyncratic reaction** to deficit of dopamine.
- Gradual onset over days to weeks[Q].
- Antipsychotics like haloperidol, metoclopramide, olanzapine, risperidone, fluoxetine, and quetiapine due to dopamine D2 receptor antagonism.
- Withdrawal of levodopa or amantadine has also produced the syndrome.

✓ *Hyperthermia,* **muscle rigidity,** and **autonomic disability.**
- *Relatively low maximal temperature (40°C) compared to patients with heat stroke and MH.*
- Raised creatine kinase, transaminase levels, and leucocytosis.
- Renal failure, hepatic failure, DIC, and seizures.

✓ *Muscle contraction is centrally mediated compared to peripherally mediated in malignant hyperthermia (MH).*

✓ NMS has higher mortality compared to serotonin syndrome.

✓ **Management:** Cooling, antipyretics, and CVS support.
- **Dantrolene** (1–3 mg/kg bolus), **amantadine** (100 mg 8 hourly), and **bromocriptine** (2.5 mg 8 hourly) have been used.
- **Electroconvulsive therapy** has been used in refractory cases.

Additional Questions

✓ **Oculogyric crises**[Q]**:** Involuntary eye deviation upward, accompanied by increased blinking and pain. It can last from second to hours.
- Typical neuroleptics, stress, and fatigue can precipitate it.

- Benztropine or diphenhydramine can be used for treatment.

RHABDOMYOLYSIS

Aetiology

✓ **Rhabdomyolysis:** Pathological breakdown of striated skeletal muscle with release of muscle cell contents into the systemic circulation.

✓ **Causes**
- **Traumatic:** Crush injuries, electrical injuries, compartment syndrome[Q] (long lie, tourniquet use, dense neuraxial block)
- **Non-traumatic:** Seizures, infections (influenza, EBV, HIV, *Streptococcus, Staphylococcus*), vigorous exercise, malignant hyperthermia, **statins**[Q], ecstasy, cocaine, **alcohol**, and DKA

✓ **Pathophysiology: ATP depletion (ischaemia) and cell wall disruption (direct myocyte injury)**
- Calcium leaks into muscle cells and activates proteases and mitochondrial dysfunction.
- Myoglobin, creatine kinase (CK), and lactate dehydrogenase (LDH) are released in the blood.
- Myoglobin can cause renal tubular obstruction and damage.

Clinical Features and Diagnosis

✓ **Clinical features:** Clinical diagnosis is made based on clinical signs and symptoms.
- **Triad of muscle pain, weakness,** and **dark "Coca-Cola"** urine along with fever, confusion, and oliguria.
- **Myoglobinuria:** Myoglobin released from muscle combines with Tamm–Horsfall proteins to form brown granular casts and can lead to tubular obstruction[Q]. Hyperuricaemia[Q] can worsen tubular obstruction.
  - ❖ **Myoglobin levels** >1,000 mg/mL are associated with kidney dysfunction.
- **Creatine kinase (CK)** >5,000 units/L is diagnostic.
  - ❖ CK levels above 5,000–10,000 U/L are associated with kidney dysfunction.

✓ **Complications**
- **Acute kidney injury**[Q] (due to dehydration, sympathetic vasoconstriction, myoglobin, and haem-blocking tubules).

- Metabolic acidosis[Q], **hyperkalaemia**[Q], ↑ uric acid, ↑ phosphates, **hypo**calcaemia (sequestered in tissues) initially, followed by **hypercalcaemia** in recovery phase[Q].
- **Disseminated intravascular coagulation (DIC).**
- **Compartment syndrome** can occur at any stage. Tissue perfusion pressure = diastolic blood pressure – compartment pressure.
  - ❖ **Pressure >30** mmHg[Q] checked with needle in tissue connected to manometer is significant.
  - ❖ Tense, swollen limb, venous congestion, arterial insufficiency.
  - ❖ Forearm (volar) and leg (anterior) compartment[Q] are more commonly involved in development of compartment syndrome.

Prevention and Treatment

- ✓ **Medical management:** Stop the offending agent. Analgesia for pain.
  - **Hydration**[Q] targeting 2–3 mL/kg/h of urine output is the treatment.
  - Thiazide is better than furosemide in adequately resuscitated patients.
  - Urinary alkalinization[Q] with sodium bicarbonate (1.26 %) is done to maintain urine pH between 6.5 and 8 to prevent formation of muddy brown casts.
  - Renal replacement therapy may be needed.
  - No role of mannitol, no pentoxifylline.
  - **Dantrolene** in selected cases like neuroleptic malignant syndrome or malignant hyperthermia.
- ✓ **Surgical treatment:** Fasciotomies for treating compartment syndrome.

Prognosis

- ✓ CK trends help in prognosis with a reduction in 20% from baseline seen as a good prognostic indicator.

POST-RESUSCITATION CARE

- ✓ **Post–cardiac arrest syndrome**[Q]
  - Myocardial dysfunction
  - Hypoxic brain injury
  - Systemic reperfusion injury

- ✓ **Post–return of spontaneous circulation (ROSC) care**
  - **Immediate interventions**
    - ❖ Advanced airway with **waveform capnography**
    - ❖ 12-lead ECG, **arterial blood pressure** monitoring with fluids, and vasopressors
    - ❖ Sedation
  - **Physiological targets**
    - ❖ SpO_2: 94–98%
    - ❖ PO_2: 10–13 kPa
    - ❖ PCO_2: 4.5–6 kPa
    - ❖ **SBP** >100 mmHg, **MAP** >65 mmHg
    - ❖ **Urine output** >0.5 mL/kg/h
    - ❖ **Glucose:** 8–10 mmol/L
  - **Coronary angiography** before CT brain ± CTPA if clinical evidence of myocardial ischaemia even in comatose patients.
    - ❖ CT brain ± CTPA before coronary angiography if clinical evidence of neurological or respiratory causes of arrest.
  - **Delayed angiography should be considered in haemodynamically stable patients without ST-segment elevation in patients resuscitated after an out-of-hospital cardiac arrest.**
    - ❖ **TOMAHAWK Trial (2021)**[Q]: No difference in 30 d mortality between the use of immediate vs delayed angiography without ST segment elevation.
  - In a pregnant patient, once return of spontaneous circulation (ROSC) is achieved, monitor fetal heart rate as well; otherwise, no need to monitor during cardiac arrest.
  - **ICU Interventions**
    - ❖ Temperature control
    - ❖ Echocardiography
    - ❖ Diagnose and treat seizures
    - ❖ Delayed prognostication for at least 72 h
- ✓ **Targeted temperature management (TTM):** Strict temperature control post–cardiac arrest.
  - **TTM2 Trial (2021):** Amongst OHCA patients, cases kept at 33°C for 28 h and then rewarmed to 37°C at 72 h vs patients kept at normothermia 36.5–37.7°C, no significant difference between mortality and morbidity was seen.
    - ❖ Hence, current evidence suggests that normothermia and actively avoiding

fever (>37.7°C) has no significant difference in morbidity or mortality.

- However, the **European Resuscitation Council (ERC) Guidelines 2021** suggests TTM with constant temperature of 32–36°C and then preventing fever for at least 72 h.

✓ **Prognostication:** Process of predicting future events. Based on medical experience and evidence-based medicine in ICU to predict a patient's outcome.

- Factors involved are acute pathology, premorbid physiology, and acceptable quality of life for the patient.

✓ **Poor prognostic signs**
- **Clinical history**
  - ❖ Initial non-shockable rhythm
  - ❖ Initial lactate concentrations and rate of lactate clearance correlate with survival[Q]
- **Clinical examination**
  - ❖ Absent pupillary and corneal reflexes even after 72 h
  - ❖ Absent motor response to pain >72 h post–cardiac arrest
  - ❖ **Confirmed myoclonic status** (≥30 min, not just the presence of myoclonic jerks) that develop ≤48 h post-ROSC; can be mistaken for intentional myoclonus, which is **Lance–Adams syndrome**
- **Neurophysiological investigations**
  - ❖ **EEG:** Unreactive baseline in response to external stimuli, presence of burst suppression, or refractory status epilepticus ≥72 h post-arrest.
  - ❖ The bilateral absence of N_2O somatosensory-evoked potentials (SSEPs)[Q] ≥24 h and ≥72 h post-arrest from those patients treated without or with TTM, respectively. In SSEP, a peripheral nerve, e.g. median nerve, is stimulated and can be detected at the cortical level normally.
- **Imaging**
  - ❖ **CT** ≤24 h showing cerebral oedema, sulcal effacement, and loss of grey-white matter differentiation.
  - ❖ **MRI** 2 to 5 d post-ROSC provides more detailed information regarding the hypoxic-ischaemic brain injury.

- **Biomarkers**
  - ❖ **Neuron-specific enolase (NSE)** and **S-100 levels** associated with poor neurological outcomes.
  - ❖ NSE can be measured in CSF and blood.
  - ❖ Evidence of NSE is better than S-100b and hence recommended.

✓ **ERC ESICM 2021 Guidelines algorithm for prognostication[Q].** Poor outcomes likely if all three of the following:
- Targeted temperature management and rewarming.
- **Unconscious, GCS motor score ≤3 at ≥72 h.**
- At least two of the following:
  - ❖ Pupillary and corneal reflex absent bilaterally
  - ❖ Status myoclonus (≤72 h)
  - ❖ NSE >60 µg/L (at 48 h and/or 72 h)
  - ❖ SSEP N20 wave absent bilaterally
  - ❖ EEG highly malignant (>24 h)
  - ❖ CT/MRI shows diffuse and extensive anoxic injury

Neurological Outcome after Brain Injury

Cerebral Performance Scale (CPC): Score 1–2 suggests good neurological outcome assessed from 6–12 months post-injury

CPC 1	Good cerebral performance (conscious, able to work, mild deficit)
CPC 2	Moderate cerebral disability (conscious, independent ADLs, able to work in sheltered environment)
CPC 3	Severe cerebral disability (conscious but dependent due to brain dysfunction like dementia or paralysis)
CPC 4	Coma or vegetative state
CPC 5	Brain death

✓ **Modified Rankin Scale (mRS):** Score 0–3 suggests good neurological outcome assessed from 6 to 12 months post-injury.
- mRS can differentiate between mild and moderate disability and hence is recommended.

mRS	
0	No symptoms
1	No significant disability (all ADLs)
2	Slight disability (not all ADLs as unable to carry out few previous activities but **works without assistance**)
3	Moderate disability (requires help, walks without assistance)
4	**Moderately severe disability** (unable to walk without assistance or care for bodily needs)
5	**Severe disability** (bedridden, incontinent, constant nursing care)
6	Dead

END-OF-LIFE CARE ON THE ICU

✓ **Frailty:** State of reduced physical, physiological, and cognitive reserve with increased vulnerability to deterioration because of relatively minor stress factors.
- *It is applicable to all age groups* but obviously is more common in older people.
- **Five conditions** often associated with frailty:
  ❖ Delirium
  ❖ Recurrent falls
  ❖ Sudden deterioration in mobility
  ❖ New or worsening incontinence
  ❖ Frequent medication side effects
- **Characteristics:** Decreased mobility, weakness, reduced muscle mass, poor nutritional status, and diminished cognitive function
- *Person's frailty can change over time.*
- **Fried frailty phenotype** score measures frailty based on aspects of physical decline, like:
  ❖ **Weight loss:** >10 pounds in last year
  ❖ **Exhaustion:** Self-reported
  ❖ **Weakness:** Grip strength in the lowest 20%
  ❖ **Slowness:** Time to walk 15 ft in the slowest 20%
  ❖ **Low physical activity:** Reduced energy expenditure (Kcal/w) in lowest 20%
- **Rockwood Clinical Frailty Scale (CFS):** 5–8 is considered frail, and 9 means

terminal illness. Used more commonly clinically. (Definitely asked in viva.)
  ❖ **Very fit:** Robust, energetic, and motivated people who exercise regularly.
  ❖ **Well:** No active disease but less fit than category 1.
  ❖ **Managing well:** Medical problems present but well controlled. Not regularly active beyond routine walking.
  ❖ **Vulnerable:** Symptoms limit activities. Tired during the day.
  ❖ **Mildly frail:** Need help for finances, transportation, heavy homework, and medications. Impairs shopping, walking outside alone, meal preparation, and housework.
  ❖ **Moderately frail:** Problems with stairs and need help with bathing. Need assistance for dressing.
  ❖ **Severely frail:** Completely dependent for personal care but are stable and are not at high risk of dying within next 6 months.
  ❖ **Very severely frail:** Approaching the end of life and won't recover even from a minor illness.
  ❖ **Terminally ill:** Life expectancy <6 months in patients who are not otherwise evidently frail.
✓ **WHO Performance Status Scale:** Used to assess a patient's ability to perform daily activities and their level of disability. Useful for deciding whether to admit a patient to an ICU.
- Also known as ECOG (Eastern Cooperation Oncology Group) performance status scale.
- **Scale**
  0: Fully active: Able to carry all pre-disease activities without restriction.
  1 Restricted in physically strenuous activity, but ambulatory and able to **carry out work of a light or sedentary nature, like light housework**, office work.
  2 **Ambulatory and capable of self-care,** but unable to carry out any work activities. Up and about more than 50% of waking hours.
  3 Capable of only limited self-care, **confined to bed or chair for more than 50% of waking hours.**

4 Completely disabled. Cannot carry on self-care. Totally confined to bed or chair.

5 **Dead.**

- **Interpretation**
  - ❖ **ECOG 0–1:** Good performance status; considered suitable for admission to ITU.
  - ❖ **ECOG 2:** Moderate performance status; require careful consideration for ICU admission.
  - ❖ **ECOG 3–4:** Poor performance status; not considered suitable for ICU admission due to high risk of mortality.

✓ **Palliative care:** Broader term that includes end-of-life care.
- It can start any time during a life-limiting illness and aims to improve quality of life and relieve pain and other symptoms.
- As a disease progresses, palliative care transitions into end-of-life care.

✓ **End-of-life care:** When patient is likely to die within next 12 months.
- Around 15–20% of patients admitted to critical care die before they leave the hospital.
  - ❖ *Up to 24% of critical care survivors are readmitted to the hospital within 90 d of discharge from the hospital.*
  - ❖ One in five critical care survivors die within a year of discharge from the hospital.

✓ **Decision-making in adult who lacks capacity**
- Take a decision based on clinical condition of the patient and acceptable quality of life to the patient.
  - ❖ Avoid using the term *futility* as it is very subjective, and take decision by determining the *potential overall benefit to the patient.*
- Check for legally binding **advanced decisions.**
  - ❖ Appoint independent mental capacity advocate **(IMCA)** in a person with no next of kin.
- Relatives can provide information about the patient's wishes, but they cannot make decisions.
- **Multiteam discussions (MDT)** if not able to come to a consensus about the decision taken.

- In case of disagreements about decisions, legal advice may be sought for from an independent court.

✓ **Organ support withdrawal in critical care**
- Non-comfort medications stopped. Can continue anti-epileptics.
- Partial/complete removal of monitoring.
- Opioids for pain and discomfort.
- Midazolam for agitation.
- Supplemental oxygen for symptomatic relief.
- Vasoactive medications are stopped.
- Extubate patient to air.
- Avoid decannulation in ECMO patients, reduce pump/gas flow in them.
- Intubation may be required for organ donation of lungs after circulatory death.
- Deactivate ICDs using magnet or by qualified personnel.

DONATION AFTER DEATH USING NEUROLOGICAL CRITERIA

✓ ***Death**[Q] is defined by the Academy of Royal Colleges as the irreversible loss of capacities for consciousness and breathing.* No statutory definition of *death* within UK law.
- **Somatic criteria:** Decapitation, rigor mortis, and decomposition. No doctor needed. Recognition of death by another person.
- **Cardiorespiratory death criteria:** Continuous apnoeic asystole for 5 min and loss of consciousness.
- **Neurological death criteria:** The complete and permanent loss of brain function as defined by an unresponsive coma with loss of capacity for consciousness, brainstem reflexes, and the ability to breathe independently.

✓ **Diagnosis of death by neurological criteria (DNC)**
- Fulfilment of preconditions: State of apnoeic coma and mechanically ventilated
- Exclusion of confounding factors
- Brainstem and apnoea testing

✓ **Age categories**[Q]
- **<37 wk:** DNC can't be confidently made.
- **37 wk–2 yr:** Criteria is same as per adults, with three conditions:

❖ 24 h before testing.

❖ 24 h between testing.

❖ No ancillary investigation.

- **2 yr and above:** Criteria as per adults.

✓ **Confounding factors**

- **Core temperature >36°C (new change)**[Q]
- **Na+ 125–160 mmol/L (new change)**
- K+ >2 mmol/L
- Mg^{2+} 0.5–3 mmol/L
- PO_4^{3-} 0.5–3 mmol/L
- Glucose 3–20 mmol/L

✓ **Preconditions**[Q]

- >6 h after loss of the last brainstem reflex
- >24 h after loss of the last brain reflex when aetiology is primarily anoxic damage
- >24 h of temperature >**36°C**
- No neuromuscular agents or neuromuscular disorders contributing to weakness
- No investigations needed for high cervical cord pathology
- No effect of depressant drugs, like prolonged fentanyl infusions
- Caution for steroids given in space-occupying lesions, like abscesses
- Caution for aetiology primarily in brainstem or posterior fossa
- Caution for therapeutic decompressive craniectomy

✓ In high cervical spine injury, apnoea testing isn't applicable[Q], so ancillary tests are required to diagnose neurological death.

✓ **Doll's eye movements**[Q] (eye movement response to head movement) **do not** form part of the formal brainstem death testing in the UK. In intact brainstem, eyes deviate to the side opposite to the head movement.

✓ Two doctors, including one consultant, both >5-yr post–full registration, are required to perform two sets of brainstem tests[Q]. No recommended minimum period between sets of tests. None of the doctors would be part of a transplant team. Completion of the second set of clinical tests is the time of death[Q].

- Time of death in case of ancillary investigation is the time at which results are available to the doctors[Q].
- Both eyes and both ears must be examinable.

Cranial Nerves II to X Are Tested[Q]

Test	Afferent	Efferent	Result in Brainstem-Dead Patient
Pupillary light reflex	CN II	CN III	Absent direct and consensual light reflex.
Corneal reflex	CN V	CN VII	No motor response to touch stimulation of the cornea.
Oculovestibular reflex	CN VIII	CN III/ IV/ VI	Absence of eye movements to 50 mL of ice-cold water injected into the external auditory meatus over 1 min, with a patient at a 30° head-up tilt. If testing is only possible unilaterally because of trauma, test is not invalidated.
Gag reflex	CN IX	CN X	No gag reflex response to stimulation of the posterior pharynx.
Cough reflex	CN IX	CN X	No cough reflex response to bronchial stimulation with a suction catheter.
Absent motor response	CN V	CN VII	Absent motor response in the cranial nerve distribution to painful stimulus (supraorbital pressure).

✓ **Apnoea test**[Q]: The pre-apnoea arterial blood gas should have a pCO_2 of at least 5.3 kPa. Apnoeic oxygenation should be done using a CPAP circuit[Q] like Mapleson C circuit. A rise in pCO_2 by 2.7 kPa and target $PaCo_2$ of at least 8 kPa along with absence of breathing confirms apnoea test as positive. A minimum of 5 min observation is a must[Q].

✓ **Indications for an ancillary investigation**
  - **Ancillary investigation required:** When a neurological examination is not possible, like extensive faciomaxillary injuries, and when effects of confounding factors on some preconditions can't be excluded.
  - **Ancillary investigation considered:** Possible spinally medicated movements causing uncertainty and to promote understanding of the clinical confirmation of death using neurological criteria to families.
  - **Cerebral CT angiography** is the recommended ancillary investigation of choice by FICM and ICS consensus guidelines. Four-point CTA criteria have 100% specificity. A diagnosis of death by neurological criteria can't be supported if the CTA demonstrates contrast opacification in any one of the four vessels.
    ❖ Cortical segments (M4 of the left middle cerebral artery)
    ❖ Cortical segments (M4 of the right middle cerebral artery)
    ❖ Left internal cerebral vein
    ❖ Right internal cerebral vein

✓ **Other ancillary investigations**
  - EEG silence of at least 30 min needed. EEG is highly sensitive modality.
  - TCD is highly specific modality but can't get signals in posterior circulation.
  - Empty light bulb sign in CT angiography.
  - Serial measurement of S-100 beta correlate closely with diagnosis of brain death.

✓ **Neurological criteria on ECMO:** If the neurological tests can't be reliably completed on ECMO, ancillary tests should be used.
  - Pharmacokinetics changes by ECMO machine can make excluding reversible causes of coma and death unreliable. Hence, specific drug levels should be performed for any concerns.
  - In VV ECMO: Cerebral CO_2 is same as peripheral venous CO_2 and can be used for assessment reliably.

- In VA ECMO: Cerebral CO_2 may differ from peripheral venous CO_2 due to variable location of mixing point between native blood flow and ECMO circuit blood flow. *Hence, multiple sites (post-membrane and systemic arterial sites farthest away from the ECMO return flow) must be sampled, and the highest pH and lowest $PacO_2$ must be used.*

✓ **Differential diagnosis:** Locked-in syndrome, hypothermia, Guillain–Barré syndrome
  - **Locked in syndrome:** Patients are conscious but can't move their limbs, grimace, or swallow.
    ❖ Blinking and vertical eye movements remain intact.
    ❖ Destruction of the base of the pons due to acute embolus to the basilar artery.

✓ **Lazarus sign**[Q]: It usually manifests with abdominal flexion, adduction, and flexion of the arms. Triggered by neck flexion. It is seen during apnoea testing due to hypoxic/hypotensive stimulation of cervical neurons.
  - It's a spinal reflex[Q] that may still be present.
  - Brain perfusion scans are conclusive for confirmation of brain death.

✓ **Donation of organs:** (1) Deceased donor: Donation after death using neurological criteria (DNC) and donation after circulatory death (DCD). (2) Living donor.
  - About 60% of deceased organ donations in the UK take place after using death diagnosed by neurological criteria and 40% after diagnosis using circulatory criteria.
  - All ITU deaths should be considered for organ donation.
  - **Specialist Nurse-Organ Donation (SNOD):** Is the local coordinator and should be involved early and before donation has been approved.
  - Only when a family has understood and accepted that death has taken place is a discussion regarding organ donation introduced.
  - Family members can refuse to authorize donation even if patient is on the organ donor register (ODR). Family members may authorize donation even if patient is not on organ donor register (ODR).

- DNC donors donated an average of 3.9 organs compared to 2.6 organs by DCD donors in 2012/2013.
  - ❖ One organ donor can save up to nine lives.
  - ❖ Three people die every day in the UK waiting for an organ.
- The donor and recipient are generally matched through the blood group (ABO system). Stem cell and kidney transplantation is through HLA–antigen matching.
- **Absolute contraindications: Age is no longer a limit for becoming a donor.**
  - ❖ Infective neurodegenerative disease (variant Creutzfeldt disease)
  - ❖ HIV disease
  - ❖ Ebola virus
  - ❖ Active cancer

✓ **Donation after death using neurological criteria**
- Coning leads to **Cushing reflex** (bradycardia and hypertension), followed by adrenergic surge, leading to tachycardia, hypertension, and often myocardial damage.
  - ❖ Pulmonary oedema in up to 18% of DBD donors due to a combination of neurogenic and cardiogenic cause.
  - ❖ After this, a period of vasodilation and relative hypovolaemia happens. Cardiac output monitoring might be needed.
- Damage to pituitary and hypothalamus can lead to **hypothermia**, diabetes insipidus (two-thirds of cases)[Q], hypothyroidism[Q], low cortisol, and insulin resistance.
- *SIRS response and disseminated intravascular coagulation (DIC) can happen in up to one-third of cases.*
- **Vasopressin**[Q] is preferred over noradrenaline as first line for these patients as they cause less pulmonary hypertension and metabolic acidosis. Also treats diabetes insipidus as well.
  - ❖ Dopamine is the preferred inotrope.
- Donor organ function usually benefits from a period of optimization following the brainstem death.
  - ❖ Correct hypotension, hypothermia, hyperglycaemia, and diabetes insipidus (vasopressin/DDAVP). Thyroid hormone may also be given.
  - ❖ **Methylprednisolone (15 mg/kg) for all donors**[Q].

- Lung protective ventilation, tidal volume 6–8 mL/kg, plateau pressure <30 cm H_2O, diuretics if pulmonary oedema.
- *Continue NG feed and LMWH.*
- Neuromuscular blocking agents may need to be given to block unwarranted motor spinal reflexes. Volatile agents abolish the autonomic spinal reflexes and contribute to ischaemic preconditioning. Volatile agents are not given to provide anaesthesia as the donor is dead.
- Laparotomy and sternotomy are done, and after a period of preoxygenation, endotracheal tube is disconnected from ventilator to prevent damage to lungs during sternotomy.
  - ❖ After adequate dissection, heparin 300 mg/kg is given and thoracic aorta, abdominal aorta, or both are clamped.
  - ❖ Organs are removed in the following order: Heart, lungs, liver, small bowel, pancreas, and kidney.

Physiological Targets		
pH >7.25	CVP: 6–10 mmHg	Glucose 4–10 mmol/L
MAP 60–80 mmHg	UO: 0.5–2 mL/kg/h	Na+ 135–145 mmol/L
Cardiac index >2.4 L/min/m²	Haemoglobin >70 g/L	pO2 >10 kPa

DONATION AFTER CIRCULATORY DEATH

✓ **Cardiovascular criteria for the diagnosis of death**
- Death may be diagnosed after a continuous 5 min period of cardiorespiratory arrest in patient in whom resuscitation has failed or deemed not appropriate.
- Absence of mechanical cardiac function can be confirmed by absence of a central pulse or absence of heart sounds.
- Apart from 5 min of confirming cardiorespiratory arrest, *the absence of a pupillary response to light, of corneal reflex, and of motor response to supraorbital pressure should be confirmed.*

- Death can be confirmed by a registered medical practitioner.
✓ UK has one of the highest rates of donation after circulatory (DCD) in the world.
  - DCD is offered to patients receiving mechanical ventilation in critical care in whom it has been decided that continuing life-prolonging treatment is no longer in patient's interest.
  - DCD should be considered in all patients who are expected to die in ICU, even in brainstem-dead patients.
  - The main limitation of DCD other than eligibility is susceptibility of organs to warm ischaemia.
✓ **Controlled donation:** Organ retrieval after expected death.
  - **Uncontrolled donation:** Organ retrieval after unexpected cardiac arrest.

Modified Maastricht Classification[Q]

Class	Arrest Type	Controlled/ Uncontrolled
I	Dead on arrival	Uncontrolled
II	Unsuccessful resuscitation	Uncontrolled
III	Anticipated cardiac arrest	Controlled
IV	Cardiac arrest in brain-dead donor	Controlled
V	Unexpected arrest in ICU patient	Uncontrolled

✓ First diagnosis of death is done using circulatory criteria (5 min), followed by family time of 5 min[Q]. Then organ retrieval is done in theatre.
  - *If the patient does not die within 30 min of the onset of functional warm ischaemia, the recipient centres will usually stand down retrieval of heart, liver, and pancreas.*
  - *If the patient does not die within 1 and 3 h of the onset of functional warm ischaemia, the recipient centres will usually stand down retrieval of lung and kidney respectively.*
  - Super-rapid laparotomy with aortic cannulation is standard in donor.
✓ **Donor functional warm ischaemic time[Q]:** *Duration of time following a sustained decrease in systolic blood pressure <50 mmHg and until the organs have been cooled with cold perfusate in theatre. Oxygen saturation below 70%*

has also been used to describe warm ischaemia time.
  - Liver: <20 min, up to 30 min
  - Pancreas: 30 min
  - Lungs: 60 min
  - Kidneys: 120 min
✓ **Graft cold ischaemia time[Q]:** Starts at cold perfusion (4°C). Ends at removal of graft from cold storage.
  - **Graft warm ischaemia time[Q]:** Starts at removal from cold storage. Ends at reperfusion.
✓ *DCD kidney transplant survival rates have 5 yr graft function and are comparable to DNC equivalents.*
  - DCD lung recipients may have even better outcome as lungs are not exposed due to catecholamine storm during DNC.
  - *DCD liver transplants have higher rates of graft failures compared to DNC liver transplants.*
✓ DCD heart and DCD kidney can be perfused ex vivo using machine perfusion.
  - DCD heart is a very fragile organ and prone to ischaemia.
✓ **DCD lung transplant:** Prevent lungs from aspiration and asphyxia.
  - Tracheal reintubation after diagnosis of circulatory death has been confirmed.
  - *Single recruitment manoeuvre (30 cm H_2O for 30 s using APL valve) at least 10 min after mechanical asystole, followed by CPAP to oxygenate the alveolar epithelium (e.g. 5 cm H_2O) and oxygen flow at 15 L/min.*

CONSENT

✓ **Consent:** Consent to treatment means a person must give permission before they receive any type of medical treatment, test, or examination.
  - For consent to be valid, it must be **voluntary, informed,** and the person must have the **capacity** to make the decision.
  - **Capacity** is an integral part of the consent process. Respect for autonomy is a key principle of medical ethics.
  - *It may not be necessary to obtain consent if a person*
    ❖ Needs emergency treatment to save their life but they are incapacitated

❖ Immediately needs an additional emergency procedure during an operation

❖ With a severe mental health condition, such as schizophrenia, and lacks a capacity to consent to the treatment of their mental health (Mental Health Act).

✓ **Mental capacity:** It is the ability to make a decision. Capacity is **time- and decision-specific.**

- Decision-making capacity can vary over time, with fluctuation even on a day-to-day basis.
- Decision-making capacity can vary based on the decision to be made (simple vs complex decisions).

Mental Capacity Act 2005 (MCA)^Q

✓ Applies to people aged 16 yr and over in England and Wales.

✓ It is designed to protect people who may lack the mental capacity to make their own decisions about their care and treatment.

- Dementia
- Learning disabilities
- Brain injury
- Temporary loss of capacity

✓ To have capacity, patients must be able to **understand** the information given to them, **retain** it, **weigh** it to make a decision, and then **communicate** the decision back^Q.

✓ **Principles of the Mental Capacity Act**

- **All patients must be assumed to have capacity, and it is the responsibility of the clinician to prove whether patient lacks it.**
- A person must be given all practicable help to make their own decision before treating as lacking capacity.
- *A person is not to be treated as unable to make a decision merely because they make an unwise decision, and a patient with capacity can take an unwise decision, even if it may result in their death.*
- All decisions about treatment and care for patients lacking capacity should be made keeping **patient's best interests.**

  ❖ Assessment of best interests must include social, psychological, and medical factors and should be informed by the patient's attitudes and opinions.

  ❖ Friends or family must be consulted.

- *Only emergency treatment can be provided without knowing patient's likely wishes for ongoing care.*
- If patient lacks capacity, information can be obtained from a patient's pre-existing advanced directive. Physicians should consult the patient's family, friends, or carers to aid identification of the patient's wishes.

✓ **Powers and bodies introduced by the Mental Capacity Act**

- **Independent Mental Health Advocate (IMCA):** An IMCA can be instructed to provide independent safeguards for people lacking mental capacity who have no one else to support them in decision-making or to be consulted.

  ❖ An IMCA is not a decision-maker. He just represents the patient without capacity, providing information to ensure whether the proposed decision is in the person's best interest.

  ❖ The patient for which an IMCA is being appointed must be above 16 yr of age.

- **Lasting power of attorney (LPA):** In case patients loses capacity in the future, they can pick someone to make decisions for them.

  ❖ The patient must be over 18 yr of age to appoint an LPA.

  ❖ *An advanced decision to refuse life-sustaining procedures must be in writing, signed, and witnessed.*

  ❖ Patients cannot insist upon futile or inappropriate treatment or unlawful procedures.

  ❖ Patient can have more than one LPA (one for health and welfare and one for property and financial affairs).

- **Court of protection (CoP):** Legal body that oversees the operation of MCA. It can:

  ❖ Decide if an LPA is reliable and official.

  ❖ Pick deputies to make decisions in your best interests.

  ❖ Make decisions in difficult cases.

  ❖ Remove deputies or attorneys who have not carried out their role properly.

  ❖ It may be the only option to authorize a DoLS where the patient is under 18 yr but more than 16 yr old and is deprived of their liberty.

- **The public guardian:** Two different jobs.
  - ❖ Register LPAs and deputies.
  - ❖ Work with other agencies, such as the police and social services, to act on any concerns about the way the attorney or deputy is behaving.
✓ **Assessing capacity**
  - Any registered professional can conduct a capacity assessment.
  - Capacity assessments are decision-specific, like care and treatment, discharge arrangements, and emergency care and treatment.
✓ **What if the person lacks capacity?**
  - Submit a DoLS application whilst they are admitted to the hospital.
  - Consult family, carers, or other close relatives.
  - Consult if needed an LMA or IMCA.

Deprivation of Liberty Safeguards (DoLS)

✓ DoLS was introduced in 2009 as part of the MCA 2005.
  - It covers people with **lacking capacity** who are **deprived of their liberty** in their best interests.
  - Applies to those who are 18 yr and over living in a hospital or care home in England and Wales.
✓ **Principle:** When medical professionals make a care plan for the patient, there is a possibility that it may amount to deprivation of liberty (e.g. sedation, restraints).
  - DoLS application may be needed in these circumstances.
  - DoLS can hence authorize the deprivation of a patient in the hospital.
  - **DoLS can't be transferred, can't be extended beyond the care home or hospital, and can't authorize the actual care of patient, which will be covered through the general authority of the MCA in best interests.**
✓ **Two key questions to ask:** Acid test.
  - Is the patient subject to continuous supervision and control?
  - Is the person allowed to leave?
✓ **Restrictive practice and restraint is lawful if:**
  - Necessary to prevent harm to the person
  - **Proportionate to the likelihood and seriousness** of the harm

- Restraint must be in the person's best interests and **a less-restrictive** alternative has been considered
- Careful considerations need to be given to whether restrictions placed on a person go beyond restraint and actually deprive them of liberty and, if so, whether those restrictions are genuinely necessary
✓ **Key bodies under DoLS process**
  - **Urgent authorization:** In an emergency, the hospital or care home (**managing authority**) can issue an urgent authorization for 7 d for itself while applying for authorization.
  - **Standard authorization:** Managing authority of the patient applies to the **local authority (supervisory body)** where the patient usually resides if the individual is at risk of DoLS within 28 d.
  - **Supervisory body:** Instructs two assessors (mental health assessors), and they will take six types of assessments to give their verdict.
    - ❖ It can give authorization for up to 12 months.
✓ **Summary of DoLS:** If a person who is lacking capacity is having restrictions in place, DoLS doesn't need to be applied for within 72 h of the adult's admission, unless there is an urgent need, such as the adult attempting to leave.
  - After **72 h,** the hospital can use urgent authorization by itself to apply those restrictions if the duration is expected to be less than 7 d.
  - Apply for standard authorization if the patient is expected to stay within 28 d.
✓ **ICU setting:** DOLS is rarely required in ICU as patients requiring ICU are not considered deprived as they are too sick to leave for their own good. (Midnight laws FICM – must read before the exams.)

Mental Health Act 1985 (MHA): Provides a legal means of treating a mental health condition without the patient's consent.
✓ **Mental disorder** is defined as any condition that affects the balance of the mind.
✓ It permits the detention of an individual and treatment of a mental illness without consent, including the physical manifestations of that illness.

- *The MHA doesn't permit the treatment of conditions unrelated to the patient's mental illness.*
- *Emergency detention of patients (usually for 72 h) until full assessment can be carried out.*

✓ **MHA criteria:** To detain a patient under the MHA, the patient must fulfil the following three criteria:
- **Criteria 1:** MHA is needed when it is necessary to detain a patient because they are **suffering from mental disorder.**
- **Criteria 2:** There must be a **recognized appropriate treatment** available for that mental disorder.
- **Criteria 3:** The patient should be suffering from a mental disorder of a nature or degree that **it is necessary for their health and safety or for the protection of others to be admitted to or remain in hospital.**

✓ **Sections under MHA**
- **Section 5(2):** Used by doctor with full GMC registration. Used when you **suspect** that the patient has some form of mental disorder and they would pose a risk to themselves.
  - ❖ Can last up to 72 h.
  - ❖ *During this, further MHA assessment is needed if progression to section 2 or 3 is needed.*
- **Section 5(4):** Used in emergencies by a nurse when a doctor is not available in the preceding situation.
  - ❖ Can last up to 6 h.
- **Section (2):** Used for **assessment** as to whether the patient is suffering from a mental disorder. It can also be used to treat a patient without consent for 28 d.
  - ❖ A section 2 is applied for by an approved mental health practitioner (AMHP) with the recommendation of two doctors. The two doctors must have seen the patient within 5 d of the application.
- **Section (3):** Used to **treat** patients with mental illness against their will.
  - ❖ It lasts for 6 months and can be renewed if indicated.

✓ Alcohol dependence and drugs are excluded from this act. Delirium tremens is not excluded.
- Patient **can have capacity** here in the contrast to DoLS.

Children

✓ Individuals aged 16 yr or above should be presumed to have capacity to consent and parental consent is not required.
- However, parents can override a competent 16-year-old's refusal of treatment.
- GMC recommends taking legal advice in these cases if treatment is in the best interests of a competent young person who refuses.

✓ **Gillick competence:** Children under the age of 16 yr can consent to their own treatment if they are believed to have enough intelligence, competence, and understanding to fully appreciate what is involved in their treatment. Otherwise, someone with parental responsibility can consent for them.
- By law, only one person with parental responsibility is needed to give consent for the treatment.

Other relevant legislations

✓ **Human Rights Act 1998:** It guarantees the right to autonomy and self-determination, including the right to make decisions about one's own healthcare. Requires healthcare providers to respect the patient's right to refuse or consent to treatment, provided they have the capacity to do so.

Additional Questions

✓ **Ethical principles in healthcare[Q]**
- Respect for autonomy: Arrive independently at decision.
- Beneficence: Do good.
- Non-maleficence: Do no harm.
- Justice: Fairness between competing claims.

✓ **Caldicott guardian[Q]**
- A person who is responsible for protecting the confidentiality of patient information.
- They uphold eight Caldicott principles.

✓ **Martha's rule**
- It is a patient safety initiative where the patient or their families can ask for an urgent review of patient's condition if they are concerned about a deterioration in their care.
- Three components of Martha's rules are as follows:
  - ❖ Patient will be asked, at least daily, about their health, and if they are

getting better or worse, the information will be acted upon using a structured pathway.

❖ Any staff member, at any moment, can ask for a review from a different team if they are concerned about the patient's deteriorating condition and they are not being responded to.

❖ This escalation rule is always available to the patient, their families, and their carers and advertised across the hospital.

CORONER'S COURT

✓ **Coroner:** *Independent judicial officer responsible for investigating a patient's cause of death in certain circumstances, like sudden, violent, or unnatural death.*

- Subject to neither local nor central government control.
- Must be a barrister or a solicitor having practiced for at least 5 yr. Appointment of medical coroners has ceased now.
- **Local authority (relevant council)** chooses the coroner and funds his functions, but coroner doesn't work under local authority.
- **Coroner** holds office under the Crown. *Lord chancellor can dismiss a coroner for neglecting his duty, committing a criminal offence, or inability or misbehaviour in the discharge of the duty.*
- The coroner is looking to establish^Q **who** the deceased is and **where**, **when**, and by **what** means the person died.
  - ❖ It is not to establish findings of blame or responsibility of the death.
- *A post-mortem or autopsy is probably the most important investigation requested by a coroner.*
- The coroner should inform the next of kin why a post-mortem is necessary and, if requested, what this involves.
- Although consent is not needed, families must be informed of any tissue, fluid, or organ retention, normally as soon as possible, after the post-mortem has taken place.
- A corpse doesn't belong to relatives or the coroner. The coroner has a right to take possession of a body for a post-mortem,

and the family has the right to disposal of the body.

❖ Coroners will be required to notify the deceased's next of kin or personal representative if the body cannot be released within 28 d.

❖ The relatives can make an application to the **high court** to overturn the coroner's decision of conducting a post-mortem by way of judicial review.

❖ The relatives if dissatisfied with the result of post-mortem can arrange another autopsy at their own expense.

- If the post-mortem examination reveals a natural cause of death, the coroner will not hold an inquest, and a Form 100B will be issued to the registrar of births and deaths by the coroner certifying the cause of death found at post-mortem.
  - ❖ The coroner can give summon to anyone to give the evidence for inquest.
  - ❖ All witnesses give evidence under oath and are first questioned by the coroner and then by anyone with a proper interest in the case either directly by them or by their legal team.
- Inquests should normally be completed within 6 months of the date on which the coroner is made aware of the death.
- Coroner should report to chief coroner any case that lasts more than a year, with reasons for delay.

✓ **Members of coroner's office:** No standard framework. Members and their roles vary from office to office.

- **Deputy coroner:** Appointed by coroner. Same qualifications as a coroner.
  - ❖ Same rights, powers, and obligations as the coroner and will sign all documentation in their own name.
  - ❖ Full authority to deputize for the coroner in his absence.
- **Assistant deputy coroner:** Appointed by coroner. Same qualifications as a coroner.
  - ❖ Same rights, powers, and obligations as the coroner and will sign all documentation in their own name.
  - ❖ Full authority to deputize for the coroner in his absence.

- **Coroner's officer:** Coroner receives information through and makes enquiry by means of his coroner's officer.
  - ❖ Traditionally are experienced police officers on permanent secondment.
  - ❖ Regular point of contact for families, funeral directors, registrars, and press.
  - ❖ No authority to sign.
- **Administrator:** Liaising with funeral directors, families, and witnesses, assisting in the listing of inquests, typing, and taking phone calls.
- **Secretary:** Standard administrative support and typing.

✓ **Potential verdicts in a coroner's court**[Q]
- **Death by natural cause:** Person died from natural causes.
- **Open verdict:** When there is not enough evidence to know the exact cause of death.
- **Misadventure:** The death was unintended or unexpected.
- **Narrative verdict:** Recording of how the deceased met his death and gives more detail of the circumstances of the death and the conclusions reached in arriving at the death.
- **Unlawful killing:** Death due to murder, manslaughter, or infanticide.

✓ **Medical examiner:** Refers a case to coroner if the cause of death is **unknown**, violent, unnatural, or in **custody.**
- Deaths from **industrial disease,** including COPD, chronic bronchitis, and emphysema, if a person worked underground as a miner for 20 yr or more, will require a post-mortem.
- Death **after anaesthesia and on table deaths** should certainly be referred to the coroner.
- There is no legal requirement to inform the coroner of deaths shortly after admission, although many coroner's offices have made arrangements that all deaths within 24 h should be reported to them.
- Any necessary autopsy is expected to be performed on the morning of the first working day after a death is reported. Hence, a case should be reported to coroner earlier in the day rather than late.

✓ **Doctor:** There is currently no statutory responsibility on a doctor to report a death to the coroner.
- The doctor's duty in strict law is to complete a medical certificate of the cause of the death (MCCD) to the best of their knowledge and belief.

✓ **Pathologist:** Does the post-mortem and determines a cause of death and gives an opinion as to whether the death was natural or not.
- Pathologists may refuse to undertake a post-mortem.
- The coroner should ideally not ask a pathologist at a hospital to undertake the examination if the conduct of any member of hospital staff may be called into question.
- The report of the post-mortem is given to the coroner in writing and with confidentiality.

REHABILITATION

✓ **Rehabilitation:** Process of returning the patient as completely as possible to the physical, social, and mental well-being.

Principles of Care (NICE CG83)

✓ **During the critical care stay**
- Rehabilitation should start as soon as possible on the ICU.
- **Short clinical assessment** on admission to determine the patient's risk of developing physical and non-physical morbidity.
  - ❖ **Physical morbidity indicators:** Anticipated long duration of critical care stay, unable to self-ventilate on FiO_2 35% of less, premorbid respiratory or mobility issues, unable to get out of bed independently, unable to mobilize independently over short distances.
  - ❖ **Non-physical morbidity indicators:** Recurrent nightmares, new or recurrent anxiety or panic attacks, hallucinations, delusions.
- **Comprehensive assessment** of patients at risk of developing physical and non-physical morbidity
- For patients at risk, **short-term** (before discharge from hospital) and **medium-term goals** (after they are discharged from

hospital) to be decided based on comprehensive assessment within 4 d of admission or before discharge from critical care, whichever is sooner.

✓ **Before discharge from critical care**
  - **Short clinical assessment** again of patients at low risk of developing physical and non-physical morbidity.
  - **Comprehensive assessment again** of patients at risk of developing physical and non-physical morbidity.
  - **Formal handover** of the individualized rehabilitation plan to the ward team.
    ❖ *Post-ICU presentation screen (PICUPS):* 14-item clinical tool to identify problems likely to require further assessment by members of the multiprofessional team and trigger appropriate referral.

✓ **During ward-based care**
  - **Short clinical assessment** again of patients at low risk of developing physical and non-physical morbidity.
  - **Comprehensive assessment again** of patients at risk of developing physical and non-physical morbidity.

✓ **Before discharge to home or community care:**
  - **Functional assessment of patient (daily functional ability)** based on two domains:
    ❖ **Physical:** Mobility problems (standing, walking, swallowing, incontinence), sensory problems (vision or hearing), communication problems (speaking, writing)
    ❖ **Non-physical:** Anxiety, depression, PTSD
  - Give information to the patient about:
    ❖ Critical care discharge summary
    ❖ Local support groups
    ❖ Driving, returning to work, housing
    ❖ How to manage activities of daily living, like diet and self-care

✓ **Two to three months after discharge from critical care:** For patients with more than 4 d of critical care admission:
  - Face-to-face **functional reassessment** of health needs and social care needs in the community or hospital by an appropriately skilled healthcare professional.
  - Refer the patient to specialist services if slower than anticipated recovery.

Post-intensive care syndrome: *New or worsening long-lasting impairments* after discharge from ITU post-serious illnesses.

✓ **Cognitive function:** Memory loss and difficulty in thinking/concentrating.
✓ **Mental function:** Anxiety, depression, post-traumatic stress disorder (PTSD).
✓ **Physical function:** Breathlessness, weakness, pain.

ICU follow-up clinics: Not standardized; 50–60% of patients attend.

✓ **PRaCTICaL Study (2009):** No mortality benefit.

Post-traumatic stress disorder (PTSD): Up to 25% of ITU patients get PTSD.

✓ **Severe anxiety disorder**, where the patient continuously relives the traumatic event and is socially impaired. Triad of symptoms.
  - Intrusive, unsettling flashbacks associated with emotional upset.
  - Avoidance of situations and stimuli associated with the trigger.
  - Increased level of alertness, irritability, chronic anxiety.
✓ **Risk factors**
  - Previous psychological condition
  - Increased duration of sedation and mechanical ventilation
  - Benzodiazepine use
  - Delirium
  - ARDS
  - Sepsis
✓ **Management:** Symptoms occur within 1 month of the event.
  - Patient with delusional memories is more at risk of PTSD.
  - PTSD is analyzed using validated tools, such as the Impact of Event Scale, PTSS-10, or PTSS-14.
  - PTSD is not reduced by a self-help recovery package given to patients on discharge.
  - Patients with severe symptoms should get a psychiatric referral. Those with moderate symptoms should be managed expectantly.

Tools for Measuring Quality of Life after ICU

✓ **European Quality of Life-5D (EQ-5D):** Assesses health-related quality of life across five dimensions:

- Mobility
- Self-care
- Usual activities
- Pain/discomfort
- Anxiety/depression

✓ **Short Form 36 (SF-36):** Measures health status.
  - **Physical activity:** How much health problems limit physical activities like running.
  - **Social activity:** How much physical problems limit social activities like visiting friends.
  - **Role activities:** How much physical or emotional problems limit daily activities like working.
  - **Pain:** How much bodily pain is experienced.
  - **Mental health:** How much psychological stress is experienced.
  - **Vitality:** How much energy and fatigue are experienced.
  - **General health:** How general health is perceived.

✓ **QALY (Quality-Adjusted Life-Year)[Q]**
  - A QALY assesses the health impact of a medical intervention or prevention program using the formula: QALY = years of life × utility value. Ranges from 0 (death) to 1 (perfect health).
  - Helps calculate cost–utility ratios for interventions and aids in resource allocation decisions.

DRUG DOSING IN RENAL AND HEPATIC FAILURE

✓ Critically ill patients have two times the risk of experiencing an adverse drug reaction compared to patients in a general medicine ward.
  - AKI is seen in up to 50% of critically ill patients.

✓ **Renal function**
  - **Cockcroft–Gault equation:** Calculates creatinine clearance and can overestimate GFR.
    ❖ Developed based on studies done on young male patients and hence may underestimate clearance in elderly patients.
    ❖ Plasma creatinine concentrations depend upon hydration, muscle mass.

❖ Creatinine clearance may not be accurate since, as GFR decreases, creatinine secretion by tubules increases.
❖ Anuric patients have a GFR less than 10 mL/min, irrespective of serum creatinine.
❖ Patients are started on dialysis when GFR is <15 mL/min.

- **Modification of diet in renal disease (MDRD):** It adjusts GFR for body surface area.
  ❖ Developed based on studies done on patients with chronic kidney disease and hence may underestimate clearance in normal patients.
  ❖ It is based on six variables: age, sex, ethnicity, serum creatinine, urea, and albumin.
  ❖ MDRD gives eGFR and has greater precision and accuracy than Cockcroft–Gault equation.

- **Chronic Kidney Disease Epidemiology Collaboration (CKD-EPI):** KDIGO recommends CKD-EPI as preferred method for GFR calculations[Q].
  ❖ Less bias and more accurate than MDRD.

✓ **Renal dosing of drugs**
  - **Directly nephrotoxic:** NSAIDs, ACE inhibitors
  - **Drugs that accumulate:** Opioids, antibiotics, metformin (lactic acidosis)
  - **Drugs that need dose adjustment:** Warfarin, LMWH, beta-blockers

✓ **Drug-induced nephrotoxicity[Q]**
  - **Altered intraglomerular haemodynamics**
    ❖ NSAIDs
    ❖ ACE inhibitors and angiotensin receptor blockers (ARBs)
    ❖ Calcineurin inhibitors (cyclosporine, tacrolimus)
  - **Acute tubular injury**
    ❖ Aminoglycoside
    ❖ Amphotericin B
    ❖ Antiretrovirals (tenofovir, foscarnet)
    ❖ Radiology contrast dyes
    ❖ Cisplatin
  - **Crystal nephropathy**
    ❖ Ampicillin
    ❖ Ciprofloxacin

- ❖ Antivirals (acyclovir, ganciclovir, foscarnet)
- ❖ Methotrexate
- **Rhabdomyolysis**
  - ❖ Statins
  - ❖ Drugs of abuse (ketamine, cocaine, methamphetamines)
- **Thrombotic microangiopathy**
  - ❖ Cyclosporine
  - ❖ Clopidogrel
  - ❖ Ticlopidine
  - ❖ Quinine
- **Interstitial nephritis**
  - ❖ Furosemide
  - ❖ Thiazide
  - ❖ Lithium
  - ❖ NSAIDs
  - ❖ Proton pump inhibitors
  - ❖ Ranitidine
  - ❖ Antibiotics (beta-lactams, rifampicin, sulphonamides, vancomycin, acyclovir)
  - ❖ Rifampicin
- ✓ **Hepatic function**
  - **Drug metabolism**
    - ❖ **Phase 1:** Oxidation, reduction, and hydrolysis. Converted to a more polar molecule.
    - ❖ **Phase 2:** Glucuronidation, sulphation, acetylation, and methylation. Turned more water-soluble.

- **Extraction ratio**^{Q}: Fraction of the drug removed from the blood after one pass through the liver.
  - ❖ **High extraction ratio (>70%)**^{Q}: Drugs depend upon hepatic blood flow rather than cellular metabolism for clearance (e.g. propofol^Q, morphine, fentanyl, midazolam).
  - ❖ **Low extraction ratio (<30%)**^{Q}: Drugs depend upon cellular metabolism for clearance rather than hepatic blood flow (e.g. phenytoin^Q, warfarin, lorazepam).

Drugs Metabolized by Cytochrome P450 System

Inducers	Inhibitors
Barbiturates	Etomidate
Phenytoin^Q	Ciprofloxacin
Carbamazepine	Erythromycin
Glucocorticoids	Fluconazole^Q
Rifampicin^Q	Metronidazole
Acute alcohol intake	Chronic alcohol intake
Smoking	Grapefruit
	Cimetidine
	Amiodarone

Guidelines for Drug Dosing in Critically Ill Patients with Renal Failure

Drug	Normal Dose	Creatinine Clearance 10–30 mL/min	Creatinine Clearance <10/min or HD	CVVHD and CVVHDF
Acyclovir	5–10 mg/kg IV q 8 h	5–10 mg/kg IV q 24 h	2.5–5 mg/kg IV q 24 h	5–10 mg/kg IV q 12–24 h
Ampicillin	1–2 g IV q 4–6 h	1–2 g IV q 8–12 h	1–2 g IV q 12–24 h	1–2 g IV q 6–12 h
Cefotaxime^Q	1–2 g IV q 4–8 h	1–2 g IV q 6–12 h	1–2 g IV q 24 h	1–2 g IV q 6–8 h
Ciprofloxacin	400 mg IV q 8–12 h	200–400 mg IV q 12–24 h	200–400 mg IV q 12–24 h	200–400 mg IV q 8–12 h
Digoxin	IV 0.25–0.5 mg loading dose, then 0.25 q 6 h (max 1.5 mg in 24 h) Maintenance dose: 0.125–0.25 mg/day	Same loading dose, then 0.0625 mg IV q 48 h	50% of loading dose, then 0.0625 mg IV q 48 h	50% of loading dose, then 0.0625–0.125 mg IV q 48 h

Drug	Normal Dose	Creatinine Clearance 10–30 mL/min	Creatinine Clearance <10/min or HD	CVVHD and CVVHDF
Fluconazole	200–800 mg IV/PO q 24 h	Loading dose (6–12 mg/kg) IV/PO, then 100–200 mg IV/PO q 24 h	Loading dose (6–12 mg/kg) IV/PO, then 100–200 mg IV/PO q 24 h, given after HD	Loading dose (6–12 mg/kg) IV/PO, then 400–1,200 mg IV/PO q 24 h
Linezolid	600 mg IV/PO q 12 h	600 mg IV/PO q 12 h	600 mg IV/PO q 12 h	600 mg IV/PO q 12 h
Meropenem[Q]	1 g IV q 8 h (2 g for meningitis)	500 mg IV q 12 h (1 g for meningitis)	500 mg IV q 24 h (1 g for meningitis)	0.5–1 g IV q 8–12 h
Metronidazole[Q]	500 mg IV q 8 h	500 mg IV q 8 h	500 mg IV q 8 h	500 mg IV q 8 h
Phenytoin	15 mg/kg IV load, then 200–400 mg PO/IV q 8–12 h	15 mg/kg IV load, then 200–400 mg PO/IV q 8–12 h	15 mg/kg IV load, then 200–400 mg PO/IV q 8–12 h	15 mg/kg IV load, then 200–400 mg PO/IV q 8–12 h
Piperacillin/ tazobactam	3.375–4.5 g IV q 6 h	2.25–3.375 g IV q 6 h	2.25 g IV q 6–8 h/2.25 g IV q 8–12 h for HD	4.5 loading dose, 2.25 g IV q 6 h
Valproic acid	10–15 mg/kg/day	10–15 mg/kg/day	Start with a low dose, adjust according to response	Start with a low dose, adjust according to response
Voriconazole	6 mg/kg IV q 12 h × 2 doses, f/b 4 mg/kg IV q 12 h	IV not recommended	IV not recommended	IV not recommended

✓ **Therapeutic drug monitoring (TDM):** Renal and liver dysfunction can add to uncertainties in drug metabolism. Apart from that, TDM is done due to various reasons:
  - Narrow therapeutic range and potential for toxicity[Q] (e.g. phenytoin, digoxin, lithium).
  - Potential for toxicity (e.g. aminoglycoside).
  - Therapeutic plasma level is important to achieve (e.g. transplant drugs like tacrolimus, valproate).

STEROIDS

✓ **Immunosuppressive and anti-inflammatory action**
  - Inhibition of cytokines and apoptosis of dendritic cells, leading to impairment of antigen presentation.

- Neutrophilia and lymphopenia (T cells more than B cells, and NK cells are not affected at all).
- Disappearance of eosinophils and monocytes from peripheral circulation.

Drug	Dose	Anti-Inflammatory Potency	Mineralocorticoid
Hydrocortisone[Q]	20 mg	1	1
Dexamethasone[Q]	0.75 mg	25	Minimal
Prednisone[Q]	5 mg	4	0.25
Prednisolone	5 mg	4	0.25
Methylprednisolone	4 mg	5	Minimal
Cortisone	25 mg	0.8	0.8

Drug	Dose	Anti-Inflammatory Potency	Mineralocorticoid
Aldosterone	n/a	0.3	400
Fludrocortisone	0.1 mg	10	300

Uses in Critical Care

✓ **Airway oedema:** Methylprednisolone 40 mg IV 4 h prior to extubation in patients who have failed a cuff-leak test (**American Thoracic Society recommendation**).

✓ **Asthma:** Prednisolone 40–50 mg daily for 5 d (**British Thoracic Society recommendation**).

✓ **COPD:** Prednisolone 30 mg daily for 7–14 d (**NICE Guidelines**).

✓ **ARDS**
  - **Dexa-ARDS Trial (2020):** In patients with moderate to severe ARDS, early use of dexamethasone decreased duration of mechanical ventilation and mortality compared to usual care.
  - **Meduri Trial (2007):** Low-dose, long-duration methylprednisolone improved lung function, duration of mechanical ventilation, ICU length of stay, and survival if used early in ARDS.
  - **LaSRS Trial (2006): Late steroids rescue for ARDS** use of methylprednisolone in persistent ARDS (7–28 d after onset) did not improve 60 d mortality but did improve ventilator-free and ICU-free days.
  - **Meduri Trial (1998):** Low-dose, long-duration methylprednisolone in unresolving ARDS improved ICU survival and lung function.

✓ **Septic shock**
  - No need to go for ACTH test to identify subset of adults that will be benefitted.
  - Hydrocortisone used and no need to wean once vasopressors are off.
  - Dose is 200 mg/day. Add steroids when noradrenaline >0.25 µ/kg/min for 4 h.
  - **ADRENAL Trial 2018:** In patients with septic shock who are being mechanically ventilated, hydrocortisone doesn't reduce the mortality but does reduce the vasopressor requirements and may shorten the duration of the ICU stay.

- **APROCCHSS Trial 2018:** In patients with septic shock who are being mechanically ventilated, **hydrocortisone with fludrocortisone** reduces the mortality and the vasopressor requirements.
- **CORTICUS Trial 2008:** Hydrocortisone doesn't reduce the mortality but does reduce the vasopressor requirements in patients with septic shock.

✓ **Chronic steroid therapy:** AAGBI Guidelines 2020
  - For patients on 5 mg prednisolone steroids beyond 4 wk, stress dose is noted.
  - **Major surgery/Caesarean section:** 100 mg IV hydrocortisone at induction of anaesthesia, followed by 200 mg/24 h.
    ❖ Post-operatively 100 mg/24 h hydrocortisone by IV infusion while nil by mouth. Start enteral steroids at pre-surgical dose if recovery is uncomplicated otherwise double the dose for up to a week.
  - **Body surface and intermediate surgery:** 100 mg IV hydrocortisone at induction of anaesthesia, followed by 200 mg/24 h.
    ❖ Post-operatively, double the dose of steroids for 48 h.
  - **Labour and vaginal delivery:** 100 mg IV hydrocortisone at induction of anaesthesia, followed by 200 mg/24 h.

✓ *Pneumocystis jirovecii* **pneumonia**
  - Prednisolone **40 mg BD** or methylprednisolone 60 mg daily IV. *Taper after 5 d.*
  - *Meta-analysis has shown significantly reduced rates of mechanical ventilation and mortality in HIV-positive patients with PJP who are treated with adjuvant steroids.*
  - In non-HIV patients, only some observational data is present, and data is not conclusive.
  - Start steroids as early as possible and not beyond 72 h after starting the PJP-specific therapy.
  - Patients who are hypoxic are most likely to benefit.

✓ **Pneumonia**
  - **CAPE COD Trial (2023):** Early hydrocortisone use in patients with severe community-acquired pneumonia reduced the risk of mortality, intubation, and use of vasopressors.

✓ **Pneumococcal meningitis and not meningo-coccal meningitis**
  - Dexamethasone **10 mg IV QDS for 4 d** if meningitis is suspected by *S. pneumoniae* and discontinued if any other cause (**Intensive Care Society recommendation**).
  - Steroids reduced mortality in cases caused by *Streptococcus pneumoniae* and reduced hearing loss and neurological sequelae in bacterial meningitis of any cause.

✓ **Covid-19**
  - **Recovery Trial (2021):** In hospitalized patients with Covid-19 requiring supplemental oxygen, dexamethasone decreases the risk of mortality, quickens hospital discharge, and reduces the risk of respiratory failure, requiring invasive mechanical ventilation.

✓ **Alcoholic hepatitis**
  - **Prednisolone 40 mg once daily for 4 wk,** followed by taper over 2 wk.

✓ **Organ donation**
  - Methylprednisolone 15 mg/kg with maximum dose of 1 g (The National Health Service Blood and Transplant Guidelines).

✓ **Addison's disease**
  - Hydrocortisone 100 mg IV followed by 200 mg/24 h (UK Society for Endocrinology).

✓ **Myxoedema coma**
  - Hydrocortisone 100 mg IV during resuscitation.

✓ **Thyroid storm**
  - Steroids reduce T4 conversion to T3.
  - Hydrocortisone 100 mg every 6–8 h or dexamethasone 2 mg IV every 6 h.

✓ **Cerebral oedema**
  - Due to intracerebral tumours and brain abscesses.
  - Dexamethasone 16 mg/day.

✓ **Autoimmune diseases**: Vasculitis, SLE, rheumatoid arthritis, myasthenia gravis, multiple sclerosis, ITP, inflammatory bowel disease, transplant rejection.

Steroids Are Not Recommended in the Following Conditions

✓ **Anaphylaxis**[Q]: The use of steroids to treat anaphylaxis is not recommended anymore (RESUS UK 2021 anaphylaxis guidelines).

✓ **Cerebral oedema**

- No steroids for traumatic head injury and spinal cord trauma.

✓ Guillain–Barré syndrome

TRANEXAMIC ACID

✓ **Tranexamic acid (TXA):** Synthetic derivative of lysine.
  - **Mechanism of action:** Competitively inhibits activation of plasminogen to plasmin[Q]. At higher concentrations becomes a non-competitive inhibition of plasminogen.

✓ **Pharmacokinetic properties**
  - Absorption: 30–50% oral bioavailability
  - Volume of distribution: 0.18 L/kg
  - Plasma protein binding: 3%
  - Route of elimination: 95% of drug excreted unchanged in urine
  - Half-life: Elimination half-life is 2 h, and terminal half-life is 11 h

✓ **Side effects:** Hypotension, headache, metallic taste, fever, nausea, diarrhoea, back pain.
  - Seizures[Q]: TXA is a competitive antagonist of GABA and glycine receptors.

✓ **Clinical trials and uses**
  - **CRASH-2 Trial (2010)**[Q]: In **trauma patients with/at risk of significant haemorrhage**, TXA had mortality benefit.
    ❖ A 1 g stat over 10 min followed by 1 g over 8 h as a continuous infusion.
  - **WOMAN Trial (2017):** TXA reduces death due to bleeding in **women with post-partum haemorrhage** with no adverse effects.
    ❖ With 1 g over 10 min. If bleeding continues after 30 min or restarts within 24 h, a second dose of 1 g IV can be given.
  - **CRASH-3 Trial (2019)**[Q]: In **traumatic brain injury patients,** TXA reduced the risk of head injury-related death in patients with mild to moderate head injury, but not severe head injury.
    ❖ A 1 g stat over 10 min, followed by 1 g over 8 h as a continuous infusion.
  - **TICH-2 Trial (2019):** In patients with acute spontaneous intracerebral haemorrhage, there was no significant difference in functional status at 90 d between the TXA and placebo groups.
  - **HALT-IT Trial (2020)**[Q]: TXA doesn't reduce death from GI bleeding and

shouldn't be used as a part of a medical approach to GI bleeding.

✓ **Other uses**
- **Cardiothoracic surgery:** 50 mg/kg IV over 30 min during theatre for reducing transfusion. (No need to check on Google – very high doses, indeed.)
- **Orthopaedic surgery:** 10 mg/kg IV loading dose during the theatre, followed by 1 mg/kg/h maintenance dose.

Aprotinin[Q]: Inhibits fibrinolysis via inactivation of free plasmin. Inhibits trypsin and kallikrein.

✓ Given before cardiac bypass to decrease blood loss but can cause increased risk of MI and stroke[Q].

EXTRACORPOREAL THERAPIES

✓ **Extracorporeal therapies:** *Blood purification techniques* that remove harmful substances from a patient's blood outside the body. Common types are as follows:
- **ECMO (extracorporeal membrane oxygenation):** Removes CO_2 and oxygenation of blood. Discussed in the chapter in the cardiovascular section.
- **CRRT (continuous renal replacement therapy):** Removes waste products when kidneys are not functioning properly. Discussed in the chapter in the renal section.
- **Plasmapheresis:** Used to remove specific toxins by separating blood components. Discussed in the chapter in the haematology/oncology section.
- **Extracorporeal liver support (ELS):** Removes toxins that accumulate in liver failure.
- **Extracorporeal cytokine removal in sepsis and septic shock:** Special filters used to remove cytokine.

Extracorporeal Liver Support (ELS)

✓ **Physiology of liver:** Toxins that accumulate in liver failure are lactate, ammonia, bilirubin, bile acids.

✓ **Indications**
- Acute liver failure: Bridge to recovery/liver transplant.
- Acute or chronic liver failure: Bridge to liver transplant/rehabilitation.

- End-stage liver disease: Bridge to liver transplant.
- Post–liver transplant graft failure.
- Post–partial hepatectomy liver failure.
- Poisoning with albumin-related drugs unrelated to liver failure (phenytoin, theophylline, and lamotrigine).
- Intractable pruritus in cholestasis.

✓ **Current use:** They have shown improvements in biochemical surrogate markers, but improved long-term survival doesn't exist yet.
- Mainstream implementation of this therapy is currently restricted due to high costs involved and limited efficacy.

✓ **Modalities used for ELS**
- **Artificial**
  - ❖ Utilize a cell-free technique to remove toxins from the blood – e.g. **molecular adsorbent recirculating system (MARS)**, single-pass albumin dialysis (SPAD), and fractionated plasma separation and adsorption (FPSA), also known as Prometheus.
  - ❖ They pass the patient's blood through a dialysis filter that has a current of exogenous albumin flowing through it. Toxins bound to patient's plasma are transferred to exogenous albumin. This albumin dialysate with toxins is then passed through an activated charcoal to regenerate the exogenous albumin again for use.
  - ❖ In **SPAD,** as the name suggests, albumin dialysate is discarded and not recirculated.
- **Bioartificial:** Living cells that detoxify blood.
  - ❖ Patient's plasma runs through a hollow-fibre network lines with hepatocytes that can be human or porcine in origin.
  - ❖ Less robust detoxifying capabilities. Still in clinical trials (e.g. **HepatAssist**).

✓ **Complications**
- Hypotension, anaemia, thrombocytopaenia, coagulopathy, sepsis

Extracorporeal Cytokine Removal in Sepsis and Septic Shock

✓ Blood is removed from the body and, through a filter, pathogens, pathogen-associated molecular patterns **(PAMPs),** damage-associated molecular patterns **(DAMPs),** endotoxins, and cytokines are removed.

✓ **Indicators of starting extracorporeal therapy:** Onset of shock in last 24 h, noradrenaline >0.3 µg/kg/min, signs of capillary leak.

✓ **Indications of stopping extracorporeal therapy:** Rapidly decreasing noradrenaline doses, deresuscitation of fluid balance achieved, normalization of lactates, reduction in ventilatory support.

✓ **Current use:** Not recommended in surviving sepsis guidelines.

✓ **Classification of modalities**
  • **Cytokine removal:** High-volume haemofiltration (HVHA), CytoSorb haemoadsorption, CPFA
  • **Endotoxin removal:** Polymyxin B haemoperfusion
  • **Combined cytokine and endotoxin removal:** oXiris membrane

✓ **High-Volume Haemofiltration (HVHA):** Standard renal-dose haemofiltration is effluent rates up to 25 mL/kg/h. *Dose above 35 mL/kg/h is called HVHA.*
  • Most of inflammatory mediators have a molecular weight <60 kDa, and a significant amount of mediators can be cleared by using higher than conventional doses.

✓ **CytoSorb:** Cytokine adsorption cartridge made of polystyrene copolymer beads.
  • Adsorbs both pro-inflammatory and anti-inflammatory cytokines, but not endotoxins.
  • Removes myoglobin, bilirubin, bile acid, PAMPs, and DAMPs as well.
  • Can be used as standalone therapy with standard blood pumps or can be used in series with CRRT.

✓ **Coupled-plasma filtration adsorption (CPFA):** Circuit contains a plasma filter, a resin sorbent cartridge, and a high-flux dialyzer for convection.
  • CPFA separates plasma from blood, and the cytokines in the plasma are then absorbed by the sorbent cartridge, and this cytokine plasma is then run through the dialyzer for renal replacement therapy.
  • No direct contact between RBCs and sorbent and, hence, less haemolysis.

✓ **Polymyxin B haemoperfusion (Toraymyxin):** Blood in direct contact with adsorbents and removes endotoxins.

✓ **oXiris membrane:** Removes endotoxins and cytokines along with CRRT, all by a single membrane.
  • Membrane is a modification of another membrane called AN69.

INTERVENTIONAL RADIOLOGY

✓ **Main indications**
  • Embolization/coiling of bleeding vessels (hepatic, splenic, pelvic, berry aneurysms, pulmonary)
  • Relieve obstruction by stenting (colonic), balloon dilatation, nephrostomy tube
  • Drain collections in abscesses
  • Insertion of devices like vascular lines (Hickman), IVC filter, PEG

✓ **Advantages**
  • Precise localization using imaging
  • Faster patient recovery time
  • Decreased morbidity and mortality
  • Minimal cosmetic effects

✓ **Limitations**
  • Remote locations anaesthesia
  • Surgical backup still required
  • Radiation exposure
  • Risk of contrast-induced nephropathy and anaphylactoid reaction

✓ **Fluid collections that can successfully be treated with percutaneous drainage**
  • **Sterile:** Ascites, pancreatic pseudocyst, haematoma, post-surgical seroma, lymphocele, urinoma
  • **Non-sterile:** Cholecystitis, enteric abscess, lung abscess, pancreatic abscess, tubo-ovarian abscess, ruptured appendicitis

✓ **Absolute contraindications**
  • None

✓ **Relative contraindications**
  • Severe haemodynamic instability
  • Coagulopathy
  • Inability of patient to cooperate
  • Lack of safe pathway to collection

✓ **Imaging guidance**
  • **Fluoroscopy:** Real-time imaging and guidance, enhanced accuracy, and less complications

- **Ultrasound:** Portable, lack of ionizing radiation, needle placement from any plane, real-time visualization of needle placement into collection, better appreciation of internal complexity of collections than CT
  - ❖ Poor visualization of deep collections and shadowing out of anatomy deep to bone or gas-filled bowel
- **CT scan:** Can visualize structures in deep pelvis and retroperitoneal space
  - ❖ Presents images mainly in the axial plane and requires time-consuming reformatting to render images in other planes
- ✓ **Complications:** Overall, less than 15% complications rates
  - **Major:** Infections, bleeding, injury to bowel
  - **Minor:** Pain, infection at skin site, malfunction of catheter

20

ITU Organization

ITU SERVICE PROVISION

✓ **National Early Warning Score (NEWS 2):**
Track and trigger scoring system used in the
UK and helps in the assessment of a patient's
risk of deterioration.
- Used for non-pregnant adults aged 16 and
  over in acute and ambulance settings.
- Score for **6 physiological measurements:**
  Respiration rate, oxygen saturation, blood
  pressure, pulse, level of consciousness, and
  temperature.
  - ❖ *The score is aggregated for all the param-*
    eters and uplifted by 2 points for people
    who require supplemental oxygen.
- **Clinical response to NEWS 2 score.**
  - ❖ **Total score 0:** 12 hourly monitoring;
    continue routine NEWS monitoring.
  - ❖ **Total score 1–4:** 4–6 hourly monitor-
    ing; inform a registered nurse, who
    must assess the patient and decide if
    escalation of care is required.
  - ❖ **Score 3 in a single parameter:** Hourly
    monitoring; registered nurse to inform
    medical team, who will decide if escala-
    tion is required.
  - ❖ **Total score 5 or more (urgent**
    response): Hourly monitoring; regis-
    tered nurse to immediately inform the
    medical team and request assessment
    by a clinician or team with core com-
    petencies in care of **acutely ill patients.**
    Provide care in an environment with
    monitoring facilities. Assessment
    expected in 60 min.
  - ❖ **Total score 7 or more (emergency**
    response): Continuous monitoring;
    registered nurse to immediately inform

the **specialist registrar** of the medical team and request assessment by a
clinician or team with core competen-
cies in care of **critically ill patients.**
Consider care in an environment with
level 2 or 3 monitoring. Assessment
expected in 30 min. *Senior clinician*
review is expected within 60 min if no
improvement.
- **Limitations:** *It doesn't account for age, pre-*
  existing conditions, or trends in vital signs. It
  may not be appropriate for use in patients
  with stroke and dementia.
✓ **Critical care outreach team (CCOT):** Group
of nurses, supported by doctors, providing
intensive care to patients outside the intensive
care unit. CCOTs are the UK version of rapid
response teams (RRTs) in the USA.
- **Purpose:** Identify and treat patients who
  are deteriorating outside of the ICU.
  - ❖ Help prevent ICU admission of these
    patients or, if needed, ensure timely
    admission.
  - ❖ Support the recovery of patients dis-
    charged from the ICU.
  - ❖ Educate ward staff.
  - ❖ Help in transfer of sick patients to ITU.
- **Core elements as per ICS framework**
  (PREPARE)
  - ❖ Patient track and trigger
  - ❖ Rapid response
  - ❖ Education, training, and support
  - ❖ Patient safety and clinical governance
  - ❖ Audit, evaluation, and monitoring of
    the patient outcome and continuing
    quality care
  - ❖ Rehabilitation after critical illness
  - ❖ Enhancing service delivery

DOI: 10.1201/9781003476214-20

- **Benefits:** Shown to reduce in hospital mortality and cardiac arrest rates.
✓ **Levels of care**
  - **Ward care:** Patients whose needs can be met through normal ward care with or without advice and support from critical care outreach team.
    - ❖ Example: Patient needing oxygen by face mask.
  - **Level 1 enhanced care:** Patients requiring detailed observations or interventions, including **basic support for a single organ system** and those stepping down from higher levels of care.
    - ❖ Patients requiring ongoing **interventions from CCOT** in their active management.
    - ❖ Example: Patient after major surgery **just for invasive blood pressure monitoring.**
  - **Level 2 critical care:** Patients requiring detailed observations or interventions, including **basic monitoring and support for two or more organ systems** and those stepping down from higher levels of care.
    - ❖ Patient needing *one organ system monitored and supported at an advanced level (other than advanced respiratory support).*
    - ❖ Patients needing long-term advanced respiratory support.
    - ❖ Patients who require level 1 care for organ support but who require enhanced nursing for other reasons, like patient severely agitated.
    - ❖ Patients with major uncorrected physiological abnormalities, whose care needs can't be met elsewhere.
    - ❖ Example: Patient needing **renal haemofiltration or inotropes and invasive BP monitoring.**
  - **Level 3 critical care: Patients who need advanced respiratory monitoring and support alone.**
    - ❖ Patient needing *two or more organ systems monitored and supported at an advanced level.*
    - ❖ Patients with *chronic impairment of one or more organ systems sufficient to restrict daily activity (comorbidity)*

and who require support for an acute reversible failure of another organ system.
  - ❖ Patients who require level 2 care for organ support but who require enhanced nursing for other reasons, like patient severely agitated.
✓ **ITU staffing ratios[Q]:** Guidelines for the provision of intensive care services (GPICS) document:
  - One consultant for 8–12 patients.
  - One resident doctor for up to 8 patients.
  - All staff on resident rota should have basic airway skills.
  - Level 3 patients: 1:1 nursing.
  - Level 2 patients: 1:2 nursing.
  - One supernumerary coordinating nurse (band 6/7) with units having less than six beds may have them at peak times only.
  - One additional supernumerary nurse per additional ten beds.
  - *<20 % temporary staff per shift.*
✓ **Standards for admission and management in critical care:**
  - Decision to admit in ITU must be discussed with on-call ICU consultant.
  - Time of decision must be documented.
  - All unplanned admissions should be within 4 h of decision.
  - All patients must have a clear and documented escalation plan.
  - ICM consultant should review in person within 12 h of admission.
  - Consultant led ward round twice a day with nurse in charge present in person.
  - Daily input from nursing, microbiology, pharmacy, and physiotherapy teams.
  - Inputs from dietetics, speech, and language therapy (SLT), occupational therapy and clinical psychology.
  - *Discharge to a general ward within 4 h of decision.*
  - **Discharge between 0700 and 2159.**
  - Review of causes for unplanned readmissions.
  - ***Repatriation within 48 h of decision.***
  - *Outpatient clinic appointment 2–3 months post-hospital discharge* for specific patients.

CRITICAL INCIDENTS

✓ **Critical incident:** Any event or circumstance that caused or could have caused unplanned harm, suffering, loss, or damage. It is a broad term and covers patient accidents/near misses, staff accidents/near misses, or security incidents.
- Steps to take if critical incident occurred:
  ❖ Ensure patient safety.
  ❖ Escalate to the responsible consultant.
  ❖ Inform patient or relative as soon as possible (duty of candour).
  ❖ Complete incident report.
  ❖ Document the event in the patient notes.
  ❖ Ensure affected staff also supported appropriately.

✓ **Never events:** Serious preventable patient safety incidents that occur despite guidance or safety recommendations which, if followed, are designed to prevent these incidents from occurring. Wrong site block/surgery was the most common never event in 2022–2023.
- **Types of never events reported**
  ❖ **Surgical:** Wrong site reported, wrong implant, retained foreign object post-procedure.
  ❖ **Medications:** Overdose of methotrexate for non-cancer patients, overdose of insulin due to wrong abbreviations.
  ❖ **General:** Transfusion of ABO-incompatible blood products, misplaced nasogastric tubes, scalding of patient.
- **Processes employed to minimize the occurrence of never events:**
  ❖ **Latent:** Standardization of processes, automated systems.
  ❖ **Active:** Barcode scanners, checklists, mandatory learning modules, guidelines, simulation training, two-person checking of drugs/blood.

✓ **Root cause analysis (RCA):** Structured, thorough investigation of a patient safety incident to find out the underlying cause and contributing factors and then to analyze these to draw out any learning point.
- To conduct RCA, **the incident is first categorized into level of harm.**
  ❖ **Level 1:** No harm/near miss/moderate harm. Handled by local person usually.

❖ **Level 2:** Severe harm or **death**. Investigated by a multidisciplinary team which was not involved in the incident.
❖ **Level 3:** Severe harm, death, or **public interest**. Investigated by an investigator external to the organization.

- **Gathering and mapping of the information**
  ❖ Medical notes, staff statements, interviews, guidelines, inspection of equipment and drugs.
- **Identifying care delivery problems (CDPs) and service delivery problems (SDPs).**
  ❖ CDPs involve failure to monitor, observe, or act (e.g. failure to observe that cannula has tissued).
  ❖ SDPs involve deficiencies in decisions, procedures, and systems (e.g. continued shortage of central venous catheters in the operating theatre).
- **Identifying the contributory factors and root factors**
  ❖ **Fishbone model used:** Equipment and resources, patient factors, working conditions, communication factors, team and social factors, education and training factors, organizational factors.
- **Generating recommendations and solutions**
  ❖ **Human actions:** Handovers, teamwork
  ❖ **Administrative actions:** Guidelines, training
  ❖ **Physical action:** Similar product packaging changed
- **Implementing solutions**
  ❖ Action plan must be **SMART** (specific, measurable, achievable, relevant, and timely).
- **Writing the report**
  ❖ **Avoid hindsight bias:** Tendency for people with benefit of hindsight to falsely believe that they could have predicted the outcome of the event.
  ❖ **Avoid outcome bias:** An incident is considered differently based on the outcome, like people are judged one way when outcome is good and another way if outcome is bad.

✓ **NatSSIPs** (*National Safety Standards for Invasive Procedures*): Based on WHO Surgical Safety Checklist in order to standardize processes and protect patients from adverse events during invasive procedures.

- **Invasive procedures:** Involving access to the inside of a patient's body.
- **NatSSIPs** can be adopted locally to form **LocSSIPs:** Local Safety Standards for Invasive Procedures.

✓ **Commonest adverse events in ICU[Q]**
- **First:** Line, drain, and catheter dislodgement
- **Second:** Medication errors
- **Third:** Equipment failure

MAJOR INCIDENTS

✓ **Major incident:** Any incident that poses **serious threat to the health of the community** or causes such numbers or types of casualties as to require **special arrangements** to be implemented.

✓ **Type of major incidents**
- **Internal:** Due to incident within a hospital, like fire or flood.
- **External:** Due to incidents outside the hospital.
  - ❖ **Rising tide:** Gradual increase in demand (e.g. epidemic of an infectious disease).
  - ❖ **Big bang:** Sudden increase in demand (e.g. a terrorist attack).
  - ❖ **Cloud on the horizon:** Predictable increase in demand ahead of time (e.g. admissions due to drug overdose during music concerts).
  - ❖ **Headline news:** Increased demand after public health alarm (e.g. people panicking after announcement of Covid-19 epidemic, rushing to hospitals).

✓ **Other classifications**
- **Natural/manmade:** Depending upon origin of disaster.
- **Compensated/uncompensated:** *Uncompensated* if load is exceeding the capacity despite additional resources.

✓ **Legislation:** Civil Contingencies Act 2004.
- **Category 1:** 999 services, local authorities, hospitals, NHS bodies, environment agencies.
  - ❖ Assess the risk of emergencies occurring, put in place emergency plans, make information available to public, coordinate with other local responders.

- **Category 2:** Energy companies, charities, telephone companies, transport companies.

✓ **Major incident standby:** Hospital is put on a standby mode after receiving a message about a major incident either from an internal source, like unusual activity within ED, or external source, like NHS England requesting a hospital to be on standby. **METHANE[Q]** model is used to record details of any alert message.
- **M:** Major incident standby
- **E:** Exact location
- **T:** Type of incident (i.e. CBRN: chemical, biological, radiation, nuclear)
- **H:** Hazards/potential hazards
- **A:** Access (*best routes for access to and exit from the hospital*)
- **N:** Number of casualties
- **E:** *Which emergency services are involved/ needed?*

✓ **Actions during hospital major incident standby**
- **Emergency department:** Start staff call-in, locate and check the pre-printed patient registration documents for a major incident, establish an **ED triage station.**
- **Critical care:** Identify patients suitable for transfer to wards; liaise with theatre coordinators for admissions to ITU.
- **Theatres:** Set up **theatre coordination point;** consider suspending all operations except for lifesaving surgery.
- **Wards:** Identify patients suitable for discharge/transfers. Prepare **trauma ward** to accept ICU step-downs/new admissions.

✓ **Major incident declaration:** Major incident is confirmed and **(H) MIMMS[Q]** (Hospital Major Incident Medical Management and Support) general checklist is used.
- Prepare areas for clinical/administrative uses.
- Call in appropriate number of staff by using a *cascade contact system.*
- Maintain internal and external communications.
- Establish a command-and-control structure for the medical, nursing, and administrative staff.
- Staff already on duty should report to their clinical areas.
- Called in staff should report to the **staff reporting areas.**

- Review mechanism of injury section of the **NHS guidelines for major incidents.**
✓ **Command-and-control framework for major incidents:** A hospital control room is designated, and the following roles are assigned to members in it
  - **Gold (strategic):** On-call **director of hospital.** Responsible for overall assessment of the effect of the major incident on the trust from human resources and financial point of view. Responsible for recovery phase planning and return to normal operation.
  - **Silver (tactical):** Responsible for **coordination of the major incident response.** Decisions about staff deployment and resource allocation.
  - **Bronze (operational):** Responsible for coordination on the **departmental level** (e.g. ED, theatres, and ICU as separate bronze commands).
✓ **Triage:** Key principle in **prioritizing the treatment of patients**, especially in situations where **resources are limited.**
  - Based on **distributive justice** at incident site.
    ❖ Performed by prehospital medics, like ambulance crew.
  - UK ambulances have used sieve-and-sort triage model usually, but that model has been replaced by the **NHS Major Incident Triage Tool (MITT) and Ten-Second Triage (TST).**
  - Priorities according to severity of injury with location of care.
    ❖ **Priority 1 (P1): Immediate** – lifesaving treatment within 1 h.
    ❖ **Priority 2 (P2): Urgent** – unwell patients with some degree of stability. Treatment within 2 to 4 h.
    ❖ **Priority 3 (P3): Delayed** – walking wounded. Treatment can be delayed for 4 h or more.
    ❖ **Dead:** Patients who have been assessed by a clinician and found not to be breathing.
    ❖ **Not breathing:** Patients who have been triaged by a non-clinician and found not to be breathing.
✓ **NHS Major Incident Triage Tool (MITT):** To be used by **NHS responders** as a single tool for

both adult and paediatric patients at the scene of a major incident.
  - **Catastrophic haemorrhage:** High priority for intervention from circulation point of view and involves tourniquet, pelvic binder, and haemostatic agents.
    ❖ Patient shifted to P1.
  - **Walking patient:** Low priority. Shift to P3.
  - **Not breathing patient:** Open airway if required, and declare dead if still not breathing when resources allow.
  - **Patient not responding to voice:** Place in recovery position and shift to P1.
  - **Responding to voice but age less than 2 yr:** Shift to P1.
  - **Respiratory rate <12/min or >23/min:** Shift to P1.
  - **Heart rate >100/min:** Shift to P1.
  - **Patient responding to voice, respiratory rate between 12 and 23/min, heart rate <100:** Medium priority, which means reassess regularly. Shift to P2.
✓ **Ten-second triage (TST):** Can be used by anyone responding (police officers/firefighters) to a major **incident before the NHS clinicians arrive.**
  - **Walking:** Shift to P3.
  - **Severe bleeding: Apply pressure, tourniquet, and packing.** Shift to P1.
  - **Talking patient with penetrating injury to chest, abdomen, or back:** Shift to P1.
  - **Talking patient without penetrating injury to chest, abdomen, or back:** Shift to P2.
  - **Non-talking breathing patient: Place in recovery position.** Shift to P1.
  - **Non-breathing patient:** CPR if resources allow.
✓ **Debriefing:** To identify lessons and provide support for staff as follows:
  - **Hot debrief:** Immediately after the incident.
  - **Cold debrief:** Within 2 wk of incident closure.
  - **Multi-agency debrief:** Within 4 wk.
  - **Post-incident reports:** Within 6 wk.
✓ **UK hospital standards in case of major incidents**
  - *All **designated level 3 critical care capability hospitals** must be able to double their normal level **3 ventilated capacity** and should be able to maintain it for up to 96 h.*

- All **nominated supporting level 3 critical care capability hospitals** must be able to double their **normal capacity for level 3 beds** and support the decant of patients from other receiving hospitals.
- All hospitals must have **action cards** for use on activation of the plan; plan to support retrieval or transfer of patients, evacuation, and shelter plan if intensive care areas become unusable for any reason; lockdown plan to prevent unauthorized access; recovery plan to ensure rapid return to normality.

SCORING SYSTEMS IN ITU

✓ **Ideal scoring system:** Easily recordable variables. Applicable to all patient populations. Core characteristics are:
- **Well-calibrated**[Q]: How well a model's predicted probabilities match the actual outcome (e.g. predicted mortality close to actual mortality rates).
- **High level of discrimination**[Q]: How well the model can separate patients into groups with and without an event (distinguish survivors from non-survivors).
  - ❖ Area under the receiver–operating characteristic curve (AUROC) is used commonly for comparing discrimination.
- **Validity**[Q]: Extent to which a test accurately measures what it is intended to measure (e.g. qSOFA is a valid tool for screening patients in ward but has limited value in ITU patients).

✓ **Types of scoring systems used in critical care**[Q]
- **Illness severity score:** SOFA.
- **Outcome prediction model:** APACHE, NELA.
- **Decision support tools:** NEWS 2.
- **Disease-specific:** MELD in liver disease, CURB-65 in pneumonia.

✓ **Area under the receiver–operating curve:** A high 100% AUROC indicates 100% sensitivity and 100% specificity. AUROC should be at least 0.7 for good discrimination.
- APACHE II = 0.85
- APACHE III = 0.9
- APACHE IV = 0.88
- qSOFA = 0.81

- SOFA = 0.79
- SIRS = 0.76
- ICNARC 2007 = 0.87
- SAPS II = 0.86

✓ **Limitations of scoring systems**
- Not designed to support decisions regarding admission to critical care unit as they are likely to be inaccurate when used on an individual level.
  - ❖ Mortality prediction tools describe risk for whole population.
  - ❖ Decision to admit in ICU should be individualized.
- Data entry accuracy is needed, and errors can generate false scores.

✓ **Measurement of quality of a critical care service**
- **Minimum standards:** Assures a minimum level of care.
- Quality indicators: Help understand the robustness of a system.

	Minimum Standards	Quality Indicators
Structure	Twice daily ward rounds Daily review and written management plan by consultant	Nurse staffing Pharmacist availability Physiotherapist availability
Process	No nighttime discharges Care bundles: VAP, CVC	Delirium screening End-of-life care policy
Outcome	Standardized mortality ratio (SMR) Morbidity and mortality meetings	Patient experience surveys

✓ **APACHE II:** Acute physiology and chronic health evaluation.
- APACHE I in 1981, APACHE II in 1985.
- Based on **12 most abnormal variables**[Q] that form acute physiological score[Q] in the first 24 h of ITU stay plus age and chronic disease. Each parameter score: 0–4.
  - ❖ **Age**[Q] and **chronic disease**[Q] (cirrhosis, NYHA stage 4 heart failure, chronic respiratory disease, dialysis-dependent CKD, immunosuppression)

❖ **Five observational variables** (RR, **MAP**, HR, GCS, and temperature)

❖ **Seven investigational variables** (Na+, K+, creatinine, haematocrit, WBCs, pH, A-a gradient)

- Maximum score is 71, with **score of >25 having a predicted mortality of >50%.**

- Score utility in neurosurgical patients in predicting mortality is low.

- *Predicted mortality figures can be used in audit or research but are not validated for use as a prognostic tool for individual patients.*

- **APACHE III:** Expanded the physiological variables from 12 to 17 and included the admission source and previous length of the stay.

- **APACHE IV:** Acute physiology makes up 65.5% of the final score.

✓ **Standardized mortality ratio (SMR)**
- Actual hospital mortality/predicted hospital mortality
- Value of 1 is normal^Q. SMR >1 is poor performance.
- In the UK, the expected mortality is calculated using ICNARC data.
- SMR is better for tracking the performance of an individual unit over time. It is not a very good tool for comparing different ITU units.

  ❖ Excludes readmissions, transfers to other critical acre units, organ donation, and palliation admissions.

  ❖ Case mix is likely to differ between hospitals/units.

- It doesn't give post-ITU mortality and assumes all pre-ICU care is homogenous.

✓ **Simplified Acute Physiology Score (SAPS)**
- Original SAPS (1984) score didn't have input on pre-existing diseases.
- Original SAPS was obtained in the first 24 h and had 14 physiological variables.
- SAPS II was developed in 1993.

  ❖ It includes 12 acute physiological parameters plus age, type of admission and chronic condition.

  ❖ Calculated once after 24 h of admission.

  ❖ Excludes burns, cardiac and juvenile patients.

- SAPS III can be modified according to region of the world.

✓ **P-POSSUM Score (Portsmouth Physiological and Operative Severity Score for the Enumeration of Mortality and Morbidity)**

- *POSSUM was introduced in 1991 and modified in 1998 due to the criticism that mortality was overestimated. Hence, P-POSSUM was formed.*

- **Twelve** physiological variables and **six** operative parameters to calculate an estimated risk for an **operation.**

  ❖ **General parameters:** Age, signs of cardiac failure, signs of respiratory failure

  ❖ **Vitals parameters:** Blood pressure, heart rate and GCS

  ❖ **Lab investigations:** Haemoglobin, WBCs, sodium, potassium, ECG abnormality

  ❖ **Operative parameters:** Operative complexity, number of procedures, blood loss, peritonitis, malignancy, emergency resuscitation possibility

- It is used to predict the risk of death and morbidity in a variety of surgical procedures.

- V-POSSUM for vascular surgery, CR-POSSUM for colorectal surgery.

✓ **Multiple-Organ Dysfunction Score (MODS)**
- **Single measure of six organ systems**: Respiratory (PO_2/FiO_2), CVS (HR × MAP/CVP), hepatic (bilirubin), renal (creatinine), haematological (platelet count), CNS (GCS).

- Each system is scored 0–4, giving a score out of 24.

- Calculated daily and can be used to calculate mortality.

✓ **Intensive Care National Audit and Research Centre (ICNARC) 2007**
- Calculated with data from the first 24 h of admission to critical care.

- Uses age, acute physiology score like APACHE II, reason for admission, CPR prior to admission, and type of admission.

- **Quality indicators^Q used in ICNARC quarterly report are:**

  ❖ **Admission risks:** High-risk admissions from the wards, high-risk sepsis admissions from the wards.

  ❖ **Acquired infections:** Unit-acquired infections in blood.

❖ **Discharges:** Out-of-hours discharges to the ward, delayed discharges (>8- and >24-h delay), and discharges direct to home.

❖ **Transfers and readmissions:** Non-clinical transfers to another unit and unplanned readmissions within 48 h.

❖ **Mortality metrics:** Risk-adjusted acute hospital mortality and risk-adjusted acute hospital mortality with predicted risk of death <20%.

✓ **Therapeutic Intervention Scoring System (TISS)^Q**
- Assessment of burden of work for ITU staff.
- Not very good for severity of disease.
- Collection of 76 items (interventions and treatments) in original TISS.
- TISS-28 version is also available based on 28 possible interventions.

✓ **SOFA (Sequential Organ Failure Assessment) Score^Q**
- **Six organ systems:** Respiratory (PaO_2/FiO_2), cardiovascular (MAP or use of vasopressors), renal (creatinine), hepatic (bilirubin), CNS (GCS), and coagulation (platelet count)
- Scored from 0 to 4 (most abnormal), giving a possible score of 24.
- An increase in SOFA score during the first 48 h in the ICU independent of the initial score predicts a mortality score of >50%.
- A score of >15 predicted 90% mortality.
- SOFA score is helpful in getting idea about progression of disease severity.

✓ **Goldman Cardiac Risk Index**
- Predictor of cardiac risk in non-cardiac surgery.
- Total of nine variables with a maximum of 53 points.
- Patients are categorized into four risk classes (I–IV), with class IV having the highest risk.
- It may overestimate the risk in the elderly.

✓ **Lee's Revised Index**
- Predicts cardiac risk in non-cardiac surgery.
- Clinical parameters used are:
  ❖ Previous TIA or CVA
  ❖ Diabetes mellitus requiring insulin therapy
  ❖ Serum creatinine ≥2 mg/dL
  ❖ History of coronary artery disease

❖ History of heart failure
❖ High-risk surgery (major vascular surgery)
- Low risk = 0–1; Moderate risk = 2; High risk ≥3.

✓ **Trauma scores** have been given in the chapter on trauma triage and initial management.

BUNDLE CARE APPROACH

✓ **Care bundle^Q:** Group of evidence-based interventions that improve the patient outcome when used in combination.

Ventilation-Associated Pneumonia (VAP) Care Bundle

✓ **Intensive Care Society–recommended bundle 2016**
- **Head elevation:** Poor quality of evidence that head end elevation was effective in reducing VAPs.
  ❖ Unclear if 45° is required or even if 15° is enough.
- **Daily sedation interruption:** Helps in reducing VAP rate, but not mortality benefit.
- Avoidance of scheduled ventilator circuit changes.
- **Oral hygiene:** Povidone-iodine is not as effective as chlorhexidine for oral care.
  ❖ About 0.12 to – 0.2 % chlorhexidine for oral care.
- **ETT with subglottic suction ports^Q:** Reduce VAP and length of stay but did not reduce mortality.

✓ **Other components of VAP bundle**
- **Oral hygiene:** Povidone-iodine is not as effective as chlorhexidine for oral care.
  ❖ Around 0.12 to –0.2 % chlorhexidine for oral care.
- **Early tracheostomy:** No benefit in preventing VAP, except sedation reduction.
- Hand hygiene.
- **Role of HME overactive humidification:** Hasn't been shown to reduce incidence of VAP.
- **Silver coating of ETT** helps in reducing the VAP rate, but no mortality benefit.
- **PPIs and enteral feeding increase the rate of VAP but are still recommended^Q.**
- **PROPHY-VAP Trial (2024):** Prophylactic antibiotic (single dose of ceftriaxone) has

been shown to be beneficial in patients post-cardiac arrest or comatose stroke or head injury to prevent early VAP.

Central Venous Catheter (CVC) Care Bundle

✓ **CDC-recommended bundle care that helped in reducing incidence of infection**[Q]
  - Strict asepsis with full barrier precautions
  - Hand hygiene
  - Use of chlorhexidine 0.5% skin preparation
  - Avoidance of femoral insertion approach
  - Daily line review with prompt removal when not required

✓ **CVC Care**
  - Transparent dressings should be changed every 5–7 d, and gauze dressings every 2 d. Site care with chlorhexidine when dressing is being changed.
  - **Disinfection of the hubs** of the CVC must be done using a chlorhexidine-based preparation or 70% alcohol.
  - **CVC removal:** In Trendelenburg position, with firm digital pressure for 5 min. Lie flat for 60 min after removal.

STOP-AKI Bundle[Q]

✓ **(S): Sepsis and hypoperfusion:** Treat sepsis and avoid dehydration.

✓ **(T): Toxins:** Stop nephrotoxic drugs like NSAIDs and IV iodinated contrast.

✓ **(O): Obstruction:** Rule out obstruction with renal tract ultrasound.

✓ **(P): Prevent harm:** Identify the cause of AKI and adjust drugs dosages.

TRANSFER OF PATIENTS

✓ **Risks and hazards of patient transfer**
  - **Patient:** Dislodged equipment, haemodynamic instability, equipment failure, nonroutine setting, loss of information during handover, patient/relative dissatisfaction
  - **Staff:** Motion sickness, disruption of shift work, injury
  - **Organization:** Disruption of normal staffing

✓ **Classification of patient transfers:**[Q]
  - **Position on care pathway:** Primary, secondary, tertiary
  - **Indication:** Clinical or capacity

  - **Urgency:** Time-critical, urgent, routine
  - **Level of care:** Levels 1, 2, 3
  - **Distance:** Intrahospital, interhospital, or international

✓ **Definitions**
  - **Primary transfer:** Patient transferred from scene of injury or illness to the nearest receiving hospital.
  - **Extended primary transfer:** Patient transferred from scene of injury to a specialist centre/trauma centre, bypassing the nearest hospital.
  - **Secondary transfer:** From one hospital to another hospital.
  - **Clinical transfer:** Transfer for specialty treatment not provided at referring hospital.
  - **Capacity transfer:** Transfer for specialty treatment normally provided at referring hospital but which is not currently available.
    - ❖ Guidance advises against transfer for capacity reasons alone. It should be the last resort with consultant agreement.
  - **Repatriation:** Transferred back to referring hospital or a hospital nearer the patient's home address.

✓ **Transfer process**
  - Decision about need to transfer the patient.
  - Agreement between referring and accepting senior doctors at the respective hospitals.
  - Handover from critical care team to transfer medical and nursing team.
  - Transfer between the care facilities using standard AAGBI equipment, and vital signs should be checked every 5 min.
  - Handover from medical and nursing transfer team to accepting medical and nursing team.

✓ **Transfer pitfalls**
  - **Airway:** Anticipate potential deterioration and intubate before the transfer if needed.
  - **Breathing:** Oxygen requirements = 2 × (patient consumption + ventilator consumption).
  - **Circulation:** At least two IV access sites should be available. *Non-invasive blood pressure monitoring in place for use in case of arterial line failure.*
  - **Disability:** Periods of increased stimuli during transfer and, hence, adequate sedation and analgesia.

- **Exposure:** All lines and drains should be securely fixed in place. Increased risk of hypothermia during transfer; hence, continuous temperature monitoring is recommended.
✓ **Specialist transfer teams:** ECMO retrieval team, paediatric critical care team, fixed-wing air transfer team.
  - **Scoop-and-run transfer**[Q]**:** Time needed for stabilization is minimized, and patient transferred straight from the scene of incident.

ARTIFICIAL INTELLIGENCE

✓ **Artificial intelligence (AI):** Technique that attempts to replicate human intelligence, analytical behaviour, and decision-making ability in machines.
  - **Machine learning (ML):** A subset of AI that allows computers to find patterns in a complex environment of multidimensional data.
✓ **Applications of AI in critical care**
  - **Disease identification** (e.g. differentiate pulmonary infiltrates due to congestive heart failure from pneumonia).
  - **Disease evolution prediction:** Tachycardia, hypotension, hypoxia, AKI, sepsis, cardiac arrest, mortality after TBI can all be predicted before their development.
  - **Disease phenotyping:** Different phenotypes of the same disease behave differently, and ARDS phenotype delineation has been done using AI.
  - **Telemedicine:** In remote areas where clinicians are not available, virtual consults can be arranged.
  - **Clinical notes and ward rounds:** AI can help summarize past history of the patient, make discharge summaries, and create referral letters.
  - **Mechanical ventilator and ventilator weaning:** AI can personalize mechanical ventilation strategies for patients with respiratory failure.
  - **Outreach and recognition of deteriorating patients:** AI-based MEWS model to predict the likelihood of deterioration and alert the primary team.
  - **Resource allocation:** Can help optimize the use of ICU beds by predicting patient needs, risk of complications, and organ support.
  - **Antibiotic stewardship:** Can help in predicting inappropriate prescriptions.
✓ **Pitfalls of AI in critical care**
  - **Interpretability:** AI uses data to reveal hidden patterns, and sometimes the rationale of the computation may not be acceptable to the clinician.
  - **Lack of robustness:** Lack of adequate clinical trials and experiments regarding their clinical readiness.
  - **Ethical concerns:** Data privacy and sharing. Data safety.

STATISTICS

✓ **Types of data**
  - **Categorical (qualitative) data.**
    - ❖ **Nominal:** No numerically significant order (e.g. hair colour, blood groups).
    - ❖ **Ordinal:** Order of magnitude (e.g. pain scores, ASA score).
  - **Numerical (quantitative) data**
    - ❖ **Discrete:** Finite values (e.g. number of children).
    - ❖ **Continuous:** Data that can take any number (e.g. height, age).
    - ❖ **Ratio:** Data series that has zero as its baseline value (e.g. Kelvin temperature scale, blood pressure).
    - ❖ **Interval:** Data series that includes zero on a larger scale (e.g. centigrade temperature scale).
✓ **Measures of central tendency**
  - **Mean:** The average value.
  - **Median:** Middle value of a data series.
  - **Mode:** Frequently occurring value in a set of data points.
✓ **Measures of spread**
  - **Variance:** A measure of the spread of data around a central point:

$$\text{Var} = \Sigma(x - \bar{x})2 \, / \, n$$

  - **Standard deviation:** *A measure of the spread of data around a central point.* ***Square root of variance.***

$$\text{SD} = \sqrt{\Sigma(xi - \bar{x})2 \, / \, n - 1}$$

- **Standard error of the mean:** A measure of the spread of a group of sample means around the true population mean.

$$SEM = \sigma/\sqrt{N-1}$$

- **Confidence intervals:** Range of values that will contain the true population mean with a stated percentage confidence. A **95.4% confidence interval is ± 2 SD**[Q].
  - ❖ 68.3% of values within 1 SD of the mean[Q]
  - ❖ 99.7% of values within 3 SD of the mean[Q]
- **Interquartile range:** The range of values that lie between the first and third quartiles and therefore shows 50% of the data points. **Best option for non-parametric data.**

✓ **Types of distribution**
- **Normal distribution**[Q] is a bell-shaped distribution in which mean, median, and mode all have the same value.
- **Positively skewed distribution:** Longer tail stretching off towards the more positive values. Mean > median > mode.
- **Negatively skewed distribution:** Longer tail stretching off towards the more negative values. Mode > median > mean

✓ **Type 1 and 2 errors**
- *p* stands for probability[Q]. Therefore, if p = 1, the event will always happen, and if p = 0, the event will never happen.
- **Null hypothesis**[Q]: Assumption is made that there is no significant difference between the means of the samples. If the result of the test gives a *p* <0.05, then there is a low possibility (5%) that the difference has

occurred purely by chance, and the null hypothesis[Q] that there is no difference between the sample is rejected.

- **Type 1 error/α-error**[Q]: It occurs when a null hypothesis is wrongly rejected.
  - ❖ The lower the *p* value and the larger the sample size, the smaller the chance of making a type 1 error.
  - ❖ A 5% chance of making a type 1 error is accepted.
- **Type 2 error/β-error**[Q]: It occurs when a null hypothesis is wrongly accepted.
  - ❖ A 20% chance of making a type 2 error is accepted.
  - ❖ Three factors that increase the chance of making type 2 error: Large variability in study population, small population size, and situation where a small difference is clinically important.
- **Power of a study**[Q]: Likelihood of detecting a difference between groups if that difference really does exist.
  - ❖ Power is probability of avoiding a type 2 error
  - ❖ Power[Q] = 1 − β

✓ **Significance tests**
- There are four considerations that should be taken into account:
  - ❖ Is the data qualitative or quantitative?
  - ❖ Is the data parametric or non-parametric?
  - ❖ Two groups or more than two groups?
  - ❖ Data paired or unpaired?

	Two Groups		More Than Two Groups	
Type of Data	**Unpaired**	**Paired**	**Unpaired**	**Paired**
Parametric (continuous)	Student's unpaired t-test	**Student's paired t-test**	ANOVA[Q]	Paired ANOVA
Non-parametric (nominal)	Chi-square test	McNemar's test	Chi-square test	Chi-square test
Non-parametric (ordinal)	Mann–Whitney *U* test	Wilcoxon signed rank test	Kruskal–Wallis test	Friedman test

- **Fisher's exact test:** It is a variation of chi-square test that is used when value of parameters in any cell is less than 5.
- **Correlation:** Degree of association between two variables

- ❖ **Pearson's correlation coefficient:** Used for normally distributed data.
- ❖ **Spearman's rank correlation coefficient**[Q]: Used for non–normally distributed continuous data, for ordinal data, or for data with relevant outliers.

❖ **Positive correlation:** r value between 0 and +1.

❖ **Negative correlation:** r value between 0 and −1.

❖ **No correlation:** r value is 0.

Change in peak expiratory flow or blood pressure[Q] can be a good example of student's paired t-test.

Odds Ratio and Number Needed to Treat

	Non-Event (People Relieved of Pain)	Event (People in Pain)
Painkiller	b	a
Placebo	d	c

- Painkiller events odd = event / non-event = a/b
- Placebo events odd = event / non-event = c/d
- **Odds ratio** = painkiller events odd / placebo events odd =
  ❖ Odds of having the outcome.
- **Relative risk** = risk of event in painkiller group/risk of event in placebo

$$= a \div a + b / c \div c + d$$

  ❖ Risk of developing the outcome
- Odds/risk ratio above 1 = Your exposure increases risk of event occurring.
- Odds/risk ratio below 1 = Your exposure increases risk of event occurring or protective effect of exposure.
- If 95% confidence interval (CI) includes value 1, then there is no statistical difference.
  ❖ Wide confidence interval = weaker inference
  ❖ Narrow confidence interval = stronger inference
- **Absolute risk reduction (ARR)[Q]** = event rate in placebo group − event rate in treatment group.

$$= c/c + d - a/a + b$$

- **Numbers needed to treat[Q]:** Number of patients that would need to be treated to prevent a single event. NNT = 1/ ARR

✓ **Sensitivity and specificity**
- **Sensitivity[Q]:** Probability that someone who has the disease tests positive.
  ❖ Numbers correctly guess positive/total number that are actually positive.
  ❖ TP/TP + FN.
  ❖ A test with high sensitivity is said to have a low type II error rate.
- **Specificity[Q]:** Probability that someone who doesn't have the disease tests negative.
  ❖ Number correctly negative/total number that are actually negative.
  ❖ TN/TN + FP.
  ❖ A test with high specificity is said to have a low type I error rate.

Both sensitivity and specificity are prevalence-independent.

✓ **Positive predictive value[Q]:** The certainty with which a positive test results correctly predicts a positive value.
- Numbers correctly positive/Total number that tested positive.
- TP/TP + FP.

✓ **Negative predictive value[Q]:** The certainty with which a negative test results correctly predicts a negative value.
- Numbers correctly negative/total number that tested negative.
- TN/TN + FN
- Both PPV and NPV are influenced by the prevalence of the disease.

✓ **Clinical trial[Q]**
- **Preclinical studies**
  ❖ In vitro studies
  ❖ Animal studies

Phase	Number of People Involved	Main Aims of Trial	Rando-mization
0	10–20 people	• Single subtherapeutic doses • Preliminary data on pharmacokinetics and pharmacodynamics • No data on safety and efficacy	No
1	20–50 people	• Finding the best dose of treatment • Assesses safety of drug • Tolerability • Pharmacokinetics • Pharmacodynamics	No

Phase	Number of People Involved	Main Aims of Trial	Rando-mization
2	Over 100s	• Checking the best dose of treatment • More about safety of drug • Some phase 2 trials randomized	Sometimes
3	Around thousands	• Comparing new treatment to the standard treatment or to a dummy drug • At least 2 randomized controlled trials for approval	Usually
4	Market	• Post-marketing surveillance • Long-term benefits and side effects	No

- Double blinding is to both investigator and participant[Q].
- Triple blinding[Q] is when investigators, participants, and people analyzing the data are also blinded.

✓ **Evidence-based medicine:** Evidence-based medicine is the conscientious, explicit, and judicious use of current based evidence in making decisions about the care of individual patients.

Level	Evidence
1a	Systemic review or meta-analysis of more than one randomized controlled trial (multiple RCTs)
1b	Single randomized controlled trial (single RCT)
2a	Non-randomized study
2b	Cohort study/quasi-experimental study
3	Case-control study
4	Case series
5	Expert opinion

Grade of Recommendations

Grade	Recommendation
A	Consistent level 1 studies
B	Consistent level 2 or 3 studies or extrapolations from level 1 studies
C	Level 4 studies or extrapolations from level 2 or 3 studies
D	Level 5 evidence

✓ **Systematic review:** It answers a defined research question by collecting and summarizing all empirical evidence that fits pre-specified eligibility criteria.

- Meta-analysis may or may not be used to analyze the results of the studies.

✓ **Meta-analysis[Q]:** A meta-analysis is the use of statistical methods to summarize the results of these studies. **Represented by forest plot[Q].**

- **Number of horizontal lines on forest plot:** Number of studies.
- **Length of horizontal line on forest plot:** Confidence interval of the study.
- **Horizontal position of square on this line:** Odds ratio.
- **Size of the square:** Power of the study.
- **Width of diamond:** Confidence interval for the combined odds ratio. If the diamond doesn't cross the Y-axis, then it represents a statistically significant outcome.

✓ **Delphi method[Q]:** Expert consensus method where a common ground is reached by gathering information from experts.

✓ **Kaplan–Meier estimator[Q]:** Used to estimate the proportion of patients surviving for a specific duration, like post-diagnosis or post-treatment.

✓ **List of guidelines[Q]**

- **CONSORT** (Consolidated Standards of Reporting Trials): For randomized trials
- **QUORUM** (Quality of Reporting of Meta-Analyses): For meta-analyses of trials
- **MOOSE** (Meta-Analysis of Observational Studies in Epidemiology)
- **STROBE** (Strengthening the Reporting of Observational Studies in Epidemiology)
- **SQUIRE** (Standards for Quality Improvement Reporting Excellence): For quality improvement

✓ **Types of biases**[Q]
- **Lead time bias**[Q]**:** When a disease is detected by a screening at an early time and hence gives the impression that survival is prolonged, but there is no effect on the outcome of the disease.
- **Attrition bias**[Q]**:** Failure to account for the withdrawals from the study group. To avoid this, data should be analyzed on "intention to treat basis."
- **Selection bias:** Avoided by using a blinded random sequencer.
- **Performance bias:** Actions of volunteers and researchers during the trial. Avoided by blinding patients and staff to the groups.
- **Detection bias:** Actions of those collecting data. Avoided by blinding of collecting and analyzing data.
- **Recall bias:** Participants enrolled in retrospective studies remember things differently and can affect the outcome.
- **Reporting bias:** More weightage on positive findings, explaining away negative findings.
- **Observation bias:** People's behaviour changes as they know they are being observed.

21

Pharmacology

ANAESTHETIC DRUGS

Intravenous Anaesthetic Agents

	Propofol	Thiopental	Etomidate	Ketamine
Chemical	• 2.6 diisopropylphenol	Sulphur analogue of oxybarbiturate	Imidazole derivative	**Phencyclidine derivative**
Presentation	• 1 or 2% emulsion (**not soluble in water**) • 10% soyabean oil • 1.2% purified egg phosphatide (lecithin: not allergic)^Q • 2.25% glycerol	• 2.5% sodium salt • Pale yellow powder • 6% Na_2CO_3 and nitrogen to prevent formation of free acid with CO_2	• 0.2% solution • 35% v/v Propylene glycol	• Only one chiral centre • **Racemic mixture** • **S (+) enantiomer 3–4 times more potent**
Mechanism of action	• Enhancing γ-aminobutyric acid (GABA)^Q–induced chloride current by binding to β-subunit • **Inhibition of NMDA receptors**	• Enhances the action of GABA by increasing conductance • Inhibition of NMDA receptors	• GABA receptor facilitation	• **Non-competitive inhibition of NMDA receptors** • **Inhibits noradrenaline uptake**
Pharma-codynamic effects	• **CVS:** ↓ HR, ↓ SVR, and ↓ contractility • **Respi:** ↓ RR, suppression of laryngeal reflexes • **CNS:** ↓ ICP, ↓ CBF, and dystonic choreiform movements • *Gut:* **Anti-emetic effect by antagonism of dopamine D2 receptor** • *Urine:* **Turns green** • *Injection:* **Pain on injection**	• **CVS:** ↑ HR, ↓ SVR, and ↓ contractility • **Respi:** ↓ RR, bronchospasm, and laryngospasm • **CNS**^{Q}**:** ↓ ICP, ↓ CBF, and ↓ $CMRO_2$ • **Renal:** Urine retention due to ↑ ADH (morphine has similar action)	• **CVS:** ↓ SVR, but HR, BP, and contractility unchanged (cardiostable) • **Respi:** ↓ RR • **CNS:** ↓ ICP, ↓ CBF, myoclonus • **Endocrine:** ↓ cortisol formation^Q by inhibiting 11β-hyd-roxylase and 17α-hydroxylase,	• **CVS:** ↑ HR, ↑BP, ↑ cardiac output, and no change in SVR • *Direct cardiac depressant effect* • **Respi:** ↑ RR, preserved laryngeal reflexes, *bronchodilation*^{Q} • **CNS**^{Q}**:** ↑ ICP and ↑ **CBF**; dissociative anaesthesia

DOI: 10.1201/9781003476214-21

	Propofol	Thiopental	Etomidate	Ketamine
			and hence not used for maintenance of sedation • Injection: **Pain on injection**	• **Gut:** Causes nausea and vomiting; salivation • **Pain:** Analgesia along with sedation
pH	**7**	10.8	8.1	3.5–5.5
pKa	11	7.6	4.1	7.5
Protein binding (%)	98	80	75	25
Volume of distribution (L/kg)	4	2.5	3	3
Clearance (mL/kg/ min)	30–60	3.5	10–20	17
Elimination half-life (h)	**5–12**	6–15	1–4	2
Metabolism	• Metabolized by **glucuronidation at position 1** and hydroxylation in **liver**^Q • Metabolism in lungs as well	• Metabolism by hepatic oxidation • Active metabolite: pentobarbitone	• Metabolized by plasma and **hepatic esterases**	• *N-demethylation and hydroxylation in liver* • **Norketamine active metabolite**
Side effects	• Propofol infusion syndrome in doses >4 mg/ kg/h (heart failure, rhabdomyolysis, acidosis) • Epileptiform movements	• Anaphylaxis 1 in 20,000 • Thrombosis if intra-arterial • Antanalgesia • **Porphyrinogen**	• Nausea and vomiting • Antiplatelet • Porphyrinogen	• Nausea and vomiting • Emergence delirium • **Porphyrinogen**
Doses	• Induction dose: 1–2.5 mg/kg • Maintenance of GA: 50–150 µg/kg/min • Sedation: 25–75 µg/ kg/min • Antiemetic action: 10–20 mg IV	• Induction dose: 3–4 mg/kg	• Induction dose: **0.2–0.3 mg/kg**	• Induction dose: 0.5–2 mg/kg IV or 4–6 mg/ kg IM • Sedation and analgesia: 0.2–0.8 mg/kg IV or 2–4 mg/kg IM • Preventive analgesia: 0.15–0.25 mg/kg IV

Opioids

Parameters	Morphine	Fentanyl	Alfentanil	Remifentanil
Relative lipid solubility	1	600	90	20
Relative potency	1	**100**	**10–20**	100
pKa	8.0	8.4	6.5	7.1
Protein binding (%)	35	83	**90 (highest)**	70
Oral bioavailability (%)	25–30	33	N/A	N/A
Volume of distribution (L/kg)	**3.5**	**4**	**0.6**	0.3
Clearance (mL/kg/min)	**16**	**13**	**6**	40
Elimination rate (min)	170	190	100	10

- **Clinical pearls**
  - ❖ Faster onset of action of alfentanil^Q is due to its lower pKa compared to fentanyl's pKa, which means that more alfentanil is available in non-ionized form and hence can cross the blood–brain barrier.
  - ❖ Patients with CYP2D6 gene duplication should not be given codeine as they are ultrarapid metabolizers and quickly convert all the codeine into morphine-6 glucuronide.

Muscle Relaxants

	Rocuronium	Vecuronium	Atracurium	Cisatracurium
Structure	Monoquaternary		10 stereoisomers	**One of 10** stereoisomers of atracurium
Intubation dose (mg/kg)	0.6 0.9 (RSI)	0.1	0.5	0.2
Speed of onset	Rapid	Medium		
Duration	Medium		Medium	
Protein binding (%)	10	10	15	15
Volume of distribution (l/kg)	0.2	0.2	0.15	0.15
Metabolism (%)	20	<5	90	95
Elimination in bile (%)	70	60	0	0
Elimination in urine (%)	30	40	10	5
CVS effects	None/↓ HR	None		
Histamine release	Rare		Highest incidence	Rare
Renal and hepatic failure^Q	Prolonged effect		No effect	

	Rocuronium	Vecuronium	Atracurium	Cisatracurium
Notes	• Unstable in solution • Three active metabolites, accumulation with repeated dosing • Can be reversed by **sugammadex**[Q]	• Rapid onset, but not enough for RSI[Q] • Can be reversed by **sugammadex**[Q]	• Hofmann elimination[Q] (30–70%) is spontaneous degradation of a quaternary ammonium to a tertiary amine **(laudanosine)** • **Epileptogenic** • **Ester hydrolysis**	• Less histamine release • Longer onset of action, **four times more potent** and longer duration than atracurium • **Hofmann degradation**

- **Clinical Pearls**
  - ❖ Neuromuscular blocking agents do not affect somatosensory-evoked potentials (SSEP).
  - ❖ Calcium channel blockers, local anaesthetics, inhalational anaesthetics, lithium, and aminoglycosides prolong the effect of non-depolarizing muscle relaxants[Q].

INOTROPES

Drug	Receptor (µg/kg/min)	HR	Contractility	SVR	DO_2	Effects
Adrenaline	$\alpha + \beta$ (0.01–0.5)	↑	↑	↑	↑	• ↑ Lactate[Q] • ↑ Renin
Noradrenaline	$\alpha_1 + \beta$ (0.05–0.5)	↓	↑	↑	↑	• Extravasation possibly causing tissue ischaemia
Vasopressin	V_1 (0.01–0.1 U/min)	↓	↑	↑	↑	• In diabetes insipidus as well
Dopamine	$D_1 + D_2$ (1–5)[Q] β (5–10)[Q] α (>10)[Q]	↑	↑	↑/↓	↑	• Splanchnic dilation • Extrapyramidal movement • Nausea and vomiting
Dobutamine[Q]	$\beta_1 + \beta_2$ (0.5–20)	↑	↑	↓	↑	• No effect on splanchnic vessels
Dopexamine	β_2, D_1 (0.5–6)	↑	↑	↓	No	• ↑ renal and splanchnic blood flow
Isoprenaline	$\beta_1 + \beta_2$ (0.5–10 µg/min)	↑	↑	↓	↑	• ↑ renal and splanchnic blood flow
Ephedrine	$\alpha + \beta$	↑	↑	↑	↑	• Indirect sympathomimetic (noradrenaline release from nerves)
Metaraminol	α_1 + some β	↓	↑	↑	↑	• Tachyphylaxis
Phenylephrine	α_1	↓	↑	↑	↑	• Used in obstetrics as better cord ABG profile
Angiotensin II[Q]	Angiotensin type-1 receptor	↑	↑	↑	No	• Can be used as an additional vasopressor
Milrinone	PDE III inhibitor (0.375–0.75)	↑	↑	↓	No	• Pulmonary vasodilation • Used in right heart failure
Levosimendan	Ca^{2+} sensitizer (0.05–0.2)	↑	↑	↓	No	• Stabilizes troponin C and actin myosin cross bridges

Important Trials Regarding Vasopressors

✓ **VASST Trial (2008):** In patients with septic shock on at least 5 mcg/min of noradrenaline, no significant mortality reduction in **vasopressin vs additional noradrenaline** use. Vasopressin may show some mortality benefit in patients with less severe vasopressor requirements.

✓ **SOAP-II Trial (2010):** Among patients with all types of shock, mortality rates were not different between **noradrenaline and dopamine**, although noradrenaline was less associated with arrhythmias.

- Noradrenaline may have a mortality benefit in a subset of patients with cardiogenic shock.

✓ **VANISH Trial (2016):** In patients with septic shock, no significant mortality reduction and reduction in renal failure in **vasopressin vs noradrenaline** use.

✓ **ATHOS-3 Trial (2017):** In patients with vasodilatory shock requiring at least 0.2 mcg/kg/min of noradrenaline, **angiotensin-II** increases the mean arterial pressure.

✓ **MIDAS Trial (2020):** In patients requiring low-dose vasopressor therapy, use of **midodrine** didn't accelerate the time to vasopressor discontinuation.

Additional Questions

✓ **Milrinone[Q]:** PDE III inhibitor and hence leads to increased intracellular cAMP.
- Increased inotropy (contraction) and lusitropy (relaxation).
- Decreased pulmonary vascular and systemic vascular resistance.

✓ **Levosimendan[Q]:** Increases sensitivity of troponin C to intracellular Ca^{2+} and, hence, increases inotropy without a significant increase in oxygen consumption.
- It also opens ATP-sensitive potassium channels and hence causes smooth muscle relaxation.

✓ **Vasopressin[Q]**
- V1: Vasoconstriction at all vessels, except pulmonary.
- V2: H_2O absorption in DCT and CD of the kidney.
- V3: ACTH release from anterior pituitary.

✓ **Midodrine:** Peripherally acting, oral α-agonist. No myocardial β activity but increases end-diastolic volume and stroke volume, decreases heart rate via baroreceptor stimulation, and causes QT prolongation.
- Approved for use as a treatment for orthostatic hypotension.
- Off-label use for weaning off vasopressors in patients on low-dose vasopressor agent.

ANTICOAGULANTS

✓ **Anticoagulants in body**
- **Antithrombin:** Inhibits thrombin, factor IXa, Xa, and XIa.
- **Protein C and S:** inhibit factor Va and VIIIa.

✓ **Prothrombin time (PT)[Q]:** Tests extrinsic pathway factors (tissue factor and factor VII) and common pathway (factor X, factor V, prothrombin, and fibrinogen).
- **Increased PT:** Warfarin, vitamin K deficiency[Q], liver failure, deficiency of extrinsic pathway, deficiency of common pathway factors.

✓ **Activated partial thromboplastin time[Q]:** Tests intrinsic pathway factors (factor VIII, IX, XI, and XII) and common pathway.
- **Increased APTT:** Heparin, haemophilia A (factor VIII)[Q], B (factor IX)[Q], C (factor X), vitamin K deficiency[Q], antiphospholipid syndrome, and von Willebrand disease.

✓ **Activated clotting time:** Measures the anticoagulant effect of heparin.
- Used to measure anticoagulation during bypass, where goal is to increase ACT to four times the pre-heparin ACT.

✓ **Coagulation tests**
- Haemophilia A (factor VIII deficiency): ↑ aPTT, PT is normal.
- Von Willebrand disease: ↑ aPTT, PT is normal.
- Subtherapeutic warfarin: ↑ PT, aPTT is normal.
- Supratherapeutic fondaparinux: ↑ aPTT and slightly prolonged PT.

✓ **Anticoagulants[Q]**
- **Parenteral**
  - ❖ **Direct thrombin inhibitor:** Argatroban, bivalirudin
  - ❖ **Indirect thrombin inhibitor:** Heparins, fondaparinux

- **Oral**
  - ❖ **Coumarin derivative:** Warfarin
  - ❖ **Direct Xa inhibitor:** Rivaroxaban, apixaban, edoxaban
  - ❖ **Direct thrombin inhibitor:** Dabigatran
- ✓ **Warfarin:** Inhibits vitamin K epoxide reductase, ↓ production of factors (II, VII, IX, and X) and protein C and S.
  - Hepatically metabolized.
  - Fluconazole[Q] is a strong, and amiodarone[Q] a moderate, inhibitor of enzyme p450, for which warfarin is a substrate.
    - ❖ Erythromycin[Q] is a CYP3A4 inhibitor as well and can increase INR.
  - **Reversal is best by vitamin K (IV 6 h, oral 24 h) and PCC[Q] (factors II, VII, IX, X, and protein C and S). Dose of PCC is 25–50 IU/kg.**
  - FFP may be given if PCC is not available.
  - Discontinue 5 d before an elective procedure, and restart 12–24 h after surgery after adequate haemostasis.
  - Bridging therapy recommended for patients at high risk of thrombotic complications (recent VTE in past 3 months, high CHADS2 score in AF patients, and prosthetic mitral valve).
    - ❖ Unfractionated heparin (UFH) and therapeutic-dose low-molecular-weight heparin (LMWH) are used for bridging.
  - **Uses of warfarin**
    - ❖ Prophylaxis and treatment of venous thrombosis and pulmonary embolism.
    - ❖ Prophylaxis and treatment of thromboembolic complications from atrial fibrillation or cardiac valve replacement.
    - ❖ Reduction in the risk of death, recurrent myocardial infarction, and thromboembolic events after myocardial infarction.
- ✓ **Dabigatran:** Direct thrombin inhibitor. Given twice daily. Where 35% protein-bound, 80% renally excreted[Q] (highest in DOACs).
  - Approved for stroke prevention in patients with non-valvular AF and for VTE prophylaxis after hip or knee replacement.
  - Avoid in patients <60 kg weight. Breakthrough VTE in patients with weight >120 kg.
  - Prolongs APTT.
  - **Idarucizumab[Q]** is the antidote available.
  - Haemodialysis may be useful.

- ✓ **Rivaroxaban:** Direct Xa inhibitor[Q]. With 90% protein-bound, 30% renally excreted. Good oral absorption.
  - Approved for stroke prevention in patients with non-valvular AF and for VTE prophylaxis after hip or knee replacement.
  - Avoid in patients <60 kg weight. Effective in patients with weight over 120 kg.
  - Can be reversed by **andexanet alfa[Q]**.
  - Haemodialysis may not be useful.
- ✓ **Apixaban:** Direct Xa inhibitor, 30% renally excreted.
  - Approved for stroke prevention in patients with non-valvular AF and for VTE prophylaxis after hip or knee replacement.
  - Lower doses in patients <60 kg in weight. Effective in patients with weight over 120 kg.
  - Andexanet is the antidote available.
- ✓ **Fondaparinux:** Synthetic **indirect Xa inhibitor** with no antithrombin activity.
  - Given subcutaneously.
  - Prophylaxis of venous thromboembolism in patients after undergoing major orthopaedic surgery of the hip or leg, or abdominal surgery, and medical patients immobilized because of acute illness.
  - Treatment of DVT, pulmonary embolism, angina, and myocardial infarction.
  - Long half-life (17–20 h), which increases to 72 h when creatinine clearance <30 mL/ min.
  - No antidote available.
- ✓ **Unfractionated heparin (UFH)**
  - Heparin occurs naturally in liver and mast cell granules.
  - Heparin binds to antithrombin III (AT-III)[Q] and increases its activity by 1,000-fold. It will inhibit factor Xa as well[Q].
  - Half-life of UFH is 45–90 min. APTT comes back to normal in 3–4 h after discontinuation. *AT-III is given in heparin-resistant cases, where desired APTT targets are not achieved.*
  - Reversal of heparin (negatively charged)[Q]: 1 mg of protamine (positively charged) for 100 units of UFH.
    - ❖ Protamine forms an inactive complex[Q] that is cleared by the reticuloendothelial system.

* ❖ **Protamine**[Q] has a short half-life (7 min). This means that rebound heparin activity can be there, and a second dose may be needed.
  * ❖ Protamine can cause anaphylaxis, bronchospasm, pulmonary hypertension, and systemic hypotension and should be given slowly.
* **Side effects:** Hypersensitivity, heparin-induced thrombocytopaenia (HIT)[Q], osteoporosis, hyperkalaemia, hypotension with fast dosing.

✓ **Low-molecular-weight heparin (LMWH)**
* Derived from UFH. More activity against factor Xa than AT-III.
* More predictable dose–response relationship, longer plasma half-lives, and a more favourable benefit-to-risk ratio compared to UFH.
* Monitoring is not usually required. Protamine doesn't fully reverse the effect of LMWH.
* Anti-Xa activity[Q] is used to measure LMWH activity. It is measured as units per mL.
  * ❖ Levels decline with time, and samples should be rapidly transported.
  * ❖ Levels increase with renal failure. Hyperbilirubinaemia interferes with results.
* **Side effects:** Less effects on platelets compared to UFH, reduced risk of HIT.

✓ **Danaparoid:** Low-molecular-weight heparinoid. More selective against factor Xa.
* Used in patients with confirmed HIT.
* No antidote available.

✓ **Bivalirudin:** Recombinant hirudin. Direct thrombin inhibitor.
* Used in percutaneous coronary interventions and cardiopulmonary bypass patients with HIT.
* Aim ACT >300 s.
* No antidote available.

✓ **Argatroban:** Reversible direct thrombin inhibitor.
* Agent of choice in HIT and renal dysfunction.
* aPTT aim of 1.5–3 times the normal.
* Use cautiously in patients with liver dysfunction and multiorgan failure. They increase PT-INR as well.
* No antidote available.

Drug	Time before Puncture/ Catheter Manipulation or Removal	Time after Puncture/ Catheter Manipulation or Removal
Unfractionated heparin	4–6 h	1 h
LMWH (prophylaxis)	12 h	4 h
LMWH (treatment)	24 h	4 h
Warfarin	INR <1.5	After catheter removal
Fondaparinux	36–42 h	6–12 h
Rivaroxaban	22–26 h	4–6 h
Apixaban	26–30 h	4–6 h
Dabigatran	Contraindicated	6 h
Argatroban	4 h	2 h

Additional Questions

✓ **Glanzmann thrombasthenia:** Autosomal recessive defect in GP IIb/IIIa receptor.
✓ **Von Willebrand's disease:** Likely diagnosis in a patient who develops prolonged bleeding after a tooth extraction[Q].

DIURETICS

✓ **Classification of Diuretics**
* **Proximal convoluted tubule (PCT):** Carbonic anhydrase inhibitors (e.g. acetazolamide).
* **Loop of Henle:** Loop diuretics (e.g. furosemide, **bumetanide**).
* **Distal convoluted tubule (DCT):** Thiazides (e.g. bendroflumethiazide).
* **Collecting duct (CD):** Potassium sparing diuretics (e.g. spironolactone, amiloride, triamterene [cause hyperkalaemia]).
* **Osmotic diuretics** (e.g. mannitol).

✓ **Ceiling effect of diuretics**
* Loop diuretics have high ceiling effect.
* Thiazide diuretics: Medium ceiling effect.
* Potassium-sparing diuretics/carbonic anhydrase inhibitors: Low ceiling.

	Furosemide[Q]	Bendroflumethiazide
Mechanism of action	• Acts on Na⁺-K⁺-Cl- contransporter on thick **ascending loop of Henle** • Inhibits absorption of Na⁺, K⁺, and Cl⁻ ions	• Acts on Na⁺-K⁺ cotransporter on **distal convoluted tubule.** • Inhibits absorption of Na⁺ and Cl⁻ ions.
Pharmacodynamic/ side effects	• **CVS:** ↓ preload, ↓ SVR • **Biochemistry:** ↓ Na⁺, ↓ Cl⁻, ↓ K⁺, ↓ H⁺, ↓ Mg²⁺, ↑ Ca²⁺, ↑ uric acid • **Renal:** ↑ GFR (used in low GFR) • Hyperglycaemia, hypercholesterolemia • **Ototoxicity:** rapid injection and reversible • ↑ lithium levels	• **CVS:** ↓ preload, ↓ SVR • **Biochemistry:** ↓ Na⁺, ↓ Cl⁻, ↓ K⁺, ↓ H⁺, ↓ Mg²⁺, ↑ **Ca²⁺**, ↑ **uric acid**[Q] **(not used in tumour lysis syndrome)** • **Renal:** ↓ GFR • **Hyperglycaemia,** hypercholesterolaemia • **Blood dyscrasias:** anaemia, leucopaenia, and thrombocytopaenia • Impotence • Pancreatitis
Pharmacokinetics	• Bioavailability: 65% • Protein binding: >95% • Excreted unchanged in urine	• Oral bioavailability: 100% • Protein binding: 96% • $T_{1/2}$: 9 h
Uses	• Congestive heart failure[Q] • Pulmonary oedema • Forced diuresis in AKI[Q]	• Hypertension • Congestive heart failure
Dose	• 20–160 mg depending upon refractory oedema	• 2.5–5 mg OD orally

✓ **Loop diuretics:** Highest efficacy amongst all the diuretics.
  - However, they increase urinary sodium, but not as high as atrial natriuretic peptide (ANP), which causes increased urinary sodium and increased urine output.
  - Furosemide is not directly nephrotoxic. It causes hypovolaemia, which can cause injury.
  - It increases PGE2 synthesis in the kidneys, which causes vasodilation; hence, they increase renal blood flow.
  - In physiological or pharmacological stress, it counters intrarenal vasoconstriction.

- Dose: Those not on furosemide, start at a dose between 20 and 80 mg, and then double if no result in 30–60 min till dose of 240 mg.
- Target urine output is 100–150 mL/h. High frequency is better than high dosage.
- No mortality benefit in fluid overload between both continuous and bolus dosage.
- Continuous infusion is superior to bolus regarding diuretic effect.

✓ **Indapamide**[Q]: Thiazide-like diuretic that causes diuresis as well as vascular smooth muscle relaxation and can be used in hypertension.

	Spironolactone	Acetazolamide	Mannitol
Mechanism of action[Q]	• Acts on DCT and collecting duct • Competitive antagonist of aldosterone	• Non-competitive inhibitor of carbonic anhydrase • HCO₃⁻ absorption at PCT decreased	• Freely filtered by glomerulus and causes osmotic diuresis • ↑ **Serum Osmolality**

	Spironolactone	Acetazolamide	Mannitol
Pharma-codynamic/ side effects	• **CVS:** ↓Preload, ↓ SVR • Biochemistry: ↑Na⁺, ↑Cl⁻, ↑K⁺ • Irregular menses and ↓ responses to vasopressors-	• **CNS:** ↓ intraocular pressure, ↓ ICP • ↓ gastric and pancreatic secretion • ↓ excretion of uric acid • Hyperchloraemic metabolic acidosis • **Urine becomes alkaline**	• **CVS:** ↓ circulating volume • **CNS:** ↓ ICP; can cross BBB post–head injury and cause worsening of ICP
Pharmacokinetics	• Bioavailability: 70% • Protein binding: >90%	• Bioavailability: 100% • Protein binding: 70–90% • $t_{1/2}$: 6 hr	• Freely filtered at glomerulus • $t_{1/2}$: 100 min
Uses	• Hypertension • Ascites • Nephrotic syndrome • Conn's syndrome	• Mountain sickness • Glaucoma	• Reduces intracranial pressure
Dose	• 50–400 mg/day	• Oral: 250 mg–1 g/day in divided doses • I/V: 250 mg–1 g 4 hourly	• 0.5–1 mg/kg bolus over 20 min

✓ **Acetazolamide**
  • Given in contracted metabolic alkalosis or a chloride-responsive metabolic alkalosis.
  • Boosts the response of loops diuretics.

Additional Questions

✓ **Pharmacodynamics Effects**
  • **Amiloride/triamterene:** Hyperkalaemia and hypermagnesaemia. Triamterene is the only diuretic which causes any direct renal injury.
  • **Furosemide[Q]:** Initially hyponatraemia, then hypernatraemia, hypokalaemia, and hypomagnesaemia. Give thiazide diuretic when hypernatraemia.
  • **Spironolactone:** Hypermagnesemia.

✓ **Spot urine sodium**
  • If it is more than 50–70 mEq/L. Then patients of heart failure have good response to diuretics.
  • Spot urine sodium has good prognostic value in acute heart failure.

HYPOGLYCAEMIC AGENTS

✓ **Insulin:** Insulin is a polypeptide of 51 amino acids formed after removal of 34 amino acids C-peptide from pro-insulin.
  • A and B chains joined by disulfide bridges.
  • Insulin binds to the α subunit of insulin receptor. Insulin receptor has two α and two β subunits.
  • Tyrosine kinase activity is on β subunit.

Insulin Type	Onset	Peak	Duration	Remarks
Rapid-acting insulin[Q] (aspart/*lispro*/glulisine)	20–30 min	1–3 h	3–5 h	5–15 min before or after meals
Short-acting insulin (regular/*soluble insulin*)	30 mins–1 h	2–4 h	5–8 h	30 min before meal
Intermediate-acting insulin (*isophane*/NPH)	2–4 h	4–12 h	12–18 h	Twice-daily regimens
Long-acting insulin[Q] (*glargine*/detemir)	1–2 h	Flat peak	12–24 h	Same time every day at any time of the day

Oral Hypoglycaemic Agents

✓ **Biguanides:** Metformin acts by enhancing uptake of glucose in muscle via GLUT-4 transporter and inhibition of hepatic and renal gluconeogenesis.
  - First line of drug in prediabetics and type II diabetics.
  - Lactic acidosis in alcohol abusers or kidney impairment.

✓ **Sulfonylureas: First gen:** Tolbutamide; **second gen:** Gliclazide, glipizide.
  - Enhances the secretion of insulin from pancreatic islet cells by binding to ATP-dependent K⁺ channels on islet cell membranes and causing release of pro-insulin.
  - Added to metformin in type II diabetics.

✓ **Meglitinides:** Repaglinide and metiglinide.
  - They block the potassium channels in beta cells in the pancreas, like sulfonylureas, but are short-acting and taken just before meals.
  - Used in patients with erratic eating habits.

✓ **Thiazolidinediones:** Pioglitazone.
  - Activates peroxisome proliferator–activated receptor γ (PPARγ) and **increases hepatic sensitivity to insulin and improves insulin resistance.**
  - Side effects: Fluid retention, liver derangement, and limb fractures.

✓ **Dipeptidyl peptidase 4 (DPP-4) inhibitors:** Vildagliptin and sitagliptin.
  - Inhibits the enzyme DPP-4, leading to increased levels of incretins.
  - Side effects: Anaphylaxis, angioedema, and Stevens–Johnson syndrome.

✓ **Glucagon-like peptide 1 (GLP-1) agonist:** Exenatide
  - Behaves as incretin and acts as agonist on GLP-1 receptor.
  - Given as subcutaneous injections.

  - Not recommended if creatinine clearance <30 mL/min.

✓ **Sodium–glucose co-transporter-2 (SGLT2) inhibitors:** Dapagliflozin, canagliflozin, empagliflozin.
  - SGLT2 inhibitors work by preventing the kidneys from reabsorbing glucose back into the blood.
  - Side effects: Can lead to euglycaemic ketoacidosis, genital and urinary tract infections.
  - Not recommended for prescribing to people with kidney disease.

✓ **Alpha-glucosidase inhibitors:** Acarbose
  - Inhibits intestinal alpha-glucosidase, resulting in delayed absorption of glucose.
  - Side effects are flatulence and diarrhoea.

Clinical Trials Regarding Glycaemic Control

✓ **Leuven I (2001):** In surgical ICU patients (mainly cardiac), use of intensive insulin therapy (BG goal of 80–110 mg/dL) **reduced mortality,** but the rates of hypoglycaemia were also higher.

✓ **Leuven II (2006):** In medical ICU patients, use of intensive insulin therapy (BG goal of 80–110 mg/dL) **didn't reduce mortality,** but the rates of hypoglycaemia were higher.

✓ **VISEP (2008):** In patients with severe sepsis or septic shock, use of intensive insulin therapy (BG goal of 80–110 mg/dL) **didn't reduce mortality,** but the rates of hypoglycaemia were higher.
  - Also, Pentastarch (HES 200/0.5) caused renal impairment and 90 d mortality.

✓ **NICE-SUGAR (2009):** In critically ill medical/surgical patients, intensive insulin therapy (BG 81–108 mg/dL) was associated with increased 90 d mortality and increased rates of severe hypoglycaemia.

22

The Endgame

GRAND REVISION

✓ **Systemic inflammation response syndrome (SIRS):** >2 of the following variables:
  - Tachypnoea >20/min
  - Tachycardia >90 bpm
  - Temperature >38°C or <36°C
  - WBCs >12 × 10⁹/L or <4 × 10⁹/L or >10% immature neutrophils
✓ **qSOFA (sepsis-related organ failure assessment):** For suspected sepsis in a non-ICU setting. AUROC of 0.81.
  - If two-thirds of criteria are positive, qSOFA is positive.
    ❖ Altered mental status (GCS <15)
    ❖ Tachypnoea >22/min
    ❖ Systolic blood pressure <100 mmHg

World Society of the Abdominal Compartment Syndrome (WSACS) Classification

Intra-abdominal hypertension^Q	• Grade I: IAP 12–15 mmHg • Grade II: IAP 16–20 mmHg • Grade III: IAP 21–25 mmHg • Grade IV: IAP >25 mmHg
Abdominal compartment syndrome^Q	IAP >20 mmHg with new organ dysfunction or failure: • **Primary:** Intra-abdominal process • **Secondary:** Illness not directly related to abdomen and pelvis.

RIFLE Criteria^Q for AKI Done in 2004: Predictive for Hospital Mortality

	Creatinine Criteria	**Urine Output Criteria**
Risk	• Increased creatinine × 1.5 or GFR drop by 25%	• UO <0.5 mL/kg/h × 6 h
Injury	• Increased creatinine × 2 or GFR drop by 50%	• UO <0.5 mL/kg/h × 12 h
Failure	• Increased creatinine × 3 • Creatinine ≥4 mg/dL • Acute rise of ≥0.5 mg/dL or GFR drop by 75%	• UO <0.3 mL/kg/h × 24 h or • Anuria × 12 h
Loss	Persistent ARF = complete loss of renal function >4 wk	
End-stage kidney disease	Loss of kidney function >3 months	

DOI: 10.1201/9781003476214-22

Staging of AKI by KDIGO[Q] Done in 2012

AKI Stage	Serum Creatinine Criteria	Urine Output Criteria
Stage I	• ↑ in s. creatinine by ≥**26.5** μmol/L within 48 h • ↑ in s. creatinine to 1.5–1.9 times from baseline within prior 7 d	• Urine volume <0.5 mL/kg/h for 6–12 h
Stage II	• ↑ in s. creatinine to **2–2.9 times** from baseline	• Urine volume <0.5 mL/kg/h for ≥12 h
Stage III	• ↑ in s. creatinine to ≥**3 times** from baseline • ↑ in s. creatinine to 354 μmol/L • **Treatment with RRT** or in patients less <18 yr, ↓ in estimated GFR to <35 mL/min per 1.73 m²	• Urine volume <0.3 mL/kg/h for ≥24 h • Anuria for ≥12 h

Grades of Encephalopathy Using West Haven's Criteria[Q]

Severity	Level of Consciousness	Cognition/Behaviour	Neurological Examination
Grade 0	Normal	Normal	May be impaired
Grade 1	Mild confusion	Reduced attention	**Mild asterixis**/tremor
Grade 2	Lethargy	Disorientation, inappropriate behaviour	**Asterixis**, slurred speech
Grade 3	Somnolent but arousable	Bizarre behaviour	Rigidity, clonus, hyperreflexia
Grade 4	Comatose	Comatose	Abnormal posturing

✓ **Modified King's College Criteria (KCC)**[Q]: Identifies patients with acute liver failure who need a liver transplant. It combines original KCC with lactate criteria.
  • It is not validated in trauma-related acute liver failure.

• Projected 5-yr survival should be >50% post-transplant. Disease mortality calculated using UK model for end-stage liver disease (UKELD).

Acute Liver Failure Following Paracetamol Overdose	Acute Liver Failure Due to Non-Paracetamol Overdose
• Arterial pH <7.3 after adequate fluid resuscitation or • A lactate level of >3.5 mmol/L (**lactate criteria**) at admission (4 h) or a lactate level >3 mmol/L after adequate fluid resuscitation (12 h after admission)[Q] or • All of the following • PT >100 s (INR >6.5) • Creatinine >300 mmol/L • Grade III-IV encephalopathy	• PT >100 s (INR >6.5) with any grade encephalopathy or • All three criteria from the following: • Age <10 or >40 yr • PT >50 s • Bilirubin >300 mmol/L • Onset of encephalopathy >7 d after the development of jaundice • Unfavourable disease aetiology: Non-A hepatitis, non-B hepatitis, halothane hepatitis, drug-induced liver failure

✓ **Myocardial infarction (MI) can be classified into five types**[Q] **based on aetiology and circumstances**
  • **Type 1:** Spontaneous MI, caused by ischaemia due to a primary coronary event (e.g. plaque rupture, erosion, coronary dissection)
  • **Type 2:** Ischaemia due to ischaemic imbalance (i.e. increased oxygen demand) (e.g. hypertension) or decreased supply (e.g. coronary artery spasm, embolism)
  • **Type 3:** Related to sudden unexpected cardiac death
  • **Type 4a**: Associated with PCI
  • **Type 4b**: Associated with documented stent thrombosis
  • **Type 5:** Associated with CABG

Contraindications to Fibrinolytic Therapy in STEMI

Absolute Contraindications	Relative Contraindications
Known brain tumour	Proliferative diabetic retinopathy
Prior intracranial haemorrhage	Known bleeding diathesis
Ischaemic stroke within last 3 months	Ischaemic stroke >3 months old
Head trauma within last 3 months	Pregnancy
Aortic dissection	Prolonged CPR >10 min
Active internal bleeding	Active peptic ulcer or recent internal bleeding
Intracranial or intraspinal surgery within 2 months	Major surgery <3 wk
Severe uncontrolled hypertension	Blood pressure >180/110 mmHg

✓ **P waves:** Checked in lead II. P wave shouldn't exceed 3 small squares. *If >3 small squares, it's right atrial enlargement.*
  • *Bifid P wave*[Q] *is seen in left atrial enlargement.*
✓ **PR interval:** To look for any AV nodal block. Normal is 0.12–2 s.
✓ **QRS wave:** Broad (>0.12 s) or narrow complex (<0.12 s), depending upon supraventricular or ventricular origin.

• **Left ventricular hypertrophy (LVH)**
  ❖ Voltage criteria, **Sokolow–Lyon criteria**[Q]: If deepest S wave in V1 or V2 and amplitude of tallest R wave in V5 or V6 is ≥35 mm.
  ❖ Non-voltage criteria: Increased R wave peak time >50 ms in leads V5/6 or ST segment depression and T wave inversion in left-sided leads.
  ❖ Voltage criteria must be used along with non-voltage criteria to be considered diagnostic of LVH.
  ❖ Most common cause of LVH is hypertension.
• **Right ventricular hypertrophy (RVH**[Q]**):** QRS <120 ms, right axis deviation, dominant R wave in V1, dominant S wave in V5/6.
✓ J point: Point in ECG where the QRS complex joins the ST segment.
✓ **QT interval:** Increased in drug toxicities.
✓ **T wave:** Normal T wave is usually in the same direction as the QRS, except in the right precordial leads. T wave is always upright in leads I, II, V3–6, and always inverted in lead aVR.
✓ **Abnormal ECG waves**
  • **U waves**[Q]: 0.5 mm deflection after T wave.
    ❖ Bradycardia (MC), hypokalaemia, severe hypothermia
    ❖ **Best seen in lead V2 and V3**
  • Tall T waves: Hyperkalaemia
  • **Osborne J waves**[Q]: Positive deflection seen in the J point in precordial and true limb leads.
    ❖ Characteristically seen in hypothermia.
    ❖ **Other causes:** Hypercalcaemia, brain injury, subarachnoid haemorrhage, vasospastic angina, *type 1 Brugada syndrome*, normal variant, idiopathic ventricular fibrillation.
  • **Delta waves:** Slurred upstroke at the beginning of the QRS complex.
    ❖ Seen in Wolff–Parkinson–White (WPW) syndrome.
  • P pulmonale (enlarged): COPD.
  • P mitrale (bifid): Mitral regurgitation.
  • **Wellens pattern A:** Biphasic T wave in V2–3. ECG pattern plus chest pain signifies critical stenosis of the left anterior descending artery.
  • **Wellens pattern B:** Deeply inverted T wave in V2–3. ECG pattern plus chest pain signifies critical stenosis of the left anterior descending artery.

- ✓ **Short PR interval:** WPW syndrome
  - **Long PR interval:** First-degree heart block, hyperkalaemia, beta-blockers, and digoxin.
- ✓ **Widened QRS:** Conduction deficits, hyperkalaemia, WPW syndrome, ventricular hypertrophy, drugs that inhibit sodium channels, like TCAs, types 1a and 1c antiarrhythmics, antimalarials, and antiepileptics.
- ✓ **ST segment changes**
  - **Reverse tick ST depression** (down-sloping ST segments): Digoxin.
  - **Saddle-shaped ST elevation** (concave ST elevation in all chest leads)[Q]: Pericarditis.
  - **ST depression:** Conduction deficits, hypokalaemia.
- ✓ **Long QT syndrome[Q] (LQTS):** Blockade of rapid potassium outward currentlt causes LQTS.
  - **QT interval:** Time taken for ventricular depolarization and repolarization.
  - Corrected QT interval (QTc): **Bazett's equation[Q]:** $QT/\sqrt{RR}$.
    - ❖ **Normal QTc for men,** <440 ms; for women, <460 ms.
  - Causes of long QT syndrome
    - ❖ **Congenital:** Romano–Ward syndrome, Jervell and Lange–Nielsen syndrome.
    - ❖ **Acquired:** Myocardial ischaemia, subarachnoid haemorrhage, hypothermia.
      - **Hypokalaemia, hypocalcaemia, and hypomagnesaemia.**
    - ❖ **Drugs**
      - **Antiarrhythmics: Amiodarone[Q],** sotalol, quinidine, procainamide, disopyramide (Vaughan Williams classes[Q] 1 and 3 drugs).
      - **Antibiotics:** Clarithromycin, **ciprofloxacin,** erythromycin, fluconazole, metronidazole, trimethoprim., and sulphamethoxazole.
      - **Antipsychotics/antidepressants: Haloperidol,** amitriptyline, citalopram, chlorpromazine
      - **Others:** Methadone**, ondansetron**, domperidone, droperidol, dexmedetomidine, protease inhibitors, organophosphates, and grapefruit juices.
  - **Presentation:** They can trigger after depolarisations, which can trigger torsades de pointes (TdP), palpitations, syncope, or sudden death.
- **Treatment:** Remove agent. Beta-blockers. ICD may be needed in high-risk patients not responding to beta-blockers.
- ✓ **Shortened QT interval[Q]:** A QT <350 ms is abnormally short and can also cause ventricular arrhythmias.
  - Hypercalcaemia, hyperkalaemia
  - Acidosis and hyperthermia
  - Digoxin
- ✓ **Brugada syndrome:** Sodium channel disorder causing sudden cardiac death in young patients.
  - **Right bundle branch block** with coved ST-segment elevation >2 mm in >1 of V1–3 and negative T wave following the ST segment.
  - Treated with **urgent implantable cardioverter.**
- ✓ **CHA$_2$DS$_2$–VASc score:** Assesses stroke risk in people with AF. Calculated in patients after >48 h of AF.
  - CHF, hypertension, age 65–74 yrs, diabetes, vascular disease, female sex score 1 point.
  - Age over 74 yr and previous stroke score 2 points.
  - Anticoagulation to be started in men[Q] with a score of ≥1 and women[Q] with a score of ≥2.

Modified Maastricht Classification for Donation after Cardiac Arrest

Class	Arrest Type	Controlled/ Uncontrolled
I	Dead on arrival	Uncontrolled
II	Unsuccessful resuscitation	Uncontrolled
III	Anticipated cardiac arrest	Controlled
IV	Cardiac arrest in brain-dead donor	Controlled
V	Unexpected arrest in ICU patient	Uncontrolled

- ✓ **American Heart Association (AHA) PE classification**
  - **Massive/high risk[Q]:** SBP <90 mmHg or drop of ≥40 mmHg for 15 min or cardiac arrest. Requiring vasopressor support; 30 d mortality risk at ~30%.
  - **Sub-massive/intermediate risk:** Presence of RV strain, dilation, or dysfunction; 90 d mortality risk at 3–15%.
  - **Low risk:** None of the above; 30 d mortality risk at ~1%.
- ✓ **ESC Classification:** Classification of patients with acute PE based on early (30 d) mortality

Early Mortality Risk		Indicators of Risk			
		Haemodynamic Instability (Cardiac Arrest or SBP <90 mmHg)	sPESI ≥1	RV Dysfunction on TTE or CTPA	Elevated Cardiac Troponin Levels (cTnI >0.05)
High		+	+	+	+
Intermediate[Q]	Intermediate high	–	+	+	+
	Intermediate low	–	+	One or none positive	
Low		–	–	–	Assessment optional; if assessed, negative

✓ **Aortic dissection: Stanford classification**[Q]
- **Type A:** Ascending aorta
- **Type B:** Descending aorta

✓ **Aortic dissection: The DeBakey classification**[Q]
- **Type I:** Ascending aorta and the descending aorta both.

- **Type II:** Ascending aorta proximal to the brachiocephalic artery.
- **Type III:** Originates in the descending aorta distal to the left subclavian artery.
  - ❖ **Type IIIa:** Limited above the diaphragm.
  - ❖ **Type IIIb:** Extends below the diaphragm.

Pacemaker Classification System: NASPE/BPEG Pacemaker Code (2002)[Q]

I	II	III	IV	V
Chambers **Paced**	Chambers **Sensed**	Response to Sensing	Rate **Modulation**	**Multisite Pacing**
O = none	O = none	O = none	O = none	O = none
A = atrium	A = atrium	I = inhibited	R = rate modulation	A = atrium
V = ventricle	V = ventricle	T = triggered		V = ventricle
D = dual (A + V)	D = dual (A + V)	D = I + T		D = dual (A + V)

✓ **Duke's criteria**[Q], definite IE: *Clinical criteria (2 major or 1 major + 3 minor criteria or 5 minor criteria).* **Possible IE:** *1 major + 1 minor or 3 minor criteria.* **Rejected IE:** Alternate diagnosis or resolution of IE, 80% sensitivity. Diagnosis is either by pathological or clinical criteria. *Pathological criteria require either surgery or post-mortem examination.*
- **Pathological criteria**
  - ❖ **Microorganism:** Demonstrated by culture or histology in either vegetations, embolized vegetations, or intracardiac abscess.
  - ❖ **Pathologic lesion:** Vegetation or intracardiac abscess confirmed by histology showing active endocarditis.

- **Clinical criteria**
  - ❖ **Major criteria**
    - **Positive blood cultures** for an organism typical causative of IE (*Streptococcus viridans, Streptococcus* bovis, *S. aureus, Enterococcus,* HACEK, *Pseudomonas*) from two sources >12 h apart or in all three cultures sent. Single positive blood culture for *Coxiella burnetii* or IgG antibody titre >1:800.
    - **Positive echocardiogram:** Oscillating intracardiac mass on valve or abscess or *new partial dehiscence of prosthetic valve* or new valvular regurgitation.

❖ **Minor criteria**
  - Predisposing heart condition or IVDU
  - Fever >38°C
  - **Vascular phenomenon:** Major arterial emboli, Janeway lesions, conjunctival haemorrhage
  - **Immunological phenomenon:** Glomerulonephritis, Osler's nodes, Roth spots, or rheumatoid factor
  - **Microbiological phenomenon:** Blood culture not meeting major criteria

✓ **Murray Score for referral**[Q] **for ECMO:** Four components with each scored from 0 to 4. Total divided by four to give a final score. *Referral criteria is a score of 3 or 2.5 with rapid deterioration.*

Score	0	1	2	3	4
Chest X-Ray Quadrants	0	1	2	3	4
Compliance	≥80	60–79	40–59	20–39	<20
PEEP	≤5	6–8	9–11	11–14	>14
PaO_2/FiO_2	≥40	30–39.9	23.3–29.9	13.3–23.2	<13.3

✓ **Light's criteria**[Q]. An exudate if:
  - Pleural fluid protein/serum protein ratio: >0.5
  - Pleural fluid LDH/serum LDH: >0.6
  - Pleural fluid LDH greater than two-thirds of the upper limit of normal range for serum LDH

✓ **CURB-65 score**[Q], 1 point for each finding.
  - Confusion, not long-standing (mini-mental test score ≤8/10)
  - **Urea** >7 mmol/L
  - **Respiratory rate** ≥30/min
  - **Blood pressure (SBP <90** mmHg **or DBP <60** mmHg**)**
  - Age ≥65 yr
    ❖ Score: 0–1: <3% mortality, 2: 9% mortality, 3–5: 15–40% mortality.
    ❖ Score 0–1: care in community; score 2–3: hospital admission; score 4–5: admission to critical care.

✓ **ARDS: Berlin Definition in 2012**[Q]
  - The four criteria for this diagnosis were:
    ❖ **Timing:** Within 1 wk of a known clinical insult.
    ❖ **Chest imaging (CXR/CT):** Bilateral opacities involving more than two quadrants – not fully explained by effusion/lobar/lung collapse/nodule.

❖ **Origin of oedema:** Respiratory failure not fully explained by cardiac failure.
❖ **Oxygenation:** PaO_2/FiO_2 <40 kPa with PEEP/CPAP >5 cm H_2O, corrected for altitude if >1,000 m.
  - **Drawbacks of this definition:** ARDS severity assessed by a single blood gas measurement without prior standardization of ventilator settings.
    ❖ Level of PEEP may have a major influence on oxygenation.

✓ **ARDS: New global definition 2024:** Included non-intubated patients on HFNO, ultrasound lung as a modality, and pulse oximetry as a mode of measuring saturation as well.
  - Acute onset within 1 wk.
  - Bilateral opacities on chest X-ray or CT scan or **B-lines/consolidations on USG**[Q].
  - Respiratory failure not fully explained by cardiac failure.
  - PaO_2/FiO_2 ratio ≤300 or SpO_2/FiO_2 ≤315 (if SPO_2 ≤97%) with PEEP/CPAP >5 cm H_2O in intubated patients or **SpO_2/FiO_2**[Q] **≤315 (if SpO_2 ≤97%) by HFNO on O_2 flow of 30 L/min in non-intubated patients**[Q].

British Thoracic Society (BTS) Classification[Q] (One of the most important tables for revision in the last few days before exam)

Moderate asthma	• Increasing symptoms • PEFR >50–75% predicted
Acute severe asthma	• PEFR >33–50% predicted • Respiratory rates ≥25/min • Heart rate ≥110/min • Inability to complete sentences
Life-threatening asthma	**Clinical signs** • Altered consciousness • Poor respiratory effort • Cyanosis • Hypotension • Exhaustion • Silent chest • Tachyarrhythmia **Measurements** • PEFR <33% predicted • SpO_2 <92% • PaO_2 <8 kPa • Normal $PaCO_2$ 4.6–6 kPa[Q]
Near-fatal asthma	• Raised $PaCO_2$[Q] • Requiring mechanical ventilation

✓ Severity of COPD is diagnosed by spirometry with **FEV_1/FVC ratio of <0.7[Q]** and FEV_1 of <80% predicted.

GOLD Spirometric Classification

Gold Stage	Severity	SpirometryFEV_1/FVC Ratio <0.7 and
I	Mild	FEV_1 ≥80%
II	Moderate	FEV_1 ≥50% but <80%
III	Severe	FEV_1 ≥30% but <50%
IV	Very severe	FEV_1 <30%

✓ **WHO classification of pulmonary hypertension[Q]**
- **Group 1** (precapillary arteries and arterioles): Pulmonary **arterial** hypertension (PAH) from *pulmonary vasculopathy* (e.g. idiopathic, connective tissue disorders, drug related [fenfluramine, methamphetamines]).
- **Group 2** (post-capillary veins and venules): Pulmonary **venous** hypertension due to **left heart disease** (e.g. LV systolic/diastolic dysfunction).
- **Group 3** (alveoli and capillary beds): Pulmonary hypertension due to **lung disease** and hypoxia (e.g. COPD, interstitial lung disease, OSA).
- **Group 4: Chronic thromboembolic** pulmonary hypertension (CTEPH) (e.g. venous thromboembolism).
- **Group 5:** Pulmonary hypertension with **unknown origin** (e.g. *sarcoidosis*, thyroid disease, *CKD*, neurofibromatosis).

✓ **APACHE II:** Acute physiology and chronic health evaluation
- APACHE I in 1981, APACHE II in 1985.
- Based on **12 most abnormal variables[Q]** that form acute physiological score[Q] in the first 24 h of ITU stay plus age and chronic disease. Each parameter score: 0–4.
  - ❖ **Age[Q]** and **chronic disease[Q]** (cirrhosis, NYHA stage 4 heart failure, chronic respiratory disease, dialysis-dependent CKD, immunosuppression)
  - ❖ **Five observational variables** (RR, MAP, HR, GCS, and temperature)
  - ❖ **Seven investigational variables** (Na^+, K^+, creatinine, haematocrit, WBCs, pH, A-a gradient)
- Maximum score is 71, with **score of >25 having a predicted mortality of >50%.**

World Federation of Neurological Surgeons Scale (WFNS)[Q]

Grade	Motor Deficit	GCS	Risk of Severe Disability, Death (%)
1	–	15	13
2	–	13–14	20
3	+	13–14	42
4	±	7–12	51
5	±	3–6	68

Modified Fisher Scale

Grade	IVH	SAH Characteristics on Admission CT Head Scan	Risk of Symptomatic Vasospasm (%)
1	–	Localized thin or diffused thin	24
2	+	Localized thin or diffused thin	33
3	–	Localized thick or diffused thick	33
4	+	Localized thick or diffused thick	40

✓ **Bamford or Oxford stroke classification[Q]** according to the stroke territory involved.
- **Total and partial anterior circulation systems (TACS/PACS):** Middle and anterior cerebral arteries involved. TACS if all three, and PACS if two out of three, are involved.
  - ❖ Unilateral weakness ± sensory deficit
  - ❖ Homonymous hemianopia
  - ❖ Higher cerebral dysfunction (aphasia and visuospatial disorders)
- **Posterior circulation syndrome (POCS):** Affects posterior cerebral circulation (vertebral-basilar system). Patient has one of these:
  - ❖ Brainstem signs, like cranial nerve palsies and contralateral motor/sensory deficit
  - ❖ Cerebellar symptoms (ataxia, dysarthria)
  - ❖ Isolated homonymous hemianopia, cortical blindness
- **Lacuna syndrome (LACS):** A subcortical stroke because of small-vessel disease. Patients have an **absence of higher cerebral dysfunction** and one of the following:
  - ❖ Sensorimotor stroke
  - ❖ Pure sensory stroke

- ❖ Pure motor stroke
- ❖ Ataxic hemiparesis
- ✓ **Nerve conduction studies**[Q]**:** No need for nerve conduction studies to diagnose it. Diagnosis of exclusion:

- CIP: Functional neuronal membrane in-excitability.
- CIM: Functional muscle membrane in-excitability.

Investigation	CIP	CIM	CINM
Creatine kinase	• Normal or slightly elevated	• **Elevated**	• Normal or elevated
CSF	• Normal cell counts • *Slightly elevated protein levels (<0.8 g/L)*	• Normal	• Normal cell counts • Slightly elevated protein levels (<0.8 g/L)
Nerve conduction studies	• ↓ CMAP amplitude • ↓ *SNAP amplitude* • **Normal conduction velocity** • **Normal conduction latency**	• ↓ **CMAP amplitude** • *Normal SNAP amplitude* • **Normal conduction velocity** • **Normal conduction latency**	• ↓ CMAP amplitude • ↓ SNAP amplitude • Normal conduction velocity • Normal conduction latency
Electromyography	• Spontaneous fibrillation potentials and sharp waves • **Long duration, high-amplitude polyphasic motor unit potentials (MUPs)**	• Spontaneous fibrillation potentials and sharp waves • **Short duration, low-amplitude polyphasic motor unit potentials (MUPs) with early recruitment**	• Features of both CIP and CIM
Direct muscle stimulation	• Nerve–muscle ratio <0.5 • **Normal direct muscle CMAP amplitude**	• Nerve–muscle response ratio ≥0.5 • **Reduced direct muscle CMAP amplitude**	• Variable
Muscle biopsy	• **Features of denervation and reinnervation** • Small angulated muscle fibres • Target and targetoid fibres, group fibre atrophy, fibre type regrouping	• **Cachectic myopathy** with myofibrillar degeneration • Thick filament myopathy with a **selective loss of myosin filaments** • Necrotizing myopathy with *muscle fibre necrosis*	• Both features of CIP and CIM
Nerve biopsy	• *Normal or **motor and sensory axonal degeneration***	• Normal	• Normal or motor and sensory nerve axonal degeneration
Creatine kinase	Normal or slightly elevated	**Elevated**	• Normal or elevated
CSF	Normal cell counts, *slightly elevated protein levels (<0.8 g/L)*	Normal	• Normal cell counts, slightly elevated protein levels (<0.8 g/L)
Nerve conduction studies	↓ CMAP amplitude, ↓ *SNAP amplitude*, **normal conduction velocity, normal conduction latency**	↓ CMAP amplitude, *normal SNAP amplitude*, **normal conduction velocity, normal conduction latency**	↓ CMAP amplitude, ↓ SNAP amplitude, normal conduction velocity, normal conduction latency

Investigation	CIP	CIM	CINM
Electromyography	Spontaneous fibrillation potentials and sharp waves; **long-duration, high-amplitude polyphasic motor unit potentials (MUPs)**	Spontaneous fibrillation potentials and sharp waves; **short-duration, low-amplitude polyphasic motor unit potentials (MUPs) with early recruitment**	Features of both CIP and CIM
Direct muscle stimulation	Nerve–muscle ratio <0.5, **normal direct muscle CMAP amplitude**	Nerve–muscle response ratio ≥0.5, **reduced direct muscle CMAP amplitude**	Variable
Muscle biopsy	**Features of denervation and reinnervation**, small angulated muscle fibres, target and targetoid fibres, group fibre atrophy, fibre-type regrouping	**Cachectic myopathy** with myofibrillar degeneration, thick filament myopathy with a **selective loss of myosin filaments**, necrotizing myopathy with **muscle fibre necrosis**	Both features of CIP and CIM
Nerve biopsy	*Normal or **motor and sensory axonal degeneration***	Normal	Normal or motor and sensory nerve axonal degeneration

- ✓ **HLH 2004 (both adult and children)**[Q]: Diagnosis of HLH can be established if either 1 or 2 in what follows is fulfilled:
  1. Molecular diagnosis consistent with HLH
  2. Diagnostic criteria with 5 out of the following 8 criteria:
     - ❖ Fever
     - ❖ Splenomegaly
     - ❖ Cytopaenia (≥2 lineages, Hb <90 g/L, neutrophils <1,000/µL, platelets <100,000/µL)
     - ❖ Haemophagocytosis in bone marrow or spleen or lymph nodes
     - ❖ Ferritin >500 µg/L
     - ❖ Hypertriglyceridaemia ≥265 mg/dL
     - ❖ Soluble CD25 ≥2,400 U/L
     - ❖ Fibrinogen ≤1.5 g/L
- ✓ **ERC ESICM 2021 Guidelines algorithm for prognostication**[Q]. Poor outcomes likely if all three of the following.
  - • Targeted temperature management and rewarming
  - • **Unconscious, GCS motor score ≤3 at ≥72 h**
  - • At least two of the following:
    - ❖ Pupillary and corneal reflex absent bilaterally
    - ❖ Status myoclonus (≤72 h)

- ❖ NSE >60 µg/L (at 48 h and/or 72 h)
- ❖ SSEP N20 wave absent bilaterally
- ❖ EEG highly malignant (>24 h)
- ❖ CT/MRI shows diffuse and extensive anoxic injury
- ✓ **Fried frailty phenotype** score measures frailty based on aspects of physical decline, like:
  - • **Weight loss:** >10 pounds in last year
  - • **Exhaustion:** Self-reported
  - • **Weakness:** Grip strength in the lowest 20%
  - • **Slowness:** Time to walk 15 ft in the slowest 20%
  - • **Low physical activity:** Reduced energy expenditure (Kcal/w) in lowest 20%
- ✓ **Rockwood clinical frailty scale (CFS):** 5–8 is considered frail, and 9 means terminal illness. Used more commonly clinically. (Definitely asked in viva.)
  1. **Very fit:** Robust, energetic, and motivated people who exercise regularly.
  2. **Well:** No active disease but less fit than category 1.
  3. **Managing well:** Medical problems present but well controlled. Not regularly active beyond routine walking.
  4. **Vulnerable:** Symptoms limit activities. Tired during the day.

5. **Mildly frail:** Need help for finances, transportation, heavy homework, and medications. Impairs shopping, walking outside alone, meal preparation, and housework.
6. **Moderately frail:** Problems with stairs and need help with bathing. Need assistance for dressing.
7. **Severely frail:** Completely dependent for personal care but stable and not at high risk of dying within next 6 months.
8. **Very severely frail:** Approaching the end of life and won't recover even from a minor illness.
9. **Terminally ill:** Life expectancy <6 months in patients who are not otherwise evidently frail.

✓ **Confusion assessment method for ICU (CAM ICU):** High sensitivity 80%.
- **Criteria 1:** First, consider whether the patient has shown an **acute mental status change** in last 24 h.
- **Criteria 2:** Check for **inattention.** If patient makes **more than two errors**^{Q}, go on to check altered levels of consciousness with the RASS score.
  - ❖ Patient is asked to squeeze the hand or blink on hearing letter A and SAVEAHAART is read before the patient.
- **Criteria 3:** Check the RASS score of the patient.
- **Criteria 4:** If RASS score is other than zero, check **disordered thinking** with four questions, like "Will a stone float on water?" "Are there fish in the sea?" "Does one pound weigh more than two pounds?" "Can you use a hammer to pound a nail?" Then, patient is told to hold two fingers with the other hand and then told to do the same with the other hand.
  - ❖ Score of more than one error on the questions or commands means there is delirium.
- Positive CAM-ICU is criteria 1 plus 2 and either 3 or 4. Can be performed on patients who are **intubated or sedated (RASS <−3).**
- Either altered level of consciousness or disorganized thinking is the criterion.

✓ **Depth of sedation:** *Richmond Agitation–Sedation Scale*^{Q} *is the most validated* and widely used tool to assess depth of sedation. Sedation-Agitation Scale (SAS) can also be used.

	Criteria	
+4	Combative	Violent and immediate danger to staff
+3	Very agitated	Pulls or removes tubes or catheters immediately
+2	Agitated	Frequent non-purposeful movements and fights ventilator
+1	Restless	Anxious but not aggressive
0	Alert and calm	
−1	**Drowsy**	Not fully alert but sustained awakening (eye opening/ eye contact >10 s)
−2	**Light sedation**	Briefly awakens (eye opening/ eye contact <10 s)
−3	**Moderate sedation**	Movement or eye opening to voice, but no eye contact
−4	**Deep sedation**	No response to voice, but movement or eye opening to physical stimulation
−5	Unarousable	No response to voice or physical stimulation

- RAAS score of −2 or higher is indicated in most patients in ITU, with RASS of −3 or −4 only for severely sick patients, like those with ARDS or raised ICP.
  - ❖ Greater depth of sedation was associated with higher duration of mechanical ventilation and in hospital mortality.

✓ **American Spinal Injury Association (ASIA) Impairment Scale (AIS)**^{Q}**:** Neurological injury score based on motor, sensory, reflex, and rectal function. *Neurological level of injury is the lowest segment with intact sensation and antigravity (grade 3 or more) motor function.*
- **Grade A:** Complete neurologic injury with no motor or sensory sensation preserved in the sacral segments (S4–S5).
- **Grade B:** Preserved sensory function but no motor function below the neurological level and includes the sacral segments (S4–S5).
- **Grade C:** Preserved motor function below the neurological level, and more than half of key muscles below the neurological level have a grade less than 3.

- **Grade D:** Preserved motor function below the neurological level, with at least half of key muscles below the neurological level having a grade more than 3.
- **Grade E:** Normal neurological function.

American Association for the Surgery of Trauma (AAST) Grade of Splenic Injury Is Used

Grade	Parenchymal Laceration Depth	Haematoma
I	<1 cm	Subcapsular haematoma <10% of surface area, capsular tear.
II	1–3 cm	Subcapsular haematoma 10%–50% of surface area, intraparenchymal haematoma <5 cm.
III	>3 cm	Subcapsular haematoma >50% of surface area, intraparenchymal haematoma >5 cm, ruptured subcapsular/intraparenchymal haematoma
IV	• 25% devascularization • Splenic vascular injury or active bleeding confined within splenic capsule	
V	• Splenic injury with active bleeding beyond spleen into peritoneum • Shattered spleen	

✓ **CT scan indications within 1 hꟴ for TBI:** Decline of GCS of 2 points, *GCS score of 12 or less on initial assessment*, GCS score of 14 or less at 2 h after the injury, suspected open or depressed skull fracture, *possible basal skull fracture*, post-traumatic seizure, *focal neurological deficits*, two or more episodes of vomiting.

- **Loss of consciousness with amnesia:** Do CT scan within 8 h *if age >64 yr* or *coagulopathy* or had a *dangerous mechanism of injury.*

✓ **Preconditionsꟴ for brainstem death testing for DNC**

- >6 h after loss of the last brainstem reflex.
- >24 h after loss of the last brain reflex when aetiology is primarily anoxic damage.
- >24 h of temperature >36°C.
- No neuromuscular agents or neuromuscular disorders contributing to weakness.
- No investigations needed for high cervical cord pathology.
- No effect of depressant drugs like prolonged fentanyl infusions.
- Caution for steroids given in space occupying lesions like abscesses.
- Caution for aetiology primarily in brainstem or posterior fossa.
- Caution for therapeutic decompressive craniectomy.

Index

For Product Safety Concerns and Information please contact our EU
representative GPSR@taylorandfrancis.com
Taylor & Francis Verlag GmbH, Kaufingerstraße 24, 80331 München, Germany